BUSINESS BASICS FOR
Dentists

BUSINESS BASICS FOR
Dentists

David O. Willis, DMD, MBA, CFP

School of Dentistry
University of Louisville
Louisville, Kentucky

⟨W⟩WILEY-BLACKWELL

A John Wiley & Sons, Inc., Publication

Editorial Offices
2121 State Avenue, Ames, Iowa 50014-8300, USA
The Atrium, Southern Gate, Chichester, West Sussex, PO19 8SQ, UK
9600 Garsington Road, Oxford, OX4 2DQ, UK

For details of our global editorial offices, for customer services and for information about how to apply for permission to reuse the copyright material in this book please see our website at www.wiley.com/wiley-blackwell.

Cataloging-in-Publication data is available through the Library of Congress.

A catalogue record for this book is available from the British Library.

Wiley also publishes its books in a variety of electronic formats. Some content that appears in print may not be available in electronic books.

Cover design by Nicole Teut

Set in 10/12pt Sabon by SPi Publisher Services, Pondicherry, India
Printed and bound in Malaysia by Vivar Printing Sdn Bhd

1   2013

Contents

Preface   vii
About the Companion Website   ix

Section 1   Personal Financial Management   1

Chapter 1   Personal Money Management   3
Chapter 2   Personal Insurance Needs   15
Chapter 3   Planning for Retirement Income   29
Chapter 4   Reducing the Personal Tax Burden   43
Chapter 5   Estate Planning   53

Section 2   Business Foundations   59

Chapter 6   Business Entities   61
Chapter 7   Basic Economics   73
Chapter 8   The Legal Environment of the
             Dental Practice   87
Chapter 9   Financial Statements   101
Chapter 10   Basics of Business Finance   111
Chapter 11   Business Taxes and Tax Planning   129
Chapter 12   Management Principles   141
Chapter 13   Planning the Dental Practice   147

Section 3   Dental Office Success Factors   159

Chapter 14   Financial Analysis and Control
             in the Dental Office   161
Chapter 15   Maintaining Production   173

Chapter 16   Maintaining Collections   199
Chapter 17   Generating Patients for the Practice   213
Chapter 18   Gaining Case Acceptance   229
Chapter 19   Controlling Costs in the Practice   241
Chapter 20   Promoting Staff Effectiveness   247
Chapter 21   Maintaining Daily Operations   277
Chapter 22   Managing Risk in the Office   319

Section 4   Practice Transitions   353

Chapter 23   Career Planning   355
Chapter 24   Employment Opportunities   361
Chapter 25   Practice Ownership   369
Chapter 26   Practice Transitions   379
Chapter 27   Valuing Practices   395
Chapter 28   Securing Financing   403
Chapter 29   The Business Plan   411

Index   419

Preface

Surveys of new dental practitioners consistently rate practice management as the area for which they were least prepared and in which they found the most problems in practice. Dental schools do an excellent job of preparing the graduate to handle the technical and patient treatment aspects of dentistry, but they do a less-than-excellent job of preparing graduates to run a dental practice.

This problem comes from several sources. Most students do not enter dental school with a business background. They have taken scientific-based courses to prepare them for the rigorous dental curriculum and have not taken a business class in their predental curriculum. Many students have never had a dental-related job in the private sector. They depend on the professional mentoring of the faculty to prepare them for the world of dental practice.

Students are concerned with the immediate needs of learning dentistry, completing clinical requirements, and passing licensing exams—and that is where their efforts should go, to their most immediate and pressing needs. They can not run a successful dental practice until they graduate dental school and earn a dental license.

For years, national boards have tested students on basic scientific and clinical knowledge and not on how to operate a successful practice. Because many dental schools teach, in part, to prepare their students to pass these boards, curriculum time and faculty efforts are heavily weighted to preparing students for this important milestone.

The economic environment of dental practice is changing rapidly, and educators have not kept up. In years past, if the new graduate knew dental techniques and treated their patients well, practice success was virtually assured. Today, new practitioners face a bewildering array of insurance plans, consumerism, corporate practices, large student debt payments, and regulatory requirements. In the face of this uncertain future, graduates want additional information to help them compete effectively in this new reality.

This book is primarily for dental students about to graduate, new graduates (both in a private practice and in other clinical settings), and recent graduates who have been out of school for five years or less. It is not written for well-established dentists who have practiced for 20 years, although they may find pearls to apply in their practices. Rather the basic business information that new practitioners can apply in their practice situation to compete effectively is presented. It is not intended to be specific management advice for every management problem—readers should consult with accountants, management consultants, or mentors about specific problems—but, if the issues can be understood, then the dentist can communicate more effectively with advisors and will understand and implement solutions and advice more effectively.

A dental practice is a small business. It responds to business concepts and rules the same as any other small business. The only difference is that dentists sell dental services, not hardware, clothing, electronics, or automobiles. So it is important to understand a business principle and then apply the principle in dental practices. In this way, a practitioner in New York City or in Mayfield, Kentucky, can use the same business principle in different-looking practices.

The numbers that are given as examples or illustrations are intended to represent the country as a whole. Some areas, especially large urban areas, have higher costs and higher fees than other, small town and rural areas. For example, typical wage rates for hygienists in large urban areas are currently in the range of $50.00 per hour; in many small to mid-sized towns, rates for hygienists are in the range of $25.00 per hour. Likewise, the fees that are charged are also generally higher in those urban areas. Therefore, the numbers that are shown may not represent a practice situation exactly, but the business concept behind the example is valid regardless of the practice area.

This book surveys the topics of operating a dental practice. As such, it is only an introduction to each of the topics. For example, although several pages are devoted to the methods of valuing a dental practice, experts have written entire manuals and even entire books on this subject alone. Other excellent texts, Web sites, and how-to manuals cover each of the topics in this book. For example, the American Dental Association produces an excellent series of books that cover practice transitions, regulatory compliance, and many other management topics in a level of detail that can not be put into one book. This book, then, is only a starting place for studying management in the office.

This book is the result of more than 25 years of teaching practice management to dental students and 20 years as a practice consultant, primarily with new and new and young practitioners. In this time, I have listened to problems that new practitioners face, helped them solve those problems, and guided them into successful careers. This book is not a spellbinding read. Instead, it is a text and a reference book. If the reader is a student, he or she may be required to read certain chapters to pass a test or course. A practitioner having a problem with staff interactions in the office may pick up the book and read the chapter on how to motivate employees. Either way, the intention is to understand how business people think about a problem and develop specific solutions to specific management problems. I hope that you find the information useful in that regard.

David O. Willis

About the Companion Website

This book is accompanied by a companion website:
www.wiley.com/go/willisdentistrybusiness

The website includes:

- Handouts
- Checklists
- Forms that can be used in the classroom setting

Section 1

Personal Financial Management

When it is a question of money, we are all of the same religion.
Voltaire

Money is central to US life. It has the power to build up or to tear down. It can grow and appreciate if properly managed or depreciate if mismanaged. Money can produce anxiety or joy—so can the lack of money. Money can lead to the gamut of human emotions, from happiness and jealousy to covet and rage. Money touches everyone in some way or another. It is used to buy power, control, and pleasure. It can easily be counted, and it becomes a surrogate for peoples' personal worth.

Money is also pervasive. There are entire broadcast networks devoted to money and investing. Daily publications and monthly magazines provide news about money and advise people how to make it and how to keep more of it. Money dominates the news. Whether the collapse of a country's economy, wars over resources, or riots and civil disturbance between those who have money and those who do not have any, money is the precipitating factor in many news stories. Money elects presidents, and financial scandal brings ruin to promising politicians and other leaders.

Millions of dollars will pass through a dental office throughout a career. Dental employees depend on a dentist for their family's financial safety and security. Dentists will pay bills and taxes and still have a significant amount of money left over for enjoyment. They then have to choose what to do with that money. It can be spent on themselves or family, gambled away, saved for retirement, or given away to churches or other worthwhile community organizations. Regardless, money needs to be managed to be spent wisely, to save it, and to invest it appropriately. A plan to manage financial affairs is needed to accomplish these ends. This is called *financial planning*. Financial planning is the development and implementation of total coordinated plans for the achievement of one's overall personal and professional objectives. It is a long-term process that requires knowledge and work and may also require the expertise of professional money managers to help a dentist establish and reach financial goals.

Concerns of the Financial Management Process

The financial planning process really is concerned with three major goals:

1. **Increasing Net Worth**   How assets are increased and liabilities are decreased so that as dentists move through their careers they increase their net worth.
2. **Balancing Family Spending**   When dentists earn money, they can either spend it or save it. Those are the only two options. If one is done, the other can not be done. An optimal mix is needed given family situations, goals, and ambitions.
3. **Planning for Emergencies**   Dentists run into financial emergencies at some point in their lives. The issue is whether or not they have prepared for these emergencies. If allowances have been made, then the emergencies will not be financially devastating.

Objectives of the Personal Financial Management Process

Given these three main concerns, the objectives of a financial plan can be grouped according to common categories. However, these categories can not be viewed in isolation because they each overlap and feed into every other

Business Basics for Dentists, First Edition. David O. Willis.
© 2013 John Wiley & Sons, Inc. Published 2013 by John Wiley & Sons, Inc.

category. The issues that dentists should examine in their own financial planning process include the following:

Chapter 1: Personal Money Management As dentists move through their career, they begin to accumulate things of value, both physical (such as houses) and financial (such as investment portfolios). Paying the principal on loans yields a similar result because eliminating a debt is equivalent to gaining a corresponding asset. These assets are then used for further investment, family purposes, or to build an emergency fund that is used for risk protection.

Chapter 2: Personal Insurance Needs Dentists face financial risks every day of their lives. These include the risk of premature death (before they have accumulated enough assets to care for their family's needs), the loss of income through a disabling condition, medical care expenses, and property and liability loses. Dentists often use insurance to protect themselves from these potential financial problems.

Chapter 3: Providing for Retirement Income No one provides business owners retirement income except themselves. The government provides several tax incentives to encourage business owners to save for their own retirement. If a retirement plan can be integrated into the office expenses, it can provide a comfortable income when business owners choose not to work.

Chapter 4: Reducing the Personal Tax Burden Taxes are a fact of life in the United States. However, personal and professional affairs can be planned to decrease tax burdens as much as possible within the laws and rules established by taxing agencies.

Chapter 5: Estate Planning As dentists accumulate wealth, they need to develop a plan for what happens to that wealth when (*not* if) they die. As small business owners, the practice may be one of the larger assets dentists own. Proper succession planning helps protect the value of this important asset. Additionally, people who have not accumulated a large amount of wealth need to be sure that their heirs are financially protected in cases of premature death.

Personal Money Management

chapter 1

Rule No. 1: Never lose money.
Rule No. 2: Never forget Rule No. 1.
Warren Buffet

Objectives

At the completion of this chapter, the student will be able to:
1. Describe common issues of personal money management for professionals.
2. Describe how personal lifestyle decisions affect the financial planning process.
3. Describe how savings affect the financial planning process.
4. Describe how to establish a personal credit rating.
5. Describe how to manage personal credit cards.
6. Describe the typical financial planning phases in a professional's life.

Key Terms

consolidation loan
credit card
credit rating (FICO score)
debit card

discretionary income
emergency fund
financial plan
identity theft

personal record management
system
safe deposit box

Goal

This chapter presents a description of the financial planning process. The relationship between practice development and personal needs will be stressed.

Many financial planning issues that young professional dentists face are the same as the general public. However, in other ways, the issues for dental professionals are unique. They often start with high debt loads but balance that with high income levels. Dentists are generally not employed by a company or organization that provides any benefits such as medical insurance or a retirement plan. They are often limited in how much income growth they can expect and must balance their income wants and needs with their desire for personal time. Because of these issues, new dentists must quickly become familiar with how to manage money.

Personal Money Management

Become a Good Money Manager

Dentists need to become good money managers, both in business life and private life. The first step is to learn all about money and how to use it. Becoming a good money manager does not just happen; it needs to be worked at, just like becoming a dentist. Dentists should study how to save, how to invest, and how to become a wise consumer. They should subscribe to *Kiplinger's* or *Money* magazine. These are the two leading personal financial magazines, and they give valuable tips for saving and making money.

Personal Records

Dentists accumulate many important personal financial records, therefore, a personal record management system, similar to the one developed for the office, should be created. Dentists should not let the paperwork pile up; they should work on records every month. They should get a safe deposit box at the bank or a fireproof safe at home for important papers. These important papers include wills, insurance policies, names of advisors, certificates of ownership, among others. Dentists should keep all tax records and related items for at least 7 years and keep insurance policies as long as they are in effect.

Getting Professional Help

As a professional, dentists have skills and knowledge that the public does not have. Dentists not only work with patients to take care of a patient's oral health but also direct and intervene as professional expertise dictates. The same is true for managing financial affairs. A dentist may have a basic level of understanding of financial management, but there are times when the guidance of a person with expert knowledge in a specific area is needed. Most dentists go first to their accountant for advice about both practice and personal finances. An accountant can be used to help with tax planning, setting up basic retirement plans, evaluating the numbers of the practice, and personal budgeting. Depending on the background and expertise of the accountant, additional help for investment planning, establishing estate plans, buying or selling or partnership opportunities, and a host of other advanced financial topics may be needed. In these areas, dentists often use a lawyer, financial planner, or management consultant. This later chapter was not included in the book. The crucial point is that dentists should become actively involved in their own personal financial management and planning but use the expertise of advisors when the situations demand it.

Personal Lifestyle Issues

Increasing Lifestyle and Income

New dentists are often like a kid in a candy store when they first start making money. They have been in school for 8 to 12 years, are often married, and have put off increasing personal spending and lifestyle while in school. Suddenly, with new-found wealth, they buy too much (often on credit) and struggle the next several years to pay increasing bills with the increasing take home pay. The tendency is for lifestyle expenses to increase along with income. Every dollar that a person makes, is spent on a bigger house, newer car, and new toys. Unfortunately, the solution is not a fun, warm process. Personal life expenses must be kept under control. It is easy to increase lifestyle to meet increasing income. Once accustomed to a certain lifestyle, it is difficult to cut back spending, for example, to start a retirement savings plan. A solution is to develop and use a family budget. If income increases, then take half the increase and use it to fund spending or investment plans. Use the other half to increase lifestyle. In this way, lifestyle increases (more slowly than without savings) and a saving or investment plan is painlessly funded. This approach does take discipline however.

Spend or Save

When money is earned, it can be spent or it can be saved. As previously mentioned, after years of training, most new dentists want to spend it immediately and enjoy it. Instead, they should get into the saving habit. Dentists should start each budget period by saving at least 20 percent of take-home pay, learning to live quite

Table 1.1 Saving (and Investing) a Dollar a Day

	5%	8%	11%	14%
1 year	$374	$380	$386	$392
5 years	$2,073	$2,244	$2,433	$2,643
10 years	$4,736	$5,592	$6,651	$7,966
20 years	$12,544	$18,036	$26,627	$40,259
30 years	$26,416	$45,728	$86,628	$171,179
40 years	$46,639	$107,351	$266,852	$701,946

adequately on the remaining 80 percent. As income increases, they should save as much of the increase as is spent. As Table 1.1 shows, saving even a dollar a day adds up to a sizeable sum over time.

Developing Personal Savings

Emergency Fund

One of the most important financial tasks is to establish an emergency fund. The emergency fund should consist of 3 to 6 months' take-home pay, depending on the amount and type of disability income insurance and other liquid assets that are available in cases of emergency. The money should be put into a low-risk liquid investment such as a money market mutual fund or checking account. (Although this is not exciting, it is safe.) It is a form of savings used for emergency needs and not as a speculative investment. Emergencies that this fund might cover include a car that dies, a short-term disability, or paying for medical treatment. It is not a vacation or Christmas savings plan. Other than emergency purchases, this fund allows one to increase deductibles on all insurance policies, which saves substantial money in premiums. Establishing the emergency fund is one of the most important *initial* financial planning jobs.

Saving versus Investing

Saving is holding onto money, stashing it away so that it can not be lost. Gain is not expected. Investing is buying an asset (possibly a stock or a share of a mutual fund) that will *possibly* increase in value over time. When one invests, gain is hoped for, but loss is also a possibility. Both saving and investing are valuable goals in the right situation. If building an emergency fund or holding on to money for a short-term purpose, then the safest bet is to make sure it is not lost. Money should be saved in a low-risk fund, such as a savings account or money market fund. If retirement is planned for in 30 years, then the long-term gains that are hoped for by investing in a mutual fund is the better route. The value of

the mutual fund may go down tomorrow, but it will hopefully (with wise fund choice) increase over the longer term.

Pay Off Debt or Build Assets

Should extra money be used to pay off debt, or should it be saved? Paying off debt as quickly as possible has become fashionable. Being debt free should be a long-term financial goal. From a purely financial standpoint, dentists should look at the after-tax return of the investment and the after-tax cost of the loan and then choose the one that gives a better return. If the interest rate is higher for the investment, then they should invest rather than pay off the loan. If the after-tax interest rate of the loan is higher, then they should pay off the loan. (See the chapter on business finance for a discussion of this topic.) From a cash flow perspective, cash may be needed for immediate necessities for the family or at the office. It is better to have an asset (the cash reserve) with a corresponding liability (the loan) than to have no cash and less of a loan. In the former case, a dentist may not need to go to a banker for an additional loan. In the latter case, when an additional loan is asked for, the banker may balk, wondering why previously loaned money was not handled properly. Once an emergency fund is built and an asset base established, then it becomes easier to put additional money into paying off debt. Again, comparing the expected return of investing with the savings from debt pay down is important. A final factor is one's personal temperament. A dentist must be a disciplined-enough investor to actually invest the money and not "blow it" on a purchase. Then the dentist must get the rate of investment return anticipated. If the loan is paid off, th dentist should have a plan for the monthly payment that had previously gone to loan payment. Finally, the dentist must invest that amount regularly or it will be spent with nothing to show for it at the end of the pay-off period.

Get Adequate Insurance

The chapter on personal insurance details the types of insurance a dentist might need. As a rule, dentists should not buy extended service contracts, which are a type of insurance. When buying a television, refrigerator, automobile, or any other major purchase, the dealer will try to sell an extended service contract. These cover most repairs needed over the term of the contract. It is better to see if the item fails and then pay to repair or replace it. The dentist should never buy additional (credit or mortgage) insurance. These types of policies insure that if one dies or becomes disabled, the policy will pay off a mortgage or car loan. These are expensive life insurance or disability policies. (Dealers sell them because they get a cut of the premium.) The dentist should have adequate life and disability insurance for his or her needs, and then remember to refuse these additional insurances when buying a major item. The dentist should never buy insurance from someone who calls because insurance policies should be investigated before being bought. As a rule, insurance should be shopped around for because it is a commodity item.

Personal Banking

Banks

Many new graduates have never had the problem and luxury of managing significant amounts of personal money. Establishing both a personal checking account and a professional (office) account are paramount. All checking accounts are not the same. Banks require different minimum amounts in accounts, charge different service fees, pay different rates of interest, and may limit numbers of checks that can be written. The dentist should shop around to find a bank that meets all his or her needs. Initially, he or she should find a checking account with low fees and low minimum balances. As assets and savings grow, the dentist should look for accounts that pay more interest and charge lower fees. Many banks allow and encourage patrons to banks electronically via the Internet. Monthly payments can be established, and transferring funds electronically to many different vendors instead of writing a physical check can also be done. If in a private practice and money was borrowed from a bank, the bank may require the dentist to keep all accounts with the bank. In this case, the "private" banking services, which add a tremendous amount of convenience to banking, can also be used.

Banking Services

Banks provide many services besides checking accounts. Most now offer e-banking, which improves convenience, and most banking can be done online. The banks loan money for small business or personal purchases and develop mortgages for large purchases. They offer credit cards for spending and often have accounts for credit card payments from patients. Many banks have special small business divisions that offer payroll and other services to the small business owner. They have safe deposit boxes for critical personal and business records. They often have investment advisors and retirement plan specialists to help a person develop and nurture these accounts. One of the first professional relationships that a dentist should make is with a banker.

Managing Credit

Credit Rating

Establishing a credit rating is another important step in financial planning. The major credit bureaus keep credit ratings on all Americans, using their Social Security numbers. This lets potential lenders quickly assess borrowers. The lender can decide if a person is a good lending risk by looking at how much he or she has borrowed before, and if the loan was paid off in a timely manner. With no credit history (i.e., someone has never borrowed money), the banker will probably deny the application for a loan. The problem is that the creditor simply does not know whether someone is a good credit risk. A credit rating can be established by acquiring a credit card and paying it off according to terms. A credit rating should also be nurtured by paying off all debts and credit cards on time. A bad credit history will haunt a person for many years. It can lead to denial of a practice, home, or other loan, denial of insurance or employment, or even the right to cash a check or open a bank or credit card account.

The lending companies commonly report a credit rating using a Fair, Isaac and Company (FICO) score, which was named for the company that developed the scoring system. (Some agencies use other, similar systems.) Scores range from 300 to 900, with most people in the 600 to 700 range. All credit scores begin at zero and a credit history is built up; it is not started at the top and subtracted down by poor credit choices. So without borrowing money or having any credit (e.g., credit card), a person does not have a credit history and is considered a poor credit risk in the eyes of the rating systems.

The higher the score a person has, the better his or her credit worthiness. A higher credit score means that it will be easier to get loans (and other forms of credit, such as credit cards), and the loans that are acquired will be at lower interest rates. Depending on the type of loan, lenders use the credit score, along with the full credit report, differently. They place more (or less) emphasis on particular components of the score, depending on their product. If a person is borrowing $200,000 for a house, the lender would obviously look at the person's score and history differently then if it was a loan for a $10,000 limit credit card.

Five major factors go into the calculation of a FICO score. They are:

1. Past delinquencies. If a person has failed to make payments in the past, he or she is more likely to repeat the pattern.
2. How has the credit been used? If a person is close to the limit on a credit card (or worse, maxed out) he or she is a greater risk.

Table 1.2 Free Credit Reports

Company	URL
Annual Credit Report	www.annualcreditreport.com
My Fico	www.myfico.com
Experian Inc.	http://www.experian.com
Equifax Inc.	http://www.equifax.com
Trans Union Corp.	http://www.tuc.com

3. The age of the credit file. A person who has had credit for a long time has a track history and is, therefore a better risk.
4. How often credit is asked for. If a person has repeatedly asked for credit over a short time, something may be awry financially.
5. The mix of credit. With only one credit card, a person is riskier than someone else who has several forms of credit, such as a home mortgage and other loans.

A person should check his or her credit history and rating on a regular (annual) basis. Each person can get one free from each of the major national credit bureaus. If a dentist is planning to buy a house, borrow for a practice, or make another major purchase, then he or she should check his or her history about 3 months in advance. If errors are found, this gives the dentist enough time to get them changed. Table 1.2 gives the Web sites of the major credit houses: Experian, Equifax, and Trans Union. They and the other sites also have a wealth of information on managing credit and debt. Depending on the study cited, 1 to 50 percent of consumer credit reports contain errors. Some may be simple and inconsequential (such as a misspelling). Others may affect a credit rating for years to come. Fraudulent activity, such as identity theft, may even be discovered. Inaccuracies can be irksome to correct. The Fair Credit Reporting Act requires bureaus to respond promptly. However, the bureaus will not necessarily change a history just because a person says so. (If they did, everyone would call and demand a clean credit history!) A person is essentially guilty until proven innocent. Proof and involving the creditor who sent in the inaccurate report are generally needed to clear a record.

Managing Credit Cards

Credit cards get more people into financial trouble than any other cause. Credit cards make it easy to buy things. When an item is purchased with a credit card, the issuing bank pays the merchant, essentially floating the credit card holder a loan for the amount of the item. The credit card holder can then "borrow" up to the limit on the credit card. (With debit cards, only the money present in an account can be used.) The credit card hold then does not have to pay the bank for the item until the end of the

month. That works well if the credit card balance is paid off at the end of each month. However, if it is not paid off, the bank charges the credit card holder interest, generally about 1 1/2 percent on the unpaid balance. That 1 1/2 percent per month, when compounded, equals nearly 20 percent per year. So paying off a credit card balance is a wise idea. The problem is that it is easy to let the balances grow to overwhelming levels, and banks are too eager to let a person amass large credit card balances. The value of a credit card is being able to borrow money for purchases (up to the card limit) and the convenience of this form of payment. The obvious down side comes if balances are not paid off regularly or if a person borrows more than he or she can afford to pay off.

There are several common-sense solutions to the credit card problem, other than using credit cards carefully and paying them off monthly. If a person has a credit card problem, use a debit card (instead of a credit card) because only the amount of money in the account can be spent. The bank will deny the merchant's authorization if there is not enough money in the account to cover the cost of a purchase. This way, a person can not overspend. Dentists should have one personal and one professional credit card. All professional purchases go on the professional card, and personal purchases on the personal card. This keeps him or her more aware of the total credit card balance and keeps the dentist from running up the total balance by having balances on several cards. (It is a good idea to have a "back-up" credit card that has no annual fee. If a primary card is lost, stolen, or for any other reason becomes inactive, the back-up card can be used.)

If using a credit card, the dentist should shop around for the best deal for the monetary circumstance. "Gold" cards have higher credit limits and more generous terms than regular cards. The catch is that a person needs to qualify by having a good credit history and income. "Platinum" cards have even higher limits and requirements. Both cards have more advantages if a person is careful and has more rope to hang a person financially if not careful. Many banks issue cards with the name of a sponsoring organization (such as an alumni association) on the card. A small amount of money goes to the sponsoring organization (instead of to the card holder as higher rebates). Dentists should avoid these cards; they are expensive. Most cards have an annual fee; this should be as low as possible. (Dentists should negotiate with a credit card issuer to eliminate the annual fee.) A low percentage interest charge is also ideal; however, there is usually a trade-off between the interest and the annual fee. Higher annual fees lead to lower interest rates. (The converse is true also.) If balances are paid off regularly, the lower annual fee is better. Interest rates should not affect this type of consumer. If balances are not paid off in full, the lower interest rates are better. The cardholder should check to see when the payment due date is on a credit balance. Some cards require payment within 10 days. Others give the credit card holder until the end of the month for payment. Finding a card that gives rebates, as either cash rebates or travel points (or miles), is also a good idea.

Family Budget

A budget is a statement of how money has been spent in the past and an estimate of future income and expenses. As such, budgets become a target for day-to-day financial living. Budgets are most frequently used when a family is having a financial problem. The family then helps set targets for spending and lets everyone know why spending is limited in one area or another. A budget can help coordinate savings and improve living standards by identifying areas of waste.

Although each budget is unique for the person, some general targets for expenditure categories can be developed. No more than 30 percent of take-home pay should be spent for housing costs, 20 percent for food (groceries and eating out), and 15 percent for other miscellaneous expenses (Table 1.3). Debt payments (including student loan payments) should total no more than 30 percent of take-home pay. The budget should also detail paying a minimum of 5 to 10 percent of take-home pay into savings (personal and retirement).

Managing Student Loans

Most new dental graduates carry a significant amount of student loan debt. This becomes a problem that affects every other area of personal financial planning. Unfortunately, there is no magic quick fix out of student debt. The rules on student loans change frequently, so no detailed advice is given here; however, the same rules apply to this as to other loans. Dentists should practice good debt management habits and be persistent to pay off the loan.

There are two general types (at present) of student loans, subsidized and unsubsidized. In subsidized loans, the government pays the interest while a person is in school, training, or certain other situations. In unsubsidized loans, the interest begins to accumulate when the

Table 1.3 A Sample Budget

Category	Percentage
Housing	30%
Food	20%
Debt Payments	20–30%
Savings	5–10%
Miscellaneous or insurance	15%

loan is secured. The interest rate is lower on subsidized loans as well. Given a choice, dentists should take the subsidized loans first and defer payment until the interest begins.

Dentists should consolidate student loans, both subsidized and unsubsidized loans. Consolidation does not work like other loan consolidations because the resulting interest rate is between the two. Given a choice, the dentist should consider paying off the high-interest loan faster rather than consolidating.

A career plan may lead to a professional opportunity that includes a given amount of loan repayment per year as part of the benefit package. Depending on debt and income levels, a person may qualify for a reduced payment scenario. Finally, student loan interest is deductible, up to an annual amount of interest. This deduction is limited for high-income earners. After a profitable practice is established, additional working capital to pay off student loan debt may be borrowed. Check the interest rates and tax deductibility of the interest before taking the loan.

Personal bankruptcy does not relieve a person of his or her student loan obligation. The only way to get out of student debt is to die. However, some unsubsidized loans become part of an estate's debt, so that even in death a person is not freed of the obligation. Dental students should check with loan services to be sure that there is a death benefit or life insurance rider that pays the loan obligation. Dentists should check the price of this insurance because it may be less expensive to buy additional term life insurance in the marketplace, rather than insuring through a loan servicing company.

Family Planning: The Cost of a Family

For many people, becoming a parent is the greatest challenge in their adult lives. These changing responsibilities, obligations, and commitments last a lifetime–once a parent, always a parent. No other life event causes people to become as thoughtful, careful, and focused on the future as having the moral, physical, and financial responsibility of raising children.

Children involve both additional direct costs and the indirect costs of increasing family size. Box 1.1 details some of these costs. No matter what people say ("Children are cheap. They hardly eat a thing!"), the simple fact is that having a family is expensive. For the dentist, these costs often come at a time when the family budget is already thin because of the need to pay off student debt and initiate a dental practice. If one parent quits work to care for children, family income gets squeezed even tighter. Some estimates place the cost of raising a child to the age of 18 at nearly $400,000. This does not include the cost of college, professional, or

Box 1.1 Extra Cost of Children

Babysitter or day-care expense
Buying (and moving) into a larger home
Remodeling or adding to an existing home
Buying a larger or more reliable car
Expanding insurance coverage
Higher insurance premiums
Moving to neighborhoods with better schools
Sending children to private schools
Paying for children's extracurricular activities
Taking family vacations
Paying increased medical bills
Buying more or different food
Buying more clothes and furniture
Buying gifts for children

Table 1.4 Car Depreciation by Year

Year	Depreciation
1	28%
2	20%
3	16%
4	8%
5	6%
6	5%
7	4%
8	3%
9	2%
10	1%

graduate schooling. Having children is an expensive proposition indeed.

What should be done to financially prepare for children? The dentist should do the same type of financial planning as was done before children, have a budget and stick to it. The dentist should have a properly funded emergency fund, more so now than before. He or she should expand savings and save for purchases, educational needs, and children's activities. The family should look closely at the impacts of having one or two working parents. One income means less money to spend and invest, but it also means that one parent will be available to care for children. Day care is expensive! Family finances will be different (costs such as day-care and work expenses), and the family dynamic will be different. The dentist should balance the trade-off in finances with the nonmaterial issues of family life.

Buying a Car

One of the first purchases a new dental graduate often makes is an automobile. However, he or she should consider driving the current car for another year; repair bills are generally less than monthly payments on a new car. If a dentist must have a new car, several strategies to maximize the dollar value of this purchase can be used. The dentist should pay cash and not finance the cost of the car. He or she should use an emergency fund to buy a new car and then replenish the emergency fund. If the automobile purchase must be financed, the dentist should not use dealer financing (unless they are running a really low interest rate promotion) because better rates can be gotten through a credit bureau or bank. The dentist should not buy a new car but buy a recent year, used

car; the savings are substantial. Table 1.4 shows the amount that the price of a new automobile depreciates each year. Buying a 2-year-old car for about half the price of a comparable new car is more financially responsible, and it is often still under manufacturer's warranty. The market is full of cars that private individuals, corporations, or leasing companies have leased. Many still have some of their initial warranty remaining; the dentist should look for one of these cars and save. The National Association of Automobile Dealers (NADA) puts out a booklet each month that gives average prices for all makes and models of used cars. The dentist should get one of these books at a local bookstore and check the prices of cars. By selling, rather than trading in an old car, he or she can get a better price. (Trading it in is more convenient but how much is that convenience worth.) The dealer may offer a high price for the trade in but not discount the price of a new car as much. A buyer should not give car keys to a salesperson. ("Give me your keys and I'll have Fred check the car out to see what we can give you on trade in.") The buyer is then a captive and can not leave; the salesperson is in control. Instead, the buyer should walk with the salesperson to view the old car but keep the keys.

Automobile Insurance

Dentists can save substantially by managing automobile insurance. (See the chapter on personal insurances.) They should always shop for automobile insurance. This is really a commodity product. Insurance from one company is the same as insurance from another. They should buy comparable policies based on price and increase deductibles as much as possible. A $500 deductible policy will pay for itself compared to a $100 policy in about 3 years. (This is an example of the value of an emergency fund.) The drive should drop comprehensive and collision insurance if the value of the car is less than $3,000. Comprehensive and collision pay to fix a person's own car. If a $3,000 car is wreck, the emergency fund should be used to buy a new one. (A liability policy should be kept. This covers the other person's losses if the wreck is not his or her fault.) The driver should drop emergency road service and rental from the policy. These can be paid for out of pocket or by joining the auto club (AAA). AAA offers free road service and free maps. Buyers should shop for special discounts. Most insurers lower premiums if for good students, an installed alarm system, or if the VIN number is etched on the glass. The buyer should check to see what special offers a company has before insuring an automobile with them. Further, the buyer should integrate an automobile policy with an umbrella liability policy to avoid duplicate insurance or any gaps in insurance.

How to Improve Spending Habits

Whatever the present financial situation, there are only two things that can be done to improve it: earn more or spend less. Assuming a person has maximized earning, several steps can be taken to improve spending habits. First, a budget must be developed. Spending patterns should be examined, looking for areas of wasteful spending or areas that can easily be cut. The plan for financial improvement should be written down; it is too easy to come up with a vague plan. Until and unless the plan is written down on paper, it does not mean anything. Credit cards should not be used. Many people get into serious financial trouble using credit cards. Checks or a debit card should be used instead. Shopping trips should be separated from spending trips. Impulse buying leads to bad financial decisions. Expensive purchase items should be compared on the Internet or a shopping-only (not purchasing) trip taken. No purchases should be made on an initial trip. When a decision has been made,

then the buyer should go on a buying trip to purchase the item; a better buying decision will be made in this way. Smoking and other costly habits should be quit. Saving a dollar a day and adding all pocket change will quickly accumulate savings.

Preventing Debt Problems

With debt management, prevention is obviously the best cure. Table 1.5 estimates what payments will be for various loans. This is important to ensure that payments fit the budget.

Keep a Reasonable Debt-to-Income Ratio

It sounds simple, but dentists should not borrow too much money. They should keep an accurate eye on the budget. Most lenders set a limit of 35 percent of total pretax income for the total debt load. This includes home mortgage, automobile loans, credit card, and other types of personal debt payment. In fact, a dentist may not qualify for certain types of loans if the debt payment-to-income ratio is too high.

Before Borrowing, Have a Specific Plan to Repay Debt

Dentists should work debt payments into the personal budget. This ensures that they will have the cash flow necessary to pay off the loan. If payments do not fit into the budget, something must be given up, either a present expense item or the anticipated purchase.

Table 1.5 Estimating Loan Payments
Multiply the loan principal (in thousands of dollars) times the factor to determine the monthly payment amount.

Monthly Payments on Each $1,000 Borrowed								
Years	4%	6%	8%	10%	12%	14%	16%	18%
1	$85.15	$86.07	$86.99	$87.92	$88.85	$89.79	$90.73	$91.68
5	$18.47	$19.33	$20.28	$21.25	$22.24	$23.27	$24.32	$25.39
7	$13.67	$14.61	$15.59	$16.60	$17.65	$18.74	$19.86	$21.02
9	$11.04	$12.01	$13.02	$14.08	$15.18	$16.33	$17.53	$18.76
10	$10.12	$11.10	$12.13	$13.22	$14.35	$15.53	$16.75	$18.02
12	$8.76	$9.76	$10.82	$11.95	$13.13	$14.37	$15.66	$16.99
15	$7.40	$8.44	$9.56	$10.75	$12.00	$13.32	$14.69	$16.10
30	$4.77	$6.00	$7.34	$8.78	$10.29	$11.85	$13.45	$15.07

Example 1: A new car is purchased for $30,000. The entire amount is financed at 8% for 5 years. What is the monthly payment?
PMT = 20.28 × 30 = $608.40/month
Example 2: A dental practice is purchased for $200,000. The entire amount is financed at 10% for 7 years. What is the monthly payment?
PMT = 16.60 × 200 = $3,320/month

Avoid Impulse Buying: Plan and Save for Purchases

Many consumers get into debt problems from their credit cards. They look at a bill at the end of a couple of months and realize that they have charged so many impulse purchases that they have reached their credit limit and now must aggressively pay down this expensive debt.

Pay Full Balances on Credit Cards Each Month

Credit card debt is one of the most expensive types of debt incurred. Most cards have a "grace period" built into payment schedules. The balance should be paid off in full each payment period so that interest payments on credit card accounts are not accumulated. If they are paid off, the borrower is borrowing the bank's money free. That is a good deal. Paying 24 percent interest per year is a bad deal.

Getting Out of Debt

If prevention has not worked, and a person has too much debt, several steps to reduce the debt load should be taken.

Understand There Are No Quick Fixes

A person can get into debt quickly, but it takes time to pay off the debt. The first step is to begin *now*. The longer a person waits, the more the interest accumulates. The person should admit having a financial problem and begin working to solve the problem. If overwhelmed, he or she should seek professional financial help. A banker, accountant, or a certified financial planner can help a person solve financial problems.

Be Ready for Lifestyle Changes

Getting out of a large amount of debt will be painful. A significant amount of money will need to be paid to lenders for an extended time. Unless income increases significantly, a person can not maintain lifestyle and pay off debt. Lifestyle may need to be reduced. A written plan should be made because until it is written on paper, it is not real. The borrower should also take on no new debt. Credit card accounts should be closed and a written accounting of all income and expenses should be maintained. A personal financial analysis should be done and this information used to budget for spending. All extra income should be put toward paying off debt.

Work with Creditors

A person should not hide from creditors. Eventually, they will find him or her. Creditors want to be repaid. They will work with a person to develop a payment plan that can be met. However, creditors must be kept informed. They may help by offering slower repayment plans or other methods that help a person get out of debt, which helps the creditor get paid the money owed.

Consolidate Debt When Necessary

Debt consolidation is when a person has several high-interest loans. It may be so difficult to make these payments that the interest accumulates faster than it can be paid off. If a person can borrow money at 10 percent to pay off an 18 percent credit card, he or she is usually better off. (Origination fees and other requirements of the consolidation loan need to be researched.) In this way, the consumer can consolidate these expensive loans and, hopefully, pay off the debt more easily. Note that this technique is primarily for people who are in debt trouble. Consolidation is not the simple panacea that some lenders make it out to be. A person now has one lender who may not be sympathetic to problems.

Use Tax-Deductible Debt, If Possible

There are times that it is to a person's advantage to use home equity loans or business loans (working capital) to pay off debt. The interest rates (effective after-tax rates) should be compared to decide which is best.

Accelerate Debt Payments, If Possible

As a rule, the faster debt is paid off, the less interest payments are made. Therefore, on the face of it, it is always a good thing to pay off debt as quickly as possible. However, there are several times when this rule of thumb may not be valid. A person may need to stretch a debt payment out to have adequate cash flow for other budget expenses. Or a person may have an incredibly low interest rate or generous terms on loans that make them attractive to keep.

A small additional payment makes a huge difference in the total loan payout. Box 1.2 shows what happens to the number of payments when the amount paid each month is increased. By simply adding $50 per month to a 10-year loan, it halves the number of payments made. (The principal paid remains the same, but it is paid more quickly and paid with less interest.) Greater savings are

---

Box 1.2 Making Larger Loan Payments

Principal = $100,000
Interest Rate = 9%
Term = 10 years

Normal Payment $1267	Additional Principal Payment			
	+$50	+$100	+$200	+$500
Payment	$1317	$1367	$1467	$1767
Years	5.0	4.9	4.6	3.9

Box 1.3 Financial Planning Phases

Phase 1
    Build the emergency fund
    Buy appropriate insurance
    Develop savings habit
    Establish family budget (spending patterns)
Phase 2
    Increase emergency fund with income
    Decrease insurance deductibles
    Begin retirement savings
    Begin children's college funds
    Begin investment portfolio
    Increase lifestyle (modestly)
Phase 3
    Maximize retirement savings
    Maximize personal savings and investment
    Increase lifestyle
    Buy toys
Phase 4
    Maximize lifestyle
    Donate wealth

---

seen with larger monthly additions. Most loans (especially mortgages) do not have any prepayment penalties associated with paying all or some principal off early. So if cash flow will support it, a person can come out ahead financially by making an extra principal payment as often as possible.

Financial Planning Phases

There is a typical order of financial tasks for young professionals to consider. These will be different for different life situations. The dentist who is single in a lucrative practice will have different constraints than a married dentist supporting a family in a start-up situation. A person will enter the phases of financial planning more or less quickly and have different emphases within the each phase than another person.

Phase 1: Increasing Debt

The first phase typically is marked by high debt levels because the graduate purchases a practice and often a home. The dentist should keep borrowing and spending under control. An initial task is that the dentist has adequate insurance. Part of personal insurance planning is to set the appropriate deductible for the circumstance. As the emergency fund is built, the dentist should decrease deductibles and decrease the cost of personal insurances. He or she should build the practice or professional situation, increasing earnings by making the practice profitable through increasing production and decreasing costs. The dentist should be sure that family spending patterns do not increase faster than income and saving increase. He or she should start funding an individual retirement account as soon as able. This helps to build a savings habit or mentality, as opposed to a spending mentality.

Phase 2: Increasing Income

During the second phase, the practice begins to generate higher income. As income increases, the dentist needs to decide what to do with the additional money. Part of the increase (half) should be used to increase savings and begin investments. As income increases, so does the amount needed for the emergency fund. The dentist should fully fund this increased emergency fund and check that insurance benefits and deductible amounts are appropriate. He or she should start a practice retirement plan and begin saving for children's higher education expenses and personal investment portfolio. The dentist should estimate personal income taxes appropriately. As income increases, loan payments remain steady, and depreciation deductions decrease (generally around year 5). At this point, many dentists find that they have not planned well for taxes and need to borrow cash to pay current taxes. Finally, once the savings habit has been developed, the rest of the increase should be used to improve lifestyle.

Phase 3: Maximum Cash Flow

During the third phase, the initial practice loan is paid off and practice income is high. When the practice loan is paid off, the dentist should reallocate half the monthly payment to increasing the retirement plan, use half the remaining half to increase personal savings and investment, and the rest to increasing lifestyle. Extra payments to retire debt to become debt free can now be made. At this point, the dentist can begin buying the toys (house on the lake, airplanes, etc.) desired.

Phase 4: Maximize Lifestyle

During the fourth phase, income is at its peak and expenses are at their lowest. A person has educated children, paid house mortgages, developed savings, and funded retirement plans. At this point, working becomes a choice, rather than a necessity. The practice and personal life can be what a person wants them to be, free of worrying about money. Many people find that they have more time to devote to social and religious causes and find additional activities to give their lives meaning.

Personal Insurance Needs

chapter 2

*I detest life-insurance agents; they always argue that
I shall some day die, which is not so.*
Stephen Leacock

Objectives

At the completion of this chapter, the student will be able to:
1. Discuss these types of insurance with respect to the purposes, types, benefits, limitations, risk management technique, features, and tax consequences:
   Medical
   Hospitalization
   Disability
   Life
   Automobile
   Homeowners
   Personal excess liability
2. Compare these types of life insurance
   Permanent (Whole)
   Universal
   Endowment
   Term

Key Terms

automobile insurance
  collision coverage
  comprehensive coverage
  damage to covered autos
  liability
  medical payments
  uninsured motorists
disability (income) insurance
  amount of monthly benefit
  any occasion policies
  "back-to-work" clause
  definition of disability
  disability insurance
  elimination period
  guaranteed renewability
  inflation rider
  length of the benefit
  noncancellability
  office overhead policy
  own occasion policies

residual clause
Social Security
substantially similar
occupation
homeowners' insurance
  homeowners coverages
  liability exclusions
  replacement cost provision
  riders
insurance
  actuaries
  adjustor
  benefit
  frequency of occurrence
  hold harmless clause
  indemnify
  independent agent
  insurer
  policy
  policy holder

premium
premium rates
proven loss
size of typical award
life insurance
  cash value
  cross-purchase agreements
  decreasing term policy
  endowment life
  loan protection insurance
  mortgage protection
  nonrenewable
  ordinary
  permanent
  pure life insurance
  renewable
  term insurance
  universal life
  variable life
  whole life

(Continued)

Business Basics for Dentists, First Edition. David O. Willis.
© 2013 John Wiley & Sons, Inc. Published 2013 by John Wiley & Sons, Inc.

Key Terms (*Continued*)

medical insurance	(HMOs)	risk management
basic coverage	independent practice associations (IPAs)	risk avoidance
copayments	limitations	risk reduction
catastrophic medical insurance	major medical	risk retention
deductibles	preferred provider organizations (PPOs)	risk transfer
excess major medical	tax deductibility	umbrella liability policies
flexible benefit plan	utilization reviews	
health maintenance organizations	personal excess liability policy	

Goal

This chapter helps the student determine what personal insurance needs will be upon entering a professional practice. It suggests methods of obtaining the best buys in insurance.

The process of risk management involves identifying and managing a person's risk exposures to protect assets and income. People can not live in a risk-free world. There is always the possibility of a loss. However, a person can protect assets against large, unexpected loses that could financially devastate others. A person needs to accept *some* risk. In analyzing risk, a person needs to separate those risks and determine which can be accepted and which need to be managed through some type of insurance. This chapter discusses forms of personal insurance. Professional insurance is discussed in a later chapter.

Box 2.1 Insurance Needs for Dentists

Personal
Medical care expenses
Loss of income (Disability)
Premature death (Life)
Property and liability losses
    Automobile
    Homeowner
    Excess liability (umbrella)
Professional
Professional liability (Malpractice)
Business liability
Loss of use
Office overhead
Required business
    Workers' compensation
    Unemployment compensation
    Social Security

Understanding Insurance

Insurance is one of the most commonly used risk-management techniques. There is insurance available to cover almost any potential loss (Box 2.1). A person needs to decide if the loss is potentially large enough or common enough to insure against. (A person may purchase flood insurance, but if he or she lives on a mountain top, why bother?) As a rule, if the loss can be self-sustained, it is cheaper, over time, not to buy insurance and to self-insure and accept the loss. For example, a dentist probably should not buy dental insurance for his or her family because the dentist can afford most dental costs incurred by family members. Should a dentist buy medical and accident insurance? Probably, because the potential loss is so great. For example, an automobile accident involving a week in the hospital for one person can easily cost $50,000, not including liability should that person cause the accident.

Insurance is a commodity. That means that the actual insurance is the same from one company to another (assuming comparable policies). Therefore, a person can shop for insurance based solely on price. Agents work for the insurer, not for the consumer. A person may pay extra for the extended insurance product, which means that the consumer may pay extra for convenience, familiarity with the agent, or broad forms of coverage. However, the insurance itself is the same. Insurance agents are all different. The dentist should shop around at least for an insurance agent. Often he or she will get better rates and better service if he or she has all types of coverage with one carrier and may also get better rates if he or she stays with an insurer for several years without a claim.

The purpose of insurance is to guard against an unexpected, large financial loss. The basic theory of insurance is that many people each pay a small amount (the premium) into a pool of funds. If any of the payers are unfortunate enough to suffer a large loss, then part of the pool of funds goes to cover that loss. For example, many people pay a small premium to an insurance company in case their home is damaged or destroyed by a disaster, such as a fire. Most people do not have any damage and therefore do not collect from their insurance company. But if a fire damages a home, the owner will receive money from the pool (as a "payout") to cover their damages. However, insurance only reimburses for a *demonstrated* loss.

Insurance companies set premium rates based on several factors that influence their expected payout from the pool of premiums. The insurer needs to cover all expected losses and make a reasonable profit along the way. Obviously, the frequency of occurrence and size of the typical award both influences the expected payout from the company. A person's history of claims, age, and other personal factors help determine the company's estimate of a particular risk as an insured party. Insurers use actuaries (similar to glorified accountants) to figure out risk tables and rates to charge their various clients. For example, the chance of an 85-year-old man dying is much greater than the chance of a 5-year old dying in a given year. The life insurance rates, based on the chance of a member of each population dying, for the 85-year-old man will obviously be higher than for the 5-year old.

Insurers face the risk that more people will die, have a house fire, or a car wreck in any given year than they anticipated. If that happens, they initially lose money, and then raise everyone's rates the following year or cancel policies of the poorer risks. Most also carry insurance themselves, through Lloyd's of London or other insurance underwriters. They call this the secondary insurance market, and it helps cover the insurers for large losses, such as natural (hurricane) or human (terrorist) disasters. Insurers use other techniques to control how much risk that they face. Copays, deductibles, limits of payment, exclusions, and other riders all help control their potential losses.

A person must decide when to use insurance. There are times when the law requires that people have insurance. (Workers' compensation and unemployment insurance are examples of required insurance for employers.) Other than these required times, a person should use insurance to help cover an unexpected, unpredictable loss that he or she cannot afford to pay out of pocket. The owner of a new $30,000 car often chooses to insure the car in case an accident causes such damage to the automobile that he or she cannot afford to have it repaired. The owner of an old $1,000 junker car may choose to carry no insurance on the vehicle. If the car is wrecked, the owner simply has lost the cost of the car. (Insuring liability, in case the owner of the junker caused the accident, is required by law in many states.) Other large unpredictable losses that may be insured against include damage to the home, hospitalization, loss of income as a result of a disability, liability as a professional (malpractice), or as a private individual (personal liability)

A person signs a contract (*policy*) with the insurance company. The contract states that the insurer (the company) will indemnify (make good a loss to) the policy holder in case of proven loss (as specified in the policy) given the restrictions written into the policy. Insurance companies usually sell policies through insurance agents. Agents may work for one company, or they may represent many companies (an "independent" agent) shopping around for the best rates for a given situation. A person's relationship with an insurance agent may be as close as that with an accountant, so a trustworthy agent should be found. The buyer should be sure that the agent explains all the options of the policies and integrates the various types of coverage for the various insurances that are purchased. The state in which a person resides, not the federal government, regulates both insurance companies and agents.

If a policy holder has a loss, the agent will be an initial contact with the company. The policy holder should understand that the agent does not decide whether the policy holder gets reimbursed for a loss. The insurance company does that. The agent is only acting as a go-between, often splitting allegiance between the policy holder and the company. An adjustor is a person hired by the insurer to decide the amount of covered loss that has been suffered. After a car accident, the adjustor will determine how much it should cost to fix the car (and therefore the reimbursable loss). The agent will act as a best friend while a person is paying premiums. If that person files a claim, things change. The agents then play "good cop, bad cop" with the adjustors and home office. Policy holders should not expect agents to go to bat for them.

Medical Insurance

Medical insurance reimburses a person for large, unexpected medical costs. At the time of the writing this book, the federal government initiated a "health care reform," which may change significantly the way people pay for health care. The government plan will use private insurers and government direct payment to pay for care. Regardless the type of insurance, it consists of several components.

1. **Basic Coverage** Basic coverage insures against losses from common medical costs, such as a doctor's office visit, minor hospitalizations, and emergency department visits. These are relatively low-cost, high-frequency medical procedures. The cost for this type of insurance is understandably high. Some policies include prescription drugs, medical devises, and therapies.
2. **Major Medical** Major medical takes up where basic coverage ends. As the name implies, it is designed to cover major medical expenses, such

as hospitalizations or surgery. It often has an upper limit over a person's lifetime. This range is typically $1 to $2 million per lifetime. If this amount is exceeded, the insurance stops paying.

3. **Excess Major Medical or Catastrophic Medical**   This insurance takes up where major medical ends. It covers catastrophic illnesses or accidents. Although these are expensive procedures, they are relatively rare, so the cost for this coverage is fairly low.

4. **Comprehensive**   Insurers often bundle these three types of insurance into a "comprehensive medical" insurance policy. In that way, they can be sure that there are no gaps in coverage and that needs are well met.

Coverage Restrictions

The insurers usually place various restrictions on payment as well. Common techniques include:

1. **Deductibles**   A deductible is an amount that an insured must pay out of pocket before the insurance begins coverage. The higher the deductible is, the lower the cost of premiums is. This is because the insurance company will pay less because the insured pays more. The trade-off for a lower deductible is higher premium payments.

2. **Copayments**   Copayments require the insured to pay part of the cost (e.g., 20 percent of the cost of the service) out of pocket. Like a deductible, this is supposed to make the insured think twice before getting medical services that may not be needed.

3. **Limitations**   Limitations exclude certain procedures or classes of illnesses. Common exclusions in medical policies include treatment for alcoholism or drug abuse, personal counseling, chiropractor, or other difficult-to-prove medical conditions. Insurance companies often limit paying for experimental drugs or surgeries. As expected, the insurer usually determines what they consider experimental.

4. **Network Providers**   Many third-party payers now have networks of providers that must be used if the insurer is to pay a portion of the cost. Other policies require that a higher portion or a higher deductible be paid if providers who are not in the network are used.

5. **Utilization Reviews**   Plans may require that the insured get a second opinion from one of the network's providers or use other methods to review the planned treatment before it occurs. Insurance companies may also review a provider's charges to see that they fall in the expected range of services.

Because of the high cost of medical insurance premiums, many employers have begun to buy cheaper managed health care contracts for their employees. These are generally not true insurance products (which indemnify, or agree to pay for a loss) but instead are forms of prepayment for care, which shifts the risk of overutilization of health services to the provider. The common forms are health maintenance organizations (HMOs), preferred provider organizations (PPOs), and independent practice associations (IPAs). These all have counterparts in the dental practice world and, like the dental products, reduce payment and increase risk for the provider. This is such a rapidly evolving portion of the insurance world that books are outdated by the time they are completed.

Purchasing Medical Insurance

Some general rules for the purchase of medical insurance coverage:

- The dentist should get adequate coverage. A $1 million comprehensive policy is a minimum.
- The better the coverage is, the higher the cost. Higher deductible, higher copayments, and required second opinions all lower the cost to the insured. The dentist should self-insure (pay out of pocket) if possible. It is usually cheaper, unless he or she *knows* the insurance coverage will be used.
- Costs to the consumer are almost always less with care using the insurer's network of providers. If a person has a particular medical provider that he or she wants to use, this might be one of the deciding factors when looking at several potential policies.
- Group policies are usually cheaper than individual policies. If a group buys a policy, the insurer spreads the risk (chance of payment) over more people, many of whom will not use the coverage. (The only people who buy individual policies are the ones who think that they will use it.) Dental society group policies or a spouse's work policy (if any) should be looked at; the savings can be substantial.
- The dentist should establish an office group policy or individual policies using a flexible benefit plan. The tax savings can be substantial.
- Almost all medical plans have some component of managed care.

Disability (Income) Insurance

The chance of a person becoming disabled at some point during his or her professional career is much greater than the chance of dying during that same time. According to the National Safety Council®, in 2008, there were 2.1 million disabling injuries caused by a motor vehicle accident, but there were 39,000 fatal motor vehicle accidents.[1] Although death is certainly a more important event than disability, too many professionals carry life insurance but do not include disability insurance as part of their financial risk management plan.

Although a simple flu can disable a person for several days, a true disability is the inability to work for at least 30 days. Less than that is considered a simple illness. Disability insurance does not insure a person from becoming disabled and does not automatically pay if a person is disabled. It protects a person's loss (of income) if disabled. So the more proper name for this type of insurance is disability *income* insurance. As with other insurable losses, a person has to show the loss to collect the benefits. For example, a dentist has to show that he or she lost $10,000 per onth in income for the policy to replace it. If he or she only had $3,000 per month of income, that is all the policy will replace, even if the policy had a $10,000-per-month face amount (limit). Disability insurance coverage, regardless the source, is designed to only replace about two-thirds to three-fourths of income. With multiple policies, the disability income insurance will generally exclude or offset payments from other policies. A common "insurance with other insurers" clause reduces payments proportional to other policies.

Disability can occur for many reasons. An automobile accident can leave a person unable to practice for the rest of his or her life. A skiing accident or simple fall in the home can render a person incapable for many months. Contagious diseases (e.g., Hepatitis B, HIV) can leave a person incapable of practice. A heart attack can disable someone for weeks or years. Modern medicine has changed many diseases, such as diabetes or cardiovascular problems, from acute deadly diseases to more chronic diseases. However, these lead to more disability claims. The Council for Disability Awareness estimates that a 35-year old female has a 23 percent chance of being disabled for 3 months or longer during her working career. Of these, there is a 38 percent chance that the disability would last 5 years or longer. For males, there is a 21 percent risk of a 3-month or longer disability during his working life, with the same 38 percent chance for a 5-year (or longer) disability. The council estimates the average duration of a disability is 13 months, and the most likely causes are musculoskeletal problems, cancer, injury, cardiovascular problems, and mental

disorders.[2] Some disability insurance only covers a person for a certain type of disabling condition. Some policies only cover accidental disability; disabling illnesses are not included under this type of policy. Occupational policies cover someone whether the disability is job related. Nonoccupational policies only cover nonwork–related disabilities. (The theory here is that workers' compensation insurance pays for occupation-related disabilities. The amount is completely inadequate for most dentists.)

Exclusions

Disability income policies do not cover every disabling condition. An *exclusion* is a condition that is not a covered disabling condition. Many are the result of individual choice. Typical policy exclusions include:

self-inflicted injuries
attempted (unsuccessful) suicide
illegal drug use
injuries that happen while flying in a noncommercial airplane
injuries that happen as a result of a war
conditions that existed before a person was eligible for coverage (pre-existing condition)

Sources of Income If Disabled

As a practicing dentist, several sources of income will be available during disability.

Accounts receivable provides an initial income flow. This flow lasts for 30 to 60 days before it dwindles. However, then a dentist has the additional problem of cash flow when starting back to work after disability is over. It takes awhile to get the cash flowing through the practice. A person should have savings or an emergency fund established for this possibility. This is the perfect use and justification for having such a fund.

Social Security provides some disability income. This will probably not be significant. It is limited to people who have 40 quarters of payments into the system, and a person also must be permanently disabled. Payments are meager compared to the lifestyle of most professionals.

If a dentist is in a group practice, he or she may have arrangements built into a contract that protects each person in case of a disability.

[1] National Safety Council®. Injury facts®. 2011 edition, p. 3. Available at http://www.nsc.org/Documents/Injury_Facts/Injury_Facts_2011_w.pdf. Accessed November 5, 2012.

[2] The Council for Disability Awareness. Disability statistics. Available at http://www.disabilitycanhappen.org/chances_disability/disability_stats.asp. Accessed November 5, 2012.

A spouse or other family member can possibly support the family without the dentist's income replacement.

Depending on the disability, a dentist may continue to own and manage the practice. For example, assume that a dentist suffers a compound fracture of the right (dominant) arm in a skiing accident. He or she can not pick up a handpiece. However, an associate dentist can be hired to keep the practice going. The owner–dentist can then come to the office to conduct staff meetings, meet and greet patients, and do other ownership duties. Most insurers consider any profit earned from these activities to be income and will decrease payments by this amount.

Disability income insurance will provide the bulk of a lost income stream. Because this income replacement is so important, a person needs to understand his or her policy and review it annually.

Factors in Choosing a Policy

Many factors affect the limitations and benefits (and therefore cost) of the individual policy. These include:

- **Amount of Monthly Benefit** Obviously, the more the benefit that is received, the more the policy will cost. Dentists need to be realistic about how much income is insured. A person *can* be overinsured. As mentioned previously, insurers will generally only pay for income that is *shown* to have been lost (i.e., the amount being made before the disability). This is to prevent fraudulent claims for disability (if a person can make more income while disabled, why work?). It also prevents malingering, or someone being exceedingly slow to return to work.
- **Length of Elimination Period** The time before the insurer's payments begin (the elimination period) affects cost. The shorter the elimination period, the more likely that a person will at some time collect from the policy. Someone may recover from a disabling condition by the time a longer elimination period takes effect. A person is much less likely to collect if he or she must wait 90 or 120 days than if he or she must wait 30 or 60 days. The shorter the elimination period is, the higher the cost of the policy. A person could theoretically buy a policy that covers him or her from the first day if disability, but it would be prohibitively expensive.
- **The Length of the Benefit Payment** How long a person continues to collect benefits if he or she is totally or permanently disabled affects the policy. Common periods include lifetime, until age 65, and for 5 or 10 years. The longer the potential payout for the insurer, the higher the cost of the policy (premiums).

The Definition of Disability

A more strict definition of the term *disability* means that fewer people will become disabled. This lowers the insurer's payout and, therefore, the cost of the policy, but it decreases protection. Is a person disabled if he or she cannot practice dentistry or if he or she cannot do any meaningful work? If someone loses a hand in an automobile accident, can he or she still pull cans of peas across the laser scanner at the local grocery store? Does this mean that a person is disabled? Some policies will pay benefits if a person is unable to perform the duties of his or her own occupation (so-called *own occupation or* "own occ" policies). This means that if a person is a practicing periodontist and cannot perform the duties of a practicing periodontist, then he or she is disabled. Other policies require that a person be unable to do the duties of *any* occupation (so-called *any occ* policies) to be disabled. This means that if someone can work in the local grocery store, then he or she is not disabled. Own occ policies have been abused by practitioners, but any occ policies do not offer enough protection. Most insurers now have language that defines disability in terms such as "substantially similar occupations," "occupational specific," or "work which a person is qualified by education, training and experience." This protects a person from having to dig ditches but does not allow him or her to claim that he or she is a periodontist, not a general dentist. Many policies also allow for the insurer to provide retraining. If a person is a practitioner, this means that under the provisions of the insurance policy a person might be retrained to review insurance claims or teach in a dental school.

Guaranteed Renewability and Noncancellability

If a person contracts a potentially recurring disease (such as a heart condition or a cancer) he or she wants to be sure that the disability policy can be renewed when renewal time comes. Otherwise, the insurer might claim that person is now a poor risk and cancel the policy or refuse to insure that person. Other insurers would also refuse to insure that person based on history or would charge such high rates that the insurance would not be affordable. Dentists should be sure that a policy is guaranteed renewable to age 65 or 70. This means that the policy can not be cancelled if a person continues to make payments. Premiums can rise if they rise for everyone (contingent on state approval). A more favorable policy is a noncancellable policy. In this type, the premium can not be increased over the term of the policy. A noncancellable, guaranteed renewable policy provides the most protection but at an added cost.

Inflation Rider

This factor helps a person maintain purchasing power if he or she is disabled for a long period by increasing benefits at the same rate as inflation. (These are often called *cost of living adjustment* [COLA] policies.)

A Residual or "Back-to-Work" Clause

These clauses really protect both the insured and the insurer. A residual clause allows the insured to continue to receive partial benefits when he or she returns to work part-time. For example, assume that a person had a heart attack. After 6 months of total disability, the physician clears that person to return to work 2 days per week, with the intention of building gradually until he or she is back a full 5 days per week as before the illness. A residual clause pays partial benefits while that person is working part-time. Without this clause, benefits end when that person returns to work, even part-time, although his or her income is much less than before the illness.

A Guaranteed Purchase Option

A person wants the right to buy additional insurance as income rises without new medical examinations or tests. This option allows a person to purchase additional insurance at specified times (e.g., each 3 years) if income warrants. This is important for dentists because their incomes often increase as a result of inflation and practitioner maturity.

Guidelines for Choosing a Policy

Given the apparent complexity of disability income policies, what should someone look for in a disability income policy? There are several general rules to consider:

- The dentist should plan for disability as if will happen tomorrow. In this way, he or she will be prepared when it does happen. The dentist should plan with a group of local practitioners to cover each other's practices in case an individual suffers a disability. He or she should let family and advisors know where policies are and who the agents are.
- Group plans are usually cheaper than individual policies. If a person is covered through a group policy through work, the dentist should take it. The coverage may not be ideal and it may need to be supplemented with another policy, but these group policies are usually a good starting place.
- The dentist should plan to replace 60 to 80 percent of pretax income. Because the benefits received will be tax free, he or she does not need to replace the income

that would have been spent on income taxes. However, with a policy that ends at age 65, retirement plan contributions should be factored in. Most insurers will limit the benefit based on proven income. This is obviously tough on beginning practitioners (who can show little income). Most insurers will write beginning policies to gain someone as a customer for their firm.

- Early in a dental career, a dentist needs shorter elimination periods and longer payment periods than later in the career. Unfortunately, this is also when a dentist can least afford the higher premiums that come with this type of insurance. The dentist should look at accounts receivable and the emergency fund to decide how long an elimination period could be weathered. Initially, a 30- to 60-day elimination period may be needed. The elimination period should be lengthened when funds have been built up. A 90- or 120-day elimination period policy will save a person a substantial amount of money in lower premium payments.
- Dentists should review policies every year. A person's needs change as income and assets change. The dentist should carry enough insurance but not overinsure. Both are costly mistakes.
- The dentist should have a residual or return-to-work clause. Many dentists are disabled by illness and return to work gradually; he or she should be sure that insurance reflects this.
- Most dentists would like to have a noncancellable policy to lock in premiums until age 65.
- This insurance covers income for personal family budget needs; a separate office overhead policy to help defray the costs of office expenses should be carried.
- The dentist should skip any riders that intend to feed a retirement plan while disabled. The riders cost a lot and often require him or her to invest only with the insurance company's affiliates. A dentist should get adequate coverage to contribute to his or her own retirement plan.
- Some insurance advisors suggest sticking with a company that has the endorsement of professional organizations (such as the American Dental Association [ADA]). They are easier to deal with if a large portion of their business is from a single, tight-knit profession. These "association policies" are packaged plans that are not as flexible as an individual policy. But if they meet a person's needs—they are designed to meet the needs of typical association members—they can provide a large cost savings.

If a person becomes disabled, he or she should not assume that the insurer or agent is a friend. It can often be a nightmare getting the insurer to agree that a person is, in fact, disabled and not just trying to scam the company. The dentist should keep excellent paper work (and copies), including all medical reports, correspondence, and phone conversations with insurers and physicians. He or she should be sure to use a physician who is knowledgeable about the particular type of disabling problem (e.g., a general practitioner should not certify an orthopedic disability). The dentist should get the best board-certified orthopedic surgeon in the area. Some dentists have had to sue their disability insurers to get the insurance company to pay benefits.

Besides basic personal disability income insurance, a person may need one additional type. Business-reducing term disability (BRTD) insurance remains in place for a certain time to cover a certain need. For example, if a dentist buys a practice that requires a monthly loan payment of $4,000 for 5 years, BRTD insurance is a good low-cost way to insure the need. A personal disability income replacement policy is more expensive and needed for *personal* income needs.

Accidental Death and Dismemberment (AD&D) Insurance

AD&D policies, although common, serve a limited need for dental practitioners. Their purpose is to provide a lump sum payment if a person dies or loses a limb in an accident. Some policies require that the limb be severed for payment to be made; others only require loss of use or function to pay the benefit. Most policies cover a person whether the accident was at work or not. The policies will not cover if a person dies or loses a limb from an illness or disease (that is not an accident). Some policies have additional discriminators that qualify the accident for coverage.

Most dental practitioners do not need AD&D policies. They should have adequate disability and life insurance to cover their special financial needs. AD&D policies are a less-expensive way to cover some of those needs, but a more comprehensive insurance plan is needed to cover most practitioners. Some dentists have AD&D policies in an insurance package for staff members as an employee benefit.

Life Insurance

Like disability insurance, life insurance is a bit of a misnomer. People do not insure against death. Everyone will die eventually. Instead, life insurance is bought to guard against premature death or death before a person has had a chance to build assets to provide for a given financial need. If life insurance is viewed as a bet or a game of chance, a person will lose. A person will lose if he or she does not collect because the company's actuaries have determined premiums that will provide a profit for the company. A person will certainly lose if he or she collects because he or she will be dead and unable to enjoy the benefits.

The terminology of life insurance is similar to other types of insurances. A person buys a contract or policy that offers certain coverage. He or she pays premiums to the insurer. If that person dies, the person that is named as the beneficiary receives the benefits or payout of the policy.

Insurance sales agents are good a making people feel obligated to buy life insurance or feel guilty if they do not have any. It is important to first think of why someone would buy life insurance. Those are the potential purposes for life insurance. If a person does not fit into one of these categories, he or she should not buy life insurance and not feel guilty about not having any.

Purpose of Life Insurance

The purposes of life insurance include:
A person may want to provide money after he or she is gone to maintain a standard of living for his or her family. If that person is the sole support or provides a significant contribution to the family budget, then he or she should plan to replace that income if he or she dies prematurely (before adequate savings and assets have been built up). On the other hand, if a spouse is an employed professional who can earn an acceptable family income if that person dies, then he or she may choose not to carry life insurance. Life insurance is not winning the lottery for the family. A dentist should plan a specific amount to replace income.

Lending agencies may require a person to carry life insurance to secure business assets. A banker may require a life insurance policy, naming the bank as beneficiary, in the amount of a practice loan. If that person dies prematurely (before the loan is paid off) then the insurance policy will pay the remainder of the loan to the bank. Practice assets then go to the person's estate for heirs to deal with.

Life insurance will fund cross-purchase agreements for practice purchase in estate planning. If a person is a member of a group practice, he or she and partners may carry life insurance on each other. (A person carries a policy on his or her partner; the partner carries one on the first person.) If one dies, the other has the money (and a contractual obligation) to buy out other's portion of the practice. (Hence the name, cross-purchase agreement.) The person's estate, and therefore the family, benefits by having a previously agreed-on purchase price and by not having to sell the person's portion of the practice at the time of death. The partner(s) benefits by knowing that the other person's heirs will not sell his or her portion of the practice to a stranger, who may not fit into the practice style that the group developed.

A person may have specific financial needs for which to plan. A spouse might provide for the family budget but cannot provide certain family benefits. A common example is providing for children's higher education. Others may be business start-up costs or paying off vacation property.

Life insurance has been touted as a savings mechanism and even a retirement planning mechanism. As a rule, there are much better savings and retirement planning techniques. The time that a person might want to use life insurance as a savings mechanism is if he or she is a terrible money manager and can not budget a savings plan any other way.

Life insurance can be used as an estate planning technique, saving estate taxes. A person simply will not need these techniques until late in his or her career. When a person gets to this point, he or she will have tax advisors to help.

Types of Life Insurance

There are two basic types of life insurance and several hybrid or combinations of the basic types.

1. **Term Insurance** Term insurance is also known as pure life insurance. This type of policy is valid only for a specific period. A person may have a term life insurance policy that is effective from July 1 through June 30 of the following year. If he or she dies at 12:01 a.m. on July 1 of the following year, the death is not covered and beneficiaries receive no benefits. If that person dies 2 minutes earlier, at 11:59 on June 30, the beneficiary receives the entire benefit amount of the policy. Many policies are renewable, which means that the policy owner has the option of paying an additional premium and extending coverage for another period. Other policies, especially ones that cover a specific event, such as a practice purchase, are nonrenewable and exist only for the insurance period. Term insurance is pure insurance because, unlike whole life policies, no cash value accumulates in the policy. A person can not save money or borrow against a term life policy. Nevertheless, term policies are much cheaper than other types of policies for comparable levels of insurance coverage.
2. **Whole Life Insurance** Whole life is also known as "ordinary," "permanent," or "cash value" insurance. Unlike term policies, whole life policies last for the whole lifetime. They allocate part of each payment to pure life insurance (like a term policy) and a portion to a savings account within the policy. A person can

then borrow against the value accumulated within the policy or cash it in at completion of payments at maturity (e.g., retirement). The value accumulates tax free within the insurance policy. This makes cash-value insurance a combination of a pure insurance product and a tax-advantaged savings vehicle. Before rushing to buy this type of insurance, consider the following. Insurance executives are conservative investors. (And well they should be. People do not want them squandering their insurance pay out by investing in risky ventures.) A return within the policy is safe but low. The company charges the policy holder interest to borrow on the account, essentially charging interest to borrow his or her own money. And finally, whole life policies are so profitable for insurers that they generally give 50 to 75 percent of the first 2 years' premium payments as commission to the agent selling the policy. That is quite an incentive for agents to sell whole life policies.

To solve problems associated with whole life policies, insurers have developed a whole group of hybrid insurance products. These have characteristics of term policies, cash-value policies, and bona-fide investments. Variable life policies take the savings portion of a whole life premium and invest it in a mutual fund or other investment vehicle that pays (potentially) more than a traditional whole-life policy. The cash value that builds up varies as the underlying investment return varies. Depending on the policy, the amount of insurance may also vary. Universal life policies are similar to whole life policies, except they pay a competitive interest rate. The underlying investment portion of the payment is tied to money market or US Treasury Bill interest rates. Endowment life policies are pay dividends as an annuity or regular payments. These policies can supplement retirement income once the retirement plan is funded.

Life Insurance Needs for Professionals

If someone is considering buying life insurance, several questions should be answered before signing any contracts or checks. These include:

• The dentist should know the reason for buying it and decide what specific financial goal will be accomplished by buying insurance. He or she should determine insurance needs based on income replacement needs. A person might not need any life insurance at all. If someone is buying insurance because an agent called on the phone and said that a young dentist needs insurance, he or she should reconsider.
• The dentist must decide how much insurance is needed. The answer to the first question will help to answer this question. He or she should estimate the cost of a college education or family income needs,

but he or she should only buy enough insurance to provide for the benefit that is needed. If buying insurance to provide a family income, the purchaser should buy approximately six to eight times annual net income. This is an amount that, if invested at 8 percent, would replace lost income.

- The dentist should decide when to buy it. If the need has been identified, he or she buy the insurance when it is needed, not before and not after.
- The dentist should decide when the insurance should end. He or she should end the insurance coverage when the need ends. Insurance to cover a practice loan can end when the loan has been paid off. Insurance to provide a college education can end when a college fund is funded or when the child completes college. As a person ages, he or she usually needs less insurance. As a person moves through his or her professional career, he or she pays off debts and builds assets. These assets can provide income in case of death. Insurance provides for loss of income if a person dies before he or she has had a chance to build an asset base. Many professionals find renewable term policies ideal for this insurance coverage.
- The dentist should decide what type of insurance should be bought. The type of policy that is bought should depend on the needs as identified previously. A 5-year decreasing term policy would be most appropriate to secure a 5-year practice loan. The insurance ends after 5 years but by then the loan has been paid off. The benefit decreases each year, but so does the principal remaining. A whole life policy in this case would be financial overkill and obligate someone to premium payments for years after the loan is paid off.
- The dentist should never buy life insurance when automobiles are purchased or when other purchases are made. Sales agents try to sell this insurance as "mortgage protection" or "loan protection" insurance that will pay off the loan if the person dies without "burdening" family. This is simply an expensive term policy. The purchaser should say "No" and mean it.
- The dentist should not buy insurance from anyone who calls on the phone soliciting business. These solicitors are generally starting agents whose sole purpose is to sell policies, regardless of someone's needs.
- The dentist should not buy whole life insurance. Whole life policies are expensive. Comparable term policies cost about 50 percent as much as a whole life policy. He or she should buy term insurance and invest the difference. If a dentist can manage a dental practice, he or she can manage the finances involved in insurance.
- Be sure to name a specific beneficiary (individual or trust) on the policy, not the estate. The beneficiary is the person who will get the proceeds of the policy if a policy holder dies. There can be enormous negative estate tax consequences if this is not done.
- If someone becomes a poor health risk (because of a disease or condition), he or she may have great difficulty buying life insurance at any cost. This is the one valid reason for buying some insurance before it is needed.

Automobile Insurance

Automobile insurance is an area in which many professionals can save significant amounts of money. Most people simply keep the same automobile insurance year after year. Yet more money is spent on this insurance annually than is on malpractice insurance. Automobile insurance policies follow a standard procedure, so comparing one policy with another is easy.

Components

Auto policies consist of four areas of insurance (Box 2.2). Some policies may not include all of the four areas.

Part A, Liability, covers a policy holder if he or she is the cause of an accident. This person also may be called on to pay for fixing someone else's property (such as their automobile) or paying them for injuries.

Part B, Medical Payments, provides some medical payment to the policy hold or someone in his or her car injured in an accident. These medical payment amounts are fairly low. The policy holder should have health and liability insurances to help cover these expenses.

Part C, Uninsured Motorists, covers the policy holder if an uninsured motorist causes an accident that damages the policy holder's car or causes the policy holder or the passengers of the policy holder harm.

Part D, Damage to Covered Autos, pays to fix the policy holder's car if it is damaged. Comprehensive coverage includes damage not caused by a collision (e.g., windshield cracks because of a stone). Collision coverage

---

Box 2.2 General Areas of Automobile Insurance Policies

Part A: Liability coverage (including bodily injury and property liability)
Part B: Medical payments coverage
Part C: Uninsured motorists' coverage
Part D: Damage to covered automobiles
      Comprehensive "all risks" coverage
      Collision (Deductibles)
      Towing and labor

pays (less the deductible) to repair the policy holder's car if it is damaged in a collision.

Cost Factors

Several factors affect the cost of an auto policy. Those affecting the liability sections include:

- The age and sex of drivers. Young males have more accidents and therefore cost more to insure.
- The uses of the automobile. The more miles and the more frequently a person drives, the more likely he or she will be to have an accident. The rates go up.
- The territory where garaged. Some areas, especially large cities, are more prone to accidents and theft. Higher rates are the norm in these areas.
- The operators' driving record. If a person has had several accidents or if he or she has received several tickets for unsafe operation (speeding, etc.), that person is a bad risk. Rates will probably go up.

One point to note: a dentist's personal automobile policy does not cover employees who are driving the dentist's car for business reasons. So if a staff member runs to the bank in the dentist's car, the dentist, not the staff member, runs the risk of being personally liable if the employee has an accident. The dentist should be sure that the office liability policy has a rider to cover employees if they regularly use the dentist's vehicle. If part of car expenses are deducted as a business expense, the dentist should let the insurance agent know. It could change the classification of the insurance, making it more expensive but more complete coverage.

Homeowner's Insurance

Homeowner's insurance protects the policy holder against loss of property and against the liability that arises from owning the property. If a neighbor's child injures themselves while in the policy holder's yard, the homeowner may be liable for damages. Homeowner's insurance covers those types of incidents. Homeowner's insurance policies are standard. Box 2.3 shows the general areas of homeowner's coverage.

There are several common riders (special provisions) that policies may contain. A "Replacement Cost Provision" obliges the carrier to replace the damaged property. Inflation can escalate the value of a home and contents dramatically over a few short years. This rider protects the policy holder from being underinsured by rising costs.

Most policies have liability exclusions. The homeowner will not be covered if the injury or damage occurred as a result of using the home for business purposes. If a spouse gives piano lessons in the home and a student gets injured

---

Box 2.3 General Areas of Homeowner's Coverage

Section I: Property coverage
  Dwelling
  Other structures
  Personal property
  Loss of use
Section II: Liability and medical payments
  Personal liability
  Medical payments to others
  Damage to property of others

Box 2.4 Types of Homeowner's Coverage

Homeowners 1 (Basic): Fire, lightning, extended coverage, vandalism and mischief, theft, glass breakage on dwellings and personal contents, and comprehensive personal liability

Homeowners 2 (Broad Form): All of basic and additional extended coverage for other specific causes

Homeowners 3: "All Risks" on buildings and Broad Form on personal property (i.e., everything is included unless the policy specifically excludes it)

Homeowners 4: Personal property only (Broad Form); for tenants

Homeowners 5: "All Risks" on buildings and personal property

Homeowners 6: Personal property and loss of use coverage (Broad Form); for condominium unit owners

Homeowners 8: Coverage on buildings and personal property somewhat more limited than Basic; for homes that may not meet underwriting requirements

---

at the home, the homeowner's insurance probably will not pay the claim because it was business related. A separate business liability is needed for that coverage. Another frequent exclusion is if the homeowner intentionally harms someone, or if there are losses from a war. Policies also exclude earthquake, floods, nuclear hazards, and many other mass disasters, although homeowners can get special (additional) coverage for many of these events.

There are eight different types of homeowner's coverage. These are standard coverage that apply to all homeowner insurance policies across the country. The purpose of requiring standard types of coverage is so that the consumer can compare different policy's coverage and the cost of each policy for the given coverage. The types of coverage are shown in Box 2.4.

The type of coverage that is required depends on what type of home the policy holder lives in and what that person feels needs to be covered.

Personal Excess Liability Insurance

The final type of personal insurance a dentist should have is a personal excess liability policy. This type of policy is also known as "umbrella liability" policies. Their purpose is to ensure that the policy holder has adequate personal liability insurance. Both homeowner's insurance and automobile insurance have liability protection, but these are limited policies, often $50,000 to $100,000 per occurrence. It is not unusual for liability cases to be settled for much more than these amounts. The excess liability policy coordinates other liability coverage and extends it to a total maximum amount.

For example, suppose a person has a $100,000 homeowner's liability policy. The neighbor's child falls off the homeowner's deck, sustaining a severe head injury. In the subsequent lawsuit, the jury awards the child $1 million in total damages. The homeowner's policy has a limit of $100,000, which is all that they are obligated to pay. The homeowner must pay the rest from their personal assets, savings, and future earnings. If the homeowner has an umbrella liability policy, it will pick up where the other (homeowner's) policy ends and pay damages up to the limits of the liability in the umbrella policy (perhaps $1 or $2 million).

Umbrella policies are inexpensive. They must be carefully coordinated with other insurance policies to ensure that there are no gaps or duplications in coverage. This is for personal liability only. Office liability and professional liability require different insurances. So a personal liability policy will not cover a person in the event of a business-related lawsuit. Given that dentists are often seen as rich members of society (and therefore able to pay large liability settlements), dentists should be sure to protect themselves and their family with this type of coverage.

Tax Consequences of Personal Insurances

As a rule, insurances for the business are a tax-deductible cost of doing business; insurances for personal affairs are not tax deductible. Most small business people want to make their insurance premium tax deductible because that decreases the total cost of the insurance. However, simply wanting them to be tax deductible does not make them so. The dentist should know the IRS rules regarding insurance premium payments to make informed decisions about insurance premium deductibility. These rules and their interpretations change frequently. The dentist should check with an accountant or tax advisor concerning the current tax consequences of insurances.

Medical Insurance

There are significant tax consequences of purchasing medical insurance. If a person (or spouse) is given medical insurance as an employee benefit, the cost of the premium is completely tax deductible to the employer and tax free to the employee. This lowers the apparent cost of the insurance coverage because the government essentially pays for some of it, through tax savings. Medical insurance premiums that a person provides for self and family through the practice are tax deductible, regardless the form of business (corporation, proprietorship, partnership, or limited liability company).

If a practice is a corporation (and, therefore the dentist is an employee) then that person qualifies for employee benefit plans, including medical reimbursement plans. Under these plans, the employer may make certain payments for medical services for its employees on a tax-deductible basis. These may be incorporated into flexible benefit (cafeteria style) plans.

Health savings accounts (HSAs) are the newest darling of health cost-containment advocates. Under these arrangements, a person may make a contribution to an HSA account on a tax-deductible basis. This must be used with high-deductible health insurance plans. The HSA then pays for costs incurred before the deductible is completed and other costs that the insured must pay (copays, etc.). Any money left over in the account is rolled over to the next year, forming a sort of savings account for healthy individuals.

These methods merely decrease the cost of insurance. They do not eliminate it. Medical insurance is one of the most expensive insurances, especially as people age. (Young people are usually healthy, and so premiums are low.)

Life Insurance

In "normal" individually purchased life insurance policies, the policy holder pays the premium with after-tax money, and a beneficiary receives the benefit free of any income taxes. Because it is all an after-tax transaction, the premiums are paid, and the beneficiary can receive the benefits without income tax consequences. The rules get more complex when someone gifts someone else a policy or pays the premiums. A tax advisor should be consulted in these cases.

Employer-sponsored life insurance policies are handled differently. The employer may provide up to

$50,000 per year of term life insurance as an employee benefit. Premiums for additional insurance provided by the employer must be included in income, based on certain IRS rules and tables. If a dentists incorporates the practice (and is, therefore, an employee) then the dentist qualifies for this benefit. The tax rules get complex regarding additional, or whole life policies. Generally, the benefit (payout) of life insurance is tax-free to the beneficiary. However, the premiums (pay-ins) may be considered taxable income to the dentist. The rules then get even more complex when life insurance is purchased through the corporation for cross-purchase, or other arrangements, depending on how they are structured. An accountant, financial advisor, and insurance agent should work out the best arrangement for the dentist's particular circumstance.

Disability Insurance

There are significant tax consequences associated with disability income policies. If a person pays premiums with after-tax dollars, then any benefits received will be tax free. If the dentist is incorporated (C corporation only) and the corporation provides disability insurance as a tax-free employee benefit, then the benefit that the dentist receives will be taxable income. The dentist will need a much higher level of coverage. It is generally better to pay for the insurance personally with after-tax money and receive the benefits tax free. If the dentist does not use the insurance (collect benefits), the corporation can reimburse the dentist (after the end of the insurance period) for the insurance premiums, thereby making them tax deductible to the corporation (and to the dentist).

Automobile Insurance

All costs associated with the use of an automobile for business purposes (including the cost of insurance) are ordinary costs of doing business and, therefore, tax deductible. The costs associated with the use of the automobile for personal purposes are not tax deductible. The problem is deciding the proportion of business use to personal use. The dentist should keep a log of use (as described in the tax section of this book) to justify the percentage of total automobile costs that are allocated for business purposes.

Homeowner's Insurance

Homeowner's insurance is generally not tax deductible. If part of a home is used as a qualifying home office, a proportional amount of homeowner's insurance premiums may be allocated to business use.

Planning for Retirement Income

chapter 3

If I'd known I was going to live so long, I'd have taken better care of myself.
Leon Eldred

Objectives

At the completion of this chapter, the student will be able to:
1. Discuss the major financial factors to be considered in retirement planning.
2. Discuss the basic components of retirement plans for dental practitioners.
3. Discuss the principles of retirement saving for dental practitioners.
4. Discuss factors that affect dentists' ability to meet their retirement goals.
5. Identify the various retirement plans available to the dentist.
6. List the major advantages and disadvantages of each type of retirement plan.
7. Discuss when, in the practice life cycle, each type of plan is most appropriate.

Key Terms

401(k) plans
after-tax money
annuity
  period certain
  single life
  joint and last survivor
composition of net worth
compounding
contribution limits
defined benefit plans
defined contribution plans
eligible employees
individual retirement account (IRA)
  back-loaded IRA
  Roth IRA
  traditional IRA

investment rate of return
Keogh plans
private savings or assets
retirement planning
  financial independence
  retirement
retirement savings
  qualified plans
  retirement plan savings
retirement savings pattern
risk
risk-return relationship
savings incentive match plans for employees of small employers (SIMPLE) plans
simplified employee pension (SEP) plans

Social Security
tax-deferred annuity
tax sheltering
  pretax contribution
  posttax (taxable) contribution
  tax-deductible savings
  tax-deferred savings
vesting
  graduated
  total (100%) vesting
Social Security
  earned income

Goal

This chapter emphasizes the general and financial planning aspects of retirement.

Business Basics for Dentists, First Edition. David O. Willis.
© 2013 John Wiley & Sons, Inc. Published 2013 by John Wiley & Sons, Inc.

Most dentists realize that they will not be able (or want) to practice their entire lives. Private dental practitioners do not have pensions or retirement income plans funded by a large employer. Instead, they are responsible for funding their own retirement savings. When they retire, they then draw down their retirement savings as they withdraw funds for living expenses. The obvious fear is that retirement will last longer than retirement funds. Retirement planning then becomes a critical personal financial planning task. Fortunately, dentists are presently some of the higher paid professionals. This makes it easier than many other vocations to set aside money for retirement planning purposes. For the simpler plans described later, a dentist can work with the office accountant or financial planner to select and carry out a plan. For the more complex plans, dentists will need to use a specialist in retirement plans. Fortunately, if a dentist starts a plan early and funds the simpler plans the maximum amount permitted, he or she should not need the more complex (and more expensive) plans. There are several types of retirement plans that a dentist owning a practice might use. Congress and the IRS change the tax implications of these plans frequently. Dentists should check with an accountant or tax advisor for the current tax laws before establishing or contributing to a plan.

This chapter describes principles of retirement planning for dental practitioners (Box 3.1). Retirement implies a gold watch and porch swing. People are living longer and healthier lives than in the past. Many dentists are retiring at a younger age than in years past. Some of them leave work entirely. Some pursue hobby or second careers. This leads to more years in retirement and a more active (and expensive) retirement as well. Others continue to work well into their later years, even working part-time for their entire lives. For these reasons, many financial planners prefer to call this process planning for financial independence rather than retirement. Financial independence is the time in life when a person can work or not. A person has adequate resources to support self and family in the chosen lifestyle.

Retiring from dental practice involves significant personal self-examination and planning. Many private practitioners have so much of their personal self-esteem committed to their practice that it becomes difficult for them to walk away. This, after all, has been a large part of their professional and personal identity. Successful retirees develop projects and interests that extend well into retirement. These tasks provide emotional and intellectual challenges that lead to high self-esteem. Playing golf every day sounds wonderful when a person works every day. After playing every day for a month, golfing loses some of its luster. Sometimes people think only the financial aspects of retirement planning. Personal emotional preparation is as important, and

---

Box 3.1 Planning for Retirement

- Have enough financial assets to last 25 to 30 years after age 65 (i.e., age 90 or 95)
- Eighty to 90 percent of preretirement income needed for retirement
- Consider inflation
- Plan, it will not "just happen"
- Tax and retirement planning laws will change; change plans several times to adapt to tax law changes.

---

often, inadequately addressed. However, this chapter examines *only* the financial bases of retirement planning.

Components of a Retirement Plan

Retirement planning for dentists is similar to a three-legged stool. Each component is necessary for the system to work, but none of them can work alone. The three components of retirement plans are Social Security, private savings and assets, and retirement savings and pensions (see Table 3.1).

Social Security

Self-employed dentists pay into the Social Security system through the self-employment tax. If a dentist is employed, either by someone else or through his or her own corporation, then the employer pays half the Social Security payments. (If a dentist owns his or her own corporation, the dentist obviously pays both halves.) Given the aging of the US population, Congress grapples with the problem of funding Social Security more or less continually. Social Security retirement payments are not large to begin with. In the future, higher income earners will pay more (both while working and in retirement) to help keep the system solvent. This effectively decreases their return. So although Social Security is not expected to disappear in the future, most dentists should *not* plan for Social Security to be a major part of their retirement income. They should plan as if Social Security will not exist in the future. Any payments received from Social Security will then be a bonus. Dentists should keep up with the news and changes that Congress makes in the Social Security system.

People should check their Social Security status and benefits regularly. The Social Security Administration provides a "Personal Earnings History and Benefits Statement." This is a history of reported earnings (throughout a person's lifetime) and an estimate of benefits at retirement. (The statement also shows

Table 3.1 Social Security Payments in Retirement Income

Preretirement Income	Needed in Retirement	Replaced by Social Security	Needed from Retirement Savings
$20,000	76%	64%	12%
$30,000	72%	55%	17%
$40,000	71%	44%	27%
$50,000	74%	37%	37%
$60,000	74%	31%	43%
$70,000	77%	27%	50%
$80,000	84%	23%	61%
$90,000	86%	21%	65%
$150,000	86%	21%	73%
$200,000	87%	9%	78%
$250,000	89%	8%	81%

Source: Georgia State University Center for Risk Management

Box 3.2 Retirement Savings

If a person invests at 5% and gets X in return; then, if he or she invests at 10%, then he or she would get X times two, right? WRONG!!

$1,000 invested, one time at the various rates and times

	20 years	30 years	40 years	50 years
5%	2,653	4,321	7,039	11,467
10%	6,727	17,449	45,259	117,390

---

estimated benefits for disability and surviving spouse and children.) The benefits are shown in today's dollars, although actual benefits are indexed for inflation, so the benefits will be higher. Form SSA-7004 can be requested by calling the Social Security Administration at 1-800-937-2000 or by visiting their Web site and applying online. A statement should follow in 2 to 4 weeks.

Private Savings and Assets

Private savings are those made with after-tax money. Examples include a dental practice, a home, and many investments. Some assets, such as a home or automobile, can not really be included as a component of a retirement plan, unless a person plans to live in a tent and walk everywhere in retirement. Financial assets (investments) are a valuable component of the total retirement asset base. These assets can be turned into immediate income, either through selling them (stock, etc.) or by using any income (such as dividends) for personal income. Private savings and investments are generally used for no-retirement purposes.

Many dentists plan on the sale of their practice to fund their retirement plan. This is a risky strategy. They may not be able to sell the practice at the time they want to sell or at a price they hoped to get. Taxes then eat a sizable portion of the proceeds. This leaves them with too small a remaining asset base to fund retirement adequately. Many dentists then find that they simply can not afford to sell the practice and retire.

Retirement Savings and Pensions

By far the most important component of a dentist's retirement plan should be his or her retirement plan savings. These are funds that are specifically earmarked for retirement savings purposes. These are designed to be a retirement savings method, not a personal savings plan. If money is withdrawn from this retirement plan savings for other uses (e.g., to buy a boat), a person will face significant taxes and penalties. "Qualified" plans receive favorable tax treatment for both the employer and employee because they comply with certain IRS code requirements. Overall, these requirements protect employees through nondiscrimination and fiduciary responsibility rules. Retirement savings are such good investments because they are funded with pretax money and grow tax free until they are withdrawn from (possibly in a lower tax bracket). However, this advantage only comes with certain stipulations, the largest of which is that the dentist (the employer) must fund his or her employees' retirement plan as well. As a rule, a dentist funding his or her tax-advantaged retirement plan to the maximum amount permitted is still advantageous. (Details about retirement plans are found later in this chapter.)

Retirement plans allow a person to save money with many tax advantages. When a person retires, he or she lives off of savings. If a person has adequate savings, he or she lives off the interest. If the savings are not adequate for this strategy, the principal amount must be gradually eroded or the retirement income expectations must be lowered (Box 3.2).

Principles of Retirement Savings

The following principles apply to all investments, but especially to tax-advantaged retirement plans.

Time

The longer the time until retirement, the more the investment will grow. The corollary of this statement is that the sooner retirement plan contributions are begun, the healthier the retirement plan will be.

Table 3.2 How to Build Retirement Savings *Investment needed to earn $1 million by age 65, assuming a 12% return*

Beginning Age	One-time Contribution	Monthly Contribution
20	$6,098	$46
25	$10,748	$84
35	$33,378	$283
40	$58,823	$527
59	$506,631	$9,456

Table 3.3 Tax Savings with and without a Retirement Plan*

	No Retirement Plan	With Retirement Plan
Gross Income	$100,000	$100,000
– Exemptions	$8,000	$8,000
– Itemized Deductions	$10,000	$10,000
– Retirement Plan (13%)	$0	$13,000
Taxable Income	$82,000	$69,000
Tax Due (25%)	$20,500	$17,250
Posttax Income	$61,500	$51,750
Tax Savings		$3,250

*Assuming 25% income tax and a 13% retirement plan contribution

Compounding

Compounding is one of the most powerful concepts to understand in retirement planning. Compounding occurs when a person earns interest on the interest already earned. The value of an investment then mushrooms as the portion of the total that a person contributed decreases. For compounding to work, many years (time) are needed, which is another reason to begin retirement plan contributions as early in a career as possible (Table 3.2).

Tax Sheltering

Retirement savings gain their advantage because they are sheltered from taxes. Tax sheltering means that a person gains an immediate tax deduction for the contribution (tax deductible), and the investment grows tax free until he or she draws it out of the fund (tax deferred). This allows for higher return (money grows tax free) and a probable lower tax rate when money is withdrawn. Note that these plans defer taxes; they do not completely avoid or eliminate income taxes.

Qualified retirement plans use pretax money for funding. If a person is in the 33-percent marginal tax bracket that means that for each $1,000 contributed, he or she gets a full $1,000 going toward retirement savings. A posttax (taxable) contribution means that for each $1,000, a person must first pay 33 percent in taxes ($333), and then invest the remainder ($667). The total return will obviously be less.

Qualified retirement plans also grow tax free. Assume a person is in the same 33-percent marginal tax bracket, and he or she earns 9 percent on an investment (i.e., $1,000 investment yields $90 per year). If the investment is in a tax-advantaged retirement plan, he or she keeps the entire $90. Next year, that person earns 9 percent of $1,090 (the initial $1,000 plus $90 earned last year) and so on (i.e., compounding). The same investment in a taxable account would only yield $60 return. A person would earn $90 but pay 33 percent in taxes ($30). Compounding is slowed significantly under this later scenario (Table 3.3).

Risk-Return Relationship

A general rule of investing is that the higher the risk, the higher the return required to get people to invest in the project. Risk is really a measure of the variability of the return of the investment. This chapter was not included in the book. The practical effect of this principle is that early in a career (and retirement plan), a person can tolerate more risk (and gain a higher return), than later in the plan (Fig. 3.1 a and b).

Factors that Determine People's Ability to Reach Retirement Goals

As a rule, a person will need 75 to 80 percent of preretirement income as a level for retirement income. This can vary, depending on the particular situation. Most retirees have lower monthly costs. This is the result of not buying work clothes, traveling to work, or other costs (such as meals) that result from work. At this time in their careers, most people have paid off the house mortgage and other loans as well. They have fewer purchases as the children grow and leave home. On the other hand, they may have higher expenses in some categories, such as travel and entertainment as they act on their retirement dreams.

Several factors determine whether a person can meet his or her retirement income goal. These include:

- **Income Level Desired** The higher the income that a person requires in retirement, the more retirement savings required. This makes intuitive sense. The difficult part is to quantify how much is enough. As with all investment decisions, the best thing to do is to make an estimate based on expected returns and inflation. One significant problem early in a career is to estimate what inflation will be by the end of that career. An income level of $10,000 per month today may be paltry when the effects of 25 years of inflation are taken into account.

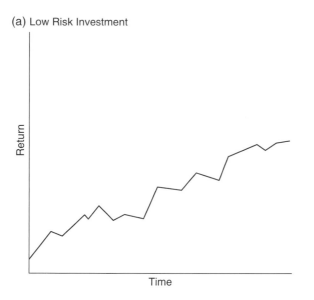

Figure 3.1 The higher the risk, the higher the return.

Table 3.4 Composition of Net Worth

	DENTIST 1		DENTIST 2	
	Book Value	Income-Producing Value	Book Value	Income-Producing Value
Home Equity	$250,000	$0	$400,000	$0
Retirement Plan	$425,000	$425,000	$225,000	$225,000
Practice	$225,000	$150,000	$225,000	$150,000
Personal Investments	$150,000	$100,000	$150,000	$100,000
TOTAL	$1,000,000	$675,000	$1,000,000	$475,000
INCOME		$4,000/mo		$3,000/mo

- **Estimated Length of Time in Retirement** How long a person will be in retirement depends on age at retirement and an estimate of longevities of the person and his or her spouse. If a person retires when he or she is 55 years old, that person should have a longer retirement than if he or she retired when age 80, all things being equal. The longer a time in retirement, the longer a person needs to be concerned about inflation eroding retirement income buying power. Another problem is if a person lives longer than retirement assets last. Some people want assets left over so that they can pass some along to their heirs. That person obviously needs more assets than the person who does not feel the need to do that.

- **Present Retirement Savings Pattern** If a person saves $1 per year, retirement goals will take a long time to be realized. Although saying that a person should increase retirement plan contributions is easy, in fact each person must evaluate personal budgets to identify areas of possible savings. To do this, a person first needs to have a budget and know where money is spent. Retirement savings must then be ranked along with other long- and short-term goals. (Once money is earned, it can only be saved or spent.) These priorities will change as stages of life and as family circumstance change.

- **Composition of Net Worth** Two people may have the same net worth, but they have different income generating potential from their assets. In Tables 3.4 and 3.5, both dentists have the same net worth. However, Dentist 2 has more assets in his or her home, which does not produce retirement income. Dentist 1 has a larger value in the retirement plan and therefore a larger monthly income in retirement.

- **Investment Rate of Return** Risk is really a measure of variability of the investment. There always some risk that the underlying company, country, or other entity will become insolvent. Then a person loses his or her entire investment. In fact, that occurrence is rare with mainstream US Wall Street investments. Instead, the greater risk is from the normal fluctuations of the economy. The primary risk is that the value of an investment will decline just when the underlying value of the investment is needed. How assets are allocated within the retirement plan then becomes important for an adequate return.

Table 3.5 Importance of the Investment Rate of Return*

	Investment Rate					
Years	1%	3%	6%	9%	12%	15%
10	$1,105	$1,344	$1,791	$2,367	$3,106	$4,406
20	$1,220	$1,806	$3,207	$5,604	$9,646	$16,367
30	$1,348	$2,427	$5,743	$13,268	$29,960	$66,212
40	$1,489	$3,262	$10,286	$31,409	$93,051	$267,864
50	$1,645	$4,384	$18,420	$74,358	$289,002	$1,083,657

*Hypothetical one-time $1,000 investment

Early in a retirement plan, a person should tolerate more risk to gain higher returns. A few percentage points can make a tremendous difference over the long haul. As a person nears and enters retirement, he or she should decrease risk exposure to protect the assets that have been built along the way.

Common Individual Retirement Plans

Individual retirement plans are not office plans. As the name implies, an individual establishes the plan. Many new dentists use these plans to begin their retirement savings. They do not have the added expense of funding staff plans, and income is lower so saving amounts are less. As the practice becomes more profitable, they may then switch to a practice-based plan.

Individual Retirement Account (Traditional IRA)

Individual plans are meant for individuals, not corporations or for business owners with employees. An IRA is an investment account that a person tells the IRS is his or her IRA. He or she can then invest in stocks, bonds, mutual funds, or many other investments within that account. IRAs can be set up through banks, mutual fund companies, or security brokers.

Saving for retirement is the primary goal when investing in an IRA. If a person takes money out of an IRA before age 59 1/2, he or she generally must pay a 10-percent penalty beyond any taxes that are owed on the investment gain. However, the IRS allows some penalty-free "special purpose" withdrawals under IRA rules. Although these withdrawals are free of the penalty, they are not tax free. A person still owes income taxes on any earnings and deductible contributions. Because IRAs are a method of retirement savings, anytime money is removed for other purposes, it will affect retirement plans and timetable.

Penalty-free distributions from an IRA are allowed for:

1. The purchase of a primary home for self or relatives (up to $10,000). (Certain restrictions apply.)

2. Certain college expenses, such as tuition, books, supplies, and room and board.
3. In an annuity fashion, where a persons make "substantially equal" payments based on life expectancy.
4. Certain medical expenses if medical bills exceed 7.5 percent of adjusted gross income (AGI).
5. Permanent and total disability or death of the IRA owner.

The traditional IRA is the prototypical defined contribution retirement account. Money that is contributed into an IRA is tax deductible (income tax is not on the money), and the account grows tax deferred (income taxes are not paid on it until the money is withdrawn during retirement). A person and his or her spouse may each have an IRA, even if the spouse does not work and earn income. However, a person must start taking out money when he or she reaches the age of 70 1/2. The IRS treats withdrawals as ordinary income. The IRS has tables that state how much (as a minimum) a person must take out of the IRA each year in retirement. If that person dies, the money in the IRA passes to the named beneficiary of the account.

Traditional IRAs are for individuals. Their advantages are ease of use, tax deductibility, and tax deferral. There are several disadvantages, including the limited amount able to be contributed, income phase outs for high-income individuals, and penalties for early withdrawals or loans. IRA money may be invested in almost any legitimate investment. These include stocks, bonds or mutual funds but not art or other personal-use assets.

IRAs are easy to set up. Simply talk to a banker or stock broker, and he or she will establish one. A more popular method is to contact any of the families of mutual funds and ask for an IRA application. They can easily be found online as well. They will require a one-page application, which essentially asks name, address, and social security number. The application contains a box to check if this is to be set up as an IRA. Send a check and the form, and an IRA is established. Contributions may be added in future years to the same IRA or another IRA can be started in a different place, as long as the total yearly contributions do not exceed the maximum amount. A person may also wait until

April 15 of the following year to make a contribution. This allows the person to compute tax liability and decide then to make a contribution for the past year.

Eligibility to deduct traditional IRA contributions from income for tax purposes depends on income, marital status, and whether a person or spouse actively participates in an employer-sponsored retirement plan. If he or she (or spouse) is not covered by an employer-sponsored retirement plan, that person may deduct 100 percent of the contribution, regardless income. If a person is married (and jointly files), he or she only looks at his or her own participation in an employee-sponsored plan to decide deductibility of IRA contributions. If income is too high for deductible contributions, a person should consider nondeductible or Roth IRA contributions instead. If a person (or spouse) participated in an employer-sponsored retirement plan, then the contribution to a traditional IRA may or may not be deductible, depending on income (AGI). The amount of a traditional IRA contribution that is deductible is phased out over certain income ranges.

Back-loaded or "Roth" IRA

Another type of IRA is a back-loaded or Roth IRA. This plan is similar to a traditional IRA, with several major differences. In this plan, contributions are not deductible, and qualified distributions are not taxable. They are, after taxes are paid on the income, used to fund the plan, truly tax free. Earnings on the account are taxable only when there is a distribution that is not qualified. A qualified distribution is one that occurs at least years after the start of the Roth IRA and meets one of the four following conditions:

1. Made after the taxpayer reaches age 59 1/2.
2. Made to a beneficiary after the taxpayer's death.
3. Made because the taxpayer is disabled.
4. Used to buy a first home.

If a person has earned income, then regardless age, he or she may contribute to a Roth IRA, provided his or her income does not exceed certain limits. Annual contributions are limited, but both taxpayer and spouse may contribute to their own Roth IRA even if both did not work. The contribution is phased out as the AGI increases, so when an AGI reaches the upper limit, a person is no longer eligible. There is no prohibition on making contributions after the age of 70 1/2. Amounts in deductible IRAs may be transferred into Roth IRAs, under certain conditions. As a rule, with several years until retirement, the Roth IRA is a better retirement investment because it essentially allows more money to be sheltered. This is because after-tax money is used for contributions.

Plans for Small Business Owners

Several types of defined contribution plans are designed for business owners. The general advantage of these plans over IRAs is the higher contribution limits. (That is, a person can shelter more income each year.) The down side (financially) to these plans is that if a dentist uses them for himself or herself, then he or she must include staff members in the plan, at the dentist's expense. This can significantly drive up the cost of the plan. When a dentist can effectively use these plans, he or she will be making enough money that the staff plan can be funded with small pain, using it as a staff recruitment and retention tool.

Rules for Office Retirement Plans

Several laws (such as the Employee Retirement and Income Security Act [ERISA]) govern how a person must conduct any tax-advantaged retirement plan. Several plans (described later) can be chosen, but some rules apply to all of the tax-advantaged plans. Generally, employees can not be required to participate in the plan or to fund all or part of their own retirement plans. There may be a minimum required participation by employees or a minimum percent of employees covered. "Top heavy" and "highly compensated employee" rules limit the amount that owners may contribute to their own retirement plans. Because these complex rules were limiting participation by small business owners, Congress developed several types of simplified plans to induce small business owners to develop retirement plans for themselves and their employees. Those rules cover the following issues: requirement, contribution limits, eligible employees, vesting, methods of contribution, and sources of contribution.

Requirement

A business owner is not presently required by law to provide retirement plans or funds to employees. (He or she is required to provide Social Security, which contains a basic retirement component.) However, most qualified retirement plans (those that are tax advantaged) require that if a qualified plan is developed for the owner, then employees must be included (at the owner's expense). The advantages of tax deferral and tax deductibility usually make it worthwhile financially to implement the plans. From an employee-management perspective, many career-oriented employees understand and value retirement plans. This helps to motivate and retain valuable employees. In this sense, it becomes a cost of doing business for the progressive dental practice.

Contribution Limits

For defined contribution plans (see the definition), an owner is limited in the amount that he or she can contribute to his or her own and to employees' plans. A person generally cannot fund his or her own plan at a higher rate (percentage of income) than he or she funds the employee's plans. There is a limit that a person can contribute to his or her own plan. The present upper limit for the owner contribution is $22,500 or 15 percent of income, whichever is less. Complex tax formulas change this number somewhat. Congress has also indexed the amount for inflation, so the maximum contribution limit changes every year with inflation and the whims of Congress.

Eligible Employees

Depending on the specific plan, an owner might define certain employees as ineligible for participation in the retirement plan. Any employee who is 21 years old, works full-time, and has at least 1 year of service (2 years if 100-percent vesting schedule) must be declared eligible for any qualified retirement plan. Because many dental office employees do not stay in long-term employment, these rules often result in decreased employee participation and contributions.

Vesting

Vesting describes whether the employee has control over the assets contributed for them. An employee who is fully vested takes the retirement assets with them when they leave employment (for any reason). Depending on the plan, an employer has the choice of one of several vesting schedules. Most plans require immediate 100 percent vesting of all funds contributed for employees. Others have graduated vesting, over 3 or 5 years. Any assets not vested return to the contributor in the event the employee leaves.

Methods of Contribution

Defined Contribution Plans

Some retirement plans, called defined contribution plans, define the amount of contribution that a person may make annually. Income in retirement varies. The contributions (assets) within the plan grow to a level determined, largely, by investment decisions. If good investment decisions are made, retirement assets will obviously grow much more than if poor decisions are made. Retirement income is unknown until it is taken out. It varies depending on how much money is in the plan at retirement, how long the income will be needed (life expectancy), and whether any assets are to be left to heirs upon death. Most retirement plans are presently defined contribution type plans.

Defined Benefit Plans

Other plans define how much income or benefit a person will have in retirement. The amount needed to contribute along the way to reach that amount varies. If a person is close to retirement, he or she needs to contribute much more than if he or she has many years left until retirement. These plans are more complex because an actuary is needed to calculate the amount needed to contribute to have a given income in the future, assuming certain investment and inflation amounts. These plans also then are more expensive. Defined benefit plans are generally used by older dentists who need to "catch up" because of inadequate early retirement funding.

Source of Contribution

Some plans require that all of the contributions come from the employer. Others allow a matching employee–employer contribution. Matching plans are useful when not all employees want to participate in a plan. They may self-exclude themselves. There are rules about how much of the contribution can go to owners or highly compensated employees, so check with an accountant to be sure a plan will comply with the regulations.

Types of Office Plans

Business can use many different retirement plans. There are defined benefit plans, money purchase plans, and employee stock ownership plans (ESOPs). However, small businesses (such as dental practices) generally use the simpler, less expensive plans. These include simplified employee pension (SEP) plans, savings incentive match plans for employees of small employers (SIMPLE) plans, and 401(k) plans.

Simplified Employee Pension (SEP) Plans

SEP plans are similar to traditional IRAs. The big differences are in the contribution limit and employees' participation. If an employer makes contributions for himself or herself, then he or she must make similar percentage contributions for all eligible employees. These contributions are 100 percent immediately vested in the employees and are treated like IRAs for the employee. They are tax deductible for the business owner. The same amount or same percentage does not have to be contributed every year, so an owner can tie contributions to practice profitability. In fact, an employer does not have to make a contribution in any given year. He or she can skip a year. An employer can contribute up to 25 percent of each employee's compensation. Self-employed dentists can contribute for themselves, up to a maximum earned income.

For a SEP plan, determining which employees are eligible is not based on full-time status. Other types of retirement plans may discriminate and cover only full-time employees but not so with a SEP. If an owner has a SEP, he or she must make equal percentage contributions to any employee who meets all of the following requirements:

1. Any employee who is at least 21 by the end of the year.
2. Any employee who has worked for the employer for 3 of the past 5 years, full- or part-time.
3. Any employee whom has been paid at least $450 for the year.

These are the most strict eligibility guidelines. An owner may be more lenient if he or she wants. Note that an owner must meet the requirements in the same manner as employees. If he or she starts a practice, the owner cannot claim immediate eligibility but require all employees to complete 3 years of service.

SEP plans are simple to establish (much like an IRA). They are popular because of the higher contribution limits and ease of establishment. Even with eligible employees, they are relatively inexpensive. For example, a $20,000 per year employee with a 5 percent contribution receives $1,000 in the plan for the year. An owner can establish these without paying large amounts for professional advice from actuaries and high-profile financial planners. The dentist should be sure to involve an accountant or financial planner in the decision, so that these professional financial advisors can help ensure that a plan is in compliance.

Savings Incentive Match Plans for Employees of Small Employers (SIMPLE) Plans

A SIMPLE plan has a specified employer contribution for employees by one of two methods:

1. A 100 percent match of first 3 percent contributed by each employee.
2. A 2 percent contribution for all employees.

This is a plan that allows employees to contribute to their own retirement account. They allow employees up to $10,000 pretax contribution per year. All employee contributions, employer matches, and earnings are immediately and fully vested in the employee. Like the SEP, all contributions are made to an IRA for the employee. SIMPLE plans are becoming the most common plan in dental practices. They are easy, flexible, allow employee participation, and offer a relatively high contribution limit, with the greatest portion of contributions going to the owner(s) of the practice.

401(k) Plans

Some incorporated dentists have a type of retirement plan known as a 401(k). These plans are similar to the retirement plans offered by many large corporations.

They were more popular before Congress established SEP and SIMPLE plans. They have similar eligibility and vesting rules as SEP and SIMPLE plans. There is additional flexibility, including the ability to borrow from the assets. They are more complex, so usually an advisor is needed (at an additional cost) to establish and administer them. Generally, large, high-income practices can take advantage of 401(k)s. The vast majority of dental practitioners can manage their retirement plans quite easily with one of the simpler plans.

Nontax–Advantaged Plans

A person should fund a tax-advantaged plan to the maximum amount possible. If he or she then has money left for additional retirement savings, then use another investment that is halfway between a retirement plan and personal savings. This is called a tax-deferred annuity.

An annuity is a series of regular payments. In a sense, a loan payment that is made is an annuity for the bank or other mortgage holder. Retirement annuities are contracts that a person purchases through insurance companies. He or she makes a series of regular payments into the annuity. (Payments should be made into the annuity with after-tax money.) At retirement, that person then receives a series of regular payments from the savings and investment growth. The advantage of annuities is that the money inside the investment grows tax deferred. (Taxes are paid on the money when it is withdrawn). The disadvantage of annuities compared with tax-advantaged plans is that the payments into the plan are not tax deductible. Also a person is generally limited in the investment options within the plan.

Some insurance sales agents claim that variations in whole life policies can replace traditional tax-advantaged retirement plans. The IRS and tax courts have consistently struck down most of these schemes. Life insurance may be a method to increase tax-deferred savings once the tax-advantaged plan is maximized, but it should not be viewed as a primary retirement planning method.

Taking Money at Retirement

When it comes time for a person to withdraw retirement assets, certain IRS rules must be followed. They change frequently, so only a primer is given here. The dentist should check with an accountant or tax advisor when that time comes. Retirement income can be received in two major ways: withdrawing from accumulations (either tax-advantaged plan or after tax savings) or buying an annuity contract from an insurance company. (Some considerations are also given for Social Security income.)

How Much Is Enough?

The first question that most people ask is "How much money do I need?" The answer depends on many factors (Table 3.6). The most obvious is income needed in retirement. If a person needs more to live on, then he or she needs a larger saving cache. As a rule, most people live on about 80 percent of their preretirement income. This is because of less need for clothing, transportation, lunches out, and other work-related expenses. Generally, by this time, a person has paid for the house, and the kids are grown. Therefore, day-to-day expenses are less. Some people's retirement income needs increase, if they have expensive hobbies or plan to travel frequently. Others may not be as great if they continue to work part-time to supplement their retirement income. People who are eligible for Social Security retirement benefits will need less than those who are not yet eligible.

The length of time in retirement is another critical factor. If a person retires at age 50, he or she will obviously have many more years in retirement than if he or she retires at age 80, all other things being equal. Each person needs to look realistically at family history and personal health and habits when estimating life expectancy. (An honest appraisal of expected lifetime is, in itself, an important exercise.) If a person has a family history of heart disease and he or she does little to address it, then he or she can plan to have a shorter time in retirement than otherwise. A person should also plan for his or her spouse's lifetime income in retirement, if that spouse is depending on that person for income. As a rule, a person should plan on living until the age of 90 if he or she has no significant health problems. This allows for a complete retirement for about 90 percent of Americans.

A person must also decide if he or she needs or wants to leave any money to heirs. Sometimes people may need to leave money. For example, if a person has a disabled adult child who dependent on the parent for income, the parent may need to provide income for the child's continued support. (This could also be accomplished through life insurance, trusts, or other methods.) A person may want to leave money to some or all children. If so, he or she will need more accumulation in a retirement account and other assets than if he or she does not. Many people want to spend all of their retirement savings, so that the last dollar in savings is spent with their last dying breath. They believe that providing a strong moral, ethical, and educational foundation early in life for their children serves them more than an inherited handout later in life.

The investment rate of return on retirement assets is another decision factor. If a person earns 13 percent consistently on retirement assets during retirement, then the money will last much longer than if the person makes 3 percent. Most people become more conservative investors as they near and enter retirement, and rightly so. People do not want to take on unneeded risk for the money on which they will be living. However, people also do not want to be too conservative with retirement assets, experiencing almost no growth. Not only does principal shrink quickly, but as withdrawals increase with inflation, the shrinkage accelerates. A person needs to grow the principal at least at the rate of inflation just to stay even. Table 3.7 shows approximately how much investment is needed for given lengths of retirement and rates of return.

Table 3.6 How Much Is Enough?
To withdraw $100 per month, a person will need:

Years in Retirement	6%	8%	10%	12%
15	$11,910	$10,534	$9,383	$8,415
20	$14,028	$12,035	$10,449	$9,173
25	$15,598	$13,043	$11,096	$9,590
30	$16,763	$13,719	$11,490	$9,819
35	$17,626	$14,173	$11,729	$9,945

Table 3.7 Extending the Lifetime of Your Assets

If principle is Earning This Rate	And You Withdraw at this Rate									
	16%	15%	14%	13%	12%	11%	10%	9%	8%	7%
12%	12	14	17	23	Here's how many years your principal will last					
11%	11	13	15	18	24					
10%	10	12	13	15	19	25				
9%	10	11	12	14	16	20	27			
8%	9	10	11	12	14	17	21	28		
7%	9	9	10	11	13	15	18	22	31	
6%	8	9	10	11	12	13	16	19	24	33
5%	8	8	9	10	11	12	14	17	20	26

A financial planning professional can run different investment and withdrawal scenarios that estimate how much money is needed at retirement given the various inputs. For rough planning estimates, there are several quick "rules of thumb" for the amount of income retirement assets can provide.

1. A person can take about 5 percent of the value per year. This assumes that a person earns 8 percent per year. Three percent of that goes to keep up with inflation, leaving 5 percent to live on. Withdrawing this amount should mean that he or she will never run out of retirement money and will leave a tidy nest egg for heirs. If a person has $2 million in retirement savings, he or she can take $100,000 per year to live on, leaving the principal intact. Real-world fluctuating returns and inflation can make this scenario attractive or not.
2. For every $1,000 (pretax) of monthly income wanted, a person needs to have retirement savings of $240,000. The math works out the same as the preceding scenario, but it focuses on income requirement. Both rules assume a moderate investment strategy of 60 percent growth stocks and 40 percent income-producing stocks and bonds (giving the 8-percent annual return).

Social Security

Social Security pays retirement income to people who have paid into the system (through Social Security or self-employment taxes) for at least 40 quarters. They also pay surviving spouse benefits, even if the spouse did not work. The amount that a person receives depends in part on the amount that paid in along the way. Even if a person pays in the maximum amount each year, the top retirement income will only be about $16,000 per year (2012 dollars). This amount is adjusted annually for inflation.

To qualify for benefits, a person must have reached a minimum age. That age changes (upward) at the whim of Congress. There is an age at which a person receives full benefits. If he or she opts to start taking benefits earlier, reduced benefits are received. There is a choice, but it is a one-time choice. The present law calls for full payments at age 70. People can receive reduced payments (80 percent) at age 65. These ages will go up as Congress tries to reduce payments to keep the system solvent.

One other quirk of Social Security payments involves earned income. If a person has earned income while collecting Social Security retirement benefits, your benefits are reduced. Presently, that reduction is about $1 for every $3 earned for people younger than 70 years of age. Older than age 70, there is no reduction. The notion here is to keep people from "double dipping" and collecting Social Security while working. The effect is to make retirees decide if it is financially worthwhile to work, even part-time, during retirement.

Tax-Advantaged Plan Withdrawal Rules

For defined contribution plans, the rules are similar to IRA withdrawals. In fact, most people place their funds into an IRA and make withdrawals from it. These are called rollover IRAs, although there is really no difference between them and other IRAs; a person simply rolls money over into one fund.

The IRS states that a person cannot withdraw funds until he or she reaches the age of 59 1/2 and must begin to withdraw them when he or she reaches 70 1/2, even if still working. The IRS requires minimum distribution of retirement funds when a person reaches 70 1/2. The IRS has tables that detail these minimum distributions. A person may take more than the minimum but not less. Any money not distributed at death goes to the named "beneficiary" of the fund.

The IRS has many other rules that govern retirement plans. Besides the minimum distribution rules, there are excess contribution, excess distribution, premature distribution, and lump sum death payment rules. At this time, there is no need to know these rules, just that they do exist and a tax advisor or tax study is needed when retirement time comes.

Annuity

As mentioned previously, an annuity is a series of regular payments. When a person retires, he or she can buy an annuity contract from an insurance company, with a one-time, lump sum payment into the annuity. These annuities are similar to a whole life insurance policy, only in reverse. A person makes a lump sum payment into the contract and receives monthly payment out of the contract. The annuity can be set up so that he or she receives payments for a certain number of years (period certain), for lifetime (single life), or the lifetime of the policy holder or spouse, whoever lives longer (joint and last survivor). Insurance companies use actuarial tables that estimate how long a person will live in combination with expected investment returns to decide the payout. Obviously, the contacts will have different payout and cost numbers depending on age, health status, age of spouse, and contract provisions.

The purpose of an annuity is to guarantee an income for a particular period. People can probably receive a higher retirement income if they properly manage their tax-deferred retirement assets. But these assets must be actively managed. When people buy an annuity for retirement purposes, they forego some monthly income for the security of known payments and an income that they can not outlive. This may be valuable for a spouse who is not financially savvy or for a disabled retiree or dependent. People are betting the insurance company that they will live longer than the insurance company actuaries estimate that the policy holder will live.

Stages in Retirement Planning

The following discussion is based on a "typical" dentist's professional financial life cycle. Each person is obviously going to be different. A person, for example, may have a working spouse who can contribute to the family and retirement budgets. Or another person may enter a salaried position that includes a retirement plan in the compensation package. Regardless, the principles involved in the life cycle remain. The cycle is described in the financial planning chapter of this book.

The sooner a person starts making maximum contributions to a tax-advantaged retirement plan, the better. However, there is an obvious trade off between present income needs (or wants) and savings (Box 3.3). Early in a career, there is a need to pay off debt. A person may have $5,000 to $6,000 per month in payments for a practice buy out or start-up loan plus student debt and personal debt for houses and other needs. Cash flow is strapped. During this phase, a person should start a retirement plan to develop the savings habit. An IRA (back-loaded) is perfect for this stage. If cash flow permits, a person can develop a SEP or SIMPLE plan, although the more important issue is to pay down the large debt load and build personal assets.

Once a person has paid off the office note, he or she enters the second, or middle, career stage. During this stage, the worry is to make the practice more efficient and profitable. He or she can apply a large portion of the previous practice loan payment to a tax-advantaged plan for the office. The person still uses time to advantage for compounding the value of the account.

Box 3.3 Stages of Retirement Planning

Early Career, Debt Payoff
  Roth IRA, traditional IRA
  SEP, SIMPLE
Middle career, maximum profitability
  SEP, SIMPLE
  401(k)
Late career, nearing retirement
  Defined benefit plan
  Target benefit plan

With increased cash flow, he or she can now comfortably make maximum contribution to the plan. SEP and SIMPLE plans can be used to best advantage. A person may also contribute to an annuity to build retirement income further. Later in this phase, if he or she has not funded the plan previously, a person should investigate a defined benefit plan to catch up with contributions.

As a person nears retirement, he or she should not need to change retirement plans, just continue to fund the existing plan. If that person decides that the plan is underfunded, then he or she should look at an age-weighted, a defined benefit, or a target income type plan. If a person has done planning properly along the way, he or she should not need to worry about these plans.

Example Strategies

Figure 3.2 shows the results of several different strategies for timing retirement savings. The results for these hypothetical doctors are based on the assumptions that they begin retirement savings at age 25 and retire at age 65. They earn an 8-percent average annual return on investment and are in a 35-percent marginal tax rate. The average return means that some years the investor earns 12 percent, and some years they lose 3 percent, but on average, they gain 8 percent. The marginal tax rate is constant over the investor's life. At retirement, it is assumed that the investor takes money out of the plan in a lump sum and pays 35 percent income tax. In fact, most investors take only as much as they need, leaving the rest to continue to grow tax deferred.

Dr. Adams makes a one-time investment. She earns $5,000, and then pays 35 percent income tax, leaving her $3,250. She invests this in a taxable account. Each year, she pays 35 percent income tax on the amount she earns for the year. This essentially decreases her earning to 5.2 percent per year (8 percent reduced by 35 percent tax). At the end of the 40 years, she has earned $25,973 and owes no taxes because she has paid them each year of the investment.

Dr. Boyd earned $5,000 and put all of it into a traditional IRA. Because IRAs are tax deductible, he did not have to pay income taxes on the initial investment, putting the entire $5,000 to work for him. The earnings are also tax deferred, which means that he gets the full value of the 8-percent annual investment return. He earns $117,312 from his initial $5,000 investment, pays taxes of $41,059 and still has three times as much ($76,253) as Dr. Adams. This shows the dramatic advantage of using a tax-advantaged retirement plan over a taxable investment account.

Example IRA Strategies

Annual investment return = 8.0%

Tax rate = 35.0%

	DR. ADAMS — Dr. Adams pays tax on $5,000, then invests it in a taxable account			DR. BOYD — Dr. Boyd puts $5,000 in a tax deferred IRA earning He pays taxes at withdrawl.			DR. CLARK — Dr. Clark waits until age 34, then put $5,000 per year in a tax deferred IRA			DR. DENT — Dr. Dent begins an IRA immediately, then stops contibutions at age 34.			DR. EDEN — Dr. Eden begins an IRA early and continues contributions until retirement age.		
Age	ANNUAL PMT	TOTAL PMTS	POSTTAX VALUE	ANNUAL PMT	TOTAL PMTS	TOTAL VALUE	ANNUAL PMT	TOTAL PMTS	TOTAL VALUE	ANNUAL PMT	TOTAL PMTS	TOTAL VALUE	ANNUAL PMT	TOTAL PMTS	TOTAL VALUE
25	3,250	3,250	3,419	5,000	5,000	5,400	0	0	0	5,000	5,000	5,400	5,000	5,000	5,400
26	0	3,250	3,597	0	5,000	5,832	0	0	0	5,000	10,000	11,232	5,000	10,000	11,232
27	0	3,250	3,784	0	5,000	6,299	0	0	0	5,000	15,000	17,531	5,000	15,000	17,531
28	0	3,250	3,981	0	5,000	6,802	0	0	0	5,000	20,000	24,333	5,000	20,000	24,333
29	0	3,250	4,188	0	5,000	7,347	0	0	0	5,000	25,000	31,680	5,000	25,000	31,680
30	0	3,250	4,405	0	5,000	7,934	0	0	0	5,000	30,000	39,614	5,000	30,000	39,614
31	0	3,250	4,634	0	5,000	8,569	0	0	0	5,000	35,000	48,183	5,000	35,000	48,183
32	0	3,250	4,875	0	5,000	9,255	0	0	0	5,000	40,000	57,438	5,000	40,000	57,438
33	0	3,250	5,129	0	5,000	9,995	0	0	0	5,000	45,000	67,433	5,000	45,000	67,433
34	0	3,250	5,396	0	5,000	10,795	5,000	5,000	5,400	0	45,000	72,827	5,000	50,000	78,227
35	0	3,250	5,676	0	5,000	11,658	5,000	10,000	11,232	0	45,000	78,654	5,000	55,000	89,886
36	0	3,250	5,971	0	5,000	12,591	5,000	15,000	17,531	0	45,000	84,946	5,000	60,000	102,476
37	0	3,250	6,282	0	5,000	13,598	5,000	20,000	24,333	0	45,000	91,742	5,000	65,000	116,075
38	0	3,250	6,609	0	5,000	14,686	5,000	25,000	31,680	0	45,000	99,081	5,000	70,000	130,761
39	0	3,250	6,952	0	5,000	15,861	5,000	30,000	39,614	0	45,000	107,007	5,000	75,000	146,621
40	0	3,250	7,314	0	5,000	17,130	5,000	35,000	48,183	0	45,000	115,568	5,000	80,000	163,751
41	0	3,250	7,694	0	5,000	18,500	5,000	40,000	57,438	0	45,000	124,813	5,000	85,000	182,251
42	0	3,250	8,094	0	5,000	19,980	5,000	45,000	67,433	0	45,000	134,799	5,000	90,000	202,231
43	0	3,250	8,515	0	5,000	21,579	5,000	50,000	78,227	0	45,000	145,582	5,000	95,000	223,810
44	0	3,250	8,958	0	5,000	23,305	5,000	55,000	89,886	0	45,000	157,229	5,000	100,000	247,115
45	0	3,250	9,424	0	5,000	25,169	5,000	60,000	102,476	0	45,000	169,807	5,000	105,000	272,284
46	0	3,250	9,914	0	5,000	27,183	5,000	65,000	116,075	0	45,000	183,392	5,000	110,000	299,466
47	0	3,250	10,429	0	5,000	29,357	5,000	70,000	130,761	0	45,000	198,063	5,000	115,000	328,824
48	0	3,250	10,971	0	5,000	31,706	5,000	75,000	146,621	0	45,000	213,908	5,000	120,000	360,530
49	0	3,250	11,542	0	5,000	34,242	5,000	80,000	163,751	0	45,000	231,021	5,000	125,000	394,772
50	0	3,250	12,142	0	5,000	36,982	5,000	85,000	182,251	0	45,000	249,503	5,000	130,000	431,754
51	0	3,250	12,773	0	5,000	39,940	5,000	90,000	202,231	0	45,000	269,463	5,000	135,000	471,694
52	0	3,250	13,438	0	5,000	43,136	5,000	95,000	223,810	0	45,000	291,020	5,000	140,000	514,830
53	0	3,250	14,136	0	5,000	46,586	5,000	100,000	247,115	0	45,000	314,301	5,000	145,000	561,416
54	0	3,250	14,872	0	5,000	50,313	5,000	105,000	272,284	0	45,000	339,446	5,000	150,000	611,729
55	0	3,250	15,645	0	5,000	54,338	5,000	110,000	299,466	0	45,000	366,601	5,000	155,000	666,068
56	0	3,250	16,458	0	5,000	58,685	5,000	115,000	328,824	0	45,000	395,929	5,000	160,000	724,753
57	0	3,250	17,314	0	5,000	63,380	5,000	120,000	360,530	0	45,000	427,604	5,000	165,000	788,133
58	0	3,250	18,215	0	5,000	68,451	5,000	125,000	394,772	0	45,000	461,812	5,000	170,000	856,584
59	0	3,250	19,162	0	5,000	73,927	5,000	130,000	431,754	0	45,000	498,757	5,000	175,000	930,511
60	0	3,250	20,158	0	5,000	79,841	5,000	135,000	471,694	0	45,000	538,657	5,000	180,000	1,010,352
61	0	3,250	21,206	0	5,000	86,228	5,000	140,000	514,830	0	45,000	581,750	5,000	185,000	1,096,580
62	0	3,250	22,309	0	5,000	93,126	5,000	145,000	561,416	0	45,000	628,290	5,000	190,000	1,189,706
63	0	3,250	23,469	0	5,000	100,576	5,000	150,000	611,729	0	45,000	678,553	5,000	195,000	1,290,283
64	0	3,250	24,690	0	5,000	108,623	5,000	155,000	666,068	0	45,000	732,838	5,000	200,000	1,398,905
65	0	3,250	25,973	0	5,000	117,312	5,000	160,000	724,753	0	45,000	791,465	5,000	205,000	1,516,218
Pretax	3,250		25,973	5,000		117,312	160,000		724,753	45,000		791,465	205,000		1,516,218
Taxes			0			41,059			253,664			277,013			530,676
After Taxes			$25,973			$76,253			$471,090			$514,452			$985,541

Figure 3.2 Example IRA strategies

Dr. Clark believes that he cannot afford to put money into a retirement plan. His current family budget will not allow it, so he waits 9 years until age 34 to begin a retirement savings program. He then puts $5,000 per year into a tax-advantaged retirement plan, such as an IRA. At age 65, his IRA is now worth $724,753 from a total investment of $160,000. After paying income tax, his plan is worth $471,090.

Dr. Dent took the opposite strategy of Dr. Clark. She put $5,000 per year into a tax-advantaged (tax-deductible, tax-deferred) IRA. However, she only invested for the first 9 years. At age 65, her retirement account is worth more ($791,465) than Dr. Clark's. This result is from a smaller total investment ($45,000) as well. Her strategy clearly shows the advantage of starting the retirement savings early, so the investor has more time for the assets to grow.

Dr. Eden combined the strategies of doctors Clark and Dent. He started putting $5,000 per year in a tax-advantaged retirement plan and continued until age 65. His account was worth more than $1.5 million before taxes and almost a million after taxes. Mathematically, it is the sum of doctors Clark and Dent.

These examples show the value of beginning retirement savings early, using tax-deductible and tax-deferred investment accounts and continuing to fund the retirement plan throughout a career. Saving for retirement is a slow-and-steady process. Through proper planning and implementation, retirement savings can be accumulated that will allow a person to choose how to spend time later in his or her career.

Reducing the Personal Tax Burden

The only thing that hurts more than paying an income tax is not having to pay an income tax.
Lord Thomas R. Duwar

Objectives

At the completion of this chapter, the student will be able to:
1. Describe the organization of federal Form 1040.
2. Define the purpose of the various supporting federal forms and schedules.
   Schedule A: Itemized Deductions
    Form 8283: Noncash Charitable Contributions
    Form 2106: Employee Related Business Expenses
   Schedule B: Interest and Dividend Income
   Schedule C: Profit or Loss from Business
    Form 4562: Depreciation and Amortization
   Schedule D: Capital Gains and Losses
3. Differentiate between deductible and nondeductible personal expenses.
4. Apply the principles of basic tax planning to the personal tax return.

Key Terms

adjusted gross income (AGI)
adjustments to income
audit triggers
business deductions
corporate practice
earned income
estimated tax declaration
federal income tax
filing status
net tax liability
occupational taxes
partnership practice
personal deductions
 standard deduction
 itemized deductions
personal exemptions
 marginal tax rate
 progressive
 regressive

personal income tax
postponing taxes
proprietorship
sECA self-employment tax
shifting income
sinking fund taxes
state income taxes
tax
tax audits
tax credits
tax elimination or
reduction
tax evasion
tax forms
 Form 1040
 Form 1065: Partnership
 Return Schedule K-1
 Form 1120: Corporate Tax
 Return

Form 2106: Employee
Related Business
Expenses
Form 4562: Depreciation
and Amortization
Form 8283: Noncash
Charitable Contributions
miscellaneous deductions
schedules
Schedule A: Itemized
Deductions
Schedule B: Interest and
Dividend Income
Schedule C: Profit or Loss
from Business
Schedule D: Capital Gains
or Losses
Scheduled SE:
Self-Employment Tax

(Continued)

Business Basics for Dentists, First Edition. David O. Willis.
© 2013 John Wiley & Sons, Inc. Published 2013 by John Wiley & Sons, Inc.

---

tax-free income	alternative minimum tax (AMT)	taxpayer compliance audit
tax rate	tax liability	total (gross) income
taxable income	tax rate	unearned income

Goal

This chapter is a general discussion of personal income taxes. The discussion focuses both on dentists who are practice owners (proprietors or partners) and those who are employees. Personal tax planning strategies will also be highlighted.

Taxes are a fact of life in the United States. As government provides more services for the population, they require more money to do those services. Government services may be thought off as primarily entitlements (such as welfare and Social Security), probably because those items are often in the news. However, governments at all levels provide many other services used by all, including military protection, the road system, basic education, the university system, air traffic safety, and restaurant safety inspections. Because of these varied services, taxes to pay for them are also varied and substantial. Table 4.1 shows how much a person might pay in total taxes (both actual and hidden). Given this huge tax liability, it is crucial that a dentist manages his or her tax liability effectively.

The single largest item of tax expense for most Americans is personal income tax. This chapter discusses personal income taxes, how the taxes are calculated, and what can be done to reduce this tax burden. The federal government levies the largest portion of income tax. Many states also have separate income taxes. Many local governments (city or county) have taxes on income beyond the federal and state taxes. Worrying about income taxes is, in a sense, a nice problem to have. It means that a person is making money.

Table 4.1 Example of Total Tax Payment*

Type	Percentage
Federal income tax	28%
Social Security tax	7%
State income tax	7%
City income tax	2%
Sales tax	5%
Property tax	3%
TOTAL	52%

*Both actual and hidden taxes. Additional (hidden) taxes include real estate transfer taxes, licenses, excise tax, gasoline tax, personal property tax, recording fees, inheritance tax, airport departure fees, corporate income tax, entertainment tax, hotel room tax, and transportation tax

Federal Income Taxes

Federal income taxes are due on any money that a person makes during the year. This income can be earned income or from investments (unearned income). Dentists who are in business for themselves determine their profit or loss from operating their business on a separate form (Schedule C) and then bring that profit or loss to the personal tax form (Form 1040). These are all due on April 15 of the following year.

If a dentist is the proprietor owner of a practice, he or she must file a long Form 1040. (There is an abbreviated version [1040-EZ] for people who do not have complex returns.) If a person owns a corporate or partnership practice, he or she will need to file returns for those entities also. If a person is a nonowner employee of a practice, he or she will have a simpler time computing personal taxes because he or she does not have to report the practice information.

Most dentists have their accountants do their taxes for them. If a person understands the basics of tax law, then he or she can give an accountant complete information and can make more informed decisions regarding his or her own individual tax status.

Income

The IRS develops and implements tax laws for the federal government. The IRS has a simple rule concerning whether money made is income or not for tax purposes. They consider any money made to be taxable income unless there is a specific waiver for that type of income in the tax codes. A few specifically designated types of income are either exempt from income taxation or taxed at a lower rate. Municipal bond income, scholarships or grants, and gifts or inheritances are exempt from income taxes. Ordinary income is the same as earned income. A person makes this money through working. Investment income (either capital gains or dividends) is unearned income. The IRS taxes it at a lower rate. Also, because a person did not earn it, he or she does not owe Social Security and Medicare (or self-employment) tax on this type of income (Table 4.2).

The form of the income is immaterial. (It does not have to be cash money.) If a person barters a crown for

Table 4.2 Tax Rates Paid for Earned and Unearned Income

Investment Income (Unearned)				Ordinary Income (Earned)	
	Capital Gain or Loss		Interest or Dividend		
	Long-term (>1 year)	Short-term (<1 year)		Wages, tips etc.	Nonincorporated business profit
Tax Rate	Lower	Ordinary Income Rates	Lower	Ordinary Income Rates	Ordinary Income Rates
Other Taxes	State, local	State, local	State, local	State, local, FICA and Medicare	State, local, self-employment tax

a house painting job, he or she has received income according to the IRS. That person should record as income the value of the house painting job. The painter should similarly include the value of the gold crown in his or her income.

Taxes are paid when the income is realized. This means that a person pays tax when value changes hands. For example, a person buys 100 shares of XYZ stock at $10.00 per share. If the price goes to $25.00 in the first year and $35.00 per share the second year, he or she pays no tax until the stock is sold. If the stock is sold in the fourth year for $55.00 per share, he or she pays tax on the appreciated value (55.00 – 10.00 = $45.00 per share) in the fourth year. By the same reasoning, a person pays no income taxes on accounts receivable because they are not income until the money is received.

Personal Deductions

Deductions are expenses that may be subtract from income before the tax owed is calculated. Some deductions are personal. Some are for business. (In this chapter only personal deductions are discussed.) The IRS has a rule similar to the "Income Rule" when looking at deductions. It considers no expense to be deductible unless they have specifically granted deductibility in the tax codes. (Just because a person believes that an expense should be deductible does not make it so.) A dentist may need to prove the amount and necessity of this expense to the IRS, so keeping excellent records that include a description of the deduction, a receipt, and a canceled check for the item is always a good idea. A canceled check, by itself, is not enough documentation.

Basic Personal Tax Formula

Box 4.1 provides a basic tax formula. Dentists need to understand the components of this formula to understand how to reduce tax liability. This is for personal (not business) tax, which will be covered later. Net income from the practice becomes personal gross income for tax purposes.

Box 4.1 Basic Tax Formula

Gross Income
 – Adjustments to Income
 = Adjusted Gross Income

– Standard Deduction or Itemized Deductions
 – Personal Exemptions
  = Taxable Income

≪Calculate Tax≫
   – Tax Credits
 = Net Tax Liability (Amount Due for the Year)

1. **Total (Gross) Income** Gross income is all the money that is made for the year. It includes income and wages, tips, profits from a business, such as a dental practice, tax refunds, rental income, or any other form of income. Earned income is income that is earned from working. Unearned income is money that is made from investments. Both are considered income for tax purposes, although the IRS treats them differently in specifics of tax code.

2. **Adjustments to Income** The tax code allows a person to adjust (or subtract) amounts that he or she paid for some specific items. Those include IRA and other retirement contributions (for self), moving expenses if he or she moved to take a new job, half of self-employment tax (if he or she is self-employed), and any alimony (but not child support) that he or she paid. Adjustments are important because they lower income, and therefore, how much tax that will be paid later.

3. **Adjusted Gross Income (AGI)** AGI is simply gross income less any adjustments. AGI is important because it is used later for setting minimums for Schedule A deductions, phase outs for exemptions, and other tax matters.

4. **Standard or Itemized Deduction** (whichever is greater) A person then may deduct valid tax deduction items from the AGI. Two methods can determine this adjustment. A person can use either one. There is a choice, but a person should use the

larger one because it reduces his or her apparent income more. This results in a lower tax liability. The two methods are:

- **Standard Deduction** A person may take a standard amount. This amount changes depending on filing status. There are four possible filing statuses. As a rule, if married, a person should file jointly. The exception is if one spouse has high itemized deductions that could not be used if using a joint filing status because of AGI limitations. The standard deduction is an amount that the IRS estimates typical filers would show. If a person owns a home or has significant medical or employee expenses, he or she is generally better off to itemize deductions.

- **Itemized Deduction** The second method that a person may use to calculate deductions is to itemize personal deductions. Box 4.2 lists the types of valid personal deductions. (These are personal deductions. Business deductions are itemized on a different form [Schedule C].) If a person itemizes, he or she must have receipts and payment proof for each deduction. This sounds like a lot of work but is really not that much of a problem if ongoing records are kept. Notice that several items are tied to the AGI. This means that, for example, a person may only deduct that portion of medical expense that exceeds 7.5 percent of AGI. If a person shows $8,000 in medical expenses with an AGI of $100,000, he or she receives a $500 deduction for those expenses ($8,000 − 7.5 percent of $100,000). The rest is lost as a deduction.

5. **Personal Exemptions** A person claims a personal exemption for self, spouse, and each dependent who lives with him or her. He or she must provide Social Security numbers for all dependents older than 1 year of age. If a person or spouse is older than 65 or blind, he or she gets additional exemptions. As income increases above a threshold, the tax code phases out personal exemptions. This is to ensure that high-income earners pay their "fair share."

6. **Taxable Income** Taxable income is AGI minus exemptions and deductions. This is the number that a person uses to calculate tax liability (or how much tax owed). From a tax planning perspective, a person wants this number as low as it can legally be made. A person can do this either by lowering income, raising adjustments, or increasing deductions and exemptions.

7. **Calculate Tax** The next step in the formula is to calculate how much tax is owed by applying a tax rate or table to the taxable income figure calculated.

8. **Credits** A credit is an allowance that Congress has provided. A credit is a one-to-one reduction of tax liability. (For every dollar of tax credit, taxes go down by a dollar.) Therefore, credits are much more valuable than deductions because they reduce tax (not just taxable income) dollar for dollar. Credits are available for child and elder care expenses, foreign taxes paid, and several other targeted expenses. A person subtracts tax credits from the tax owed.

9. **Net Tax Liability** (**Total Tax Due**) The balance is the net tax liability. At this point, the IRS requires that a person adds other, nonincome taxes, such as Self-Employment Tax and Alternative Minimum Tax. When added, this becomes the net tax liability. That is the total amount of tax owed for the year. Any estimated payments made or any amounts withheld during the year offset this tax liability. At this point these amounts are reconciled. If a person has paid in too much throughout the year, he or she gets a refund. If a person has not paid in enough along the way, he or she owes additional money to make up the difference.

Box 4.2 Tax Deduction Items from AGI*

Medical expenses (excess of 7.5 percent of AGI)
State and local income taxes
Real and personal property taxes
Mortgage interest (primary or secondary residence)
Gifts to charity (cash or property)
Casualty and theft losses (excess of 10 percent AGI)
Miscellaneous or job expenses (excess of 2 percent AGI)

*AGI, adjusted gross income

Tax Rates

A tax rate is the specified percentage that the law stipulates what is paid on taxable income. Some taxes (such as federal income taxes) are "progressive," which means that the rate increases by a series of percentages as the taxable income increases (Table 4.3). Other taxes are "flat" taxes, in that the rate remains flat despite the income. Still others are "regressive" taxes that tax lower incomes higher than higher income tax entities.

The tax system developed in this country is a graduated or progressive system, which is to say that the more that a person earns, the higher a rate of tax that he or she pays. This increased rate is only for the amount above the threshold. When income takes a person into the next higher bracket, he or she does not pay the

Table 4.3 A Fictional Illustration of Progressive Tax Rates
This is a simple illustration of fictional progressive tax rates. The actual tax rates are different.

Taxable Income	Marginal Tax Rate
$300,000	30%
$200,000	25%
$100,000	20%
$0	10%

Table 4.4 Marginal Rate and Tax Savings

Amount Of Deduction	Marginal Tax Rate	Cost	Tax Savings
$1,000	15%	$850	$150
$1,000	35%	$650	$350

higher percentage on all of the income, only on the amount above that bracket cutoff. This marginal tax rate is one of the more powerful concepts for the tax-payer to learn. The marginal rate is the tax that a person will pay on the next dollar earned. If he or she earns enough to qualify for the next higher tax bracket, only the amount above the bracket is charged the higher rate, not all of the income. For example, using the fictional tax table, if a dentist earned $250,000, he or she would pay 10 percent on the first $100,000 of income ($10,000), 20 percent on the next $100,000 of income ($20,000), and 25 percent on the remaining $50,000 of income ($12,500) for a total of $42,500. He or she would be in the 25-percent marginal tax bracket, which means that if he or she earned an additional $25,000 this year, he or she would pay 25 percent (or $6,250) in additional tax.

The marginal rate is also important because it deter-mines the value of the tax savings that result from tax planning strategies. If a person has a business deduction that costs $1,000 and he or she is in the 15-percent marginal tax rate, the after-tax cost is $850. (There is a $150 savings on taxes.) If, however, a person is in the 35-percent marginal tax bracket, the after-tax cost is only $650 because there is a $350 savings on taxes (Table 4.4).

Every tax-paying entity has specific tax rates. Congress changes these rates frequently to meet changing fiscal and social moods and responsibilities. They also change the rules regarding income exclusion, deductions, and many other tax-sensitive issues. Therefore, only concepts are discussed in this chapter, not specific numbers or rates.

Components of Form 1040

Form 1040 is the basic tax form that all individuals must file with the federal government. It reports their income for the previous year, allowable deductions, taxes already paid, and the tax owed. If a person uses certain items or lines on Form 1040, he or she may need to complete a supporting schedule or form that give the details of the transactions involved on that line. For example, if a person operates a sole proprietorship business, such as a dental office, he or she reports the profit or loss from operating that business on one line of 1040 (business income or loss). He or she then attaches a completed Schedule C: Profit or Loss from Business that details all income and expenses from running a business. Some common forms and schedules that many dentists use are described here.

Form 1040 Itself

The Form 1040 comes in several levels of complexity. Most dentists complete the full Form 1040 rather than the abbreviated Form 1040-EZ.

Schedule A: Itemized Deductions

This form is used to detail allowable personal deductions. If a person does not have enough personal itemized (specific) deductions, then he or she may opt to take the standard deduction, whichever is larger. If a person is an employed (nonowner) dentist, then he or she must take professional expenses as miscellaneous deductions on this schedule. This is a problem because there is a 2-percent of income threshold that must pass with these deductions.

- **Form 8283: Noncash Charitable Contributions**   This form is used to detail all donations to charitable organizations. Old clothing, toys, discarded appli-ances, old books, out of style neckties, old cars, and many other items will be collected by organizations such as the Volunteers of America. They will come to pick up the donated items, and then leave a receipt for them. The total value of the donation should be put on Schedule A. Later in a career, when a person wants to donate more valuable assets to charities, the rules get more complex.
- **Form 2106: Employee Related Business Expenses**   If a person is an employee, he or she will detail business expenses on this form, then put the total on Schedule A. Expenses that qualify include organization dues (e.g., American Dental Association [ADA]), automo-bile operating and depreciation expenses, continuing education, and professional books and journals. If a person is a business owner, he or she will put these expenses on Schedule C or the corporate return because there is no 2-percent threshold for expenses on Schedule C as there is on Schedule A (Personal Itemized Deductions).

Schedule B: Interest and Dividend Income

When a person has an investment portfolio, he or she should receive interest and dividends from those investments. That income (if more than $400) should be itemized on Schedule B and then entered on the "Income" section of Form 1040. One advantage to this type of income is that because it is unearned, a person does not need to pay FICA or Medicare taxes on it.

Schedule C: Profit or Loss from Business

If a person is a sole proprietor, this is the form that will be used to report business income. Business-related expenses are subtracted from gross income to arrive at a net income for the business. This amount is carried over to Form 1040 in the "Income" section.

- **Form 4562: Depreciation and Amortization** A person must keep a running tally of equipment age and depreciation status, so that he or she can determine the amount of that value that is claimed as a depreciation expense in any given year. This form determines the amount of that deduction, which is entered as a business expense on Schedule C.

Schedule D: Capital Gains or Losses

Like Schedule B, this schedule is generally used when a person has an investment portfolio. He or she may also need this form when selling a dental practice. The amount of the gain (or loss) is detailed on this sheet and then carried to the "Income" section of Form 1040.

Schedule SE: Self-Employment Tax

This schedule determines the amount that a person must pay in self-employment (FICA and Medicare) tax. Because a person had to pay his or her own matching Social Security, he or she can deduct half this amount from taxable income. (Other wage earners did not have to pay tax on that amount either.) This is done by entering half of this tax as an "Adjustment to Income" on Form 1040. If a person practices as a corporation, the corporation takes the deduction for matching Social Security and Medicare taxes, which is the employee equivalent of the self-employment tax.

Schedule K-1

If a practice files taxes as a partnership, the partnership will file a form for the entity and give each partner a Schedule K-1 to help them report his or her individual income from the partnership. Because a partnership is not a separate taxable entity, these are information-only forms for the IRS. No one files a K-1 with Form 1040 but instead keeps it with their records. A person may carry the amounts on K-1 to several places on Form 1040, depending on the type of income or expense.

Form 1120: Corporate Tax Return

If a practice is a corporation, the corporation will file this return. A person will be an employee of the corporation and so will receive a W-2 for services like any other employee (entered on Form 1040.) If a person is an owner or part owner, he or she may also have dividends from the corporation to report.

Other Income Taxes

State Income Taxes

Some states have taxes on income that are beyond federal income taxes. As a rule, states that have these income taxes follow the format of federal forms fairly closely. Some states, in fact, simply use the same form, applying different percentages for the taxes. Most states have a few differences relating to state-specific municipal bonds and other state-specific initiatives.

Local Income Taxes

Some cities, counties, and other municipalities also have income taxes. These vary tremendously. Some cities call them "occupational taxes"; some call them "sinking fund taxes" (because they often retire sinking fund debt). Regardless the name, they are a form of income tax.

Alternative Minimum Tax

The tax laws give special treatment to certain types of income and deductions. In the past, taxpayers who used these special rules aggressively could substantially (or completely) avoid paying income tax. Some people saw this as unfair and tantamount to abusive use of the system. To assure that everyone pays their fair share, Congress developed the Alternative Minimum Tax (AMT). They intend this to ensure that everyone pays a certain minimum amount in taxes, even if they have used the rules correctly to reduce their tax burden. The AMT calculations require a person to figure tax the normal way and then refigure it without the special income and deductions (so-called tax-preference items). The person then pays taxes based on whichever method leads to higher taxes.

AMT often hits start-up dentists who have relatively high incomes (because of the high depreciation) and mid-career high income dentists (because of the loss of exemptions and deductions). Dentists should be aware of the problems of AMT and work with an accountant to reduce the impact on taxable income. (A dentist might, for example, not accelerate depreciation deductions if it causes him or her to be subject to the AMT.)

Issues for the Self-employed Dentist

Estimated Tax Declaration and Payment

Anyone whose income does not have tax withheld by their employer must estimate federal and state income for the upcoming year and make four equal quarterly payments instead of withholdings. This includes proprietors, partners, and employees who receive dividends and other forms of unearned income. The date that these federal payments are due is:

April 15	Declaration and first payment
June 15	Second payment
Sept 15	Third payment
Jan 15	Fourth payment

A person does not have to file an estimated return if his or her total federal income and self-employment taxes will be less than $500. There are penalties and interest if he or she underestimated tax liability by too much. An accountant will help calculate estimated tax payments.

Self-Employment Tax (Social Security and Medicare Tax)

An additional tax that the federal government levies on all earned income is the Social Security and Medicare Tax, also known as the Federal Insurance Contributions Act (FICA). This is actually composed of two taxes, one on the employee, and an equal one on the employer. Together, they fund Social Security benefits and the Medicare program. Everyone who has earned income pays this tax. Employees pay it as Social Security and Medicare taxes, self-employed individuals as Self-Employment Tax. Self-employed individuals must pay not only the employee portion of the tax but also pay their own matching portion as well. They do get some deduction for their self-employment tax on Form 1040. Self-employment tax is figured on Schedule SE and attached to Form 1040.

Tax Planning for the Individual

Tax planning is a lifetime work for many individuals, so this section barely begins the process. The section on business taxes and planning interweaves with this section for practicing dentists.

Most accounting firms send their clients a tax information organizer at the end of the year. This contains the information from the previous year's tax returns and gives prompts for the current year's information. Sometimes they have separate organizers for personal and office information. If a person has done proper bookkeeping along the way, this should not be a huge burden. If a person gets the information to the accountant well before the deadline, then the accountant can examine the upcoming return and make suggestions to lessen the tax burden for both the current and next year.

Many firms also distribute a tax planning workbook that summarizes current tax laws. These are an excellent source to begin learning about individual tax planning. These workbooks point out that there are really only five strategies to (legally) reduce the tax burden. Tax planning goals are to increase spendable, after-tax income and to increase wealth. (Business taxes are covered later.) They are tax elimination or reduction, recharacterizing income, shifting income, postponing taxes, and using business expenses judiciously.

Tax Elimination or Reduction (Avoid or Reduce the Tax)

The most important thing a person can do here is to know the tax laws so that he or she can communicate effectively with an accountant or tax preparer. If a person does not take a deduction to which he or she is entitled, the IRS generally does not call it to that person's attention. The federal tax code is so complex and ever-changing that it is not worth a person's time to know all of the details, amounts, and nuances of the laws. By learning about and using the general rules, such as the proper filing status, personal deductions, and charitable giving, a person can keep taxes as low as possible. A person can earn some income that is free from federal income tax, such as municipal bond income.

Recharacterizing Income (Turn Earned Income into Unearned Income)

All income is subject to income tax. Only earned income is subject to FICA or self-employment tax. If a person can take some earned income and make it unearned, then he or she can save the FICA or self-employment tax, which is 15.3 percent (or 2.9 percent on income above the threshold). Unearned income includes rent (for the office), lease income (for equipment), and dividends from corporations. By establishing separate tax entities for these activities, a person can take income that would be earned and make it unearned, with the associated tax savings.

Shifting Income (Income Taxed at a Lower Rate)

A person can shift income to family members who are in lower tax brackets, thereby decreasing the tax that the family unit owes. A person only does this if the child is financially responsible or if he or she controls the income that the child earns. This helps to fund college plans and even IRAs for the child. A person can employ family members through the practice or establish a family entity that earns and distributes some income that a dentist would normally earn, taking it from his or her high tax bracket to family members' lower tax bracket. These strategies are briefly discussed in the section on business taxes. A dentist should have advisors establish these plans to be sure they meet current tax laws.

Postponing Taxes (Wealth Accumulation without Current Income Taxes)

The most common way of using this strategy is to fund a tax-deferred retirement plan for a person, himself or herself. This takes money out of current taxable income and allows it to grow without paying taxes until it is withdrawn at retirement. If a person hires family members in the practice, he or she can contribute to their retirement plan, increasing the value of this strategy. A person can also postpone taxes by using some forms of life insurance, annuities, and family gifting programs.

Using Business Expenses Judiciously (Shifting Expenses to the Business Unit)

The IRS does not allow some expenses as full deductions for an individual, but the same expense is deductible from a business if it is a valid cost of doing business. As many of these costs as possible should be shifted to the business to take full deduction. Examples here include continuing education courses, business use of the car, and professional dues. If a person does not, have a practice, he or she should consider moonlighting or setting up a consulting business so that he or she can be sure that these expenses are fully deductible.

Tax Audits

The IRS examines (audits) tax returns to verify that the tax reported is correct. The IRS intends audits to ensure that people report taxes honestly. They really do not make a lot of money for the government. (Some large cases make significant sums for the treasury.) Instead, the government attempts to scare a person into reporting accurately. With sizeable penalties and interest, a person should take this threat seriously. If a return is selected for examination, this does not mean necessarily that a person has made an error or been dishonest. Often the IRS needs additional information to verify numbers. Other audits may be more onerous.

The IRS levies significant penalties and fines for cheating on taxes, if they catch the person. If someone makes a simple mistake, he or she will probably only have a fine, back taxes, and interest on the taxes to pay. If a person knowingly cheated the government (e.g., not claiming income or not filing taxes), he or she may be found guilty of tax evasion and spend time in prison, as well as the fines, interest, and back taxes due.

How Returns Are Selected for Audit

There are several reasons a return may be chosen for an audit. The most common are computer scoring, large corporations, information matching, related examinations, and taxpayer compliance audit.

Computer Scoring

Most returns are selected for examination based on a computer scoring system. A computer program (the Discriminant Function System) compares a return to accepted averages or norms for the same type of return. (They compare dentists' offices to other dentists, not physicians' offices or hair stylists.) The program scores every individual and many corporate tax returns. IRS agents then review the highest-scoring returns. They select some for an audit based on which they feel are most likely to need review and which items are commonly reported incorrectly. They call these audit triggers. Common audit triggers include office expenses, meal and entertainment expenses, and home office deductions. So if a return is out of line with norms for the same type of return, the IRS will possibly contact that person.

Large Corporations

The IRS examines many large corporate returns annually. Dental professional service corporations (PSCs) are not part of this program but may be subject to audit through any of the other programs.

Information Matching

The IRS examines returns when payment reports, such as W-2 forms or interest statements from banks, do not match the income reported on the tax return. This often happens to dentists because insurance companies report to the IRS how much money they pay a person each year. If income numbers do not match the numbers reported by the insurers, a person will likely get a call (or a letter) from the IRS. This is especially a problem in group practices in which insurers may make payment in one doctor's name but credit them to another's.

Related Examinations

Returns may be selected for an audit when they involve issues or transactions with other taxpayers, such as business partners or investors, whose returns were selected for examination.

Taxpayer Compliance Audit

This is a particularly odious audit procedure. In this audit, the IRS requires the taxpayer to come to the IRS office to justify and document every income and expense item on the return. These are then used in developing the database for comparison in the computer scoring type of audit. The IRS has reduced the number of these audits significantly in the past several years because of taxpayer outrage and, therefore, political resistance.

Audit Methods

The IRS may conduct an audit by mail or through an in-person interview and review of the taxpayer's records. The IRS conducts most audits (at least initially) through the mail. If a person receives a letter from the IRS, it will generally claim that they have recomputed his or her tax based on the enclosed reasons or information. Generally the tax will be higher as a result, although occasionally they may reduce it. The letter then states that if he or she wants to dispute the IRS's findings, reply within a certain time. (The IRS takes their deadlines seriously.) At this point, contact an accountant and reply quickly to the letter. If the IRS requires an interview, it may be at an IRS office (an office audit) or at the taxpayer's home, place of business, or at the accountant's office (a field audit). Regardless, a person will need to have records to prove his or her claims.

Estate Planning

chapter 5

A man's dying is more the survivor's affair than his own.
Thomas Mann

Objectives

At the completion of this chapter, the student will be able to:
1. Describe the purposes of estate planning.
2. Identify the primary techniques of planning an estate.
3. Discuss common methods of estate transfer.
4. Discuss the use of a testamentary letter.
5. Discuss issues of personal competency and common methods of addressing competency problems.

Key Terms

codicil
community property
contract beneficiaries
estate planning
estate taxes
executor
federal unified gift and
estate tax
gifts
guardian
intestate
joint tenants with rights of
survivorship (JTWROS)

lifetime transfers
living will
personal outline
(testamentary letter)
powers of attorney
  agent
  general
  limited
  present
  springing
probate administration
probate court
requisites of a valid will

revocation
right-to-die statement
surviving spouse exemption
trustee
wills

Goal

This chapter examines the basic principle of estate planning.

Business Basics for Dentists, First Edition. David O. Willis.
© 2013 John Wiley & Sons, Inc. Published 2013 by John Wiley & Sons, Inc.

Planning one's estate is not thought of as a pleasant task. After all, it forces a person to face his or her own mortality. It is, however, a useful and necessary task. It can also be personally satisfying. Estate planning is not about the person planning because he or she will not be around to know the difference. Instead, estate planning is a task that is done for family, for heirs, and for those that a person loves and cares about. An estate plan can be as simple as a will or can involve a will, trusts, contracts, and named beneficiaries. It depends on how much a person owns and how complex his or her wants are.

People should probably dust off their estate plan every 3 to 5 years or whenever they have a major life change. As their estate gets more valuable and complex, people will seek out lawyers who deal with estate planning issues. People often forget what they put into their plans. Circumstances also change quickly. Their retirement savings or value of a practice may have blossomed over the past several years. They may have had additional children, divorced or remarried, received another inheritance, or changed insurances significantly. All these can affect how a will and estate plan are structured.

Purpose of Estate Planning

Planning an estate will accomplish several purposes.

To Be Sure Who Gets What

A person may have a special gold watch or Aunt Tillie's flower vase that he or she wants to go to a particular child. Although not trivial (in fact, these decisions are often the most contentious), the decision takes on added importance when significant amounts of money are involved. This money may be from assets owned, proceeds from insurance policies, retirement plan proceeds, practice sales, inheritances, or countless other sources. If a person properly plans his or her estate, he or she will resolve conflicts, reduce squabbles between family members, and assure that assets will be distributed the way intended.

To Give Beneficiaries Protection and Guidance

A person may be the primary source of family income and financial expertise. If he or she dies, beneficiaries may need help in managing the family finances or other affairs. A person may want to appoint a banker or other trusted advisor as the trustee until family members are old enough to mange their own affairs. Through estate planning, a person can assure that beneficiaries are protected from fraudulent advisors and kept from squandering the money earmarked for a particular purpose.

To Provide for the Welfare of Minor Children

If a person has minor children, he or she has a special estate planning problem. If the spouse is still alive, he or she will naturally take care of any minor children. However, if both die (e.g., in an accident), then the problem suddenly becomes enormous. Not only does the child have to cope with the parents' deaths, but they also must forge new parent ties. A parent needs to ensure that someone will be the guardian for the children until they reach the age of majority, when they can legally manage their own affairs. If a person does not have someone selected ahead of time, then the state will appoint someone. That may not be someone in whom the parent has trust or confidence. This person needs to provide both the emotional and financial guidance that would have been provided. (The potential guardian should be asked before named.) Unmarried siblings or couples may not be the best choice if they are not tuned into raising children. Elderly parents may want the responsibility but may not be physically able to parent children now and until the youngest child is 18. If a person is divorced, remarried, or part of a blended family, additional legal problems develop concerning visitation and support. The more that can be ahead of time, the more service will be providing for the family.

To Help Guide the Executor (Administrator)

An executor (sometimes called the administrator or personal representative) is the person responsible for collecting information, paying bills and expenses, seeing that assets are distributed properly, and generally marshaling an estate through the probate process. Being an executor is a thankless job. Relatives and creditors all try to influence the executor. In addition, there is simply much hard work to do, selling assets, having other assets appraised, paying bills, closing credit card and other accounts, and keeping everyone informed of the process. Executors can be paid (from the estate) for their work. The executor is named in the will. The estate planner should think about who would do these duties best and should ask that person ahead of time.

To Eliminate Delays and the Expense of Probate Administration

Probate administration takes many months, or even years, to complete. This happens especially when the estate is not well planned. Lawyers then bicker over who gets what and who deserves which assets. A well-planned estate reduces these delays and expenses. During the time that the estate is in probate, the assets are essentially "locked up" until they are distributed. This can be a problem if family members or other heirs need that money to live on. In this case, a person needs to be sure to provide sufficient liquid assets outside the probate process for their support.

To Plan for the Business Transition

If a person is the owner of a dental practice or other business, he or she has another special estate planning problem. That problem is that the value of the practice drops quickly if the owner is not present seeing patients. An owner should have a plan for what happens to the practice in case of death or disability. If a person is in a group practice, he or she may have cross-purchase agreements to cover the eventuality. If a person is a solo practitioner, he or she should have an accountant or other trusted advisor with a plan for continuing and selling the practice. A spouse, significant other, executor, or agent should have enough information immediately available to deal with the practice immediately. Any delay can be financially devastating. Often the spouse does not even know how to get into the office, much less how to look for a buyer or how to sell the practice. This should be taken care of for their peace of mind and financial security (Box 5.1).

To Reduce Estate Taxes

Depending on the value of an estate, taxes can take a significant amount that might otherwise go to heirs. The estate pays any taxes that are due and then distributes the assets. Whoever receives the asset then, receives it free of income tax because taxes have already been paid (by the estate). However, if the estate contains a large amount of nonliquid assets (e.g., real estate), then the estate may have to sell some of those important assets to pay the estate taxes. Many professional people have estates that are large enough to trigger significant estate taxes. Proper planning will reduce those taxes and allow for the maximum amount to flow through for the heirs' support and enjoyment.

What Constitues an Estate Plan

At a minimum, there are three primary elements of an estate plan.

Will

A will is a written instrument or legal document that takes effect on a person's death (Box 5.2). It disposes of a person's right to real or personal property that he or she owns at death. Everyone has a will. Some are written by the person who owns the property; others are written by the state. If a person dies without a written will, he or she has died *intestate*. This means that the state will determine who receives property. Here, the state essentially writes a will for the person. These "state-made" wills vary tremendously from state to state. They allocate assets to various family members. These may include spouse, surviving children, parents, brothers and sisters, and grandparents. If the person has no heirs, the estate is generally turned over to the state. Many states have a "Surviving Spouse Exemption," which declares that if a person dies intestate, a certain amount (such as the first $10,000) of personal property goes to the surviving spouse (ahead of all creditors and funeral expenses). Some states also have "dower and curtscy" rights. This antiquated term says that the surviving spouse is entitled to one half the real and personal property as "dower" and not as heir. Obviously, the smart thing is to write a will to avoid all these legal problems. The will can also set up other methods of property transfer (such as trusts) as described later.

Box 5.1 Items to Consider during a Business Transition

Location of the office keys
How to use the office security system
Computer security codes
Home phone numbers of office staff
Names and numbers of major suppliers and labs
Combination to the safe
Name of doctor to refer patients
Plan for practice continuation
Plan for practice sale

Box 5.2 Items to Consider when Creating a Will

1. Selection of executor
2. Selection of guardians for children
3. Creation of trusts for children or incapable
4. Orderly payment of debts
5. Right to sell real estate
6. Potential tax savings

A Durable Power of Attorney

A Power of Attorney allows a person to make financial decisions for some other person if the latter is incompetent. The person holding the power does not hold title to any of the property. It allows another person (the agent) to handle the financial and business affairs if of the incapacitated person. This is especially important if the person is the owner of a dental practice (or other business), and he or she has sole access to the finances of the business. Depending on how personal finances have been structured, the durable power of attorney may be necessary here as well. A limited power of attorney allows the agent to act only in a certain area, for example, selling a house or paying bills for a dental practice. A general power of attorney gives the agent broad authority to transact almost any matter that the person could, such as selling personal property and financial assets or filing tax returns. A present power of attorney takes effect immediately. A springing power of attorney lies dormant until it "springs" into action, generally when the person becomes disabled. (Often a physician or other third party is required to certify that the principal lacks capacity.)

Traditional power of attorney ends when the incapable person dies or becomes competent again. Formalities of establishing a durable power of attorney vary from state to state. Some states require that they be filed with the register of deeds.

A Living Will

A living will designates someone to make medical decisions on a person's behalf, if the latter becomes incapacitated. A living will is also known as a right-to-die statement. It establishes a legal method for a person to provide affirmative direction to medical personnel for medical decisions when the subject is incapable of making medical decisions. This occurs, for example, when the person is in a coma. States are different in their interpretation of the validity of such living wills. So if a person spends significant time in more than one state, he or she may need more than one living will. Although living wills may not provide legal direction, they give moral direction in difficult decisions for caregivers in case of incapacitation.

Personal Outline (Testamentary Letter)

A personal outline, or testamentary letter, is not a legal document. It is a convenience for the person who is the executor of the will (or the administrator of the estate). The outline details information that the executor will need to properly process and probate an estate. The letter should be prepared for a person who is totally unfamiliar with the personal situation. This makes the process easier for an outside someone who does know the person. A testamentary letter should include the following information:

1. **Personal Information** Social Security number, birth certificate, etc.
2. **List and Location of Assets** Real estate, stocks, automobiles (title location), mortgage information, retirement accounts, safe deposit (lock) boxes, and combinations to safes
3. **Practice Information** Accountant, location of deeds, leases, computer back ups, buy-out provisions, etc.
4. **Names of Advisors** Attorney, accountant, investment advisor, insurance agent, and stock broker
5. **Personal Wishes** Burial/cremation, funeral wishes, distribution of personal property, etc.
6. **Insurance Policies** (especially life insurance policies) Company, agent, policy number, and location
7. **Liquidity** For taxes and expenses, living costs until distribution of estate

Methods of Property Transfer

There are three basic methods of transferring property. They are wills, estates, and lifetime transfers (gifts and trusts). A person can also transfer some property outside the probate process. This is done through jointly held property (which passes to a survivor) and through life insurance or pensions, which pass directly to a named beneficiary.

Wills

Wills are the basic and most common form of asset transfer. They are legal documents, although many states do not require that a lawyer write them. A person should have several copies of his or her will. One should be kept at home; one in a safe deposit box (in case of a house fire); and one with a lawyer as a back up. When a person dies, a probate court will settle the will. These are special courts that handle estate cases. They establish the validity of the will, "read the will," and distribute assets according to the will or intestacy law.

Each state has requisites of a valid will. They vary by state. Some more common requirements include:

1. The will must be in writing and signed by the will writer.
2. The will must show testamentary intent (i.e., the person recognizes that this is his or her will).
3. A person must have testamentary capacity (18 years old or older, sound mind, not acting under fraud or influence, etc.).

4. The will must be witnessed by credible witnesses.
5. Some states allow handwritten (in testator's handwriting) or "holographic" wills.

Because each state's requirements are different, it is a good investment to have a lawyer draft the will. Lawyers can help to be sure that the will complies with the state's rules. They can also be sure that the estate plan has been designed to meet a person's needs and desires.

Wills may be revoked. This revocation may be intentional (on the person's part) or unintentional. Reasons for revocation include physical destruction, writing a subsequent will, or through operation of law (such as marriage or divorce). So if a person gets married or divorced, he or she should be sure to write a new will. A codicil is simply a written modification to an existing will. A codicil does not revoke the original will. It just amends it.

Trusts

There are two kinds of trusts, living (revokable) and nonrevokable trusts.

Living Trusts

A living (or revokable) trust is a legal entity into which a person can transfer assets during his or her lifetime. The will can also stipulate that certain assets should be transferred into a living trust at death. The trust takes ownership of the assets. However, a person can cancel or change (or revoke) the trust anytime before his or her death. A person retains control (but not ownership) of the assets.

A person can use a revokable trust much like a will, by instructing how assets will be distributed in the trust after death. These assets are distributed without probate, so the assets will be distributed more quickly and less expensively. A person can also name a bank or financial advisor as the trustee (the person who "runs" the trust), or he or she can act as trustee. Revokable trusts do not present any tax advantage that cannot be achieved in a will.

Nonrevokable Trusts

Nonrevokable trusts are, as the name says, not revokable. That means that once a person sets them up and place assets in the trust, he or she cannot get them back. The trust takes ownership of the assets. The person does not retain either the control or ownership of the assets.

Nonrevokable trusts have a distinct tax advantage over revokable trusts. Because a person does not retain any control, the assets placed into the trust are removed from the person's estate. Depending on how the trust is set up, a person may even gain a tax deduction for the contribution. These trusts get complex. A lawyer and tax planner will be needed to maximize the effect of these trusts.

Lifetime Transfers

A person can arrange for estate transfers by gift or sale during his or her lifetime.

Joint Tenants with Right of Survivorship (JTWROS)

This method of transfer says that upon death, the asset passes to the other owner(s). There is no testamentary control. Therefore, these properties are not included in the person's estate or probate. However, a person must be sure when establishing the account that it is listed as JTWROS.

Community Property

Some states have community property laws. This means that spouses have a one-half vested interest in all property owned in the marriage. There are no survivorship rights of the part not owned.

Gifts

Anyone may give up to $11,000 per year (2011) to any other person, without a tax liability. (More than this triggers a gift tax liability.) This means that a husband and wife may give (through gifts) to each of their children a total of $22,000 each year. These lifetime transfers can obviously decrease the amount of the estate. The transfers can be in cash, securities, property, or other items of value.

General Estate Planning Issues

1. There is a federal unified gift and estate tax that is of most concern. Most states have additional taxes on estates. The federal limit on estates is presently (2012) about $5 million. (That limit has been scheduled to change yearly.) There are also generation-skipping taxes, excess retirement accumulation taxes, and sometimes transfer taxes. If a person's estate is more the unified gift and tax limit, he or she will need to plan carefully to avoid taxes as much as possible. The more the estate grows above this cut-off point, the more the person needs professional estate planning help.
2. Each estate situation is unique. A person's will and estate plan will also be unique. There are computer

programs that can generate basic wills. Most dentists, especially practice owners, have complex estates and potential problems if the estate is not properly structured. A person probably needs a lawyer to draft a will and to ensure that the estate plan gives heirs maximum benefit. He or she should review the estate plan any time he or she has a significant life event such as a family birth or death, a divorce or marriage, or a practice purchase or sale. Other than that, he or she should review the estate plan every year or two to ensure that it meets current needs.

3. Insurance has been called the "poor man's estate." The policy holder should name a beneficiary for life insurance proceeds. If he or she does not name a beneficiary, the proceeds will be included in the estate for tax purposes. Whoever receives those benefits, receives them tax free. A person can split beneficiaries, naming several people, each to receive a part of the benefit.

4. Any pension, profit sharing, IRAs, or other retirement accounts should have named beneficiaries.

5. If a person owns a dental practice, he or she should make sure that survivors know that time is important. The longer the survivors wait to sell the practice, the less valuable it becomes. They should not be surprised if dentists call inquiring about the practice soon after the news of the death. Survivors should take names and return the calls as soon as possible. The planner should have a detailed plan to sell the practice (who advisors are, who will value the practice, who will run the practice until it sells, etc.) and arrange to maintain the practice until the sale is completed.

6. There is an unlimited marital deduction for estate taxes. This means that someone can give his or her spouse the estate, tax free. However, the remaining spouse may have a huge tax liability when he or she dies. A person can avoid many of these taxes with proper planning.

Section 2

Business Foundations

I have seen how the foundations of the world are laid, and I have not the least doubt that it will stand a good while.
Henry David Thoreau

A dental practice is a small business that sells dental services. As such, it is subject to the same laws, community forces, and business principles as any other business. Business owners and operators have studied, applied, and refined these principles over the years. There is a common language of business; some words carrying specific meanings that are different from common usage. Businesses act and report information to interested outsiders (such as bankers or the IRS) in commonly accepted ways. These all become the foundation or building blocks of a successful business.

A dental practice exists in a social environment of the community in which people practice. Patients come from the community. Staff members live and raise their children in the community. Dentists are a visible, active, and esteemed members of the community. So the entire fabric of the practice is drawn from the community it serves. The two become inseparable. This is not only the immediate community but also the larger state and national communities. Many external factors influence practitioners and small business operators, but some of these factors can be controlled. Others, such as the economy, are factors that can not be controlled, only responded to. So dentists must learn to be members of the community to prosper. They should not define their job as sitting in an office fixing teeth. Instead, they must see themselves as important providers of care and purchasers of goods and services in the community.

Some dentists believe that applying hard business logic to a professional practice is unprofessional or undignified. However, there is nothing sinister in establishing an efficient business framework in which a person practices the art of patient care. Certainly the two intersect in many places, but by keeping patient care as the focus of every patient interaction, the two can be equally served.

Major Goals of the Business Foundations Sector

Business foundations relate to three major goals:

1. **Make the Practice Responsive to the Community** To understand the forces in the community that affect small business and use the same forces to improve a dental practice.

2. **Make the Practice Act Like a Business** To understand basic business principles so that dentists can make a dental practice more efficient and effective.

3. **Make the Practice Act Legally** The regulatory environment demands that all businesses, especially those delivering personal or medical services, such as dentistry, act legally and keep patient care and safety as their top priority.

Objectives of the Business Foundations Section

Given these three main goals, the objectives of the foundations of business for a dental practice are given here. These are the blocks that are used to build the foundation of a strong business.

Chapter 6: Business Entities Dentists should establish a business entity that protects and enhances their business purpose.

Business Basics for Dentists, First Edition. David O. Willis.
© 2013 John Wiley & Sons, Inc. Published 2013 by John Wiley & Sons, Inc.

Chapter 7: Basic Economics   Dentists need to understand how the economy affects their practice so that they can respond appropriately. By making correct decisions that depend on the economic environment, they can maximize profit and their net worth.

Chapter 8: The Legal Environment of the Dental Practice   Dentists need to be sure that the practice operates according to the laws that regulate businesses.

Chapter 9: Financial Statements   Financial statements are part of the common language of business. Dentists need to understand these statements so that they can converse effectively with their bankers and advisors.

Chapter 10: Basics of Business Finance   Businesses borrow and use money. The entire banking system is based on the time value of money and its outgrowths. If dentists understand this building block, they can maximize their return.

Chapter 11: Business Taxes and Tax Planning   As part of the greater community, people must pay taxes. Dentists need to know which taxes to pay and how to plan legally to reduce the tax burden to increase profitability.

Chapter 12: Management Principles   When dentists structure a business, they need to address several common areas.

Chapter 13: Planning the Dental Practice   Dentists should develop an effective plan to help guide themselves to a successful practice.

Business Entities

chapter 6

*Any business arrangement that is not profitable to the
other person will in the end prove unprofitable for you.
The bargain that yields mutual satisfaction is the only
one that is apt to be repeated.*
B. C. Forbes

Objectives

At the completion of the chapter the student will be able to:
1. Understand the various forms (business entities) of dental practices
    Proprietorship
    Partnership
    Corporation
    C corporation
    S corporation
    Limited liability company

Key Terms

board of directors
business entity
C corporation
corporation
dividends
employee status
joint and severable liability

limited liability
company (LLC)
ownership interest
partnership
partnership agreement
pass-through entity
piercing the corporate veil

professional service
corporation (PSC)
S corporation
shareholders
sole proprietorship
stock

Goal

Make students aware of the various business arrangements that are available to dentists.
The student should be able to define his or her desires regarding participation in such an
arrangement.

Business Basics for Dentists, First Edition. David O. Willis.
© 2013 John Wiley & Sons, Inc. Published 2013 by John Wiley & Sons, Inc.

Business entities in dentistry can take any of several forms. There is no "right" business arrangement for dentists. Many physical, financial, managerial, and legal considerations will influence their decision. Because a dentist's circumstance is unique, his or her resolution of these issues will be similarly unique. Understanding the differences between these arrangements will help match a dentist's needs with the particular type of entity. A business arrangement should maximize factors that are important in a person's particular situation. A dentist will work with an accountant, lawyer, and management consultant to decide which business entity is best for his or her circumstance.

The business entity that is chosen has almost no bearing on the day-to-day operations of the practice. A dentist still sees patients, hires staff, collects payments, and pays expenses regardless the form of business.

Entity Decision Points

Dentists should consider four main factors when deciding which business entity to use for a practice (Box 6.1).

1. The tax liability can be different between the various types of entities. Because each circumstance is unique, some practitioners can take advantage of taxes differences that others can not.
2. Business entities also differ in liability protection. Some entities provide general liability protection (though not professional protection) that others do not. Along with adequate insurance protection and a personal level of risk tolerance, the choice of the business entity contributes to the office risk management plan. As with taxes, each circumstance is different, so no one business entity is best for all dentists.
3. Some types of entities limit the number of owners. Some require that owners be US citizens.
4. Finally, some entities (particularly corporations) require additional administrative burdens in tax forms, meeting minutes, and officer elections. If dentists are not willing to put in the extra time and effort to comply with the regulations, then choose a different, less burdensome entity. The owner(s) of the practice must understand and evaluate the advantages and disadvantages of each form of business, given their particular circumstance. Lawyers, accountants, and management consultants can give valuable advice, but it is up to the owners of the practice to decide the form of business the practice should take.

Types of Entities

A general business (such as a hardware store or building contractor) can take any of the five types of entities listed in Box 6.2. Each state defines these types of businesses (or entities) in state laws and the tax codes. The federal government has tax rules regarding the entities as well. These basic forms of business each have a unique combination of advantages, disadvantages, ownership, and compensation issues.

There are special rules for health professionals and others who perform professional services for the community (e.g., architects, accountants, and lawyers). These businesses (including dental practices) must take one of the four types of entities given: sole proprietorship, general partnership, professional limited liability company, or a PSC. The actual business entity is the same as those for general businesses, but special liability and tax rules govern these professional associations. State laws generally require incorporated health care providers to use a special form of a corporation. Different states have different names for them (Professional Corporation [PC], PSC, Professional Service Association [PSA], or Professional Associations [PA]). Each state has a professional association act that governs these entities. Some states require that only practicing providers be shareholders; other states allow corporate or nonprovider ownership of PCs. Dentists should check with an attorney to be sure of the state's rules on the entity types for professional businesses.

Box 6.1 Four Business Entity Decision Factors

Liability protection
Tax implications
Owner characteristics
Administrative burdens

Box 6.2 Types of Entities

Types of General Business Entities
    Sole proprietorship
    General partnership
    Limited partnership
    Limited liability company (LLC)
    Corporation
Business Entities for Professionals
    Sole proprietorship
    General partnership
    Professional corporation (PC)
    Professional limited liability company (PLLC)

Sole Proprietorship

A sole proprietorship is the simplest form of business. It exists any time an individual earns money on his or her own. In this form of business, the owner is the business. Profits and losses are therefore personal. The person who has day-to-day responsibility for running the business usually owns the business. There are advantages and disadvantages to a sole proprietorship (Box 6.3).

Advantages

Proprietorships are easy and inexpensive to establish. If a person operates a business and does not declare another type of entity, he or she is by default a proprietorship. There are no administrative requirements other than filing a doing business as (DBA) form if the practice has a name. There are no special accounting rules to follow except general IRS rules and rules of good accounting practice.

Disadvantages

Because a person is the business in a proprietorship, he or she cannot be isolated from legal or financial responsibility and liability of the business. A person must sign personally for loans, pledging personal collateral. He or she can use personal assets to satisfy any debts or judgments against the business. This liability is both personal and unlimited. Because the person is an owner, he or she is not considered an employee. This limits, to a degree, the tax-advantaged employee benefits that the owner can provide for himself or herself.

Ownership

As the name implies, sole proprietors are the only (sole) owner (proprietor) of the business. If there are two or

more owners, then by definition the business is not a proprietorship, but it is instead a partnership (or other form of business).

Compensation

A proprietorship builds up assets (including cash) in the business. Because a proprietor is the owner rather than an employee, he or she does not pay himself or herself a salary or a wage. Instead, he or she takes a draw (withdraw) from the assets of the business or practice. In the short run, he or she can borrow money and then withdraw it from the practice to live on. Over time, he or she can only take compensation from the practice's profits. If a person does not make a profit, then he or she cannot take a draw.

Taxation

A proprietorship is not a separate tax entity. The owner reports all profits or losses on his or her personal Schedule C. He or she must estimate their income tax liability and prepay it quarterly. He or she must also pay self-employment taxes (SETA)—the equivalent of Social Security (FICA) and Medicare taxes—for the self-employed. From a tax perspective, it does not matter how much a person takes out of the business as a draw. The issue is how much money (profit) the business made. This defines the income tax due. If a person does not take a draw, then the asset (cash) remains in the practice but has already been taxed.

Dental Practice Implications

Proprietorships are the most common form of individual dental practices because they are so easy and inexpensive to set up. Dentists typically protect themselves from liability through adequate insurance. There used to be advantages, such as retirement plan funding, for other forms of business, but tax codes have ended most of those advantages.

General Partnership

A partnership is a business entity in which two or more people have a common interest and share ownership, profits, and losses from a business. Although the partnership is a separate legal entity from its owners, it is conceptually similar to a multiowner proprietorship. If two people join to own and operate a business, they are a partnership, unless they explicitly state that

> **Box 6.3** Advantages and Disadvantages to Sole Proprietorship
>
> Advantages
>   Easy and inexpensive to form
>   Complete control of the business
>   Income taxed once to owner
>   No separate tax returns required
>   Loses flow through to owner
>   Easy to form or dissolve business
> Disadvantages
>   Unlimited liability for owner
>   Fringe benefit deduction lost for owner

> **Box 6.4** Advantages and Disadvantages of a Partnership
>
> Advantages
>   Combined resources of partners (financial, managerial, or personal)
>   Easy and inexpensive to form
>   Income taxed once to owners
>   Losses flow through to owners
> Disadvantages
>   Unlimited liability for owners (joint and severable)
>   Profits must be shared with others
>   Tax return (informational) must be filed
>   Fewer fringe benefits for owners

they are establishing another form of business. This arrangement combines the abilities, energies, and financial risk of each participant. Partnerships have no limits as to the number of partners. (However, there must be at least two.) From a practical standpoint, large groups often take a corporate structure for reasons that are discussed in this section. There are advantages and disadvantages to a partnership (Box 6.4).

Advantages

A partnership is perhaps the most versatile method of group dental practice organization. It allows varying degrees of ownership, income distribution, and cost allocation. Compensation, for example, may be based on fixed dollar amounts or percentages of production or collections. Partnerships can make allowance for including new partners or for partners who leave the partnership. There are few paperwork and technical requirements in setting up and operating the partnership. Start-up costs and technicalities are low because each member has a personal investment in the partnership, their combined credit worthiness may make securing loans easier.

Disadvantages

Several significant disadvantages to the partnership form of a group practice exist. First, partners share "joint and severable liability" for partnership debts. That means that a person is personally liable for debts of the partnership or the acts of other partners. For example, if one of the partners, acting for the partnership, buys a piece of property, other partners are responsible for the debt as if they had purchased it themselves. If a partner is guilty of malpractice, the court may require other partners to help pay any judgments not covered

by insurance. Another disadvantage may occur when one partner wants to leave the partnership. Lacking a properly constructed partnership agreement, ownership in the partnership may be more difficult to transfer if one partner decides to leave. Finally, management of the partnership may be more complicated because each partner has a voice in the decision making. A well-written partnership agreement that lists responsibilities, provisions, and requirements of the members of the group helps to overcome these problems. Another disadvantage concerns employee benefits. Like a proprietorship, a partner is an owner, not an employee. Therefore, partners are limited in what they can provide to themselves as tax-advantaged employee benefits.

Ownership

Partnerships involve more than one owner. These do not need to be equal owners. One person can provide more of the start-up capital and have more say in the operation of the business. Also classes of partners, each with different rights and responsibilities, can be set up. Because partnerships can take so many forms and can exist on a handshake, dentists should always have a written partnership agreement when entering a partnership. A written partnership agreement clarifies each partner's role and identifies the rights and responsibilities of each partner. The written agreement compels the partners to define their relationship in advance. With this exchange of ideas, partnerships can have a greater chance of success. Most states have enacted some form of the Uniform Partnership Act that generally defines the rules of a partnership for that jurisdiction. For these reasons, consult an attorney familiar with the law in this area before an arrangement is completed.

Compensation

Partners are compensated like proprietors. They take a draw on the assets of the partnership. Partners do not necessarily need to divide income from the business evenly, but whatever the method of income distribution, the partnership agreement should state it clearly. For example, dentist partners may decide to divide income according to production levels for the month or may allocate specific payments to specific dentists.

Taxation

The partnership is similar to the proprietorship from a tax perspective. The IRS does not tax the partnership itself, but the partnership must still determine its profit or loss and file an information tax return. Like a proprietorship, a person must estimate individual income taxes and prepay them quarterly, and pay SETA. Once the partnership determines the profit or loss, they pass it through to the individual partners for taxation purposes based on their profit-and-loss ratio. For example, if a person has a 50/50 partnership with an income of $10,000, a partner would receive and pay tax on $5,000 in compensation. If losses occur, these apply to the individual partners' tax returns as well. The partner might offset income from other sources with the loss from the partnership. The partnership files an information return with the IRS, and each partner that tells the IRS how much income each partner has for the year. The IRS then runs a computer match to be sure that each partner has reported income properly.

Dental Practice Implications

True partnerships are not common in dentistry. Most practitioners prefer the independence of an individual practice or the protection of a corporation or limited liability company (LLC).

Corporations

A corporation is third common business form a dental practice may take. Incorporated dental practices operate similarly to other business corporations. Owners form corporations under applicable state law. They issue stock or shares in the ownership of the corporation. They may issue one, or millions, of shares. The number of shares that a person owns is proportional to his or her ownership interest. People who buy stock buy a share in the assets of the company. If the value of the company increases or decreases, the value of each share of stock also changes. If the corporation makes a profit, the board of directors may elect to pay out some (or all) of the profits to the owners of the stock as dividends. Changing ownership of a corporation is easy; a person simply sells shares of stock. There are places where a person can buy or sell shares of publicly traded stock called stock exchanges (e.g., NYSE, NASDAQ). No one publicly trades shares of individual dental practices, so the sale takes place between two private citizens. (In the real world, dental practice transfers get more complex.) Some of the larger networks of dental practices do trade on the public stock exchanges.

A corporation functions as a separate legal entity. It has an unlimited life, unless the shareholders dissolve it. It pays tax on its profits. A corporation owns the practice assets and hires the staff and dentists. The individual dentists may be owners of the corporation, employees of

Box 6.5 Advantages and Disadvantages of
    Corporation

Advantages
    Limited shareholder liability
    Separate entity for tax purposes
Disadvantages
    Time and cost of set up
    More paperwork and legal formalities
    Federal and state securities law compliance
    Possible double taxation

the corporation, or both. Those who are employees receive a salary or other compensation that they pay tax on individually. If the dentists are also owners (stockholders) in the corporation, they also pay tax on any profit (earnings) that the corporation distributes to its shareholders. There are advantages and disadvantages to corporations (Box 6.5).

Advantages

Corporations provide the major benefit of liability protection for the owner(s). Liability is of two types, either professional liability (malpractice) or general business (slip and fall) liability. If someone sues a person as a health care provider for professional negligence (malpractice), then he or she will be sued as both as the owner of the business and personally, as the provider of care. Because the corporation is a separate entity, the owners are not *personally* responsible for acts of negligence by other shareholders or employees. Owners can only lose the money they have invested in the corporation. Therefore, they protect their personal assets in case of a shareholder's professional negligence but not from acts of their own negligence. If a corporate shareholder is guilty of an act of professional negligence, someone may sue them both as an individual practitioner (personally) and as an owner the corporation. The plaintiff may sue another shareholder as well but only as an owner of the corporation. They can only recover what the shareholder has invested in the corporation, not his or her personal assets.

Corporate practices have a decreased tax audit frequency. Accountants complete most corporate returns; individual dentists complete many Schedule C forms. Some auditors may assume that a Schedule C (proprietorship) return may hide many personal expenses not found in a corporate return. Although these may or may not be true, the result is a lower audit rate for corporations (based on IRS audit statistics).

Disadvantages

Corporations are more costly to initiate and require significant amounts of paperwork to maintain. A person in a corporation must be sure to act like a corporation (hold annual meetings, formally elect officers, have minutes, etc.). Otherwise, during a legal action, the courts may rule that if a group has not acted like a corporation, they should not be treated like a corporation and will remove the corporate protection. Once formed, corporations are difficult to dissolve. Because it is a separate business entity, a person may pay tax on income twice, once as earnings of the corporation and again when as distributions to the shareholders or employees as dividends or bonuses. As an employer, the corporation must also pay FICA, federal unemployment taxes, and state unemployment taxes on an employee. However, these are similar to self-employment taxes. Transfer of the shares in case of a dental practice corporate sale can cause tax problems because the stock is neither depreciable nor deductible to the buyer and is a gain (over basis) to the seller.

Ownership

In corporations, the shareholders are the owners of the corporation. They own the individual shares (or ownership rights) of the corporation. The shareholders elect a board of directors that makes the major management decisions for the corporation. These people serve at the pleasure of the stockholders, and the stockholders can remove them under the articles of incorporation and bylaws. The board then elects officers (such as a president) to manage the day-to-day operations of the corporation. The officers then hire employees to work for the corporation. In a practical sense, this means that dentist shareholders elect people (employees, others, or themselves if a solo practitioner corporation) to the board of directors. The board then appoints the corporate officers, including the president of the corporation. In an individual-incorporated practice, the dentist may be the sole stockholder, the chairperson of the board, president of the corporation, and dentist–employee all at the same time. Only "qualified professionals" (dentists) can be shareholders in a PC in some states. Being an owner does not necessarily mean being an equal owner. A dentist may only own 5 percent of the stock of a corporate practice and, therefore, only have a minority (5 percent) say in management decisions.

Compensation

Two forms of compensation exist in a corporation. In the first, a person earns money for the work he or she does as an employee of the corporation. This is the more common compensation method and may take the form of a salary, commission, or wage. The corporation withholds FICA, federal income, state income, and any local taxes from the wages, the same as other employees of the corporation. This person, therefore, does not have to estimate income taxes and file them quarterly as in a partnership or proprietorship.

In the second form, a person earns money for the ownership of the corporation (if he or she is an owner). Corporations pay dividends out of their earnings (profits) to the owners as a payoff for investing in the corporation (owning shares).

Taxation

A corporation is a separate tax-paying entity. Therefore, the corporation files its own tax return and pays taxes on any profits earned by the corporation. Corporations take two forms (or "flavors") from a tax perspective: the regular (or "C" corporation) and the pass-through (or "S" corporation). The IRS assumes that a corporation is a C corporation, unless the owners elect or declare themselves to be an S corporation. These other forms affect how the IRS taxes the corporation's profits but really do not affect corporate structure or day-to-day function. General (nonprofessional) corporations have a graduated tax rate, in which lower earned income is subject to lower tax rates. PCs lose the graduated tax rates that nonprofessional corporations enjoy. This causes all of the practice income to become taxed at the same rate, eliminating the income shielding that is available in "normal" corporations.

Dental Practice Implications

After proprietorships, corporations are the most common form of business that dental practices take (although LLCs are increasing quickly). Several good reasons exist for incorporating a dental practice. In group practices, especially high-risk groups, the liability shielding is worth the costs of incorporation. If a person is practicing in a group that does many high-risk procedures (such as surgeries and implants), the corporation shields his or her personal assets from the professional negligence of other providers in the corporation. Practice transfers become easy in corporate practices, especially in large groups in which owning dentists may enter or leave the practice frequently. Depending on the tax form of the corporation (C or S corporation), tax savings may result from the corporation. Special ownership rules (such as no foreign owners) apply to S Corporations.

Types of Corporations

There are two types of corporations that professional service corporation (PSCs) may take.

Regular "C" Corporations

C corporations are formed under applicable state law and are subject to Subchapter "C" of the Internal Revenue Code. There are many advantages and disadvantages to a C corporation (Box 6.6). Because this is a separate tax entity, it pays income tax on any profits. If the C corporation then chooses to pay dividends, it pays them from after-tax profits. Dividends are taxable income for the individual who receives them. So dividends are taxed twice, once at the corporate level and again at the individual level. PCs generally must pay a flat (non-graduated) rate (currently 35 percent) on all profits retained in the corporation. Individual state and federal income tax rates may add an additional 45 percent (depending on applicable dividend tax rates) to the previously taxed dividends. For these reasons, prudence dictates that PCs pay out all of their profits for the year as bonuses to the providers and owners, showing no corporate profit for the year (and therefore declare no dividends). This is not only legal, but the tax code encourages it through the flat 35-percent tax rate on PCs.

In the C corporation, the dentist files his or her wages and earnings on his or her personal Form 1040 based on the W-2 provided by the corporation. Employees of the corporation are eligible for many employee benefits offered by the corporation that pass-though owners are not. These may include cafeteria plans, dependent care allowances, or certain insurances. Depending on a person's needs, this may be an important decision factor.

Most of the disadvantages of the C corporation may be overcome with proper planning. By reducing the corporations profit to zero, a double tax on annual corporate earnings can be avoided. Paying bonuses to owner–dentists at the end of the year and retirement plan contributions usually accomplish this. Double taxation in the sale of the corporation through restrictive covenants, consulting agreements, or deferred compensation can also be managed. Finally, most dentists who are used to the need for proper documentation and formal paperwork in their dental lives can manage the paperwork requirements.

Pass-Through (Subchapter "S") Corporations

S Corporations are formed under applicable state law and are subject to Subchapter "S" of the Internal Revenue Code. That is to say, the corporation follows all of the regular corporation rules about incorporation, shareholders, and liability protection. However, the owners have elected to be treated like a partnership for tax purposes, so the S corporation becomes a hybrid tax entity. There are many advantages and disadvantages to S corporations (Box 6.7). These corporations do not pay a tax on their corporate profits. Instead, the income, expense, and credit items of the corporation pass through to the shareholders. The shareholders then report them on their personal income tax returns. This election allows business expenses, such as depreciation, tax credits, and losses to flow through to the owners, just like a partnership. The S corporation washes all income, losses, credits, and deductions through the S corporation at the end of the year. The individuals carry them directly to their personal tax returns. Because these are emptied each year, the S corporation has no retained earnings. This eliminates any possibility of double tax on corporate earnings because they tax all earnings on the doctor's individual tax return, whether actually received or not.

Like a partnership, the S corporation, files an informational return for the IRS. The individual owners receive a form from the corporation that describes the how much income they should declare

---

Box 6.6 Advantages and Disadvantages of a
      C Corporation

Advantages
  Maintain full deductibility of employee benefits
Disadvantages
  Possible double taxation of corporate profits
  Lose flow though of losses and tax credits

Box 6.7 Advantages and Disadvantages of as
      S Corporation

Advantages
  Maintain liability protection
  Early losses become personal deductions
  Profits are passed through without double taxation
  Family income shifting is possible
  Easier accounting and paperwork than C corporation
Disadvantages
  Lose tax deductible employee benefits for owner(s)
  Must follow corporate rules and regulations
  Profits are taxable based on ownership percentage

on their personal taxes. Owners (shareholders) may also receive distribution of profits of the corporation. The corporation distributes profits as corporate dividends. Unlike the C corporation, the S corporation does not pay taxes itself but passes through tax items to the owners. So the S corporation does not tax profit, and therefore, dividends at the corporate level. When the individual receives a dividend payment, this payment is considered unearned income because it was earned through investment, not through sweat and toil. Because this income is unearned, the individual does not pay Social Security or Medicare taxes on the dividend payment as they would have on earned income. The IRS rules require that the corporation compensate owner–dentists for the dentistry they do at a "reasonable" level. (Owners can not claim all income as dividends.) However, significant tax saving may be available for S corporation owners who use this strategy.

In an S corporation, a person loses many of the fringe benefit advantages of being an employee of a C corporation. Many special rules concern converting to and from a subchapter S corporation. As a rule, this election is especially valuable for start-up corporations that have many deductions and show a loss for tax purposes. This loss can offset "ordinary" income of the shareholders, up to the amount they have invested in the corporation ("basis"). (The accounting for this is complex, so dentists should check with an accountant.) Tax credits flow through to the owners' personal returns as well. The IRS taxes all of the income of S corporations, whether from earnings or the sale of assets, directly to the shareholders in proportion to their interest, even if the income is not actually distributed. This can lead to "phantom income" that shareholders must pay income tax on.

If a person is planning to sell a corporate practice, the S corporation election has an advantage over the C corporation status. The IRS will tax the capital gain from the sale of a corporation's assets at the corporate level and again at the individual level, leading to another form of double taxation. With the sale of an S corporation, the IRS taxes the gains once (to the former owner's personal income), eliminating the double taxation of the capital gain from the sale.

Piercing the Corporate Veil

Piercing the corporate veil is a legal doctrine that allows the courts, when justified, to ignore the corporate structure. The courts then hold the shareholders of the corporation personally responsible for the actions carried out in the name of the corporation. States differ somewhat in their interpretation of this doctrine.

Generally, piercing the corporate veil is justified when someone does one or more of the following:

1. Professionally injures someone.
2. Personally and directly injures someone.
3. Undercapitalizes the corporation.
4. Fails to deposit taxes withheld from employees' wages.
5. Fails to observe the formalities of corporate existence, such as annual meetings and minutes.
6. Siphons funds to the dominant shareholder(s).
7. The majority shareholder(s) guarantee corporate liabilities in their individual capacity.
8. Intentionally does something fraudulent, illegal, or reckless that causes harm to the company or to someone else.

To protect a PSC from being "pierced," dentists should practice good preventive business practices. They should maintain adequate insurance and corporate assets and follow all corporate formalities. Shareholder and director meetings should be held as required, and directors and officers should be elected as called for in the charter. Dentists should keep accurate and timely minutes of all corporate meetings, noting all personnel issues, such as changing salaries or benefits in the corporate minutes. Each state views this differently, so dentists should check with a lawyer and an accountant for local preventive business practices.

Limited Liability Company

LLCs are relatively new forms of business organizations. This legal entity combines the best aspects of the corporate entity (i.e., limited liability) and the partnership entity (i.e., pass-through tax flow). In addition, the LLC has greater flexibility than the S corporation in adapting to various forms of ownership. In the past, the most common use of an LLC was to replace limited partnerships, notably, to hold and operate real estate investments. The LLC is becoming more common in the dental practice world. Like the corporate form, professional practices are generally professional limited liability companies (PLLCs), subject to those state laws.

Advantages

LLCs are flexible. There may be one or many (even unlimited) owners, known as members. It is a separate legal entity from its members. LLCs are easy to establish. Like a corporate entity, the LLC has an unlimited life unless dissolved, and LLC members have limited personal liability. There are few administrative requirements. Members set the level of these requirements through the

LLC's operating agreement. They can run the business themselves or elect or appoint one (or more) of the members to operate the business. The members may elect the tax status of the LLC.

Disadvantages

There are few disadvantages to the LLC form of business. The members are generally subject to SETA tax (depending on the entity's tax choice), similar to a proprietorship. Most states have a nominal annual fee for LLCs.

Ownership

The owners of the LLC are the "members." There may be one or many members. They may each own equal or different shares in the LLC. The operating agreement, which is similar to a partnership agreement or corporate bylaws, defines how the LLC operates. LLCs may be managed by the members or a manager.

Compensation

Members are compensated according to the LLC's operating agreement. This leads to great flexibility in methods of compensation.

Taxation

Taxation for LLCs is flexible. The members may elect how they want the LLC to be taxed.

Single-member LLCs by default are treated as a sole proprietor for income tax purposes. In this form, they are considered a "disregarded entity" so the individual does not have to file a separate LLC return, only a personal federal Schedule C. The member may elect to be treated as a corporation (either C or S corporation) and file appropriate tax forms and information.

Multimember LLCs by default are treated as a general partnership for income tax purposes. They must file informational returns similar to a partnership. The members may elect for the LLC to be taxed as a corporation (either C or S corporation) and file appropriate tax forms and information.

Generally, then, profits and losses pass through to the individual members for income tax determination. In this form, LLCs are pass-through entities and have only one level of income taxation (unless they have elected to be taxed like a C corporation).

Dental Practice Implications

PLLCs are the newest form of business entity for professional practices. They are rapidly becoming the most popular. They have the limited liability of the corporate form, the ease of set up of a proprietorship, open ownership rules, few administrative requirements, the pass-through tax characteristics of an S Corporation, and flexibility to change the structure.

When to use the Various Entities

There are some common instances when dentists use the various business entities for their practice formation (Table 6.1).

Proprietorship

Proprietorships are the simplest form of business, so they are often used for start-up practices. Because the owner is personally liable for his or her acts of professional negligence, the form of business does not give much protection in this regard. Many established individual practitioners that do not use tax-planning strategies (such as renting space or equipment from themselves), use this simple form of business their entire professional careers.

Partnership

Partnerships are not common in dentistry because of the shared liability. They are often seen in family limited partnerships that lease space or equipment to the practice. These are frequently set up to have different ownership and management rights (limited partnership) in the family situation. Limited partnerships in real estate ventures, in which one partner (the general partner) has expertise that the contributing (limited) partners do not, are also frequently seen.

C Corporation

C corporations may be used for established practitioners that need the employee benefits that are available to employees of this form of business. They are sometimes used for group practices to shield the owners from liability, but tax advantages of the S corporation or simplicity of the LLC often are an important deciding factor.

Table 6.1 Characteristics of Different Business Entities

Characteristic	Sole Proprietor	General Partnership	C Corporation	S Corporation	Limited Liability Company
Separate tax entity?	No	Yes	Yes	Yes	Yes
Number of owners	One	Two or more	Unlimited	Limited to 75; limited foreign ownership	Unlimited
What a person owns	Assets	Portion of assets	Shares of stock	Shares of stock	Membership interest
Required documentation	None	Should have a partnership agreement (not required)	Articles of incorporation, bylaws, minutes of annual meeting, employment agreements	Articles of incorporation, bylaws, minutes of annual meeting, employment agreements	Should have operating agreement
Personal liability of owners	Unlimited	Unlimited, joint and severable	Limited, except for an individual's professional errors	Limited, except for an individual's professional errors	Limited, except for an individual's professional errors
Management	Owner is the manager	Managed by partners	Board of directors and officers of corporation	Board of directors and officers of corporation	Managers or members, by agreement
Transfer	Sale of assets (or portion) may be limited by state law (e.g., only to dentists)	Sale of assets (or portion) may be limited by partnership agreement or state law (e.g., only to dentists)	Sale of stock (ownership interest); usually limited by shareholder agreement and state law (e.g., only to dentists)	Sale of stock (ownership interest); usually limited by shareholder agreement; complies with Subchapter S requirements	Sale of assets may be limited by state law
Taxation Level	Individual, reported on Schedule C; no practice income tax	Individual reports share of income/expenses; partnership information return	Individual earnings taxed as wages/salaries; corporate income tax on corporate profits	Individual reports share of income/expenses; taxed like a partnership; corporate information return	Single owner: withhold or estimate depending on election. Multiowner: information return, depending on election
Individual Taxes	Estimate, prefile quarterly	Estimate, prefile quarterly	Corporation withholds taxes as employee	Corporation withholds taxes on earnings, estimate on distributions	Estimate, prefile quarterly

S Corporation

S corporations are common in dentistry. Start-up practices enjoy the flow through of start-up deductions and losses while keeping the liability protection of the corporate entity. High netting practices (above $250,000 per year) can distribute some profit as a dividend, reducing Medicare taxes. Group practices can use this form for liability protection. Practice sales have more favorable tax implications than C corporations. However, there are rules about S corporation ownership (such as only US citizens may be owners) that might limit the usefulness of this entity.

LLC

Rules for LLCs vary by state, so the value may change depending on specific state rules. Generally, they are easy to establish. They hold the limited general liability of the corporate form without many administrative requirements. They are a separate business entity, so dentists may set the practice, and a real estate or leasing company up as an LLC so that they can do business with the separate entity.

Basic Economics

chapter 7

*If you teach a parrot to say "Supply and Demand,"
you can get him a Ph.D. in economics.*
Thomas Carlyle

Objectives

At the completion of this chapter, the student will be able to:
1. Discuss the economics of dental care delivery, specifically supply-and-demand issues as they relate to practicing dentists.
2. Discuss the factors that influence the supply of dental services.
3. Discuss the factors that impact the demand for dental services.
4. Discuss the effect of managed care in the economics of dental practices.
5. Discuss the role of technology in the economics of dental practices.
6. Discuss the use of dental auxiliary personnel the economics of dental practices.
7. Discuss the predominate social trends that impact economics of dental practice.
8. Differentiate between public and private consumption goods.
9. Discuss gross domestic product and its effect on dental practices.
10. Discuss the business cycle and its effect on dental practices.
11. Discuss inflation and its effect on dental practices.
12. Discuss how the Federal Reserve Bank influences dental practices.
13. Discuss haw the federal budget influences dental practices.

Key Terms

business cycle
composition of GDP
consumer confidence index (CCI)
consumer price index (CPI)
contraction phase
deflation
demand for dental services
  apparent price
  availability of substitutes
  determinants of demand
  nonprice considerations
  price
discount rate
expansion phase
Federal Reserve System (Fed)
fiscal policy
Federal Open Market Committee (FOMC)

general economic prosperity
  primary industries
  secondary industries
  tertiary industries
government borrowing
government spending
gross domestic product (GDP)
gross national product (GNP)
inflation
laws of economics
  economic goods
  opportunity cost
  private consumption good
  public consumption goods
leading economic indicators
market equilibrium
  market
  market price
  market shortage

market surplus
monetary policy
open market operations
recovery phase
reserve requirement
supply and demand
  demand
  elasticity
  demand curve
  law of demand
  market demand
supply
  barriers to entry
  elastic supply
  law of supply
  market supply
  supply curve
supply siders
tax law changes

Business Basics for Dentists, First Edition. David O. Willis.
© 2013 John Wiley & Sons, Inc. Published 2013 by John Wiley & Sons, Inc.

Economics deals with human wants, needs, behaviors, and responses. As such, economists can never "prove" anything. That is, there are always confounding factors in real-life economics that makes all economic ideas "theories" that must applied in individual circumstances.

Dental services respond to the laws of economics like any other good or service. Understanding the basic notions of supply-and-demand economics accurately to respond to changing economic conditions is, therefore, important for practitioners. The study of economics is usually broken into two general areas: *macro*economics and *micro*economics. The difference in the two is a difference in scope. Macroeconomics looks at the whole economy and forces that affect it. If forces that affect the entire dental industry, such as national economic policies, changing demographic patterns, bank interest rates, inflation, and labor supply issues, are examined, this is a macro view of economic conditions. Microeconomics looks at the individual business, person, or practice and how he or she responds to changing conditions. It examines how prices are determined, and how much goods and services each individual produces and consumes. Each has major implications for how a person practices dentistry.

Microeconomics: The Individual Buyer and Seller

Microeconomics examines the individual firm (or practice) and individual consumers that purchase goods and services from those firms. It attempts to answer questions of why people buy, at what price they will buy, and what producers are willing and able to do to influence their buying decisions. Several microeconomic theories and their effects on dental practices are described.

Public and Private Goods

Any time economists speak of economic "goods" they refer to anything that is both desirable and limited and for which people will give up something else to obtain. A good may be physical items for sale (e.g., cars, televisions, or shampoo) or services that consumers buy and use immediately (e.g., hair cuts, dance lessons, or massages). In this sense, dentistry sells goods consisting of both the physical products such as dentures, partials, and restorations, and the less tangible service "good" such as prophylaxes, endodontics, whitening procedures, or extractions. Some people even view intangible items such as leisure time and health as goods because people are willing to sacrifice to "buy" these commodities.

Economists often speak of public or private consumption goods. A private consumption good is purchased and consumed by an individual in the society, rather than the whole society. (A whole group may individually purchase and consume the good, but it is not done as an act of the whole, rather as acts of individuals.) When individuals purchase DVD players, vacations, automobiles, and food, they are consuming those goods privately. If a person cannot pay the price required, he or she is excluded from having the use and benefit of the good. Public consumption goods benefit the whole of society, or at least many people. National defense, the road system, and police and fire protection are examples of public goods enjoyed equally by most people in society. Society cannot legitimately exclude those who cannot pay from enjoying the use and benefit of these goods.

Because private suppliers cannot exclude nonpayers from enjoying public consumption goods, they generally will not provide these goods on a for-profit basis. Instead, government is expected to provide public consumption goods. (Government may contract with private suppliers to provide the good or service, but the government is still ultimately responsible.) There is a significant ongoing debate in this country over what a public good is and what level of those services should be provided. Different people believe that health, and therefore medical and dental care, "fit" as either private or public goods. Depending on the answer, a different set of financing, access, delivery, and pricing policies will result.

Presently, US society considers dentistry a private consumption good. People will purchase as much of the service as they want and can afford. Although the government provides some dental services, people do not have unlimited and equal access to the service. Because dentistry is a private consumption good, it follows the economic laws of supply and demand.

Economic Choices

Economists believe that all economic resources are limited. That is to say that everything people use to produce or purchase economic goods and services that they desire are limited or scarce. Because these resources are limited, people are forced to make choices between alternatives that provide satisfaction. The choice not taken is lost, and therefore sacrificed. This sacrifice is called an "opportunity cost." For example, a family may have a given income. They want to purchase both a new car and a larger home. Because of their income limitations, they cannot purchase both goods (the car and the home). Instead, they are forced to decide between the two. If they choose to buy the car, they lose the enjoyment of the new home (an opportunity cost). However, if they decide to make a down payment on a new home, they forego the satisfaction from the car.

The notion of economic choice applies to both producers and consumers. Different people weigh the values of goods and services, and therefore the opportunity cost of forgoing those goods, differently. A consumer with limited resources may need to decide between a vacation and extensive dental work. The opportunity cost associated with foregoing each option will help to decide. As a producer, a dentist needs to decide the value of economic goods such as leisure and recreational time. Although a person may have the opportunity to make additional income by working longer hours, he or she will weigh the opportunity costs associated with foregoing time for personal and family enjoyment.

Laws of Supply and Demand

The basic issue of economic is choice making. Both society as a whole and individuals within that society decide what to produce and consume. The way that people decide to use their limited resources determines both the supply of and demand for goods and services within a market economy. This free choice leads to the US capitalistic, market-driven economy. Other systems (Communism, and to a degree, Socialism) plan the economy and determine how much of each good and service is provided and at what price.

Demand

To the economist, *demand* means the quantity of a good or service that individuals are willing and able to buy at each and every possible price. Demand then defines a relationship between price of a commodity and the number of units the buyer is willing to purchase. It implies that consumers both want the product and can pay for it. The resulting law of demand states that "as the price of any good decreases, the quantity of that good that consumers are willing and able to purchase will increase. As price increases, consumers will demand a smaller quantity of the good." This is an inverse relationship; as one factor gets larger, the other gets smaller. Evidence of this law in action can be seen by looking at everyday buying habits. Clothing stores lower the price

at the end of season to clear their racks of goods. Unscrupulous contractors and building suppliers increase prices after a natural disaster, when demand is high. Automobile dealers stimulate demand through rebates and other discount offers.

Demand has the important characteristic of elasticity. A demand that is very elastic means that the quantity demanded (and bought) is sensitive to price. Here, the demand curve is much flatter. For example, as the price of coffee rises, consumers buy less and less coffee, instead buying substitutes, such as tea and colas. Inelastic demand means that the quantity demanded is insensitive to the price of the good or service. For example, diabetics will buy the same amount of insulin despite the price. Their demand for the good is inelastic and the curve is steeper.

A demand curve is a graphical representation of this relationship between price and quantity demanded. A demand curve can be drawn for any good or service in the market, and the curve always slopes down and to the right. Although many actual demand curves have been determined for various products, they are more useful for understanding the concepts of economics. Figure 7.1 shows a typical, hypothetical demand curve, in this case for crowns. As the price of crowns increase, fewer people are willing and able to afford this service; the quantity demanded then decreases. Any individual buyer will reach a point at which they refuse to buy any additional units because they have fulfilled their needs or because their opportunity costs are too high. Their demand is essentially satiated. However, as the price decreases, more buyers come into the market and are willing to purchase the good, although other consumers may have dropped out of the market.

An individual consumer's demand for services will vary depending on factors such as income level, future

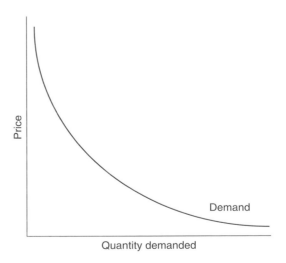

Figure 7.1 A demand curve

expectations, and personal wants and desires. Demand curves are then generally determined for the entire market. A market demand is simply equal to the sum of all the individual demands. This realizes that some consumers will never buy the product (e.g., gold crowns) at any price, others may buy many products at unlimited price, and most fall onto a continuum between the two extremes.

Supply

To this point, only one side of the economic exchange, the buyer, has been looked at. The behavior of the seller or producer (the "supplier") is equally important to the transaction.

To the economist *supply* means the quantity of a good or service that the supplier is willing and able to offer for sale at every possible price. Suppliers are usually thought of as the people who own factories, shoe stores, or dental offices. These are the suppliers in the product market for final goods and services. However, there is a similar market for resources to produce the goods. Producers must compete in the open market for wheat for bread, steel for cars, and an hour of the hygienist's time.

Supply then defines a relationship between price of a commodity and the number of units the seller is willing to supply. The resulting law of supply states that "as the price of any good increase, the quantity of that good that suppliers are willing and able to offer for sale will increase. As price increases, suppliers will supply a larger quantity of the good." This is a direct relationship; as one factor gets larger, so does the other. Supply displays the characteristic of elasticity similar to demand. Elastic supply means that a change in the price of the good leads to a large change in the quantity supplied.

A supply curve is a graphical representation of this relationship between price and quantity supplied. A supply curve can be drawn for any good or service in the market, and the curve always slopes upward and to the right. Figure 7.2 shows a typical, hypothetical supply curve, in this case also for gold crowns. As the price of gold crowns increase, dentists are willing to work harder and produce more of the products; the quantity supplied then increases. Any individual seller will reach a point at which they refuse to produce any additional units because they have fulfilled their needs or because their opportunity costs are too high. Their supply is essentially satiated.

An individual producer's supply of services will vary depending on factors such as the cost of production, degree of profitability, future expectations, and personal wants and desires. Supply curves are also determined for the entire market. A market supply is simply equal to the sum of all the individual supplies. The market

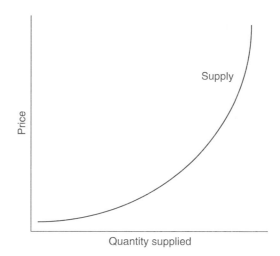

Figure 7.2 A supply curve

supply is determined largely by the obtainable profits. If supplying the good or service is lucrative compared with other forms of income generation, then more people will attempt to become suppliers. The size of the market, social climate, and barriers to entry limit the numbers of successful suppliers. Dentistry, for example, has steep barriers to entry in that there are academic dental school entrance requirements, limited number of dental school places, licensure requirements, and high start-up costs. These barriers keep the supply curve for dentistry stable.

There is little support for the idea that more providers of health services lowers the cost to the public. In fact, the opposite may be the case. It is well established that the number of surgeons in an area determines how much surgery is done in that area. Dentistry may follow a similar pattern. Rather than competition stimulating price reductions, it may increase prices in an area. One explanation for this apparent paradox is that practitioners may need to generate a certain amount of money to meet expenses and have a targeted income for themselves. According to this "target income hypothesis," fees in an area will increase until practitioners meet those needs.

Market Equilibrium in Demand and Supply

A "market" occurs when suppliers and demanders (consumers) exchange value (money). In a dynamic market, changes are expected to take place in both supply of and demand for services as the underlying conditions change. When the forces of supply interact with the forces of demand, a market price is established, which is an equilibrium point where the supply of goods and the demand for those same goods is equal. Graphically, this occurs where the upward-sloping supply curve and the downward-sloping demand curve intersect (Fig. 7.3).

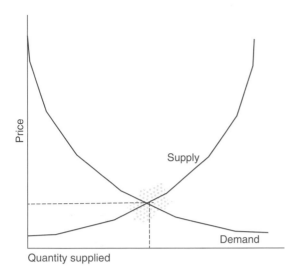

Figure 7.3 Market equilibrium

A market is never in exact equilibrium. Instead, there is fluctuation as producers and consumers adjust to changing conditions. A market shortage is a condition in which the demand for a good or service is greater than the supply of that good or service. The price then rises as consumers bid up the price. More dollars then chase fewer goods until suppliers produce either more goods or service or more suppliers enter the market (increasing production) to take advantage of excess profits. A market surplus is a condition in which the supply of a good or service is greater than the demand for that good or service. Prices drop as suppliers accept less to sell products. Profits for producers decrease as the price falls. Eventually, inefficient producers are forced from the market as profit margins decrease.

If a good is freely traded, shortages and surpluses do not last. The forces of market competition cause a readjustment of prices and it establishes a new equilibrium. Those who are willing to pay more will get what they want, pushing up prices and eliminating the shortage. Those who are willing to sell for less will gather sales, driving down prices and eliminating surpluses.

Resource markets behave similarly to final goods and services. Businesses become the demanders and households (and the people who make them up) are the suppliers. Dentists compete not only with each other for the services of staff but also with alternative forms of employment. If dentists, as a group, do not pay a wage comparable to similar forms of employment, given similar background, training requirements, and working conditions, then a shortage will occur. This drives the price of staff members up. If an individual dentist wants to hire a hygienist at less than the market rate for hygienists, he or she probably cannot hire one, unless other nonwage factors (e.g., benefits, time off, convenience) balance the hygienist's opportunity cost of a lower wage.

The Economics of Dental Services

Given that dentistry is a private consumption good, it would be expected to react to the forces of supply and demand in the marketplace as any other consumer good. And in fact, that is what happens. These macro forces occur through an aggregation of individual micro choices. So when thinking about the overall demand for services, more (but not all) of dental patients respond as the macro theory predicts.

Demand for Dental Services

Demand for dental services follows the classic downward-sloping demand curve. However, many social factors affect the shape of the demand curve. These are called the determinants of demand.

Price

Price is, by definition, one primary determinant of demand. Equally important to the true price is the apparent price for the consumer. Third-party plans, in effect, reduce the apparent price to the consumer by 50, 80, or even 100 percent. If a patient's insurance pays 50 percent, the procedure which in reality costs $300 apparently only costs $150. Consumers will obviously buy many more services at this lower price. A person's higher income makes the opportunity costs lower because they will not have to forego as many purchases in trade-off for dental services. The person with the higher income then buys more dental services because his or her out-of-pocket expense appears smaller. Physicians' services, on the other hand, are not nearly as sensitive to family income. In fact, lower-income families use physician services more than their wealthy cohorts.

Nonprice Considerations

Many nonprice considerations affect demand for dental services. An individual's tastes, wants, needs, and desires play a role in the individual's demand. Society as a whole generates tastes and wants as trends, fads, and fashions. To the extent that these trends affect the core of the business of dentistry, or alternative forms of discretionary spending, they will affect demand for dental services. If, for example, society values preventive health behaviors or aesthetics more highly over time, then logically the demand for related dental services would be expected to increase. The large demand for tooth whitening and other cosmetic services points to this increase. Consumers also place a value to attributes of the product or service other than the face attributes. These extended features, such as guarantees, convenience, or availability can increase the demand as well. If a practitioner stays open extended hours, this convenience may generate additional demand for their particular services.

Availability of Substitutes

If lower priced substitutes exist, consumers will migrate to those substitutes as the price of the good increases. Tea is a good substitute for coffee. As the price of coffee increases, more consumers drink tea. When the price of coffee declines, those tea drinkers migrate back to their original drink coffee. Diabetics have a more difficult time finding substitutes for insulin. Their dependence makes the demand for insulin almost perfectly inelastic. If the price of insulin increases, they will pay for it because there are no reasonable substitutes. There are no legal substitutes for dentistry. The only people who can legally "sell" dental services are dentists. However, to the extent that dentists compete with each other, other dentists act as substitutes. Dentists who can differentiate themselves from other dentists in the area have few substitutes. Their patients are more reluctant to leave to find substitutes if prices rise. This loyalty may be generated by specialty work or by the interpersonal skill and behaviors of the dentist and their staff members.

General Economic Prosperity

Primary industries are those that bring money into a region. This is generally in wages paid for workers or for natural resources used. Examples include manufacturing plants, mining and forestry, agriculture, and tourism. Secondary industries, such as computer support and subassembly plants, support the primary industries and the people who work in those industries. Tertiary industries provide services for the workers in the higher-level industries. Grocery stores and dental offices are examples. General economic prosperity affects personal incomes. Personal income in turn affects the individual's demand for discretionary services, such as dentistry. If the economy is robust, workers have more money as producers compete for workers, bidding up the price. The workers in turn spend their wages at the automobile dealership and shoe store. The automobile dealer and shoe salesperson have higher incomes and buy more discretionary services, such as dentistry. A dollar, then, flows many times through the economy as workers purchase goods and services from neighbor businesses.

Demographics of the Demand for Dental Care

Several factors point toward long-term growth in demand for dental services. The increasing educational level of the population and increasing disposable income, caused in part by the increase in two-wage earner

families, leads to higher demand. Increases in dental third-party coverage leads to a lower apparent cost for the service and a higher demand. The public has an increased awareness of dental health caused in part by professional efforts and in part by advertising messages for dental care products such as toothpastes. Overall health consciousness of population is increasing as evidenced by fitness centers, dietary changes, and a decrease in alcohol consumption. There is an increase in the senior segment of the population who has higher disposable incomes and more teeth at risk for a longer time. Prime users are young adults with above-average incomes, living in suburban metropolitan areas. Usage patterns have begun to merge over various demographic groups (e.g., age, sex, income, and census tracts).

Supply of Dental Services

Supply of dental services follows the classic upward-sloping supply curve. However, like the demand side, many social factors affect the way the supply curve acts. These are called the determinants of supply.

Number of Producers Is Limited

The dental profession holds a monopoly in the dental care market, including steep barriers to entry (e.g., educational requirements, licensure). The cost of starting dental schools and the pressure from the profession work to hold the number of new practitioners stable in the future. New dental schools and increasing enrollment of existing schools work to increase the number of practitioners. Given an aging population of practitioners, no one is sure what to expect regarding the supply of dental services in the future.

Productivity of Producers

The productivity of individual producers varies tremendously depending on the dentist's age, educational currency, business interests and skills, personal tastes and desires, use of auxiliary personnel, and use of new technology. There is presently a small excess capacity in the system. This is more pronounced in some areas. Overall, many experts expect the excess capacity to decrease over the next several years as more practitioners retire or decrease practice size.

Technological Improvements

Changing technologies are increasing how much dentistry can be produced. They are also increasing the number and types of services provided. Changing the types of services provided increased demand for those services. Changing technology affects the materials that dentists use, making more materials available and also materials that are easier and faster to use, leading to more services being provided. Technological improvements also allow the office to process the paperwork associated with treatment more quickly and efficiently. Computerized, electronic claim processing, for example, frees receptionist time.

Regulations

Regulatory bodies can significantly affect the supply of dental services. Licensing of independent paraprofessionals (such as denturists and hygienists), state regulations regarding delegation of intraoral duties, laws regarding foreign-trained dentists, and laws regarding corporate ownership of practices all affect the aggregate supply of dental services. Significant regulatory pressures exist to maintain existing supply patterns of dentists. Although government will not pay to increase the number of dental schools, entrepreneurs see a market in developing private dental schools. However, there may be pressure from practitioners and the public to change the laws regarding delegation of duties, allowing dentists to more easily leverage their time, energies, and knowledge.

Demographics of Supply for Dental Services

Most dental practitioners in the United States are individual general dentists. The supply of new practitioners is stable and under the general influence of dental practitioners through various accrediting and licensing bodies. The population of dentists is aging, with a large group in the 45- to 60-year-old cadre. As dentists age, their productivity decreases significantly. They often continue to practice on a part-time or reduced basis as they enter retirement.

Economic Characteristics of the Dental Care Market

Given the previous discussion, the following can be said in regard to the dental care marketplace in the United States.

- The purchase of dental care follows traditional supply and demand economics. Dentistry is a private consumption good.
- Not all consumers purchase dental services for the same reasons, at the same prices, or with the same convictions.
- The supply of practitioners does not change abruptly but instead ebbs and flows as conditions change. Significant barriers to entry exist for dentistry. No one expects this to change significantly in the near future.

The supply of dental practitioners is relatively steady. Demand fluctuates more quickly.

- Demand for dental service is tied closely to disposable income. As such, it varies with general economic conditions, third-party coverage, and alternate forms of spending. Presently, demographic factors point to an increasing demand for dental services across all population groups.
- Increasing demand for services with relatively tight constraints on the supply of services leads to higher prices for services and resulting higher income for providers. Recent trends show dental incomes to be steadily rising, both on a current dollars and on an inflation-adjusted basis.

Macroeconomics: The Big Picture

Macroeconomic looks at the economy in total. It is not concerned with how the individual consumer, firm, or business acts, except as it contributes to the whole. There may be individual differences (any single company may be growing during an economic slowdown). Regional, local, sector, or specific products may not follow the overall, national trend. Economic effects ripple through the economy. If a business slows production, their suppliers and the suppliers' suppliers (and all of their employees) feel the slowdown as well. So all parts of an economy are interconnected and interdependent. Dentists depend on a strong economy to give consumers spendable income and employee benefits to help pay for the services dentists offer. What follows is a primer on macroeconomics and how changes in the economy affect dental practices.

Gross Domestic Product (GDP)

Definition of GDP

GDP is a measure of general economic prosperity for a country for a given period. It is the sum of the market value of all goods and services produced. When GDP is increasing, the economy is growing. People are then producing more goods and services, and more people have jobs and can afford to purchase those goods and services. Money ripples through the economy as it passes from hand to hand. General economic prosperity is increasing. Conversely, when GDP is decreasing, production of goods and services slows. Unemployment and lower paychecks increase as businesses lay off workers to keep costs in line with lower production. This general economic slowdown then spreads through the economy as fewer people have extra money to spend on goods and services.

Table 7.1 Contribution to GDP*

Domestic consumption	70%
Investment in plant and equipment	16%
Government spending	20%
Net exports	–6%
Total	100%

*Estimates of 2012 expenses

Composition of GDP

GDP is composed of four large categories (Table 7.1). Consumption by individuals is the largest single component of GDP, accounting for approximately 68 percent of the US economy. Consumption is driven, largely, by the confidence consumers have in the economy. If they believe that their jobs are secure and economic prosperity will continue, then they buy more goods and services, often borrowing money to finance their purchases. The consumer confidence index (CCI) is a measure of these consumers' attitudes. It is often used as a leading indicator of consumer purchases. Investment in inventory, plant, and equipment (and houses) is the second largest component of GDP at 18 percent. When businesses purchase equipment for their factories (or dental practices), they do not consume that equipment but expect it to contribute to productive capacity of the firm for many years. Businesses buy business assets in anticipation that they will need additional products to sell, that is when they believe that the economy will improve (or remain strong). When GDP is decreasing, businesses do not invest in new plant and equipment, exacerbating the GDP decline, until they believe the economy is ready to improve. Houses are a long-term asset that individuals purchase similarly to businesses' equipment and plant purchases. Government spending, at the federal, state, and local levels is the third component of GDP, at 18 percent, which is approximately the same as the investment category. Government spending comes from the taxes that they collect. The federal government may also borrow money, so that they can spend more than they bring in through taxes. (This is known as deficit spending.) State and local governments cannot issue money, so by law, most must operate in a balanced budget mode, spending only what they bring in. The final component of GDP is net exports. This is the difference between total exports (all goods and services sold to or in foreign countries) less all imports (foreign goods and services sold here). If the nation imports more goods and services, then net exports are negative, decreasing GDP. If the nation exports more than imports, then the difference raises GDP in this country (Box 7.1).

Gross national product (GNP) is similar to GDP but does not include net imports. Most economists believe that the inclusion of net imports makes the GDP a better indicator of the national economy than GNP, although

Box 7.1 Composition of GDP

$$GDP = C + I + G + NE$$

Where,
C, consumption by individuals of durable and non-durable goods and services
I, investment in inventory, plant, equipment, and new homes
G, government (federal, state, and local) spending
NE, net exports (exports – imports)

they commonly report both. Increasing GDP is different from inflation. Inflation is a general increase in prices of goods and services. GDP is an increase in the amount of goods and services produced. (Real GDP is adjusted to remove the effects of inflation.) So the economy can experience rising GDP without inflation, inflation without rising GDP, or even deflation (a general decrease in prices) with rising or falling GDP. However, as a rule, inflation increases as GDP rises.

Why GDP Is Important for Dental Practices

Dentistry is, largely, a discretionary service. That is to say, people (in total) have the option of purchasing dental services or not. If they have extra discretionary income, they may choose to spend it on elective (and expensive) dental services, keeping dentists busy with high-margin services. When the economy slows (decreasing GDP) then people have less money and are less willing to spend what they have on expensive, elective services. The dental marketplace then slows; the services that dentists provide are often less complex, less expensive, and therefore, lower margin items. So a dentist may end up working harder but making less profit.

The Business Cycle

The business cycle is a way of describing the typical increases and decreases in economic prosperity. It is also used to decide when to purchase certain investments and when many business decisions are appropriate. Although the idealized cycle is shown in Figure 7.4, no cycle perfectly fits the curve. Slight changes occur because of regional economic differences, different responses of government and the Federal Reserve System (Fed), and different expectations of consumers and business leaders. Given these caveats, the business cycle still provides a valuable framework for understanding economic change.

An entire cycle may take a few to many years to complete. The United States recently (1992–2000) went through a prolonged period of economic expansion, followed by a period (2001–2005) of slowing GDP growth. Predicting the future direction of the cycle is obviously vital to many rational business decisions. To help their prediction, economists use a series of indicators that usually lead the actual economy by several months to years. Some of those key leading indicators are given in Table 7.2.

Expansion Phase

During the expansion phase, GDP is increasing. Businesses buy more raw goods, parts, and supplies. Employment is high as companies hire more people to keep up with the increasing demand for goods and services. Workers' incomes increase as they demand higher wage rates. Inflation then begins to rise as wealthy workers buy more goods and services at higher and higher prices. Business capacity use nears a high point. Loan demand is strong as families buy houses and companies borrow to finance their expansion plans. The Fed then tightens the money supply, to keep inflation in check, causing interest rates to rise. The higher cost of borrowing, in concert with the decreasing profits from higher wages and supply cost, causes GDP growth to slow, forming a peak. Investors

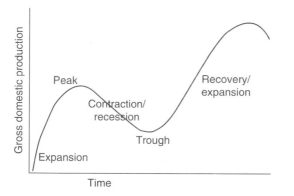

Figure 7.4 The business cycle

bail out of stocks as expected company profits decline, often buying real assets or commodities, hoping for stable values in these markets.

Contraction (Recession) Phase

As the economy enters a contraction phase, GDP growth slows or declines. Government increases its spending in an attempt to offset the slowdown in the private sector. They often must finance this spending with deficit spending (borrowing) because tax revenues are also falling as profits and incomes decline. Because of lower demand and high inventories generated during the expansion phase, businesses buy fewer parts and supplies, leading to slowdowns in those suppliers' industries. Unemployment rises as business lay off idle workers. Even those who are working are reluctant to spend much money as their confidence in the future economy wanes. Business and personal borrowing decline, along with consumer and business purchases. Inflation subsides as consumers become much more selective shoppers. The Fed expands the money supply, lowering interest rates to promote borrowing. Eventually, the economic recession ends as consumers and businesses take advantage of lower interest rates, and businesses begin to gear up for the upcoming expansion. (A recession occurs when GDP declines for two consecutive quarters. A depression is a severe and prolonged recession.) The trough formed becomes a new base for the next round of recovery (or expansion) of the economy.

Recovery Phase

During the economic recovery, consumers begin to spend for goods and services that are at depressed prices. This drives the GDP higher. Businesses spend down their previously built up inventories. Unemployment is high but steadily declining as businesses begin to hire back workers. Business profits recover sharply. Demand for

Table 7.2 Economic Indicators

Gross Domestic Product (GDP)	**Consumer Confidence Index (CCI)**
Gauge the health of the economy	Public's confidence in economy
Fed's monetary policy; government fiscal policy	Leading indicator of consumer spending
www.bea.gov	www.consumerresearchcenter.org
M2 (Money Supply)	**Current Employment Statistics (CES)**
All the money in circulation	Employment, wage, and earnings data
Fed's monetary policy	Health of labor force (economy)
www.federalreserve.gov/releases/h6	www.bls.gov/ces/home.htm
Consumer Price Index (CPI)	**Retail Trade Sales**
Changes in prices (inflation and cost of living)	Retail and food service sales
Fed's monetary policy	Consumers' personal retail consumption
www.bls.gov/cpi/home.htm	www.census.gov/cgi-bin/briefroom/briefrm
Producer Price Index (PPI)	**Standard and Poor's 500 Stock Index (S&P 500)**
Changes in prices at the wholesale level	Benchmark of a market basket of stocks
Early inflation indicator	Stock capital and economic expectations
www.bls.gov/ppi/home.htm	www.spglobal.com

credit and borrowing increase. However, the Fed holds monetary policies steady as both inflation and interest rates remain low. Investors begin to buy stocks in anticipation of future profits. As the general economic recovery continues, the economy enters a new phase of expansion, leading to higher levels of GDP.

What Effect the Business Cycle Has on Dental Practice

Dental practices are businesses and are, therefore, subject to the same economic forces as other, larger businesses. Although the economic climate can not be controlled, dentists can respond to it appropriately. Remember, there are overall trends. Some people will buy the finest dentistry even during a profound depression, and others will not, even when the economy is expanding rapidly.

During the expansion phase of the business cycle, more patients to be ready and willing to purchase more complex care can be expected. Often workers receive better benefit packages (including dental benefits), which further help them to pay for extended dental care. The mature practice can tighten credit and collection policies as demand for services remains strong. (Growing practices do not have as much discretion in their policies. They tend to be locked into the convention for the area.) Staff will expect increasing raises, as alternative employment opportunities bid up the price of labor. Inflation means that a dentist needs to manage fee increases aggressively, to keep up with rising costs and general price increases. Before the Fed tightens the money supply, a dentist should lock variable rate loans into fixed rates, in anticipation of higher interest rates to come.

As the economy peaks and enters a contraction phase, expect consumer spending to decline. Patients generally will be more reluctant to spend large amounts of money for "big ticket" items, such as reconstructive work. Instead, many will be more cautious, buying essential and less costly service such as routine prophylaxes and fillings. Often even established practitioners find that they need to extend easier credit terms to patients, extend the duration of treatment, or offer discounts as inducements to have more expensive work completed. Costs remain steady. Staff members want to keep their jobs and so are not in a strong bargaining position for wages or benefit packages. Suppliers have inventory to sell down. If a dentist has a ready supply of money as the economy nears a trough, he or she can find, and negotiate, significant major equipment bargains. Interest rates begin to fall, lowering the cost of financing a purchase and stimulating the dentist to invest in plant and equipment. Stock investors move away from growth stocks to stable consumer products, such as food,

clothing, and cleaning products that people continue to buy instead of discretionary products.

During the early part of the recovery, if a dentist plans to expand the practice physically, he or she should set them up to be ready for the coming turn around. As pent-up consumer spending begins to pick up, he or she needs to have the capacity to see the additional patients and do the additional work. This is easy financially because interest rates continue to be low, but competition for suppliers may lead to a wait to have the work completed. Once the recovery is in full swing, the practice responds again to the expansion phase of the cycle.

Inflation and Deflation

Inflation

Inflation is a general increase in the price of goods and services. Inflation occurs in a healthy economy when "too many dollars chase too few goods," thereby bidding up the prices of those goods. Modest (1 to 2 percent per year) inflation is acceptable if growth in GDP leads the inflation. Inflation raises the prices for goods and services that are purchased and produced. It also makes borrowing easier because people will pay off loans in the future with dollars that are worth less than today's. If prices rise faster than the economy expands (inflation is greater than GDP growth), economic planners will generally try to cool off inflation while maintaining growth, a tricky proposition at best.

Deflation

Deflation is a decrease in the general price of goods and services. The United States has not experienced a significant period of deflation since the Great Depression in the early 1930s. Although falling prices sound good from a consumer's perspective, several collateral problems arise when prices fall. Businesses do not make as much money because they now sell their goods at a lower price. They have produced them with an expectation of higher margins, so money is lost on each item sold. Businesses then have trouble making their debt payments, so investors dump stocks, decreasing the value of individual portfolios and the companies themselves. Layoffs then result, and the economy spirals downward. So deflation is a more significant worry for economic planners than hyperinflation. (Disinflation means inflation, but at a decreasing rate. It is different from deflation.)

Two economic indices are often used to gauge inflation. The consumer price index (CPI) is the cost of a representative "market basket" of urban consumer goods (including food, clothing, and energy costs). The federal government has tracked and reported the change in the price of this market basket monthly. (They also have special variations of the CPI, such as health care–related costs.) A second index is the producer price index (PPI). This is similar to the CPI but looks at the cost of raw materials and labor for producers. They conduct and report it similarly to the CPI. Although both are leading indicators (i.e., they predict future economic trends), the idea is that the PPI leads more than the CPI.

What Effect Inflation and Deflation Have on Dental Practices

People cannot control inflation, but can monitor and respond to it. If prices are rising rapidly, dentists should raise fees to keep pace. (If underlying GDP is not growing, dentists may not have much freedom to raise fees because patients will not purchase the same amount of dental service at the higher fees.) Otherwise, the cost of materials and labor will rise, decreasing a dentist's profitability. Lower inflation means that dentists need more modest increases to keep profitability up.

Inflation usually means that the Fed and member banks will raise interest rates. Higher rates mean that people will be paying more to the bank and taking less home as profit, squeezing a family budget. In fact, if rates rise too much, dentists may be priced out of the market for borrowing money. This is especially common with new practitioners who are not excellent credit risks (high existing student loans, low net worth, and low demonstrated income). If dentists have a fixed rate loan, they will be paying with inflated dollars (a good thing). If dentists have a variable rate loan, the interest rate (and therefore payments) will soon rise (a bad thing).

Fiscal Policy

Fiscal policy is the combined action of the federal government uses to help manage the economy. A combination of the Congress and the president initiates fiscal policy. Political rhetoric to the contrary, it takes both sides to have any effect. Congress passes legislation (such as tax cuts) and the president signs them into law. The president may propose tax changes (such as

decreasing the capital gains tax rate). However, if Congress does not pass the enabling legislation, the proposal cannot ever become law. Neither side can act unilaterally, so for either side to blame the other is pure nonsense but makes good political fodder.

The purpose of fiscal policy is threefold, namely to (1) maintain full employment, (2) keep prices stable, and (3) continue economic (GDP) growth. Because this deals with politicians, they will often use these actions to promote social goals as well as purely fiscal (financial) ones. For example, Congress decided that helping existing business to make their facilities more accessible to disabled individuals was important. So they passed a law signed by the president that created tax credits for small business owners who spend money remodeling their facilities to make them more accessible (part of the Americans with Disabilities Act). Here, Congress did not intend a change in tax law to stimulate the economy but to meet a socially desirable goal.

The government only has three tools at its disposal in initiating fiscal policy. They are tax law changes, government spending, and government borrowing. Congress and the president use these tools to keep the economy strong and to get reelected.

Tax Law Changes

Changes in tax law can stimulate expansion or contraction (Table 7.3). Any change that leaves more money in the hands of private businesses or the public is considered expansionary. For example, if the government increases depreciation deductions for business or adds a tax credit for children, more money will remain in the hands of individuals and businesses to be spent, thereby boosting the economy. (This also means that less tax revenue is in the hands of the government. They must either cut their spending or borrow to maintain current levels of expenditures.)

Tax changes are often viewed from the supply-and-demand perspective. A tax cut stimulates demand, moving the demand curve to the right. More people buy more goods and services at higher prices. Depending on the amount of the increased demand, this may lead to

Table 7.3 Fiscal and Monetary Policy

Issue	Fiscal Policy	Monetary Policy
Who is responsible	Congress and president	Federal Reserve Board
Authority	Congress passes legislation; president signs into law	Federal Reserve Board acts independently and implements decisions
Tools available	Change in tax laws	Change reserve requirements for banks
	Increase or decrease government spending	Change the discount rate
	Finance deficits through borrowing by issuing new government securities	Conduct open market operations

inflationary pressures. Tax cuts can also lower the cost of doing business, stimulating the supply curve to move upward (an increased quantity at lower prices). Supply siders believe that this then stimulates further demand for these lower priced goods and services. Tax increases move the supply and demand curves in the opposite direction as tax cuts.

Changes in tax law come in many forms. They may be across the board rate reductions or changes targeted at special groups or business sectors. Remember that politicians who want to reward their cronies and get reelected bring tax changes. So issues of tax fairness always enter these decisions. Should changes favor the "fat cats" and businesses (where most of the money is) or be spread across the board? Tax cuts for higher income individuals often go to savings or investment. Cuts for lower income individuals are usually spent immediately. If so, who benefits more and less and is that fair? Political rhetoric on the issue increases with proximity to elections.

Government Spending

When consumer and business spending are low, such as during a contraction or recession, government tries to stimulate the economy by spending more money. Although the government sector cannot fully make up for lack of consumer and business spending, they try to "prime the pump," hastening economic recovery. Often this spending surpasses revenues from taxes. When this occurs, they must finance the deficit through government borrowing or Federal Reserve actions. As an economic expansion occurs, government can reduce its spending, paying down its deficit. This hardly ever occurs because politicians are running this system.

Government Borrowing

When the federal government spends more than it takes in through taxes, it must finance the difference by borrowing money. It does this by issuing Treasury bonds, bills, and notes. (They differ based on the length of maturity). In these, the Treasury borrows a certain amount of money, promising to pay it back in a certain period at a given interest rate. This interest rate (so called "risk-free" rate) is low because it is backed by the full faith and confidence of the federal government. (If the federal government defaults on its loans, the financial markets would be in total chaos.) This borrowing increases the nation's total deficit, which must be paid back in the future from tax revenues. (Inflation helps to soften the cost of a pay back by the government.)

There are several side effects of government borrowing. Issuing federal debt securities causes a general increase in interest rates because lenders lend money to the federal government. Increases in interest rates lead to decreased borrowing, decreased buying, and therefore decreased economic activity. Borrowers that are riskier than the federal government must pay higher rates to offset the increased risk. This "crowding out" of businesses in the debt security market leads to a decrease in corporate borrowing and a resulting decrease in economic activity.

Monetary Policy

Monetary policy is concerned with the amount of US money that is in circulation. The Federal Reserve System (the central bank of the United States) controls the supply of money. Its customers are not consumers like the common person but are instead the country's banking system and the federal government.

The Federal Reserve System

The Fed is composed of a board of governors, the Federal Open Market Committee (FOMC), and twelve Federal Reserve district banks. The Fed is an independent branch of the government. It is not a profit-making institution and must periodically report its actions and plans to Congress. The Fed controls the monetary policy, and therefore the money supply of the United States. It is not the US Treasury, but it does issue debt securities for the government to finance budget deficits. The Federal Reserve bank issues money (Federal Reserve notes) and makes loans to commercial banks, who then lend money to US businesses and individuals.

The Federal Reserve System has four functions (Table 7.4). It conducts the nation's monetary policy, regulates the banking industry, supervises the financial system and markets, and provides financial services to the US government. The Fed uses three tools to accomplish its functions. They can set the reserve requirements for banks, set the discount rate changed to banks, and buy (or sell) US government securities on the open market.

The Fed Tools

The Fed requires member depository institutions (banks and savings and loans) to keep a certain percentage of the money deposited with them on "reserve." This means

Table 7.4 Fed's Monetary Policy Actions

Desired Effect	Federal Reserve Board Action
Expansionary (expand the money supply)	Purchase government securities Lower reserve requirement Lower discount rate
Contractionary (reduce the money supply)	Sell government securities Increase reserve requirement Raise discount rate

that they may not lend that money. The higher the required reserve, the less there is to lend out and the higher the interest rates rise in response. (Supply and demand dictates that more borrowers push up the rate on scarce loans.) The Fed requires banks to keep in reserve 8 to 14 percent of transaction (checking) accounts and 0 to 9 percent of savings (CD and savings) accounts. Changing this requirement a few percentage points (within the range) can profoundly affect how much money is available to borrow. The Fed does not change this often, so it is unimportant on a daily basis. If the Fed changes the reserve requirement, something big is going on in the economy.

The discount rate is the rate charged to member banks to borrow money for them to issue loans. By changing this discount rate, the Fed encourages (or discourages) banks from lending money, affecting the liquidity in the banking system. The discount rate is for short-term loans only. Long-term interest rates change consequently. Changing the discount rate also affects stock and bond prices because required rates of return change in response to changing interest rates.

The most powerful tool that the Fed uses to accomplish its purpose is open market operations. The FOMC meets periodically (usually monthly) to assess and change its policy. These meetings are so important that the daily and financial press report them. Open market operations consist of the sale or purchase of government securities (bonds, bills, and notes), which then expands or contracts the nation's money supply. If the Fed sells securities, it receives cash, which they remove from the banking system (therefore there is less to lend or invest), slowing the economy. When the Fed buys securities, it pays cash, which is added to the banking system (therefore there is more to lend or invest), stimulating the economy. Because the Federal Reserve prints money, it can never run out.

The Fed has a target (sustained, noninflationary) for GDP growth. Growth above this target it considers inflationary and so it steps on the "brake," slowing the economy. Below the target, the Fed presses the "accelerator," trying to stimulate the economy. In the past several years, the Fed has tried to smooth the business cycle from a boom-or-bust mode to one of slower growth and "soft landings" by using a gentler foot on both the brake and accelerator.

Table 7.5 Effect of Interest Rate on Loan Payments

Annual Interest Rate	Monthly Payment
3%	$1,321
6%	$1,461
9%	$1,609
12%	$1,765

This shows the difference in monthly payment of a $100,000 loan over 7 years, based on different interest rates. In the real world, the economy is a difficult system to manage. Politicians (who control fiscal policy) want to have prosperity (people employed) just before an election. They want aggressive, expansionary monetary policies. The Fed, on the other hand, wants to keep economic stability. They want slow, steady (even unspectacular) growth. If the growth is too rapid, they may face an economic crash as a result. Consumer confidence affects spending and, therefore, GDP. Politicians, the news media, and world events all affect consumer confidence, consumer spending, and the economy. Finally, economic policy is established based on forecasts (such as leading economic indicators). The policy is only as good as the forecasts.

What Effect the Fed Has on Dental Practice

Fed actions do not affect a dental practice directly, but their indirect effects make them an important component of the economic environment. The Fed indirectly sets the interest rate that a person pays for a loan. It profoundly affects the growth in GDP and therefore, the business cycle.

Interest rates have a dramatic and immediate effect of new dentists. When a dentist borrows money to establish a practice, buy into or buy out an existing practice, or purchase a new home, car, or other consumer good, then the prevailing interest rate will determine his or her monthly pay back and, therefore, the amount that an be borrowed. Table 7.5 gives the pay back for an example loan, given several different interest rates. The amount needed to pay back the loan increases dramatically as the interest rate rises. If a person has a certain amount of money budgeted for monthly loan payments, he or she may be limited in the amount that a banker or other lender will be willing to lend.

The Legal Environment of the Dental Practice

chapter 8

What do I care about the law? Hain't I got the power?
Cornelius Vanderbilt

Objectives

At the completion of this chapter, the student will be able to:
1. Describe the sources of laws.
2. Describe the common methods of resolving legal disputes.
3. Define criminal law and give examples of both felonies and misdemeanors.
4. Describe the principle elements of contracts.
5. Describe the common types of contracts seen in dental practices.
6. Define torts and give examples of intentional torts.
7. Differentiate between negligence and liability.
8. Describe the common labor laws and describe how they affect dental practice.
9. Describe the common consumer protection laws and describe how they affect dental practice.
10. Describe elements commonly found in state dental practice acts.

Key Terms

administrative regulation
Americans with Disabilities Act
  disability
antitrust laws
arbitration
bankruptcy
  Chapter 7
  Chapter 13
  general (unsecured) creditors
  involuntary petition
  secured creditors
  voluntary
civil law
common law
consumer protection
contracts
  offer
  acceptance

assignment
breach of contract
consideration
capacity of the parties
legality of purpose
court precedent
criminal law
  felonies
  misdemeanors
debtor protection laws
  Fair Credit Billing Act
  Fair Credit Reporting Act
  Fair Debt Collection Practices Act
  Truth-In-Lending Act
employment at will
Equal Employment Opportunity Commission (EEOC)
Employee Retirement Income Security Act (ERISA)

Fair Labor Standards Act (FLSA)
  child labor laws
  exempt employees
  minimum wage laws
  minimum wage rate
  overtime laws
Federal Trade Commission (FTC)
lawyer's inquiry
legislative mandates
legislatively enacted statutes
litigation
mediation
Occupational and Safety Health Administration (OSHA)
personal inquiry
public accommodation
reasonable accommodation
Social Security

(Continued)

Business Basics for Dentists, First Edition. David O. Willis.
© 2013 John Wiley & Sons, Inc. Published 2013 by John Wiley & Sons, Inc.

Key Terms (*Continued*)

state dental practice acts	intentional torts	strict liability
summons and complaint	liability	vicarious liability
torts	negligence	unemployment compensation Insurance
absolute or strict liability	plaintiff	Federal Unemployment Tax Act (FUTA)
attractive nuisance	principal–agent relationship	State Unemployment Tax Act (SUTA)
comparative negligence	punitive damages	unjust (or unfair) dismissal
compensatory damages	respondeat superior	workers' compensation system
contributory negligence	sole remedy	exclusive remedy rule

Goal

The goal of this chapter is to familiarize students with the common legal issues faced by dental practitioners.

This chapter gives the new dentist an overview of common legal issues that affect dental practices. It is only intended as an introduction. Any time a dentist faces legal issues, he or she should gain competent legal advice, preferably from a lawyer who is knowledgeable about the specific concern. Laws exist for many aspects of people's daily lives, from operating motor vehicles to divorce. This chapter is concerned with laws as they relate to the small business owner. Dental malpractice law specifically will be covered in another chapter.

The Source of Laws

Governments make laws to protect the citizens or to help settle disputes between them. The US Constitution is the "supreme law of the land." Along with state constitutions, it sets the framework for how governments are formed and how they exercise their powers.

The method most people think of in forming laws is a legislatively enacted statute. In this type of law, a legislative body (either local, state, or national) passes a statute or law for the jurisdiction that they cover. There are often additional hurdles to pass before the statute carries the true force of law (e.g., executive branch endorsement), but the basic form of the law originates in the legislative branch. Legislatures often pass legislative mandates, which are not laws, but carry the same force as a law. For example, they require employers, by law, to carry unemployment and workers' compensation insurance on all of their full-time employees. This mandate results in an added expense to the employer, equivalent to a tax on employees. Although the government does not run it, it has the equivalent force of law as if it were.

Laws may also be enacted by administrative regulation. Legislatures may establish agency boards and commissions to oversee and enforce particular

legislation. For example, Congress has not written specific workplace rules and regulations, but instead established the Occupational Safety and Health Administration (OSHA). Congress then charged that organization with developing and implementing rules and regulations to guide workplace safety. These regulations carry the same force and effect as legislative statute.

The final way that laws are formed is through the court system or court precedent. Legislatures cannot pass laws to cover every possible circumstance. The courts may give a judgment as to the legality of a certain action or who should prevail in a certain circumstance. Future courts then may use that initial ruling as a precedent and apply that ruling as a basis for making a new ruling. The gradual accumulation of these rulings and precedents becomes part of the common law of the land.

Resolving Disputes

Often people have a differing opinion concerning how to apply the law in a particular case. This may be the result of different views of facts or circumstances or differing notions of guilt or innocence, right or wrong. Nevertheless, the dispute must be resolved. Two common methods exist for resolving disputes: litigation and some form of alternative dispute resolution (ADR). Litigation occurs when one person (or government) takes another person to trial in a court of law. The person who initiates the proceeding (sues or takes the other to court) is the *plaintiff*; the person he or she takes to court to defend against the suit is the *defendant*. The trial may be decided by a trial judge or by a jury, depending on the type of dispute and desires of the participants. To avoid the cost and time involved in trials, many contracts may call for ADR through mediation or arbitration. Mediation and arbitration happen when both sides agree to present their case to a knowledgeable third party. In mediation, the mediator tries to resolve the problem through discussions and assisted negotiation. Mediation is a voluntary process; either side may still take the other to court if they are not satisfied with the results. In arbitration, the arbitrator makes a decision that is binding; the decision of the arbitrator is final.

Criminal Law

Criminal law is concerned with wrongs against society. These wrongs may be violent acts, deceit, concealment, or wrongful use of force. They are prosecuted by an agent of the government, such as the district attorney (DA) on behalf of the state, not the victim. Criminal law is divided into felonies and misdemeanors. This classification is based on the severity of the punishment. Felonies, the more serious crimes, are punishable by death, fine, and imprisonment for more than 1 year. Misdemeanors, the less serious crimes, are punishable by fines and jail sentences of less than 1 year. Some lawyers add the classification of petty offenses, for minor violations of traffic ordinances, building codes, or other municipal ordinances. Punishment for criminal conduct is imposed for two reasons: to punish the guilty person and to deter others from committing similar crimes. Table 8.1 gives some common examples of crimes.

Civil Law

Civil law is concerned with rights, duties, and wrongs against individuals, rather than against society. If another individual wrongs a person, he or she is entitled to a "day in court." Civil law defines the legal relationship between individuals in three general areas: contracts, torts, and property. This chapter discusses the first two, which contain the bulk of issues important for practicing dentists.

Table 8.1 Criminal Acts

Felonies	Misdemeanors
Assault	Battery
Arson	Gambling
Bribery	Petty larceny
Burglary	Littering
Embezzlement	Prostitution
Forgery	Public disturbance
Grand larceny	Simple assault
Kidnapping	Traffic violations
Manslaughter	Trespass
Murder	
Price-fixing	
Rape	
Robbery	

Contracts

A contract is a legally enforceable agreement involving the mutual promises of two or more parties. Most states require that some contracts (e.g., real estate contracts) be in writing to be enforceable. As a rule, all contracts *should* be in writing to record the true understanding among or between the parties. People hear what they want to hear and understand what they want to believe. Their perception of an agreement may be entirely different from someone else's. Oral or verbal contracts are usually enforceable. The problem is to define what either party truly said. Written contracts avoid this problem. A contract does not need to be written by a lawyer to be legally binding, but a person should be careful if he or she tries to negotiate and enter a contract without competent legal advice. He or she can be bound to a bad contract as easily as by a good one.

A contract states the rights and responsibilities of the parties. It has five principal elements. They are:

1. **Offer** The offer is a specific promise to do something in exchange for the other party doing something in return. For example, the buyer will promise to pay the seller $300,000 for the assets of the seller's dental practice if the seller promises to sell them to the buyer.
2. **Acceptance** The acceptance says that there is agreement to the terms and conditions of the offer. In the proceeding example, the seller agrees to sell the buyer the seller's practice assets according to the terms of the buyer's offer.
3. **Consideration** Consideration is the value exchanged between the parties for performance of their mutual promises. In the example, the buyer and seller exchange $300,000 as consideration (or value) for the assets.
4. **Capacity of the Parties** All parties must have the mental and legal capacity to enter a contract. Someone who is underage or who is mentally impaired cannot enter contracts without the consent of the guardian.
5. **Legality of Purpose** A contract must have a legal purpose to be enforceable. As an example, an employment contract made with an unlicensed person in a regulated profession (dentistry) would be void because a person cannot legally employ another who has no license.

Common contracts in dental practice include the following:

1. Office lease
2. Employment (associate) agreement
3. Insurance (managed care) plan participation contracts

4. Promissory note
5. Partnership agreement
6. Buy-sell agreement
7. Bill of sale
8. Contract for practice purchase

Some contracts may be assigned, which means one party has the right to transfer the promise to a third party who was not part of the original agreement. For example, a person might assign the lease for office space to another person. Most personal contracts cannot be assigned.

As stated previously, a contract is a promise by two or more parties to do something. If one party fails to fulfill the contractual obligations, a breach of the contract has occurred. The nonbreaching party can attempt to receive monetary damages to compensate for his or her loss through the contract not being fulfilled. When someone breaches a contract, there are four common alternatives for reaching a remedy: negotiation, arbitration, mediation, or litigation. Some contracts state how any disputes will be handled.

Torts

A *tort* is a civil wrong, other than a breach of a contract, committed against a person or their property for which the law gives the right to recover damages. Torts are different from crimes, which are wrongs against society (Table 8.2). Some acts, such as assault, may be both a wrong against a person (a tort) and a wrong against society (a crime). Intentional torts involve deliberate actions that cause injury. Unintentional torts are not deliberate.

Negligence is a tort that involves injury that results from the failure to use "reasonable care." Negligence is the most commonly discussed tort in dentistry. The four elements needed to prove negligence are given here. (Professional negligence is a special type of negligence, which is discussed later.) One critical element of this tort is duty. Without a duty (or obligation or relationship) to another person, one does not owe that person reasonable care. Duty arises from a person's conduct or activity.

Someone who is doing something has a duty to use reasonable care so as not to injure others. Whether a person is driving a car or practicing dentistry, he or she has a duty not to injure others through unreasonable conduct. Usually, people do not have a duty to avoid injury by nonconduct. A member of the public has no obligation to warn someone else of a possible problem, even if he or she has seen the problem. (There may be a moral call to warn the other but no legal requirement.) A sunbather, then has no legal obligation to warn swimmers of a shark in the area. However, if there is a special relationship between the parties, the situation changes. A business that rents surfboards has a special relationship with the renter and probably does have a legal responsibility to warn of sharks in the area. The business is potentially liable if it negligently rents the board without proper warning. Consequently, many professional office buildings are justifiably concerned with security and other protection measures.

Negligence is the failure to behave as a reasonable and prudent person in a similar situation would behave (Box 8.1). A person a duty not only to recognize a potential problem, but also to do something to prevent the problem (a duty to act). This is not an absolute differentiation. Instead, the individual's actions (or inactions) must be compared to a norm that changes over time and for which different people may have different values. For example, assume a person has a dental office in a northern state that has steps leading to the front door. If it snows, most people would say that a reasonable and prudent person would sweep the snow from the steps and apply a salt to melt any remaining ice to prevent people from slipping and injuring themselves. If the dentist fails to sweep the snow, he or she has probably not acted as a reasonable and prudent person would have acted in a similar situation. If a patient or anyone else who has a reason for being there slips on the ice or snow and gets injured, he or she would probably sue the dentist for damages (and win) claiming that the dentist was negligent in not sweeping the snow and ice from the steps. This example is obvious. The problem comes when juries are asked to decide cases in which it is not clear whether or not a prudent person would have recognized a danger in a similar circumstance and acted

Table 8.2 Common Torts

Assault	Placing another in apprehension for his or her physical safety
Battery	Illegal touching of another person
Libel	Written defamation of another to ridicule his or her character
Slander	Verbal defamation of another to ridicule his or her character
False arrest	Unjustified confinement of a nonconsenting person
Trespass	Entering another's property without consent or refusing to leave

Box 8.1 Elements of Negligence

1. Existence of a duty of care owed by one person to another
2. Unreasonable care that breaches the duty
3. The defendant's behavior caused the plaintiff's injury
4. There was an actual injury

to prevent the accident. Lightning strikes a golfer. Should the golf course superintendent have warned the golfers (by sirens or other devices) that there is lightning in the area and to take cover, or should the golfers have known, without warning, to take cover during a thunderstorm? A doting elderly patient trips on the door threshold while entering a dental office and sustains injuries. Was the threshold loose or in another way hazardous or a potential problem? If so, would a reasonable and prudent person have previously fixed the threshold? Did the person's impaired condition contribute to the accident? Obviously, juries need to make judgments concerning both the degree of hazard presented by a problem and what is a reasonable and prudent response to a potentially hazardous situation.

There are several instances in which negligence is further defined. Contributory negligence says that the failure to use reasonable care by the plaintiff (or injured party) in a negligence suit contributed to the injury. In the past, cases in which the plaintiff's own actions contributed to the injury "in any degree, however slight," were dismissed. The trend today, however, is to move from this strict interpretation toward one that compares how much of the fault is the plaintiff's and how much is the defendant's. Juries award damages based on the proportionality found. Comparative negligence then allocates the fault (and damages) between plaintiff and defendant.

Vicarious liability is imputed liability. The negligence of one person makes another liable. A common example is the legal doctrine of respondeat superior ("let the master reply"). This doctrine assumes that if an employee is liable for acts committed while on the job, then the employer (or business owner) is also liable. This is as a result of the principal–agent relationship, which says that the employee is advancing the interests of the employer. Once the employee is found negligent, the owner is strictly liable. Warning a staff member to be careful when driving cases to the lab does not prevent the owner from being vicariously liable when the employee runs a red light and has an accident while doing so. Or consider a case in which a hygienist drops an instrument in the eye of a patient, causing significant and permanent visual damage to the patient. The hygienist is personally liable for the patient's negligence. Similarly, the dentist is personally negligent for failure to supervise the hygienist adequately, and the employer is liable to the full extent of its assets, under the doctrine of respondeat superior. As a rule, the corporate structure does not protect a person from the professional negligence caused by that person or one of his or her employees. The limited liability purportedly given to shareholders of professional service corporations is illusory. Any liability protection is for business liability only, not professional liability.

Absolute or strict liability assesses negligence without a fault. Juries award damages, although there was nothing wrong with what the liable person was doing. This is the one case given in which negligence does not need to exist for there to be a liability. A common example, besides the one in the preceding paragraph, is in workers' compensation cases. The juries assume that the owner is liable, although the employer may not have been negligent. The worker, then, collects compensation from the business owner's workers' compensation insurance carrier. In these cases, this is the sole remedy, which is to say that the worker cannot sue the owner for any damages above those compensated by the insurance carrier, even if the owner was negligent or had an unsafe work place or work practices. This is the trade-off for requiring employers to carry state-approved workers' compensation insurance.

An attractive nuisance is an event or item that might attract and injure someone, especially a child. The owner or occupier of the property must use due care to discover children on property and then to warn or protect them from injury or death. A swimming pool in a crowded neighborhood will attract many children who live nearby. The owner should, besides using reasonable methods of protection, such as nonclimbable fences, find children and warn them against the dangers of being around an unsupervised pool. Pets, especially wild animals, can attract children, with dangerous consequences.

Liability is the legal responsibility to make good a loss or damage that has occurred because of a person's actions or inactions. It is important to note that, except strict liability cases, liability occurs only if negligence is proven. If a person is found negligent and therefore liable, the courts usually will require that person to compensate the injured party for repair of the injuries suffered. (To indemnify is to make whole or make good for a loss.) These compensatory damages include the following general categories:

1. past and future medical expenses,
2. past and future economic loss, including loss of property and loss of earning power, and
3. past and future pain and suffering.

Determining the actual amount awarded for each of these categories creates significant problems and many horror stories from those who love to bash the legal system. Often juries decide by sympathy as much as true financial loss.

Courts and juries may also require punitive damages of liable individuals. They levy these punitive damages to punish the defendant for grossly negligent or "willful and wanton" behavior. A key element of punitive damages is to decide the motive of the defendant. If the jury determines that the motives were malicious or intentionally damaging, then punishment is in order. The amount and appropriateness of punitive damages are presently being debated in the courts and congresses of this country.

Employment (Labor) Law

Congress has developed many statutes that address the relationship between owners of business and their employees. Most of these laws are intended to protect workers from unfair practices by business. They give few privileges to the owners of businesses.

Workers' Compensation Acts

The workers' compensation system was designed to provide a way to pay workers or their families if the worker is accidentally injured, killed, or contracted an occupational disease because of employment. Two simple tests determine whether an employer must pay workers' compensation:

1. **Was the injury accidental?**   Although the laws apply only to workers who are accidentally injured, proving that employers acted intentionally to injure a worker is difficult. Most states have an exclusive remedy rule, which states that these compensation laws are the only remedy of a worker against an owner for injuries on the job. They may not sue the owner separately for negligence in the workplace.
2. **Was the injury during employment?**   The courts have taken a broad interpretation of the meaning of the term "in the course of employment." Generally, if the injury were in any way related to work, it might be a workers' compensation issue. An employee may have a heart attack or chronic fatigue syndrome, claiming the cause was a stressful job. Because the states are involved heavily in the administration of the workers' compensation system, there is a wide variation nationally on qualification and awards.

The effect of the Workers' Compensation Act on dental practice is seen when an employee is injured while on the job. These injuries may be physical, such as a cut or an eye injury; they may be infectious, such as contacting hepatitis through an inadvertent needle stick; or they may be mental or emotional. (Each state administers their own workers' compensation system and so has different definitions of qualification for these injuries.) The injured worker will generally receive medical care for the injury, compensation for lost wages while recuperating, and often disability payments if the injury causes long-term disability. Because this program is an "insurance," a person pays for these benefits indirectly through insurance premiums.

Wage and Hour Laws

The Fair Labor Standards Act (FLSA) is a federal law that is administered by the states. It defines the rules regarding wages and hours in the workplace. Because each state administers the laws, there is some variation in their interpretation. However, these all have some provision for the following issues:

- Minimum wage laws define the minimum hourly rate you may pay an employee. Congress periodically changes this base rate. Although technically this only applies to businesses in "interstate commerce," nearly all firms have a customer or supplier in another state and therefore fall under these rules. If Congress increases the minimum wage rate, firms often raise the wage rates of all the employees at the lower end of the wage scale as they try to maintain pay differences among classes of jobs and employees.
- Overtime laws describe how overtime work must be treated. Overtime is considered all work more than 40 hours per week. Note that this is not based on 8 hours per day or 80 hours per 2-week pay period but on a 40-hour work week. (There are a few states that define overtime as more than 8 hours of work per day.) If an employee works more than 40 hours in a given work week, the law requires the employer to pay the employee's base pay plus a 50 percent premium (i.e., "time and a half") for all hours worked beyond the basic 40-hour work week. Compensatory time the following week to make up for the overtime worked may not be offered or required.
- Certain employees may be exempt from overtime laws. They are generally professional or managerial people. Owners do not have to pay these exempt employees overtime, which is why entry level managers at the local fast food restaurant may work 60- or 80-hour work weeks. Few dental office employees qualify as "exempt" employees. Associate dentists are professional personnel and therefore exempt. True office managers (who supervise several people and have hiring authority) probably would qualify as exempt. Dental assistant, hygienists, and receptionists are not exempt from the overtime laws in most states. If they are paid a "salary," the employer must still pay overtime more than 40 hours.
- Child labor laws define how much a child can work and the types of jobs he or she may hold. As a rule, children (younger than 18 years of age) may not work in any occupation that is physically demanding or dangerous. The hours that they may work are also limited. The number of hours allowed is often based on whether or not schools are in session.

FLSA has significant effects on the dental practice through minimum wages, overtime rules, and exempt employee status. Dentists should be sure to keep excellent time records both for accurate wage determination and to guard against claims by disgruntled present or former employees.

Unemployment Compensation

The government requires that employers carry unemployment compensation insurance on all their employees. This is a joint federal–state program and is composed of both the Federal Unemployment Tax Act (FUTA) and a State Unemployment Tax Act (SUTA). Although this is technically a tax, from a perspective as an employer, unemployment compensation behaves more like insurance. The more claims that former employees collect on an employer's "account," the higher the premium that the employer will be charged.

Unemployment compensation is designed to help people who have lost their job through no fault of their own. They must actively look for another job while they are collecting unemployment compensation and the government limits the length of time a person can collect unemployment. The laws disqualify an employee from collecting any unemployment compensation if any of the following three events happen:

1. The employee refuses other similar work.
2. The employee was discharged for proper cause.
3. The employee quit employment voluntarily.

If a former employee files for unemployment compensation listing an employer as a former employer, he or she will receive information regarding the claim. If an employers wants to dispute the claim, he or she should initially complete the paperwork without delay. A hearing may be held, where the employer, former employee, and a hearing officer sit together. The hearing officer may ask for records (such as time sheets) or other documentation from the employer. After hearing from both sides, the hearing office makes a decision. Without proper documentation, an employer does not stand a chance of winning. Even with proper documentation, hearing officers often lean toward the side of the former employee. The moral of this story is that an employer should always keep excellent employee records.

The Occupational Safety and Health Administration (OSHA)

The federal government requires that employers provide a safe workplace for their employees. They enforce this requirement is through OSHA. Congress established OSHA under then President Richard Nixon. Congress has expanded it from high-risk industries, such as construction and mining, to include nearly all employment situations, including dental offices and other health care settings. OSHA works closely with other governmental organizations, such as the Center for Disease Control and Prevention (CDC), when it establishes regulations that pertain to their particular area of expertise.

OSHA is concerned only with worker safety. It does not have authority over patient safety in the dental office. If a dentist practices as a corporation, the dentist is an employee of the corporation (although also an owner) and then OSHA regulations apply to the dentist in the workplace. If a dentist is a proprietor or a partner owner of a dental practice, OSHA has no regulatory authority over the dentist in the workplace (because he or she is an owner, not an employee); but the regulations apply to all other office employees regardless the form of business. However, other regulatory organizations (such as the state board of dentistry) may apply standards (such as the CDC standards) to you as a health care provider.

In the dental office, OSHA is concerned with three general areas. They are:

1. infectious diseases and their spread to workers,
2. hazardous chemicals in the work environment, and
3. general work conditions which include problems such as fire safety, office ventilation and ergonomics.

OSHA standards are discussed in more detail in another chapter of this book.

Americans with Disabilities Act

The American with Disabilities Act (known as "the other ADA" in the dental profession) is intended to ensure that disabled people are not discriminated against in the US commercial world. The ADA defines a disability as "a physical or mental impairment that substantially limits one or more major life activities." The law stipulates that disability includes hearing and visual impairments, paraplegia, epilepsy, past drug use, alcoholism, HIV, and AIDS. The law does not, however, define what "major life activities" are. The ADA has the potential to affect dentistry in the two following ways.

Businesses may not discriminate against any customers or patrons based on any disabling condition. The provisions of this part of the law apply to all places of "public accommodation," which includes dental offices. It is, therefore, illegal to treat any disabled person differently (from a dental standpoint) than a dentist would treat a nondisabled person. If a dentist routinely does anterior endodontics, then he or she may not refuse to do anterior endodontics on a person simply based on the disabling condition. If a dentist routinely refers anterior endodontics to the endodontist, then a dentist may refer a disabled person who requires this treatment to the endodontist. Any new building or major remodeling must be prepared to allow the disabled access to the office. If a dentist treats a disabled person, he or she must make reasonable accommodations for the disabled person's treatment and he or she must be sure that the disabling condition does not compromise the quality of the care provided. If a hearing-impaired person is a patient, a dentist must ensure that the person understands treatment options and make a full informed consent to the treatment. This may require the use of written notes, sign language, or a professional signer. (Dentist must bear the cost unless other provisions have been made with the patient.)

Businesses must also make reasonable accommodations to protect the rights of individuals with disabilities in all aspects of employment. There is no absolute rule about what makes an accommodation reasonable. It depends on the size of the employer, the cost of any changes, and the impact on others. Possible changes may include restructuring jobs, altering the layout of workstations, modifying equipment, or providing special equipment. Employment aspects include the application process, hiring, wages, benefits, and all other aspects of employment.

Presently, dental practices that employ fewer than fifteen people are exempt from two federal statutes, Title VII of the Civil Rights Act of 1964 (which prohibits discrimination based on race, religion, etc.) and the ADA (which prohibits discrimination based on disabling conditions). Most individual dental offices, therefore, are exempt from the federal legal statute. Whether a dentist chooses to abide by the moral imperative of the federal statute is a personal choice, if a dentist has fewer than fifteen employees. Be aware, however, that many states and local governments have similar laws that apply to smaller employers. In addition, many lawyers will attempt to hold a person to the standard despite the number of employees. So the best strategy is to follow the law, even if a person does not think it applies. A job description and open communication (and documentation) should be used during the interview process.

Social Security

Social Security provides income when a family's earnings are reduced or stopped because of disability, death (survivor protection), or retirement. The government requires an employer to participate in the Social Security system through matching contributions on employees' wages. This is covered in more detail in the chapter concerning business taxes.

Pension Plan Incentives and Protection

To participate in most tax-deferred, tax-deductible ("qualified") retirement plans), an employer must include employees in the plan and fund their retirement contribution at a level equal to the employer's. Employee Retirement Income Security Act (ERISA) has set guidelines for participation and contribution. Because there are so many types of plans and because this area of tax law changes frequently, it is only mentioned here that there are provisions of law that affect the way a person can structure a retirement plan. Retirement planning is considered in depth in a different chapter.

Unjust Dismissal

In the United States, people generally practice the doctrine of "employment at will," which states that the employer hires the employee at the employer's will, and the employee works at his or her will. Either can end the relationship at any time (unless there is a contract that states otherwise). (The converse is the fire-at-will doctrine, which states that the employer may fire an employee "for good cause, for no cause, or even for cause morally wrong" unless prevented by agreements or contracts.) However, the days when an employer can exercise the fire-at-will doctrine and fire an employee without fear of retribution are quickly fading into the history books. Unjust (or unfair) dismissal occurs when an employee is forced to accept termination of employment in circumstances that are harsh, unreasonable, or unjust. Examples of unreasonable firings include firing a person because they are pregnant, because they will soon be vesting in a pension plan, or because of a discriminating factor, such as race, age, or religion. An employee whom is unfairly dismissed may seek reinstatement or compensation from the previous employer through the courts. (Firing issues are dealt with in more detail in the chapter on personnel policies.)

An employer might face consequences for firing an employee despite the justness of the firing. The employee may collect unemployment compensation, which may affect the employer's unemployment tax rates. The former employee may attempt to retaliate, either through legal or illegal methods. A former employee who has a key to the office can easily cause havoc by disrupting utilities, disturbing materials, records, or computer files. He or she may cause problems by calling OSHA, the IRS, the Wage and Hour Cabinet, board of dentistry or other regulatory agencies claiming that an employer has acted illegally. Although these organizations all understand employee retaliation, law requires many to investigate all complaints brought to their attention.

There is no single law that regulates dismissal of employees. But the effect of this concept on the dental office is that an employer should be careful when firing an employee. He or she should check the date when the employee vests in a pension plan (if any) and be aware of any other potential reason for a former employee to sue (e.g., pregnancy, race, age) claiming *that* was the reason for the dismissal rather than their job performance. If the employee falls into any of these protected groups, the employer should be sure to have excellent documentation before firing. Otherwise, it may appear, on the face of it, that the employer is firing this employee unjustly (because of the discriminating factor). It would be up to the employer to prove that this is not so.

Discrimination and the Equal Employment Opportunity Commission (EEOC)

The EEOC enforces federal laws that prohibit employment discrimination based on an individual's race, religion, sex, national origin, age, or disability. The EEOC coordinates the enforcement of several different laws related to employment discrimination. These include Title VII of the Civil Rights Act of 1964, the Age Discrimination Employment Act of 1967, Title I of the ADA, and the Equal Pay Act (EPA) of 1963.

Overall, these laws prohibit hiring discrimination, workplace harassment, or firing preferences based on any of the listed discriminating factors. (In this sense, sexual harassment in the workplace is a form of unlawful sex discrimination.) In fact, most of these laws apply only to larger employers (15 or more employees). However, as with the ADA, many states have similar laws that apply to all employers. Just because a law does not apply, this does not absolve anyone of the moral imperative to treat people fairly and equally, no matter their external characteristics.

Consumer Protection Laws

Another body of law concerns the relationship of the business with its consumer and the public, as a whole. These can be grouped into the general heading of consumer protection and include debtor protection, antitrust laws, and price-fixing–related laws. Consumer protection is an idea that has really only emerged since the end of the Second World War. Although there were limited consumer protection laws in force before this time, the rise in consumerism accompanied by an increase in the number of consumer protection laws has blossomed as the US consumer has become wealthier (Table 8.3).

Table 8.3 Consumer Protection Laws

Law	Duty
Truth-in-Lending Act	Requires lenders to fully disclose all credit terms before a loan is made or an account is opened
Fair Credit Reporting Act	Regulates the consumer credit reporting industry
Fair Debt Collection Practices Act	Prevents debt collection agencies from abusive or deceptive collection practices

The Federal Trade Commission (FTC) was created in 1914 as an independent regulatory body whose purpose was to protect consumers and keep competition free and fair. The FTC enforces competition through the various antitrust laws and enforces consumer protection through trade practice regulations. In fact, these two charges overlap considerably.

Debtor Protection Laws

Fair Credit Reporting Act

Congress designed the Fair Credit Reporting Act to ensure that credit bureaus and clearing houses keep accurate credit histories. Credit histories are important for consumers because businesses use them to qualify individuals for loans, mortgages, and other forms of credit. They also are often used in insurance ratings and even job decisions. A damaging credit history may mean that an individual pays higher interest rates or does not qualify for a loan or credit card. Because a credit bureau posts information given to them by lenders and other creditors, they are unaware if inaccurate, and potentially damaging, information is placed in someone's credit history. The Fair Credit Reporting Act requires that credit bureaus allow an individual to challenge the completeness and accuracy of information in the credit file. If the credit reporting agency cannot verify a disputed item, it must delete or correct it. If a reinvestigation does not resolve a dispute, the Fair Credit Reporting Act permits the consumer to file a statement of up to 100 words to explain his or her side of the story.

In the dental office, the effect of this act is most noticeable if the employer is a member of a credit bureau and regularly verify clients' credit history before extending credit to them. Here, an employer may find incorrect information that the individual will want to correct. If an employer uses a collection agency to help collect overdue accounts, he or she will find that the agencies will inform the various credit reporting agencies of the patient's poor payment history. This then affects the patient's credit worthiness. Individuals, even dentists, should check their credit history regularly. (The process for that is given in the personal financial management chapter of this book.)

The Truth-in-Lending Act

Congress designed the Truth-in-Lending Act to ensure a meaningful disclosure of credit terms so that the consumer can compare various sources and forms of loans. This act does not limit the charges imposed but requires that the lender fully show all charges before the completion of the credit. They accomplish this disclosure through two ideas: the finance charge and the annual percentage rate (APR). The finance charge is the sum of all charges by the debtor (or someone else) to the creditor as a condition of credit extension. These include interest charges, service charges, loan fees, points, credit report fees, and any other charges for extending credit. The law also requires that the lender show the finance charge, expressing it as an annual percentage rate, and even specifies how this rate should be computed. The finance charges and lending rates must be shown to the borrower on a financing statement, which also includes any delinquency charges, late payment charges, and securities.

In dental practice, the effect of this law is to require a business owner to make full disclosure any time he or she plans to charge interest for any unpaid balances. The owner may be subject to both civil and criminal penalties for violating this law. It is perfectly within his or her right to charge interest on unpaid balances. However, if the person does so, he or she must be sure to abide by the spirit and the letter of the truth-in-lending laws. (Model disclosure forms will help keep a business owner on the fair side of the law.) An owner's confidence in following the law will partly make this decision. The rest is what similar practitioners in a particular community customarily do. If no other dental practitioners charge interest on unpaid balances, it becomes problematic, from a marketing perspective, for one practitioner to charge interest. Service charges (a fixed amount per month, rather than a percentage of the remaining balance) are not interest and therefore, not included in this law.

The Fair Debt Collection Practices Act (FDCPA)

Congress designed the FDCPA to prohibit debt collection agencies from using abusive or deceptive collection techniques (Box 8.2). The act only applies to agencies and individuals whose primary business is to collect debt for others, unless a person represents himself or herself to be a debt collector or make the debtor believe that the person is. Creditor collections (such as a dentist or the dentist's staff collecting on his or her own accounts) are exempt from the act. They assume that most creditors will want to maintain the goodwill and patronage of the patron (or the patient) besides collecting the amount owed. However, many people assume

---

Box 8.2 Fair Debt Collection Practices

The collector may *not*:

1. Physically threaten the debtor
2. Claim to be an attorney, if they are not
3. Use obscenities
4. Telephone before 8:00 a.m. or after 9:00 p.m.
5. Telephone repeatedly, in an attempt to annoy
6. Place collect calls to the debtor
7. Threaten with arrest or garnishment, unless a person can legally and intends to do so
8. Use any "unfair or unconscionable means" to collect the debt
9. Continue collection efforts after written notification to stop by the debtor; sole remedy is to sue
10. Limits contact with third parties

---

that these collection requirements apply to all collection efforts and will try to hold the individual creditor to the same standards.

The effect of this law on dental practice is twofold. First, a dentist should understand the limitations placed on a debt collection agency's efforts to collect money owed to the dentist. If a dentist has conducted "in-house" collection efforts effectively, a collection agency cannot do much more to collect the debt. Second, although no one holds a dentist to the collection act standard, consumers may hold the dentist to the standard in their minds. Many states also have laws that place creditors (dentists) on the same ground as collection agencies regarding collection practices. So it is a good idea to follow the same rules when a dentist or staff attempt to collect overdue accounts as collection agencies must follow.

Bankruptcy

Bankruptcy is a common and confusing occurrence in modern US society. Bankruptcy laws apply to both consumers and incorporated businesses. The intent of bankruptcy is to give the debtor some protection from creditors to make a fresh start and to treat creditors fairly. This discussion limits itself to individual consumers' bankruptcy, the type that a dentist might encounter if a patient files for bankruptcy.

Bankruptcy proceedings begin upon the filing of either a voluntary (filed by the debtor) or involuntary (filed by one or more creditors of the debtor) petition to a special bankruptcy court. Two outcomes are possible in bankruptcy proceedings against an individual. This is the individual's decision, not the creditor's. The first option (called Chapter 7) occurs when the individual's nonexempt property is liquidated (sold) and the money realized goes to pay off as many debts as possible. The court then discharges or eliminates all of the debts (paid and unpaid). The second option (called Chapter 13) occurs when the individual's finances will be reorganized. The debts will be adjusted, not eliminated. In this latter case, the court will rearrange the amount and repayment schedule of the debts to allow the debtor to pay them off. Most debtors choose to have their debts discharged (wiped off the books) and their property liquidated, rather than to seek an adjustment because they would remain obliged to pay some of the debt. Even when an individual's property is liquidated, federal and state laws allow the individual to exempt certain portions of their property from the process. This often includes the person's personal house and certain retirement accounts.

The effects of the bankruptcy laws on dental practice are minor. (If a dentist is declaring bankruptcy, the effects are obviously major and an attorney experienced in bankruptcy law is needed.) When a patient files for bankruptcy and owes a dentist money, he or she will list the dentist as a creditor. There is a hierarchy or priority for paying debts off from liquidation proceeds. General (or unsecured) creditors (like a dentist) are the last group paid, after secured creditors such as business creditors, governments (taxes), estate administrators, and others. The debtor's trustee may contact a dentist asking him or her to forgive or reduce the person's debt. As a rule, a dentist will not get much either way, except a case of ulcers from the anger engendered. The best cure for patient bankruptcy is active prevention. Be sure to qualify patients financially before doing large cases on them.

Antitrust Laws

Antitrust laws began in this country in the late 19th and early 20th centuries. The purpose of this series of laws is to promote healthy economic competition and all of the benefits supposed to result from that competition. Congress aimed the original laws at large corporations who formed "trusts" or conglomerates to gain monopolistic control over a given industry. Once they gained monopolistic control, they eliminated competition, established common business policies, and controlled territories and price levels to prohibit any new competitors from gaining a start in the market. Consumers paid higher prices and lost control of markets as a result.

There are many different laws that are collectively known as antitrust laws. They deal with price fixing, exclusive contracts, mergers, acquisitions, and interlocking directorates. The Federal Trade Commission (FTC) and the Department of Justice are primarily charged with ensuring a competitive marketplace through enforcement of these various laws. The important fact to note in antitrust laws is an attempt by more than one person or firm to influence the marketplace. Nothing prohibits a person from setting any price he or she chooses for fees or participating (or not) in any managed care plan. However, if a dentist gets together with other practitioners and agree to make similar business decisions to influence the marketplace, there are potential antitrust violations in that scenario. If guilty, fines are large. Guilty or innocent, legal fees are huge. The simple solution is to avoid any group or association activity that even appears to attempt to influence the marketplace.

Antitrust laws do not affect dentistry often, but when they do, the effect can be profound. The following are general categories and examples of possible antitrust violations in dentistry:

1. Agreeing with competitors not to participate in a certain reimbursement program (such as a capitation plan) is restraint of trade.
2. Forming a trade group that has an exclusive contract (such as an Independent Practice Association [IPA]) would be a restraint of trade, if that group controls the local marketplace.
3. When there are discussions of price with competitors and parallel pricing decisions result, price fixing is assumed to have happened.
4. State boards of dentistry or dental organizations that prohibit advertising by members or dentists are decreasing competition and are, therefore, acting illegally.
5. Any attempt by organized dentistry to limit participation in or eliminate a third-party payer (such as a managed care plan) is strictly illegal, even if the restriction is based on a professional ethical standard.

Laws Regulating the Dental Profession

Each state has its own set of laws that regulate the practice of dentistry in that state. They are known as the "Dental Practice Act" for the particular state. Note that no national law governs the practice of dentistry. Because it is left to each state, each state's laws will be unique. Each state's dental practice act is unique. However, most have many common legal issues for dentists that they discuss. Many consist of a shell of the law, followed by an interpretation by the regulatory agency responsible for interpreting and administering the law. Different states give different amounts of authority in these areas to the representative board.

Definitions

Most acts begin with a series of definitions. What is "practicing dentistry" or "dental hygiene?" What is a dental laboratory, a dental student, or university? What is the Board of Dentistry and where does it gain its power? The answer to these questions affects the interpretation of the rest of the law that follows.

Board of Dentistry

Often the next section of the law discusses the board of dentistry. It details the source of the board's authority, its powers, and its duties. A section on membership, qualifications for members, and terms of office follow.

Licensing for Dentist and Dental Hygienist

Generally, the acts have separate sections that describe the laws and regulations aimed at licensing dentists and dental hygienists.

Practicing without a License

What happens to a person who practices without a valid and current license? This section describes the fines and other punishments levied against someone who breaks this portion of the law. This section intends to protect the public from unlicensed practitioners.

Student Licenses

How can students learn to do dentistry if they are unlicensed and therefore cannot do dentistry? This section of the law grants students the privilege of doing dental procedures. There are often strict requirements, such as enrollment in an accredited program, not gaining personal financial benefit from the procedure, and being under the direct supervision of a licensed instructor.

Qualification for License

What are the qualifications for gaining an initial dental license in the state? Are there any reciprocal agreements with other states? Many states accept license by credential. This means that if a person has practiced in another state for a certain number of years, this state will review his or her record and grant a dental license. Generally, the dentist must have a "clean" record and show a history of continuing education. Reciprocal agreements will allow a dentist in another state to gain licensure in this state if the other state grants the same privilege to dentists from this state. Many states may grant special licenses. These may be for educators, dentists who are working in charitable or public health settings, or residents in postgraduate educational programs. There are

often special agreements that they have contracted with these licenses.

Renewal of Dental License

What are the requirements for license renewal, once the dentist or hygienist has gained initial licensure? Many states have continuing educational requirements, and all have fees associated with renewal. This section may also detail grounds for refusal of relicensure.

Revocation or Suspension of License

What are the grounds for revoking or suspending a dental license? This act carries significant financial implications for the dentist, so these sections are usually specific in granting the authority to the board. It will usually describe the procedure they will follow and what records (public and private) they will keep. They will describe the method and procedure of appeal as well.

Auxiliary Personnel

What may a dentist legally delegate to auxiliaries within the practicing state? Some states allow hygienists to practice independently, but others require general supervision. (This means that a dentist must have seen the patient and written orders but do not have to be physically present while the hygienist does the procedure.) Other states require direct supervision, which means that the dentist must be physically present when the hygienist (or other auxiliary) works on a patient. Some states allow assistants to function in an expanded role. They often call these auxiliaries *expanded duty dental assistants* (EDDAs) or *expanded function dental auxiliaries* (EFDAs). Some states require formal training. Different states allow these EDDAs to do different intraoral procedures, from taking intraoral radiographs, rubber cupping a patient's teeth, placing fillings, constructing temporaries to filling endodontics. Because each state is different, the dentist must carefully review the state practice act to learn what procedures auxiliaries are allowed (positive law) or not allowed (negative law) to do.

Anesthesia, Deep Sedation, and Conscious Sedation

Many states have regulations concerning who can put patients under general anesthesia and deep sedation. They often impose additional education and certification requirements on those dentists who do these procedures. Many states have educational requirements that they must meet before a dentist may use conscious sedation (e.g., nitrous oxide oxygen analgesia).

Complaint Procedures

If someone has a complaint against a practicing dentist, this section describes how he or she should handle complaint. It will tell if an investigation is allowed or required, what the procedures are, and what are the possible outcome of a hearing.

Specialties

The states all define who may act, advertise, and promote themselves to be a dental specialist. This section will also describe the educational and experience qualifications required, the limits of practice for declared specialists, and the examination procedures required for designation.

Dental Laboratories

Some states set limits on dental laboratories, requiring registration and certification. Dentists may then only use register and certified dental laboratories. This section of the law describes that process.

What to do if Sued

There are several levels of legal maneuvers that people may call "being sued," including personal inquiries, legal inquiries, and a summons and complaint. Most legal inquiries will relate to patients and a person's role as a dentist. However, other issues, such as general business liability, may also trigger legal inquiries. Whatever the legal problem, the most important line of defense is to contact a lawyer as soon as practical.

If the problem involves liability, then the dentist should also contact his or her liability carrier (professional, personal, or business) when the dentist is aware of a potential problem. Besides providing coverage for certain claims made against the dentist, most policies have provisions for paying for all or part of the legal fees involved in defending the suit. The specific carrier and policy determines if they allow a dentist to choose (or contribute to the choice of) a defense attorney. If the carrier is not notified of a problem in a "timely" manner, this may allow the carrier to refuse coverage for loss or defensive costs. If a person has a question about whether to report a particular issue, err on the safe side and inform the carrier. It is in the carrier's interest to ensure that a person does not get hit with a loss.

Personal Inquiry

A patient may make a personal inquiry, asking to see or copy "his or her" record. The dentist owns the physical record, but the patient owns the information contained in the record. So in most states, a dentist has an obligation to provide the patient a copy of his or her record (free of cost to them). Any additional copies may carry a reasonable fee for copying and handling. A dentists should never give up the original record (unless by court order) and should only give copies of paper or radiographs. Other people might lose records. The dentist needs to keep the original. The dentist should not make up, alter, or forge any paper or computer records.

An obvious question for a dentist (or staff) is to ask the person who requested a copy of their records why they are wanted. If the patient is dissatisfied, the dentist might satisfy the patient then and defuse a developing problem. If the action is a malpractice action, the dentist should immediately contact his or her carrier whenever he or she becomes aware of a potential malpractice action. If the issue is as simple as the patient moving and needing to transfer records to a dentist out of town, then there is no problem.

Lawyer's Inquiry

A lawyer may request information or a copy of a patient's record. This is generally a more serious matter than a patient making an inquiry. If a lawyer contacts a dentist, the dentist should find out the information requested and the reason and then agree to contact the lawyer later. This gives the person a chance to gather thoughts, contact a lawyer, make appropriate copies, and gather other material. Besides contacting a lawyer, a dentist should immediately contact his or her liability insurance carrier.

Summons and Complaint

A dentist may be served with a summons and complaint either in person or through the mail. (The summons says that someone has sued, and the accompanying complaint gives the allegations made against the person and begins the suit.) Generally, the person then only has 20 days to file an "Answer" or formal response to the complaint. Failure to meet this deadline often results in a default judgment against the person who was served. Time is critical in this situation.

Immediately upon receiving a summons, a dentist should contact an attorney. The dentist should never try to answer the complaint because he or she does not know the law and may cause problems, such as making a procedural error, giving the other side unnecessary information, or unknowingly admit facts alleged.

A dentist should also begin immediately to collect any documentation that may relate to the issue. (The dentist should not make up, alter, or forge any paper or computer records.) He or she should also list anyone who may have information about the lawsuit, although the dentist should not speak to anyone other than an attorney or insurer about the suit. All of this information will be useful to an attorney in the defense of a suit.

A lawsuit is never a pleasant experience for anyone involved. The dentist should contact a lawyer and liability carrier early in the process and keep excellent records and notes. A dentist should not tell the opposing lawyer or patient any more than his or her lawyer says so, and he or she should not talk with staff or other people about the suit. By following these guidelines, the dentist will help to ensure that the legal process is as easy as possible.

Financial Statements

In business a reputation for keeping absolutely to the letter and spirit of an agreement, even when it is unfavorable, is the most precious of assets, although it is not entered in the balance sheet.
Lord Chandos

Objectives

At the completion of this chapter, the student will be able to:
1. Differentiate between the following financial tools:
   Family budget
   Corporate balance sheet
   Corporate profit-and-loss (income) statement
   Cash flow statement
   Personal balance sheet
   Personal income statement
   Pro forma statements
2. Describe how each of the financial statements are used in dental practice.
3. Describe cash flow and its importance to the dental practice.
4. Describe working capital and how it is used in a dental practice.

Key Terms

actual	financial statements	operating statement
assets	income	pro forma statements
balance sheet	income statement	profit
budget	liabilities	profit-and-loss statement
cash flow statement	loss	statement of financial position
expenses	net worth	variance

Goal

The goal of this chapter is to define the common financial statements that are used in dental practice and to describe the information that they contain and how dentists use the statements.

Business Basics for Dentists, First Edition. David O. Willis.
© 2013 John Wiley & Sons, Inc. Published 2013 by John Wiley & Sons, Inc.

Business has a vocabulary that is as specific and descriptive as any other written or spoken language. Words have meanings in the language of business that business people the world over recognize. The first of those words are the different types of financial statements.

Financial statements are the way that businesses commonly express their financial transactions and history. They take the same, standard format, regardless the type or size of business. In this way, banks and other financial institutions can easily assess financial health and compare one operation to other, similar organizations. Dentists need to understand how to develop these statements, what each component is, and how to use them. Bankers will probably call a dental practitioner to develop each of these forms if he or she requests a loan for practice purchase or start-up.

Two forms of financial statements, personal and corporate, are shown in this chapter. Because most dentists must personally guarantee loans and other practice finance options, bankers generally require a personal financial statement for these guarantees. The proprietor practitioner is inseparable from the practice, so personal statements are especially appropriate for them. With large or networked practices, bankers may request the corporate form of these statements because the personal involvement of a dentist is less critical for their success. The format of the forms is similar, though not exactly the same.

The forms discussed are:

Personal Forms
    Personal Income Statement
    Personal Balance Sheet
Corporate Forms
    Corporate Income Statement
    Corporate Balance Sheet
    Corporate Cash Flow Statement

Personal Financial Forms

Personal financial forms show the state of a person's personal financial health. If a person owns a dental practice, he or she finds it difficult to separate himself or herself financially from the businesses. These financial forms will help to examine that difference.

Personal Income Statement

The personal income statement is a moving picture of a person's personal cash inflows and outflows (Box 9.1). The income statement examines money flows over a specific period, generally a month or year. It is often used as the basis for developing a budget, which aims to use past income and expenditures to plan for the future.

Box 9.1 Personal Income Statement

Income − Expenses = Difference

This statement looks at the sources and uses of personal family money. Exact categories of income and expense will be different depending on a person's personal situation. If, for example, a person is not married, then a spouse's income is meaningless. If a person is divorced, then a line for alimony or child support payments might be added to the income or expense section (depending on whether a person is paying or receiving these payments).

Expenses are usually grouped by type on the personal income statement. Savings and investments are payments that a person really makes to himself or herself. The payments still represent cash flowing through to the savings or investment vehicle, so they must be accounted for. They then appear on the personal balance sheet, making that statement more positive. Fixed expenses are those that generally cannot be changed over the short term. A person can buy a smaller home, decreasing the payment in the future, but for the immediate concern, a person cannot change a home mortgage payment. (Most debt service is a fixed expense.) A person may have some control over expenses such as food (buying hamburger instead of steak), but he or she still must spend money on these fixed expenses. Discretionary, or variable, expenses are those that a person consciously chooses to make. A person doe not need to go out to a restaurant for dinner. He or she can save money by staying in and cooking, so the dining experience is a discretionary financial decision. (There is obvious personal choice in deciding which of these expenses are discretionary and which are fixed.) The difference between income and expenses tells whether a person is living within his or her means.

Many people use the personal income statement as the beginning point for developing a budget for personal financial planning. A budget is a statement of how a person has spent money in the past and an estimate of future income and expenses. Budgets are used for planning the financial needs of a family by setting expected goals for income or expense by explaining and evaluating spending patterns. As such, they become a target for day-to-day financial living. Budgets are most frequently used when a family is having a financial problem. They then help set targets for spending and let everyone know why spending is limited in one area or another. A budget can help coordinate savings and improve living standards by identifying areas of waste. Bankers may require that a person develops an income statement or family budget when borrowing money to set up or buy out a dental practice. The bank wants to make sure that the person has assessed how much money needed for family living expenses so that the bank can evaluate whether the business can support all of the cash needs (operating, tax, financial, and personal).

Example Personal Income Statement

The sample statement in Table 9.1 shows a personal income statement for John and Mary Doe for the year given. It shows family income from Mary's practice, John's work, and other sources. The total of each category is in the next column to the right of the last entry for the category. Family expenses for the Does are broken into three categories: savings, fixed, and variable expenses. In the example statement, John and Mary are close to living within their income. They are making substantial deposits into savings, investments, and retirement plans. Most of their discretionary expenses are well under control, which in turn allows for the high savings rate.

Table 9.1 Example Personal Income Statement

Personal Income Statement John and Mary Doe for the Year January 1 – December 31, 201X		
INCOME		
Practice Income (after taxes)	$99,338	
Spouse's Income	$67,200	
Investment Income	$2,570	
Other Income	$1,250	$170,358
EXPENSES		
Savings and Investment		
Credit Union Savings Acct	$5,800	
Stock Investments	$4,067	
Retirement Plan Contribution	$10,000	$19,867
Fixed Expenses		
Home Mortgage Note Payment	$18,250	
Practice Note Payment	$28,500	
Student Loan Payment	$12,000	
Auto Note Payment	$4,800	
Credit Card Payments	$800	
Food	$6,400	
Medical	$1,600	
Insurances	$6,500	
Utilities/Household	$8,000	
Dependent Care	$6,000	
Taxes	$29,000	$121,850
Discretionary (Variable) Expenses		
Entertainment/Dining	$3,900	
Clothing/Personal Care	$5,500	
Stewardship/Donations	$3,000	
Auto Expenses	$5,200	
Miscellaneous	$6,000	
Cash	$5,200	$28,800 $170,517
DIFFERENCE		(159)

Box 9.2 Net Worth Equation

Assets – Liabilities = Net Worth

Personal Balance Sheet

The statement of financial position (balance sheet) shows what a person owns (assets) and what a person owes (liabilities) at a specific point in time. The balance sheet then is a "snapshot" of a person's financial position at a declared date. It will be different tomorrow as assets change value and as loans are paid off. In fact, bankers and financial planners like to examine changes in a balance sheet to learn how well a person is doing financially. (Total net worth should be growing.)

The balance sheet should become more positive over time. This shows that a person is accumulating wealth and paying off loans. There are really only two ways for net worth to grow (Box 9.2). A person can increase assets by either saving money or increasing the value of an asset. Or a person can decrease liabilities by paying off debt. If a person borrows and then uses the money to purchase an asset, net worth remains unchanged. This happens, for example, when a person buys a dental practice. He or she takes on debt but also now owns an asset of equal value. The net worth remains unchanged. As the debt is paid down or the value of the practice increases, net worth becomes more positive.

It is possible to have negative net worth. This happens to young professionals who have significant educational debt and few assets. Their total liabilities (educational and other debts) are more than the total of what they presently own (assets). Although not an enviable position, it is common.

Bankers generally ask a person to prepare a personal balance sheet when he or she applies for a loan or to borrow money for a business or personal purchase. It is also good practice for the person to prepare one each year to assess his or her financial status. If a person is a proprietor, he or she will use a personal balance sheet (because all assets and debts are personal) and include the practice as an asset on the statement. If a person belongs to an incorporated business, he or she may need to develop two statements, one for the practice (a corporate balance sheet) and the other a personal statement of financial position. Often banks have specific forms that need to be completed. These forms are usually the bank's particular versions of the generic balance sheet.

Example Personal Balance Sheet

Table 9.2 is a personal balance sheet for John and Dr. Mary Doe. These are things that they own as husband and wife. The balance sheet is for the date given. It

Table 9.2 Example Personal Balance Sheet

Statement of Personal Financial Position John and Mary Doe as of December 31, 201X			
ASSETS			
Cash/Cash Equivalents			
Checking Account	$3,050		
Credit Union Savings	$4,000		
Money Market Account	$7,500		
Life Insurance Cash Value	$8,000	$22,550	
Personal Use Assets			
House	$135,000		
Automobiles	$28,000		
Personal Property	$52,000	$215,000	
Business Use Assets			
Dental Practice	$467,500	4$67,500	
Investments			
Stock Portfolio	$7,800		
Mutual Funds	$6,500		
SEP/IRA	$18,980	$32,280	$738,330
LIABILITIES			
Short-Term Liabilities			
Credit Card Balances	$950	$950	
Long-Term Liabilities			
Auto Note Balance	$4,920		
Home Mortgage Balance	$87,900		
Student Loans	$175,000		
Dental Practice	$270,300	$537,820	$538,770
NET WORTH			$199,560

will be different as the Does' investment change value or as they pay off loans or buy new assets. Each type (or class) of asset or liability is grouped together. The value of each asset is in the first column, and the sum of the value of the assets in the class is in the second column, next to the last individual asset value. The assets class values are then summed similarly to develop a total of all assets (in the third column).

The first asset class is "Cash" (or items that we can quickly convert that into cash). Cash is needed for routine, daily purchases, and for an emergency. Investments are not considered "near cash" because a person might lose a large portion of his or her value if he or she were forced to sell the investments at the "wrong time." Personal-use assets are not important from a financial planning perspective. Most people will not sell their house or car when they retire, for example, so these assets are not used for retirement or investment planning purposes. Business-use assets should generate income at a level that gives a reasonable return on the investment. These assets are often sold at retirement and can become a part of the retirement portfolio. The personal balance sheet shows personal items owned and amounts owed. One of those business assets may be a dental practice. Investments are long-term assets that should generate a reasonable return

(over time). They become the backbone of retirement, personal, and business planning efforts.

Liabilities are similarly grouped. Short-term liabilities are debts that a person owes that are due in 1 year or less. In Table 9.2, credit card balances are due immediately. This might also include signature loans, bridge loans, or other short-term borrowing. Long-term liabilities are debts that will take more than one (or many) years to pay off. The example shows an auto loan, home mortgage, student loan, and a practice loan. Each of these long-term liabilities should have a capital (or other large) asset on the list for which the liability paid. The auto, home, and dental practice notes are each associated with an obvious asset. The one questionable item is the "Student Loan" entry. The student loan payment purchased a "hidden" asset that does not appear on the balance sheet (a dental degree), but the associated liability must be included. In a sense, a person has invested in his or her human capital when he or she borrowed money for education. Unfortunately, the IRS does not allow this as a depreciable asset for tax purposes.

Table 9.2 shows a total of $738,330 in assets (things that the Does owned) and $538,770 in liabilities (or things that the Does owed). The difference ($199,560) is their net worth. In other words, if they sold everything they own and paid all of their debts, they would have (less commissions, sales fees, and taxes) $199,560. As they build their asset base and pay down loans, their net worth will become more positive.

How the Personal Financial Statements are Related

The easiest way to understand how the personal financial statements are related is to look at the previous examples. On the income statement, a person earns money either through work or through investment return. One of two things can be done with that money: spend it and it goes way or invest it and purchase an asset which the person then owns. Some of the money has to be spent. People need food, utilities, and clothing. Other items may be required by contract or facts. People need to provide day care for the children so that they both work. Taxes and student loan payments are required by law or contract. The financial value of these payments evaporates when they are paid. Other payments buy assets (physical or financial) that appear on the balance sheet. If a person "spends" $1,000 in savings, he or she now has an additional $1,000 as a financial asset on the balance sheet. The underlying asset that is purchased may increase in value over time (such as a savings account) or decrease in value (such as when an automobile is purchased). So saving (investing) improves the balance sheet and therefore personal wealth (making them more positive), while spending does not affect a balance sheet (or personal wealth).

Using debt is a bit more complex. Assume that a person purchases an automobile. If an asset is purchased for cash, the balance sheet is unchanged. A person has decreased cash, but he or she increased the personal use asset by an equal amount. As the car ages and decreases in value, the balance sheet declines by an appropriate amount. Any future expenditures for savings go onto the balance sheet as a financial asset. If the automobile is purchased with debt (borrowing the money for the purchase), the balance sheet also remains unchanged. Now the value of the asset (the car) and a corresponding increase in liabilities (the amount owed for the car) is reported on the balance sheet. Payments for the automobile loan are part interest, which goes away to the bank, and part principal, which decreases the loan liability, improving the balance sheet. However, the asset decreases in value as it ages, cancelling out most of the decrease in the liability.

In the example statements, the Doe family is increasing their balance sheet by saving $29,867 last year. These payments improve their financial assets. The various loan payments in part decrease the corresponding liability (the principal portion of the payment) and in part do not affect the balance sheet (interest portion). Some assets increase in value (e.g., the house, dental practice, and investment portfolio), whereas some decrease in value (e.g., automobiles and personal property). Discretionary spending does not affect the balance sheet.

Corporate Financial Forms

Corporate financial forms describe the financial condition of a business entity. The entity may be a proprietorship, corporation, or limited liability company. Generically "corporate" forms can be used, although they may describe a different business entity.

Profit-and-Loss Statement

The profit-and-loss (P&L) statement is similar to the personal income statement used for personal financial analysis (Box 9.3). One is personal and one business related. This statement shows income and expenses and the resulting net income or net loss for a specific period. In corporate forms, it is commonly called a P&L statement

---

Box 9.3 Profit and Loss Equation

Income – Expenses = Profit (Loss)

---

or an operating statement because it shows the results of the business operations over a given period. These forms detail taxable income and expense items, not cash flow as in the personal statement. If the income items that flow are more than the expense items that flow out, there is a profit. If the outflows are greater, then a loss is registered.

The income statement forms the basis of income taxes. The items placed on a business profit and loss statement are tax items. If a person is a proprietor, he or she reports taxes on the IRS's Schedule C, which is nothing but a P & L statement. Many income statements are arranged according to this Schedule C format (where the expenses occur alphabetically). Others attempt to organize the information better by categorizing items of expense for analysis. Both types are given as examples.

Sample Income Statement (Schedule C Format)

Table 9.3 is a P&L statement because the bottom line (literally and figuratively) is the profit or loss from operating the business. Where the balance sheet is a

Table 9.3 Sample Income Statement (Schedule C Format)

Corporate Profit and Loss (Income) Statement (Schedule C format) for the Year Ending December 31, 201X		
INCOME		
Gross Collections	$298,723	
Returns and Allowances	$875	
Net Collections		$297,848
EXPENSES		
Advertising	$854	
Auto Expense	$1,928	
Commissions	$0	
Depreciation	$23,047	
Employee Benefit Program	$3,640	
Insurance	$1,650	
Interest Expense	$12,487	
Legal and Professional	$1,790	
Office Expense	$3,817	
Pension/Profit Sharing	$3,048	
Rent or Lease	$12,000	
Repairs and Maintenance	$270	
Taxes and Licenses	$9,108	
Meals, Travel and Entertainment	$139	
Utilities	$8,955	
Wages	$60,950	
Other Expenses		
Temporary Services	$340	
Bank Charges	$120	
Office Supplies	$1,000	
Office Cleaning	$3,055	
Dental Supplies	$17,010	
Dental Lab	$29,754	
Dues and Publications	$1,050	
Continuing Education	$1,808	
Postage	$690	$198,510
PROFIT (LOSS)		$99,338

snapshot at a particular time, the P&L shows money flows over a given period, in this case for the calendar year ending on December 31. This form lists income, then expenses, by category. This format lists those expense items alphabetically because the IRS tax form Schedule C (Profit or Loss from Operating a Business) lists them this way. It makes year-end tax accounting easier. The income statement is a tax statement. It shows items (such as depreciation), which are not a cash expense but a calculated amount. Loan payments consist of a part interest and part principal. The interest portion is an expense, but the principal portion is not. Instead, the principal is accounted through depreciation of the asset. The statement does not have a cash infusion from a loan nor a loan principal payment because these are not generated from business operations.

Table 9.3 shows that Dr. Mary Doe collected $298,723 in the dental practice last year. She wrote return checks for $875, leaving a net collection of $297,848. She recorded a total of $198,510 in valid business expenses for the practice. She categorized them as shown. (The chapter on taxes gives details about these tax expense categories.) Because income was greater than expenses, Mary showed a profit of $99,338 for the calendar year.

Sample Income Statement (Categorized Format)

Table 9.4 shows the same information as the previous statement (Table 9.3). The difference is that this form collects the information into logical categories. These forms can be used to analyze the business better than a simple alphabetical listing. For example, the total staff costs include not only wages but also benefit plans, temporary services, pension plan contributions, and any commissions paid. Although this number seems large, it represents 23 percent of collections, which is within the normal range for a general dental practice. By grouping similar items together, where expenses occurred can more easily be seen.

Corporate Balance Sheet

Most businesses develop a balance sheet each year. This way, they can compare their previous year's financial snapshot with the current one. This "running tally" allows them to see progression over time.

The corporate balance sheet is different from the personal sheet in that there is no net worth. Instead, the sheet lists the owner's equity, which is, in a sense, the net worth of the entire corporation for the owners. When a person begins a business, he or she borrows money to buy equipment and finance operation of the business. This creates a liability on the business as capital because the business is a separate entity from its owner(s). From an

Table 9.4 Sample Income Statement (Categorized Format)

Exhibit 3a
Corporate Profit-and-Loss (Income) Statement
(Categorized Format) for the Year Ending December 31, 201X

INCOME			
Gross Collections	$298,723		
Returns and Allowances	$875		
Net Collections			$297,848
EXPENSES			
Staff Costs			
Commissions	$0		
Employee Benefit Program	$3,640		
Pension/Profit Sharing	$3,048		
Wages	$60,950		
Temporary Services	$340	$67,978	
Office Space Costs			
Depreciation	$23,047		
Rent or Lease	$12,000		
Repairs and Maintenance	$270		
Utilities	$8,955		
Office Cleaning	$3,055	$47,327	
Office Expenses			
Insurance	$1,650		
Office Expense	$3,817		
Postage	$690	$5,157	
Marketing Expenses			
Advertising	$854	$854	
Bank Expenses			
Interest Expense	$12,487		
Bank Charges	$120	$12,607	
Variable (Production) Expenses			
Dental Supplies	$17,010		
Dental Lab	$29,754		
Office Supplies	$1,000		
Professional Expenses			
Legal and Professional	$1,790		
Taxes and Licenses	$9,108	$10,898	
Owner's Expenses			
Auto Expense	$1,928		
Meals, Travel and Entertainment	$139		
Dues and Publications	$1,050		
Continuing Education	$1,808	$4,925	$198,510
PROFIT (LOSS)			$99,338

Box 9.4 Assets Equation

Assets = Liabilities + Equity

---

accounting perspective, a business is the sum of its liabilities and assets. So after these liabilities are subtracted from the value of the assets, the positive remainder is the owner's interest or equity, in the business (Box 9.4). This format also lets someone see how assets were financed. A person can either borrow money (incurring a liability) or use his or her own money (owner's equity) to purchase an asset. Corporate balance sheets usually show assets in one

Table 9.5 Corporate Balance Sheet

Corporate Balance Sheet Dr. Mary Doe, PLLC December 31, 201X			
ASSETS			
Current Assets			
Cash Accounts	$32,000		
Accounts Receivable	$53,500		
Inventory (Supply)	$6,000		
Prepaid Expenses	$2,000	$93,500	
Long-term Assets			
Equipment	$85,000		
Goodwill	$130,000		
Real Estate	$160,000	$375,000	$467,500
LIABILITIES			
Current Liabilities			
Accounts Payable	$15,000	$15,000	
Long-term Liabilities			
Mortgages	$240,300		
Other Debt	$15,000	$255,300	$270,300
OWNERS EQUITY			$197,200
TOTAL LIABILITIES AND OWNER'S EQUITY			$467,500

section and liabilities and net worth in the other. The two sections must be equal ("balance").

The corporate balance sheet is used less for proprietorships, such as individual dental practices because the proprietor is the business. It becomes more valuable for larger companies, especially those owned by stockholders. This shows their equity interest, or share value, in the company. As more large group and network practices evolve, more interest and emphasis will be placed by bankers and other financiers in dental corporate balance sheets.

Sample Corporate Balance Sheet

Dr. Doe's corporate balance sheet shows the financial position of the practice as of December 31, 201X. (As a proprietor, she would not usually prepare a corporate balance sheet because she owns the practice personally. It is presented here for illustration.) It lists total assets of $467,500. Current assets are those that are liquid. That is to say, they are cash or can be quickly and easily converted into cash. Long-term assets are physical equipment and real estate and the intangible asset of goodwill. Large corporations value their assets at the time of purchase, regardless the gain or loss in value of the asset. Many smaller businesses (such as dental practices) value the assets using a current fair market value. Liabilities are similarly broken into current and long-term categories. Current liabilities are due immediately or within 1 year. Long-term liabilities are due in more than a year. They are generally used to buy long-term (capital) assets.

Box 9.5 Corporate Cash Flow

Inflows = Outflows

Corporate Cash Flow Statement

This statement is similar to a P&L statement, with a few important differences. This statement shows the cash receipts and cash disbursements for a specific period and the resulting cash balance changes (Box 9.5). In the proprietorship (and other cash-based businesses), it essentially describes the office checkbook. In large businesses that use accrual-based accounting methods, it highlights important changes in the balance sheet.

For example, if cash is moved from a savings account to a checking account, a person has made a cash transaction, although this is not a taxable event. (The money was his or hers; he or she had already paid taxes on it.) A loan payment requires a cash flow, although it accounted for differently from a tax perspective. The cash flow statement shows cash changes. The P&L statement shows taxable income.

There are several important differences between the cash flow represented by the checkbook and the P&L statement. Some transactions involve tax events but not cash. Others involve cash transfers but not tax events. The checkbook contains cash items. The P&L statement contains tax items. The major differences are:

- Depreciation is a noncash expense on the P&L statement. It does not occur in the checkbook.
- A loan payment is composed of part loan principal and part interest. The entire payment (principal and interest) is recorded in the checkbook, but only the interest portion is on the P&L statement.
- When a person borrows money, cash flows into the checkbook but does not show on the P&L statement as taxable income. Likewise, savings paid from the office checkbook is a cash event, but not a tax event and so does not show on the P&L statement.
- When a person pays money back (principal on a loan), cash flows from the checkbook but does not show on the P&L statement.
- A draw is a cash flow from the checkbook but does not occur on the P&L statement. The same is true for any money for personal use taken from the checkbook. (It is also considered a draw.)
- If a person pays personal income taxes from the office checkbook, the taxes are not a deductible expense. It is the same for any personal insurance paid from the office checkbook. (Business taxes and insurances are deductible on the profit and loss statement.)

Three major sources of cash flow into or out of the practice. Cash flow from operating activities is the result of daily practice operations. That is to say, these are payments from patients, insurance companies, and credit cards for the dental services done. Offsetting this is money spent to pay suppliers and employees, which decrease cash from operating activities. Bankers are interested in operating cash because it shows the cash flow from the core business. Cash flow from investment activities relates to cash spent for property, plant, equipment, and other capital assets. As a proprietor, a business does not hold investments because those are personal and do not appear as a cash flow. Generally cash is spent for office equipment and improvements when production is expected to increase. Finally, cash flow results from financing activities related to borrowing or repaying loans. If a person borrows money for the practice, cash flows into the checkbook, although this is not taxable income. Conversely, paying back the principal on a loan results in a decrease in cash in the office checkbook but does not result in a tax deductible expense. Net free cash flow is the total of cash flows from operations, investing, and financing. Many large corporate cash flow statements break these sources and uses of cash into their separate categories. Most dental practice cash flow statements combine these categories.

Note than some outflows (such as savings) actually go to self. In a sense, this is "taking money from one pocket and putting it in the other." In reality, savings are an asset that increases on a balance sheet. This improves a person's overall financial position. Cash flow statements are often used to decide if a person has enough money flowing through the practice to make recurring mortgage and other loan payments. Any excess cash can pay down the principal on a mortgage. Any cash shortage must come from savings or borrowing. Therefore, cash flow statements must balance. That is to say, cash inflows must equal cash outflows.

Cash flow is important because it shows a person's liquidity and solvency (ability to pay immediate bills). These include regular office expenses, payroll, and loan payments. Banks are concerned that a person can make these payments. If a person cannot pay them from operating income, then that person should plan to borrow enough money to pay them while the practice is growing to the point where it can sustain the payments. The only way to decide this is to do a cash flow projection.

A person should leave enough cash in the office checking account for 2 to 3 months' expenses. This changes over time as cash flows into and out of an account. A dental practitioner needs enough cash for:

- All monthly expenses (bills paid, credit cards paid, salaries)
- Routine purchases (lab, rent etc.)
- Unexpected loss of income (office closed, vacations etc.)

- Annual ebb and flow of business
- Minimums required by banks (for no fees)
- Future obligations (employee taxes withheld, personal tax payments, insurance owed, etc.)
- Special needs (injury, disability, savings)

The cash flow projection shows how a person expects the cash to flow through the practice for a given time, often the critical first year. When a procedure is done on a patient, a dentist may not receive the entire amount as a cash payment. Instead, some may come in the future as a payment from an insurance company or from a patient who did not pay a bill in full at the time of the service. This accumulates over many patients and many procedures. Accounts Receivable is the cumulative amount that patients owe a dentist for services already done. The dentist's expenses (owed) to suppliers, landlords, and staff are due immediately. However, if a person has not received full payment for those dental services billed, this leads to a "cash flow problem" or cash flow crunch," in which the office will be profitable but cash is flowing in so slowly from patients that immediate bills for suppliers, staff, and other expenses are unable to be made. The solution is to borrow money (called "working capital") to cover these cash flow shortages. The cash flow projection estimates how large is the cash shortage, and therefore how much working capital that a person will need. Typically, dentists need from 3 to 6 months' expenses as working capital for a startup practice in a moderately competitive environment. If the area is more competitive, growth and cash flow will be slower, and therefore the working capital needs will be more.

Sample Cash Flow Reconciliation

Table 9.6 compares the corporate income statement with the office checkbook. This sample shows that Dr. Doe had $297,848 flow into practice income (from patient and insurance payments). She borrowed no money, so none flowed into the checkbook from this source. She claimed a depreciation expense of $23,047 on her income

Table 9.6 Cash Flow Reconciliation

Corporate Cash Flow Reconciliation Dr. Mary Doe (proprietor) for the Year ended December 31, 201X		
Cash Inflows		
Net Practice Income	$297,848	
Borrowing	$0	
Depreciation Expense	$23,047	$274,801
Cash Outflows		
Net Operational Costs	$175,403	
Draw	$78,460	
Personal Expenses Paid	$4,925	
Loan Principal Payments	$16,013	$274,801

Table 9.7 Sample Cash Flow Projection

Cash Flow Projection

	Month 1	Month 2	Month 3	Month 4	Month 5	Month 6	Month 7	Month 8	Month 9	Month 10	Month 11	Month 12	Year #1
Doctor Production	$7,621	$8,764	$10,079	$11,590	$13,329	$15,328	$17,627	$20,271	$23,312	$26,809	$30,830	$35,455	$221,016
Hygiene Production	$1,732	$2,078	$2,494	$2,993	$3,591	$4,310	$5,172	$6,206	$7,447	$8,937	$10,724	$12,869	$68,553
TOTAL PRODUCTION	$9,353	$10,842	$12,573	$14,583	$16,920	$19,638	$22,799	$26,478	$30,759	$35,746	$41,554	$48,324	$289,569
TOTAL CASH RECEIPTS	$4,676	$7,946	$11,084	$12,855	$14,912	$17,304	$20,086	$23,322	$27,088	$31,473	$36,580	$42,531	$249,859
Dental Laboratory	$842	$976	$1,132	$1,312	$1,523	$1,767	$2,052	$2,383	$2,768	$3,217	$3,740	$4,349	$26,061
Clinical Supplies	$561	$651	$754	$875	$1,015	$1,178	$1,368	$1,589	$1,846	$2,145	$2,493	$2,899	$17,374
Office Supplies	$187	$217	$251	$292	$338	$393	$456	$530	$615	$715	$831	$966	$5,791
TOTAL VARIABLE COSTS	$1,590	$1,843	$2,137	$2,479	$2,876	$3,338	$3,876	$4,501	$5,229	$6,077	$7,064	$8,215	$49,227
Staff Wages	$5,265	$5,265	$5,265	$5,265	$5,265	$5,265	$5,265	$5,265	$5,265	$5,265	$5,265	$5,265	$63,183
Employment Taxes	$684	$684	$684	$684	$684	$684	$684	$684	$684	$684	$684	$684	$8,214
TOTAL STAFF COSTS	$5,950	$5,950	$5,950	$5,950	$5,950	$5,950	$5,950	$5,950	$5,950	$5,950	$5,950	$5,950	$71,397
Office Rent/Lease	$1,500	$1,500	$1,500	$1,500	$1,500	$1,500	$1,500	$1,500	$1,500	$1,500	$1,500	$1,500	$18,000
Utilities	$800	$800	$800	$800	$800	$800	$800	$800	$800	$800	$800	$800	$9,600
Repairs	$100	$100	$100	$100	$100	$100	$100	$100	$100	$100	$100	$100	
TOTAL OFFICE SPACE COSTS	$2,400	$2,400	$2,400	$2,400	$2,400	$2,400	$2,400	$2,400	$2,400	$2,400	$2,400	$2,400	$28,800
Office Expenses	$317	$317	$317	$317	$317	$317	$317	$317	$317	$317	$317	$317	$3,800
Insurance, Business	$416	$416	$416	$416	$416	$416	$416	$416	$416	$416	$416	$416	$4,992
TOTAL OFFICE COSTS	$733	$733	$733	$733	$733	$733	$733	$733	$733	$733	$733	$733	$8,792
Bank Charges	$50	$50	$50	$50	$50	$50	$50	$50	$50	$50	$50	$50	$600
Mortgage Payment (Practice)	$3,041	$3,041	$3,041	$3,041	$3,041	$3,041	$3,041	$3,041	$3,041	$3,041	$3,041	$3,041	$37,098
TOTAL BANK COSTS	$3,091	$3,091	$3,091	$3,091	$3,091	$3,091	$3,091	$3,091	$3,091	$3,091	$3,091	$3,091	
Marketing & Promotion	$583	$583	$583	$583	$583	$583	$583	$583	$583	$583	$583	$583	$7,000
TOTAL MARKETING COSTS	$583	$583	$583	$583	$583	$583	$583	$583	$583	$583	$583	$583	$7,000
Management Consulting	$0	$0	$0	$0	$0	$0	$0	$0	$0	$0	$0	$0	$0
Accounting	$200	$200	$200	$200	$200	$200	$200	$200	$200	$200	$200	$200	$2,400
TOTAL PROFESSIONAL COSTS	$200	$200	$200	$200	$200	$200	$200	$200	$200	$200	$200	$200	$2,400
Draw	$4,000	$4,000	$4,000	$4,000	$4,000	$4,000	$6,000	$6,000	$6,000	$6,000	$6,000	$6,000	$60,000
Personal Insurances Paid	$300	$300	$300	$300	$300	$300	$300	$300	$300	$300	$300	$300	%3,600
Continuing Education	$50	$50	$50	$50	$50	$50	$50	$50	$50	$50	$50	$50	$600
Professional Dues and Journals	$83	$83	$83	$83	$83	$83	$83	$83	$83	$83	$83	$83	$1,000
TOTAL OWNER'S COSTS	$4,433	$4,433	$4,433	$4,433	$4,433	$4,433	$6,433	$6,433	$6,433	$6,433	$6,433	$6,433	$65,200
TOTAL CASH OUTFLOWS (COSTS)	$18,981	$19,234	$19,528	$19,870	$20,267	$20,729	$23,266	$23,892	$24,620	$25,467	$26,455	$27,606	$269,913
NET CASH FLOW	($14,304)	($11,287)	($8,444)	($7,015)	($5,355)	($3,425)	($3,181)	($570)	$2,469	$6,006	$10,126	$14,925	
CUMULATIVE CASH POSITION	($14,304)	($25,591)	($34,035)	($41,050)	($46,405)	($49,830)	($53,011)	($53,580)	($51,111)	($45,105)	($34,980)	($20,054)	($20,054)

statement. Because she never wrote a check to the IRS for "Depreciation" but claimed a tax deduction, this noncash item is added back into the reconciliation. Her cash outflows include net operational costs for the office, the amount that she took as a draw on the assets (for living expenses), personal tax-deductible expenses paid through the office, and loan principal payments. (She included the interest portion as a deductible expense in net operating costs.) Cash inflows equal outflows.

Sample Cash Flow Projection

Table 9.7 shows an example cash flow projection for the first year of Dr. Doe's dental practice. It gives good faith estimates of how much doctor and hygiene will produce each of the first 12 months and an estimate of how much the resulting collections will be. (Obviously, these are only as good as the estimates that form the basis of the projection.) It contains cash expenditures, including a "draw" and personal expenses, such as insurances and continuing education expenses. Because it is a cash statement, it contains loan payments but no tax items such as depreciation.

The most important lines are at the bottom of the form. The "Net Cash Flow" shows how much cash can be expected to flow through the practice each month. In the first month, collections of $4,676 and cash expenses (actual checks written) of $18,981 for a cash deficit of $14,304 are estimated. The second month, the cash deficit is $11,287 for a total cumulative for the 2 months of $25,591 is estimated. Monthly cash flow are expected to be negative through month 8, when a total cumulative deficit of $53,580 is expected. It is not until month 9 when the monthly cash flow is projected to be positive, and the cash deficit starts getting paid down. Using this analysis, more than $53,500 of working capital is needed to get through the first year of practice. If the cash inflows with outflows were balanced, the needed cash from loan proceeds would be entered as an inflow similar to collections.

How the Corporate Statements Are Related

The corporate balance sheet lists what Dr. Doe's practice owns and owes. As a single owner limited liability company, the practice is a disregarded entity and she pays income tax as a proprietorship. The income statement (which becomes her Schedule C) shows the result of operating her practice. The cash flow reconciliation shows the actual cash transactions for the year. In the example, practice operations resulted in a taxable profit of $69,338 for the year. She drew $78,460 cash from the office checkbook. This was not a taxable event.

Pro Forma Statements

Pro forma statements are projected statements. They can be any of the four types described in this chapter. The essential element of a pro forma is that it is a guess of what the statement will be at a given time in the future. If a person is preparing a pro forma income statement for the practice, he or she needs to estimate numbers of patient visits, average charges, number and pay rate of staff, and many other items of expense. Obviously, a pro forma statement is only as accurate as an educated guess about the future. Often, banks will ask a person to develop a pro forma cash flow (to assess whether he or she has adequate cash to meet expected expenses) and income statement (to determine expected income and tax situations).

Basics of Business Finance

chapter 10

> *The safest way to double your money is to fold*
> *it over once and put it in your pocket.*
> Frank McKinney Hubbard (Kin Hubbard)

Objectives

At the completion of this chapter, the student will be able to:
1. Describe how the time value of money affects dental practice management decisions.
2. Use the time value of money formulas to solve common dental office finance problems.
3. Describe the elements of loan amortization.
4. Describe common lease–purchase decisions in dental practices.
5. Describe advantages and disadvantages of leasing assets.
6. Discuss common issues in leasing office space.
7. Discuss common issues in leasing automobiles.
8. Discuss common issues in leasing office equipment.

Key Terms

amortization schedule	IRS useful lifetime	present value of a future
compounding	leasehold improvements	dollar
down payment	leverage	principal
economic useful lifetime	loan amortization	property lease
equipment replacement plan	loan conditions	residual value
future value	money factor	sublease
future value of a present	net lease	term of a loan
amount	operating lease	time value of money
gross lease	payment	triple net lease
interest	present value	value of an annuity

Goal

The goal of this chapter is to present concepts of business finance. It presents specific examples of how these ideas are used in dental practice.

Business Basics for Dentists, First Edition. David O. Willis.
© 2013 John Wiley & Sons, Inc. Published 2013 by John Wiley & Sons, Inc.

Business finance looks at how dentists use money in the dental practice to gain or improve profitability. Dentists use it to purchase equipment and materials, hire staff members, and pay costs of the business. Applying finance principles properly maximizes the profit from the practice.

Time Value of Money

A basic premise of finance is that money has a time-associated value, and time has a money-associated value. A dollar in the future will be worth less than a dollar received today, just as paying a dollar in the future is less costly than paying a dollar today. There is a psychological reason for this, given that most people prefer the certainty of having a dollar now to the uncertainty of having a dollar in the future. That future dollar will be worth less because of the likelihood of inflation eating away at its buying power. In addition, a dollar invested wisely will bring a positive return, increasing the value of that present dollar in the future. Time value of money calculations let a person evaluate how much less that future dollar is worth so he or she can make informed financial decisions. This is done by bringing cash flows to a present value for comparison. The higher the assumed interest rate, the more important these calculations become.

These calculations all depend on the idea of compounding. This is the financial process in which a person earns interest on the principal amount, and then he or she earns interest on the interest and the principal. That person then earns interest on an increasing amount over time. The total amount compounds as the interest portion becomes larger and larger.

For example, a person feels that he or she needs $3 million (in today's money) to retire comfortably in 30 years. If a 3-percent annual inflation is assumed, how much will need to be saved each year to meet the goal? A person agrees to buy a dental practice for $350,000 in 5 years. How much is that in today's money? The answers to these questions have an obvious, important financial impact.

These numbers can easily be calculated with a financial calculator (e.g., HP 12-C), by using spreadsheet with financial functions (Excel), or by using the tables that included with this chapter. Although these tables do not give the precise results that a banker may have, they are more than adequate for planning purposes. Throughout the chapter, several common examples of using these important techniques are given.

Future Value of a Present Amount

The future value of a present amount is the future amount of an initial deposit when compounded for a given number of periods at a given rate. This calculation is important when planning future expenditures or savings. To compute this amount, the first three of the four values is needed:

PV present value, the amount in today's dollars
i interest rate, the compounding rate for each period
n number of periods, number of compounding periods
FV future value, the amount in future dollars

Using Table 10.1, find the future value factor (FVF) for the given i and n. Multiply the PV by the FVF to figure out the FV.

$$PV \times FVF = FV$$

Example Problem 1
A person invests $2,000 in a CD earning 8% interest, compounded annually. What will the CD be worth when it matures in 5 years?

PV = $2,000
FV = ??
i = 8%
n = 5

Looking at the table, find the FVF at the intersection of 8% and 5 periods (1.4693). Multiply this FVF by the PV ($2,000) to find the FV $2,938.60.

Example Problem 2
A person needs $3 million (in today's money) to retire comfortably in 30 years. If a 3% annual inflation is assumed, how much will be needed in today's dollars to meet the goal?

PV = $3,000,000
FV = ??
i = 3%
n = 30

Looking at the table, find the FVF at the intersection of 3% and 30 periods (2.4273). Multiply this FVF by the PV ($3,000,000) to find the FV $7,281900.

Example Problem 3
A person wants to start a college fund for a newborn daughter. He or she believes that $120,000 ($30,000 per year times 4 years) in today's dollars is needed, and this money in will be needed in 20 years. Assuming a 3% annual inflation, how much will be needed in today's dollars for the daughter's college fund?

PV = $120,000
FV = ??
i = 3%
n = 20

Looking at the table, find the FVF at the intersection of 3% and 20 periods (1.8061). Multiply this FVF by the PV ($120,000) to find the FV $216,732.

Table 10.1 Future Value of a Single Present Amount

	2%	3%	4%	5%	6%	7%	8%	9%	10%	12%	15%	20%
1	1.0200	1.0300	1.0400	1.0500	1.0600	1.0700	1.0800	1.0900	1.1000	1.1200	1.1500	1.2000
2	1.0404	1.0609	1.0816	1.1025	1.1236	1.1449	1.1664	1.1881	1.2100	1.2544	1.3225	1.4400
3	1.0612	1.0927	1.1249	1.1576	1.1910	1.2250	1.2597	1.2950	1.3310	1.4049	1.5209	1.7280
4	1.0824	1.1255	1.1699	1.2155	1.2625	1.3108	1.3605	1.4116	1.4641	1.5735	1.7490	2.0736
5	1.1041	1.1593	1.2167	1.2763	1.3382	1.4026	1.4693	1.5386	1.6105	1.7623	2.0114	2.4883
6	1.1262	1.1941	1.2653	1.3401	1.4185	1.5007	1.5869	1.6771	1.7716	1.9738	2.3131	2.9860
7	1.1487	1.2299	1.3159	1.4071	1.5036	1.6058	1.7138	1.8280	1.9487	2.2107	2.6600	3.5832
8	1.1717	1.2668	1.3686	1.4775	1.5938	1.7182	1.8509	1.9926	2.1436	2.4760	3.0590	4.2998
9	1.1951	1.3048	1.4233	1.5513	1.6895	1.8385	1.9990	2.1719	2.3579	2.7731	3.5179	5.1598
10	1.2190	1.3439	1.4802	1.6289	1.7908	1.9672	2.1589	2.3674	2.5937	3.1058	4.0456	6.1917
15	1.3459	1.5580	1.8009	2.0789	2.3966	2.7590	3.1722	3.6425	4.1772	5.4736	8.1371	15.4070
20	1.4859	1.8061	2.1911	2.6533	3.2071	3.8697	4.6610	5.6044	6.7275	9.6463	16.3665	38.3376
25	1.6406	2.0938	2.6658	3.3864	4.2919	5.4274	6.8485	8.6231	10.8347	17.0001	32.9190	95.3962
30	1.8114	2.4273	3.2434	4.3219	5.7435	7.6123	10.0627	13.2677	17.4494	29.9599	66.2118	237.3763

Table 10.2 Present Value of a Future Amount

	2%	3%	4%	5%	6%	7%	8%	9%	10%	12%	15%	20%
1	0.9804	0.9709	0.9615	0.9524	0.9434	0.9346	0.9259	0.9174	0.9091	0.8929	0.8696	0.8333
2	0.9612	0.9426	0.9246	0.9070	0.8900	0.8734	0.8573	0.8417	0.8264	0.7972	0.7561	0.6944
3	0.9423	0.9151	0.8890	0.8638	0.8396	0.8163	0.7938	0.7722	0.7513	0.7118	0.6575	0.5787
4	0.9238	0.8885	0.8548	0.8227	0.7921	0.7629	0.7350	0.7084	0.6830	0.6355	0.5718	0.4823
5	0.9057	0.8626	0.8219	0.7835	0.7473	0.7130	0.6806	0.6499	0.6209	0.5674	0.4972	0.4019
6	0.8880	0.8375	0.7903	0.7462	0.7050	0.6663	0.6302	0.5963	0.5645	0.5066	0.4323	0.3349
7	0.8706	0.8131	0.7599	0.7107	0.6651	0.6227	0.5835	0.5470	0.5132	0.4523	0.3759	0.2791
8	0.8535	0.7894	0.7307	0.6768	0.6274	0.5820	0.5403	0.5019	0.4665	0.4039	0.3269	0.2326
9	0.8368	0.7664	0.7026	0.6446	0.5919	0.5439	0.5002	0.4604	0.4241	0.3606	0.2843	0.1938
10	0.8203	0.7441	0.6756	0.6139	0.5584	0.5083	0.4632	0.4224	0.3855	0.3220	0.2472	0.1615
15	0.7430	0.6419	0.5553	0.4810	0.4173	0.3624	0.3152	0.2745	0.2394	0.1827	0.1229	0.0649
20	0.6730	0.5537	0.4564	0.3769	0.3118	0.2584	0.2145	0.1784	0.1486	0.1037	0.0611	0.0261
25	0.6095	0.4776	0.3751	0.2953	0.2330	0.1842	0.1460	0.1160	0.0923	0.0588	0.0304	0.0105
30	0.5521	0.4120	0.3083	0.2314	0.1741	0.1314	0.0994	0.0754	0.0573	0.0334	0.0151	0.0042

Present Value of a Future Dollar

The present value of a future amount is how much must be deposited today to have a given amount in the future, when compounded for a given number of periods at a given rate. This calculation is not used as much as the other calculations, but it is still important when planning future expenditures. To compute this amount, the first three of the four values are needed:

FV   future value, the amount in future dollars
i   interest rate, the compounding rate for each period
n   number of periods, number of compounding periods
PV   present value, the amount in today's dollars

Using Table 10.2, find the present value factor for the given interest and number of periods. Multiply the FV by the PVF to figure out the PV.

$$FV \times PVF = PV$$

Example Problem 1
A person wants to save $30,000 in 5 years for a down payment on a vacation home. How much should be deposited today to have $30,000 in 5 years? It is believed that 8% can be earned after taxes on the investment.

FV = $30,000
i = 8%
n = 5
PV = ??

Looking at the table, find the PVF at the intersection of 8% and 5 periods (0.6806). Multiply this PVF by the FV ($30,000) to find the PV ($20,418). That is to say, if a person deposits $20,418 in an account and earns 8%, after 5 years it will be worth $30,000.

Value of an Annuity

An annuity is a series of regular, periodic payments. When a person buys a car and sets up a loan, it is repaid as an annuity. If a savings plan is established in which a certain amount is set aside each month, an annuity has been established. Because an annuity compounds (i.e., earns interest on the interest earned) a table is needed to determine how much the annuity earns, or costs. Two annuity tables will be used. One determines how much a regular savings plan will be worth in the future. The other determines how much the payment on a loan will be.

Determining Payments

When a person repays loans as an annuity, the loans are usually compounded monthly. Table 10.3 determines a monthly payment based on compounding the interest monthly. If the interest is 12 percent per year compounded monthly, the actual interest rate is 12.68 percent (1 percent compounded monthly). This amount will be more than an annual compounding amount, but it is more accurate. (The tables have this conversion built into them.)

To compute the payment amount, the first three of the four values is needed:

PV   present value, the amount of the loan principal
i   interest rate, the annual interest rate charged on the loan
n   number of years, number of years you will pay on the loan
PMT payment, amount of the periodic payment

Use the table to determine the annuity monthly payment (AMP) factor for the loan's interest annual interest rate and term (number of years). Multiply the resulting AMP by the number of thousands of dollars of loan principal. Remember this is a monthly payment per $1,000 borrowed. Be sure to multiply by 12 for an annual amount.

$$PV / 1,000 \times APF = FV$$

Example Problem 1
A person is buying a new car. The price of the car is $28,000. A $2,000 down payment is made, and the loan is at 9% for 4 years. What is the monthly payment?

PV = $26,000 ($28,000 – $2,000)
i   = 9%
n   = 4
PMT = ??

Looking at the table, find the AMP at the intersection of 9% and 4 years ($24.89). Multiply this AMP by the number of thousands borrowed (Present Value/1000=26) to find the monthly payment amount $647.14 ($7,766 per year).

Example Problem 2
A person is buying a dental practice. The price of the practice $350,000. The entire amount will be financed. The loan is fixed at 10% for 7 years. What is the monthly payment for the practice?

PV = $350,000
i   = 10%
n   = 7
PMT = ??

Looking at the table, find the AMP at the intersection of 10% and 7 years ($16.60). Multiply this AMP by the number of thousands borrowed (Present Value/1000=350) to find the monthly payment amount $5,810 ($69,720 per year).

Table 10.3 Annuity Monthly Payment Factor

	2%	3%	4%	5%	6%	7%	8%	9%	10%	12%	15%	20%
1	84.24	84.69	85.15	85.61	86.07	86.53	86.99	87.45	87.92	88.85	90.26	92.63
2	42.54	42.98	43.42	43.87	44.32	44.77	45.23	45.68	46.14	47.07	48.49	50.90
3	28.64	29.08	29.52	29.97	30.42	30.88	31.34	31.80	32.27	33.21	34.67	37.16
4	21.70	22.13	22.58	23.03	23.49	23.95	24.41	24.89	25.36	26.33	27.83	30.43
5	17.53	17.97	18.42	18.87	19.33	19.80	20.28	20.76	21.25	22.24	23.79	26.49
6	14.75	15.19	15.65	16.10	16.57	17.05	17.53	18.03	18.53	19.55	21.15	23.95
7	12.77	13.21	13.67	14.13	14.61	15.09	15.59	16.09	16.60	17.65	19.30	22.21
8	11.28	11.73	12.19	12.66	13.14	13.63	14.14	14.65	15.17	16.25	17.95	20.95
9	10.13	10.58	11.04	11.52	12.01	12.51	13.02	13.54	14.08	15.18	16.92	20.03
10	9.20	9.66	10.12	10.61	11.10	11.61	12.13	12.67	13.22	14.35	16.13	19.33
15	6.44	6.91	7.40	7.91	8.44	8.99	9.56	10.14	10.75	12.00	14.00	17.55
20	5.06	5.55	6.06	6.60	7.16	7.75	8.36	9.00	9.65	11.01	13.17	16.99
25	4.24	4.74	5.28	5.85	6.44	7.07	7.72	8.39	9.09	10.53	12.81	16.78
30	3.70	4.22	4.77	5.37	6.00	6.65	7.34	8.05	8.78	10.29	12.64	16.71

Determining Savings

When a regular savings plan is established, an annuity is essentially being set up. A series of regular payments is made into an account. That account earns interest on the money deposited each period and earns interest on interest earned in the account.

To compute the payment amount, the first three of the four values is needed:

i   interest rate, the annual interest rate earned on the annuity

n   number of years, number of years you will pay into the annuity

PMT   payment, amount of the annual payment into the annuity

FV   future value, the future amount the annuity will be worth

Use Table 10.4 to determine the future value annuity (FVA) factor for the annuity's annual interest rate and term (number of years). Multiply the resulting FVA by the amount of the regular annual payment (in dollars).

$$PMT \times FVA = FV$$

Example Problem 1

A person is saving for a down payment on a vacation home. The home will be purchased in 5 years and can save $1000 per month. It is believed that 8% can be earned in the market (after taxes) on the investment. How much will the person have for a down payment in 5 years?

i   = 8%
n   = 5
PMT = $12,000 (this is $1,000 per month times 12 months)
FV   = ??

Looking at the table, find the FVA at the intersection of 8 percent and 5 years (5.867). Multiply this FVA by the annual payment amount ($12,000) to find the value of the annuity at the end of the time ($70,404).

Example Problem 2

A person is saving for retirement. He or she can put $15,000 per year into a tax-deferred retirement account, and he or she estimates earning 12% in the market on the investment. How much will have been accumulated in 30 years?

i   = 12%
n   = 30
PMT = $15,000
FV   = ??

Looking at the table, find the FVA at the intersection of 12% and 30 years (241.333). Multiply this FVA by the annual payment amount ($15,000) to find the value of the annuity at the end of the time ($3,619,995).

Example Problem 3

A person previously decided that he or she needed $216,732 in 20 years for a newborn daughter's college fund. If this person believes that 9% (after taxes) can be reasonably earned in the market, how much will need to be saved each year to fund the daughter's college savings fully?

i   = 9%
n   = 20
PMT   = ??
FV   = $216,732
PMT × FVA = FV
PMT   = FV/FVA

This problem is different in that the future value is known and the payment must be solved for. Looking at the table, find the FVA at the intersection of 9% and 20 years (51.161). Divide the FV ($216,732) by the FVA to figure out the annual savings needed ($4,236) to fund the plan fully.

Capital Budgeting

Capital assets are things that the practice owns that last for several to many years. Examples include dental chairs, computers, curing lights, and furniture. These long-term assets are usually purchased with a loan that last for a long time as well. In fact, most corporate finance officers try to match the term of the loan with the approximate expected lifetime of the asset. A person does not want to extend the term of the loan for a longer period than the useful lifetime. (No one wants to still be paying for a piece of equipment after it has been disposed of.) Capital assets are usually large, expensive pieces of equipment. The decisions about financing these assets carry a large price tag. So planning for the purchase of these assets becomes an important managerial function.

There are several reasons a person might make capital purchases in a dental practice. When buy an existing practice, the person buys the assets of the practice. These may be hard assets (such as dental equipment) and soft assets, such as goodwill and ongoing concern value. The equipment will need to be replaced in a practice periodically as older equipment wears out. A facility might need to be modernized as newer equipment and technology becomes available. An existing facility might need to be expanded. Each of these should be done with a definite plan and timetable for paying for them.

Asset Types

Supplies are things that the practice buys and uses up quickly, usually in less than a year. Assets are things

Table 10.4 Future Value Annuity

	2%	3%	4%	5%	6%	7%	8%	9%	10%	12%	15%	20%
1	1.000	1.000	1.000	1.000	1.000	1.000	1.000	1.000	1.000	1.000	1.000	1.000
2	2.020	2.030	2.040	2.050	2.060	2.070	2.080	2.090	2.100	2.120	2.150	2.200
3	3.060	3.091	3.122	3.153	3.184	3.215	3.246	3.278	3.310	3.374	3.473	3.640
4	4.122	4.184	4.246	4.310	4.375	4.440	4.506	4.573	4.641	4.779	4.993	5.368
5	5.204	5.309	5.416	5.526	5.637	5.751	5.867	5.985	6.105	6.353	6.742	7.442
6	6.308	6.468	6.633	6.802	6.975	7.153	7.336	7.523	7.716	8.115	8.754	9.930
7	7.434	7.662	7.898	8.142	8.394	8.654	8.923	9.200	9.487	10.089	11.067	12.916
8	8.583	8.892	9.214	9.549	9.897	10.260	10.637	11.028	11.436	12.300	13.727	16.499
9	9.755	10.159	10.583	11.027	11.491	11.978	12.488	13.021	13.579	14.776	16.786	20.799
10	10.950	11.464	12.006	12.578	13.181	13.816	14.487	15.193	15.937	17.549	20.304	25.959
15	17.293	18.599	20.024	21.579	23.276	25.129	27.152	29.361	31.772	37.280	47.580	72.035
20	24.297	26.870	29.778	33.066	36.786	40.995	45.762	51.160	57.275	72.052	102.444	186.688
25	32.030	36.459	41.646	47.727	54.865	63.249	73.106	84.701	98.347	133.334	212.793	471.981
30	40.568	47.575	56.085	66.439	79.058	94.461	113.283	136.308	164.494	241.333	434.745	1181.882

Table 10.5 Types of Assets

Asset	IRS Useful Lifetime	Economic Useful Lifetime (Estimated)
Hard Assets		
Furniture	7 years	10 years
Dental Equipment	7 years	15 years
Computers	5 years	6 years
Buildings	39 years	50 years
Leasehold Improvements	15 years	10–50 years
Soft Assets		
Goodwill	15 years	5 years
Covenant Not to Compete	15 years	2 years

Table 10.6 Matching the Term to the Type of Loan

Type of Debt	Term of Loan
Credit card debt	Immediate
Auto purchase	5 year max
Dental practice	5–7 years
Dental equipment	2–5 years
Dental building	20 years
Home mortgage	30 years
Education loans	30 years

the practice buys that last for more than a year (often many years). These assets are usually broken into soft and hard assets and are then further categorized by their expected useful lifetime (Table 10.5). Two types of "useful lifetimes" are used. The IRS declares a useful lifetime for tax purposes. This determination states how many years must be used in determining the tax depreciation for the asset. Economists are interested in establishing an "economic useful lifetime," which is an estimate of how long the asset is expected to serve its function for the business before it will need to be replaced. So although the IRS states a 7-year useful lifetime for a dental chair (meaning the chair can be depreciated in no fewer than 7 years), in fact, a dental chair should last for 15 to 20 years, if it is well cared for and well maintained. Its economic useful lifetime (for practice planning purposes) is probably 20 years.

Mortgage Types

A mortgage is an installment loan (a series of equal payments) secured by a hard asset that it has been used to purchase. As a rule of thumb, the payment for an asset should be extended over its useful lifetime. This keeps the cash need for the payment at the lowest possible amount.

The term of the loan then has a large impact on cash flow. Many corporate finance managers will match the term of the loan to the expected lifetime of the asset purchased. This allows the lowest safe cash requirements to pay off the loan before the asset completely depreciates, increasing how much cash is freed for other purposes. A person wants to be sure that the term of the loan is no longer than the lifetime of the asset so that he or she is not paying for the asset when it has no more value. Table 10.6 shows the typical term for loans for various types of assets.

Equipment Replacement Plan

If assets lasted forever (or entire professional lifetime), they would be purchased once and forgotten about. In fact, assets wear out from use. New and better equipment becomes available. Developments in the industry make some equipment obsolete. Other equipment continues to be useful. To prepare for large asset purchases, many practices budget a certain amount of income for equipment update and replacement. In this way, they can be assured of having modern methods and techniques available. Especially with the reliance on computers and software (which are expensive and have relatively short economic useful lifetimes of 3 to 7 years), an equipment replacement plan becomes a near necessity. During the practice payoff phase, most dentists spend from 8 to 10 percent of gross revenues on a loan payoff (capital and interest). Although not usually necessary in the mature practice, it is prudent to budget half this amount (1 to 2 percent of revenues) for replacing and updating equipment.

Borrowing Money

Almost every business borrows money to purchase equipment or expand facilities. The businesses usually pay this off through the process of loan amortization. This becomes a an important topic for financial mangers.

When a person borrows money and purchases a large asset (e.g., car, house, or dental practice) he or she owns the asset. It is titled in his or her name, which means that he or she must pay for upkeep and repairs and can (with certain restrictions) sell it whenever desired. The banker (or other lender) will file a lien with the county in which the asset resides. This is a legal document that says that the lender has an interest in the property (they have lent money to buy it) and it can not be sold until the loan is paid in full. If all payments are completed as agreed, then the lender will "release" the lien, so that the owner has no more restrictions. If a person wants to sell the asset while still owing money on it, then he or she must use the sale proceeds to satisfy the loan. The lender will then release the lien on the property.

Leverage

Financial leverage occurs when a person takes a loan, and then reinvests the proceeds with the intent to earn a greater rate of return than the cost of the loan (interest). That asset may generate money (a dental practice or piece of dental equipment) or may be sold later (real estate or other investment). If the rate of return on the assets purchased is higher than the rate of interest on the loan, then the return on equity will be higher than if it was not borrowed. However, if the return on the asset is lower than the interest rate, then the return on equity will be lower than if it was not borrowed. Leverage allows greater potential returns but greater potential losses to the investor. If the investment declines significantly or becomes worthless, the loan principal still needs to be paid to the lender.

Loan Security

A banker makes a "secured" loan when the borrower pledges, or promises, certain assets or things of value if the borrower defaults on the loan. An automobile loan is secured. If a person defaults on the loan, the lender can repossess the automobile, selling the car to satisfy the unpaid portion of the loan. Here, a person pledges the automobile as "collateral" for the loan. When the bank (or other lending agency) lends the money to purchase the automobile, they file a lien in the local courthouse. Therefore, the loan is secure, from their perspective. Unsecured loans have no assets pledged as collateral. These are obviously more risky loans for the banker, so they generally carry a higher interest rate. A "signature loan" is guaranteed only by a person's signature, guaranteeing to repay the loan. It is obviously in a person's best interest to repay it so that a he or she can borrow again with an unblemished credit history. The banker can still take that person to court to satisfy an unsecured loan, but if he or she has no assets (or have lost them all), the bank probably could not collect. A person may use signature loans to pay tax bills or other short-term obligations, if a person is short of immediate cash.

A loan may be secured in several ways. As previously mentioned, the borrower may pledge certain assets as collateral. This might include the car for a car loan, business assets for a practice loan, or stocks or investment accounts. A mortgage is a loan secured by a large fixed asset, such as a dental practice or a home. A cosigner can secure a loan by pledging specific assets (e.g., their house, stocks, or bonds) or may take on general obligation, by signing and personally guaranteeing that the borrower will pay the loan. (The banker will obviously investigate the cosigner carefully before doing this!) Young professionals may not qualify to borrow money by themselves but may gain financing if a parent or other relative cosigns the loan, often pledging specific assets. If the loan payment goes as planned, the cosigner has no cost from cosigning the loan. On the other hand, in the primary borrower defaults on the loan, the bank can (and generally will) institute legal proceeding to ensure payment from the cosigner.

Principal Amount

The principal of a loan is the amount borrowed. It is the value of the asset or property, less any down payment, with fees possibly added. A down payment is an amount of money that a person pays as an initial, upfront portion of the total amount due. It is usually given in cash at the time of completing the loan. The larger the down payment, the lower the amount financed. Bankers often require some loan value (often 10 to 25 percent) as a down payment. This does several things. It qualifies the person as having enough money to participate in the venture. It makes the person more interested in the success of the venture because he or she has some of money at stake in the deal. That person therefore has an interest in seeing that the asset remains in good repair and condition. It protects the banker, to a degree, from default. For example, assume a person has a 25 percent down payment. If the cost of the asset declines 10 percent and it is sold, the banker gets all of their money back. The 10 percent loss comes from the owner's portion. Because little of the initial payment goes to reducing principal, the asset can decrease in value faster than it is paid off, resulting in "negative equity," in which the borrower owes more than the asset is worth. (This is known as being "upside down" in the loan.) If the owner then tries to sell the asset, they must pay the difference ("bring money to the table") to sell. If the owner defaults ("walks away from the loan"), the value lost comes first from the owner (down payment) and then from the lender (borrowed capital). It protects the lender if the asset does not decrease in value more than the down payment.

Interest

Interest is the money that the borrower pays the lender for the privilege of using the principal. Interest is usually expressed as an annual percentage. This is then applied to the remaining loan principal to decide the interest

Table 10.7 Comparison of Term and Rate for a Loan*

		8%	9%	10%	11%	12%
5-year term	Annual payment	$24,332	$24,910	$25,496	$26,091	$26,693
	Monthly payment	$2,028	$2,076	$2,125	$2,174	$2,224
7-year term	Annual payment	$18,703	$19,307	$19,921	$20,547	$21,183
	Monthly payment	$1,559	$1,609	$1,660	$1,712	$1,765

*Principal = $100,000
The amount of the payment is related to both the term and the interest rate. The longer the term, lower the payments. The lower the interest rate, the lower the payment.

owed. Although the rate is expressed as an annual amount, it is usually compounded monthly. For example, a rate of 12 percent per year compounded monthly is the same as 1 percent per month. However, 1 percent compounded 12 times is actually 12.68 percent. The difference in these two rates applied to a $100,000 loan is more than $682 the first year.

An interest rate might be a fixed rate. This means that the percentage charged during the loan will remain fixed throughout the loan. If the borrower negotiates the loan for 6 percent, then 6 percent it will remain. Lenders have often lost money by charging fixed rates for their loans. For example, if a loan is at 4 percent fixed and the inflation rate climbs to 8 percent per year, the bank is losing money by lending it. If they could, instead, offer that loan to someone else, they would now get 8 percent, or twice the interest they are presently charging. To solve this problem, most lenders have some type of variable, or "floating," interest rate loans. In these type loans, the interest rate changes depending on some agreed on economic indicator. If the economic indicator rises, the loan's interest rate goes up. Conversely, if the indicator drops, the loan's rate decreases. This protects both the bank and the borrower (but especially the bank) from locking in unfavorable interest rates.

As a rule, banks use the "prime interest rate" in determining the specific variable rate for business loans. "Prime" is the rate charged by the biggest banks to their best customers (e.g., Ford, General Electric, etc.). The prime rate is published daily in the business press and in the business section of most metropolitan newspapers. The banks often charge an additional 1½ to 2 percentage points above prime for a new professional's loan. So if a loan is at prime +2, that person is paying two percentage points above the prime interest rate. The rate is usually recomputed monthly based on changes in the prime rate. There are often limits to the frequency of change or the amount of increase or decrease in the rate that can be applied.

Some banks and most mortgage lenders offer the choice of either a fixed or variable rate loan. The fixed rate loan usually carries a higher nominal interest rate, to protect the lender from the possibility of rising rates. All the loan factors, not just the interest rates, need to be considered if the bank offers a choice of fixed or variable rate loans (Table 10.7). What are the rates? How often are the variable rates adjusted? Are there maximum or minimum changes allowed? Are there different closing costs or other hidden cost of a particular loan? What is the estimate of the future economy? Will interest rates will be rising or falling soon? Does the higher fixed rate lead to unacceptable payment schedules?

Term of a Loan

The term of a loan is the number of payments required to pay off the loan principal under normal conditions and with no changes in any other loan factors. Most dental business (start up or buy out) loans have terms of 5 to 7 years.

There is a trade-off between the term of the loan and the amount of the payment. The longer the term (the greater the number of payments) the lower the regular payment, but the greater the total amount of interest paid. As a rule, a shorter term is desired, so that the loan will be paid off sooner. However, a person may not be able to afford the higher regular payment required of the shorter term loan and may need, instead, to lengthen the term of the loan to decrease the payment to a manageable amount. If a person has a large student debt load, some bankers will allow him or her to stretch the practice loan out to 10 years. This lowers the practice loan payment amount so that the person can meet all cash needs more easily. However, more in total interest cost is paid by using the longer term.

So the loan decision then is a balancing act between the interest rate and the term to keep the payment amount (cash flow) within the budget. Because interest rates are less negotiable, many people extend the term of the loan to get the payment down to a level that fits the budget. The problem with this approach is the higher cost of the debt through increased total interest payments. Table 10.8 shows the effect of interest rates and terms on a loan principal of $100,000.

Table 10.8 Amortization Schedule*

Year	Payment	Principal	Total Interest	Principal Remaining
1	$54,773	$9,773	$45,000	$490,227
2	$54,773	$10,653	$44,120	$479,574
3	$54,773	$11,612	$43,162	$467,962
4	$54,773	$12,657	$42,117	$455,306
5	$54,773	$13,796	$40,978	$441,510
6	$54,773	$15,037	$39,736	$426,473
7	$54,773	$16,391	$38,383	$410,082
8	$54,773	$17,866	$36,907	$392,216
9	$54,773	$19,474	$35,299	$372,742
10	$54,773	$21,226	$33,547	$351,516
11	$54,773	$23,137	$31,636	$328,379
12	$54,773	$25,219	$29,554	$303,160
13	$54,773	$27,489	$27,284	$275,671
14	$54,773	$29,963	$24,810	$245,708
15	$54,773	$32,659	$22,114	$213,049
16	$54,773	$35,599	$19,174	$177,450
17	$54,773	$38,803	$15,970	$138,647
18	$54,773	$42,295	$12,478	$96,352
19	$54,773	$46,102	$8,672	$50,251
20	$54,773	$50,251	$4,523	$0
	$1,095,465	**$500,000**	**$595,465**	**$119,093**

*Dr. Jones buys a house, securing a mortgage for the amount shown. Her annual payments are given. (This loan would actually be compounded monthly, but would be too large to show.)
Principal = $500,000
Term = 20 years
Rate = 9.0% per year
In this example, Dr. Jones pays a total, over the 20-year life of the loan, of $595,465 in interest, as well as the total principal of $500,000.

Payment Schedules

When the banker decides a loan, he or she will develop a schedule for the borrower to make payments. These payment schedules take any of several basic forms. There are, of course, hybrids and combinations of the basic forms. As a rule, borrowers must make monthly payments, unless specifically negotiated otherwise. If additional payments or payments that are larger than required by the loan contract are made, the extra amount *should* go toward the reducing the principal. Make certain in the negotiation that this is the case.

Amortization Schedule

A typical loan is paid off, or amortized, over time in a series of regular, equal payments, called *installments*. An amortization schedule shows these installments and the amounts that are allocated to principal and interest within each payment. (Table 10.9 is an example of an amortization schedule). Amortization schedules are usually done on a monthly basis. Because of space constraints, an annual reporting is shown.) The

Table 10.9 Example of Interest Only for First Year
Dr. Jones buys a dental practice, securing an installment note for the amount shown. She has an option to pay "interest only" during the first year. Her annual (estimated) payments are given. (This loan would actually be compounded monthly.)

Year	Total Payment	Principal	Interest	Principal Remaining
1	$27,000	$0	$27,000	$300,000
2	$77,128	$50,128	$27,000	$249,872
3	$77,128	$54,639	$22,489	$195,233
4	$77,128	$59,557	$17,571	$135,676
5	$77,128	$64,917	$12,211	$70,759
6	$77,128	$70,759	$6,368	$0
	$412,640	**$300,000**	**$112,639**	

"Normal Payment" Option

Year	Total Payment	Principal	Interest	Principal Remaining
1	$77,128	$50,128	$27,000	$249,872
2	$77,128	$54,639	$22,489	$195,233
3	$77,128	$59,557	$17,571	$135,676
4	$77,128	$64,917	$12,211	$70,759
5	$77,128	$70,759	$6,368	$0
	$385,640	**$300,000**	**$85,639**	

Principal = $300,000
Term = 1 year (Interest only)
     = 5 years (Normal schedule)
Rate = 9.0% (Interest-only option)

amortization schedule points out several important things. The interest portion of a business loan is deductible as a normal business expense in the year in which it occurs. During the initial payment portion of the loan, most of the payment satisfies the interest needs rather than principal. This creates a much larger tax benefit early in the amortization. As the borrower moves through the lifetime of the loan, a higher proportion of the payment is applied to the principal. The principal portion is not directly deductible. It is an asset that improves the balance sheet. The value of the asset can generally be deducted through depreciation. (To the extent that principal represents the value of the asset purchased, the entire cost of the loan then is deductible, either directly through the interest deduction or indirectly through depreciation of the asset.) Most depreciation methods load more of the depreciation expense earlier in the asset's lifetime. So tax deductions decrease while a loan is amortized, although cash flow remains steady.

Interest Only

Some loans require interest only payments for a certain period. Bankers often offer this to professionals and other new business owners. The bankers realize that it may take several months to get the business (or practice) up and running, producing enough cash to pay the bills and the start-up loan. To solve this problem, it can probably be negotiated to pay the interest portion of the normal payment for the first several months to a year. The person still eventually pay the entire principal, but the principal is put it off until the person is, hopefully, better able to afford the cash flow needed for the entire payment.

Balloon Payment

A second type of payment schedule is called a "balloon payment." In this schedule, the borrower pays the entire principal at the end of the loan period. Often the person must still pay interest monthly. Using a balloon payment allows the borrower to keep the payments as low as possible, although there is additional risk at the end of the term that the borrower cannot make the entire balloon payment.

Accelerating Debt Payments

As a rule, the faster debt is paid off, the less interest payments are made. Therefore, on the face of it, it is always a good thing to pay off debt as quickly as possible. However, there are several times when this rule of thumb may not be valid. A person may need to stretch a debt payment out to have adequate cash flow for other budget expenses. A person may have an incredibly low interest rate or generous terms on loans that make it attractive to keep.

A small additional payment makes a huge difference in the total loan payout. Table 10.10 shows what happens to the number of payments when the amount paid each month is increased. By simply adding $50 per month to a 10-year loan, the number of payments made is halved. (The principal paid remains the same, but it is paid more quickly and so less interest is paid.) Greater savings are seen with larger monthly additions. Most loans (especially mortgages) do not have any prepayment penalties associated with paying all or a portion of the principal off early. So if the cash flow will support it, a person can come out ahead, financially, by making an extra principal payment as often as possible.

Table 10.10 Accelerating Debt Payments
What effect does making a larger payment have on the length of the loan?
Principal=$100,000
Interest rate=9%
Term=10 years

		Additional Principal Payment			
		+$50	+$100	+$200	+$500
Normal payment	$1267	$1317	$1367	$1467	$1767
Years	10.0	9.4	8.9	8.0	6.2

Paying off Debt Early or Investing

From a purely financial standpoint, a person should compare after-tax interest rates of the loan and the investment. If the interest rate is higher for the investment, then invest rather than pay off the loan. If the after-tax interest rate of the loan is higher, then pay off the loan. There are several times when this rule does not apply. If a person needs to save for a particular purpose, then save (or invest) rather than pay off the loan. For example, if a person has adequate cash flow, he or she should establish an emergency fund, even if he or she has remaining debt on which payments are being made. A solid emergency fund is more important. He or she may be saving for a down payment on a house or other cash needs. Here the person may make the savings/investment rather than extra debt payments. Although many people have the admirable goal of being debt free, balancing the value of readily available cash asset and more debt with the position of no ready cash and less debt is more important. As a rule a person is better off with the available cash.

Lease–purchase Decisions

If a practice needs an asset (e.g., a piece of new equipment, office space, or an automobile), there are a couple of ways to pay for it. It may be purchased outright with existing cash. Money can be borrowed to buy the asset and then pay back the lender over time, or the asset can be leased, often with an option to purchase the asset at the end of the lease period. Each carries advantages and disadvantages.

If an asset is leased, the total cost of leasing is usually more than purchasing the same asset. The landlord or leasing company must borrow money, buy the asset, and then charge a higher interest rate for them to make a profit. If a person leases (or rents) the asset the entire lease payment is (with certain exceptions) a tax deduction. The person does not own the asset at the end of the lease (unless it is then purchased).

If money is borrowed to purchase the asset, the person owns the asset, but he or she also incurs a balancing liability (debt) to purchase the asset. The asset value may grow, remain the same, or decrease while the loan is being paid off. The cost of the interest for the loan is deductible. The cost of the asset is deducted through depreciation. If a person has enough cash to purchase the asset outright, he or she does not have any finance charges (interest) to pay, but he or she loses any investment gain that could have been made with the money. For example, assume a person can reasonably expect to make 10 percent after taxes on the investment, and a loan to buy the asset costs 6 percent after taxes. In this scenario, the person should borrow the money, earning the difference of 4 percent (10 − 6). If, on the other hand, is a person is earning 4 percent and a loan is at 10 percent, he or she is better off buying the asset outright and avoiding the finance charges.

Leasing by Asset Type

There are three common areas in dentistry where the lease-or-buy decision occurs. This section discusses each of those.

Automobiles

Leases and purchase loans are two different methods of automobile financing. Each has its own benefits and drawbacks, depending on the circumstances, wants, and needs. Loans finance the purchase of a vehicle. A person owns it and can drive it as many miles as desired, with only the cost of additional maintenance and wear and tear to consider. The loan is based on the interest rate negotiated, generally based on credit history. A person can sell the vehicle anytime for its depreciated resale value, taking the gain or loss.

A lease finances only the use of a vehicle for a specified time. In a sense, a person only pays for the portion of the cost of that he or she uses during the term of the lease. He or she pays a financial rate (the money factor or lease rate) that is similar to interest on a loan. It is generally a couple of percentage points higher than the prevailing rate, so that the leasing company can make a profit on the difference. Credit requirements for leasing (e.g., credit score) are somewhat more strict than for purchase loans because of higher risks to the financial company. At the end of the lease, the automobile can be returned to the leasing company or it can be purchased for its depreciated resale (residual) value.

For example, if a person leases a $30,000 car that has an estimated resale value of $20,000 after 24 months, he or she only pays for the difference, $10,000 (depreciation), finance charges, and fees. If, on the other hand, the same automobile was purchased, the person pays the entire $30,000, finance charges, and possible fees (Table 10.11). This is the reason that leasing offers much lower monthly payments than buying. Leasing does not build equity, buying does. Leasing has lower monthly payments but no equity. In the short term, a person is better off financially to lease. In the long term, a person is better off buying.

When an automobile is leased, there are several considerations. The person still pays for routine maintenance and any major repairs (such as wrecks) not covered by the automobile's warranty. (Therefore, insurance must be kept on the vehicle.) The lessee may have to make a down payment (an origination fee) and

Table 10.11 Leasing versus Borrowing for an Automobile
A person wants a $30,000 automobile. He or she can lease it for 3 years (7.5% money factor) with an $18,000 residual value or can purchase it at 6%.

	Lease	Loan
Car price	$30,000	$30,000
Down payment	$2,000	$2,000
Residual value	$18,000	N/A
Amount financed	$10,000	$28,000
Months	36	36
Interest rate	7.5%	6.0%
Monthly payment	**$311.06**	**$851.81**

other start-up costs for the lease. Leasing companies give a certain number of miles to the lease, for example, 2 years and 25,000 miles. That means that if a person drives more than 25,000 miles during the 2-year lease, he or she pays a hefty penalty (such as 20 cents per mile above 25,000 miles) when the lease ends. If a person drives less, he or she does not get a rebate. A lease can not generally be canceled early without substantial penalties. If the person does not like the car, too bad; he or she is stuck with it for the term of the lease. Even if a person's needs change or he or she decides the car is junk, unless the person is willing to pay substantial penalties, the car is his or hers for the term of the lease. New cars are generally the only ones leased. Automobiles that hold their value as used cars are better lease candidates than those that depreciate quickly. (The leasing company has less residual value to sell at the end of the lease with a quickly depreciating type of automobile.) A person can drive a nicer car for a smaller monthly payment than purchasing, although he or she has nothing at the end of the lease term. Despite leasing company hype, tax savings are the same for leasing or buying. The person has the option of buying the car at the end of the lease for the residual (remaining) value, but if that is what he or she wants to do that, simply buying the car from the beginning saves money. Dentists should buy or lease through the practice. (See the chapter on taxes for a discussion.)

There really are two situations in which a person should consider leases. If a person gets a new car every 2 or 3 years, then it is financially better to lease. This way, he or she always has an automobile under warranty and do not have to worry about buying and selling used cars. If a person plans to own the car for many years (or even run it until the "wheels fall off") then it is financially advantageous to buy. The other time when leasing may be an advantage is when a person simply can not afford the down payment or regular payments required of an automobile purchase. Here, a person can lease a better car for a lesser monthly payment. However, at the end of the lease, he or she does not have any equity and has to start over. The person never gets to the point when he or she does not have an automobile loan payment. Consider driving a less expensive type of car as an alternative.

Office Space

Many dentists lease office space. In this arrangement, the person or company that owns the property (lessee, landlord) sells the right to use the property (lease) to the tenant (lessee). In return, the lessee pays rent to the landlord. Leases have a term, or length associated with them, which may be one to many years. Although a short-terms lease allows a person to move at the end of the term, most dentists have trouble simply picking up the office and moving it because of equipment, plumbing, and other office design needs, and because patients get used to a particular location. So most dentists negotiate longer term leases (more years) often with options to renew. This also gives him or her a known future cash flow.

In theory, all lease arrangements are all negotiable. Mostly, negotiating power is based on the local market conditions. If there are many empty commercial properties similar to the one being negotiated, the lessee has more leverage. A tighter local market favors the landlords. Often with larger developments, landlords are reluctant to allow an individual lessee privileges, for fear that other lessees will ask for similar considerations. In the ideal world, a person will have two or more acceptable office spaces and can negotiate with each potential landlord over specific terms and items of the lease. In the real world, a person must be prepared to walk away if the landlord does not meet the bottom line terms.

When leasing office space, there are several common types of commercial lease arrangements. They are named based on how the landlord charges tenants. A gross lease is a property lease in which the lessee pays the landlord rent. The landlord then pays all expenses associated with the property, such as utilities, repairs, insurance, and (often) taxes. A net lease requires the lessee to pay some cost associated with the property. (The landlord only receives, as rent, the portion of the payment that is net of expenses.) Several versions of net leases exit, the most common being the triple net lease. In a triple net lease, the lessee pays rent to the landlord, all taxes, insurance, and maintenance expenses associated with the use of the property. The landlord then passes all expenses of ownership onto the lessees, protecting himself or herself (in part) from loses. Where there are several tenants in a property (such as an office building) the costs are usually prorated among the tenants based on square footage leased. In this type of lease, the rent amount will change as the landlord's taxes, insurance, and maintenance costs change (usually increase). One contentious issue is often heating and air-conditioning

repair or replacement. These can be large-ticket items that landlords often assign to tenants in net leases.

A person should check out the local market so that he or she can negotiate the lease amount effectively. They quote most leases on a dollar amount per square foot leased per year. For example, a landlord may quote a 2,000-square-foot office at $15.00 per square foot. This means that the lessee will be $30,000 per year (2,000 sq. ft. × $15.00) or $2,500 per month ($30,000/12 months) in rent. Most landlords want to include an annual price increase in the lease. If so, they should cap the increase so that the lessee will know how much will be paid in the future.

Tenant improvements are a large expense with most dental office leases. Those include interior walls, cabinets and counters, special plumbing (e.g., vacuum, compressed air, nitrous oxide, oxygen, etc.), special bracing for wall-mounted equipment and routine carpet, paint, and lighting. The cost of these improvements, even in a modest office can easily run into the hundreds of thousands of dollars. As a rule, the tenant pays for these "leasehold improvements." Often landlords will offer a modest amount of leasehold improvement cost in the lease term, not realizing the extent of the improvements needed to establish a dental office. (If a person is looking at a site that was a previous dental office, many of these improvements may have already been done.) A negotiation point may be to have the landlord provide some or all these improvements, writing their cost into the price of the lease. This saves a person form having to borrow money for improvements, taking their costs from capital and putting their cost instead into operating costs (the lease). This also allows the lessee to expense these costs over the term of the lease (say 5 years) instead of depreciating them over 15 years if he or she provides them. Dentists should note that if the lease is extended beyond the initial term that they have the cost of these improvements negotiated out of the cost of the ongoing lease.

Try to get the right to sublease the space written into the lease. If a person wants to leave, he or she can then lease the space to someone else for the duration of the contracted lease. (This gives the person more flexibility but is not a required term.) A person should be sure to check the ability to put up visible signs that identify his or her office. Many developments restrict the size or types of signs permitted by lessees. A person may also negotiate other terms, such as the lessee being the only dentist in the development, if that is an advantage.

An obvious finance issue for dentists then is when office space should be leased and when it should be bought or built. There are both financial and nonfinancial issues at work. From the financial perspective, purchasing is usually better than leasing, if the person stays in the same location for many (10 or more) years.

Mortgage payments are usually fixed over time, unlike lease payments. The person can depreciate the cost of the building and contents (but not land) over 39 years and deduct the cost of interest associated with office real estate. Although the entire cost of the lease is deductible, it may be more than the total cost of purchase. At the end of the time, with the purchase option, the person has an asset (the real estate) that can be sold, hopefully at a profit.

Other considerations relate less to financial tradeoffs. One is personal choice. Many dentists do not want the headaches of property ownership. Others want the control and independence associated with ownership. Especially young dentists may not have the financial resources needed to buy commercial real estate. Most banks will lend 75 to 90 percent of the appraised value of a property. The person must then come up with 10 to 25 percent as a down payment. If he or she can not, purchasing is simply not an option. Availability is always a question. There may not be acceptable properties for either rent or purchase when and where a person is looking. In larger cities, there may not be any acceptable property for sale. (Unless he or she buys an entire high rise office building!) Leasing is then the only alternative. With the purchase option, a person can find the right place and make changes to make it exactly what is desired. Especially with stand-alone dental offices, the eventual sale of the building and practice can be a problem. Because of the extensive remodeling, the building can only be used as a dental practice without a large expense. Selling a dental practice without the location lowers the value of the practice considerably.

If a person can not find a qualified buyer, he or she may be in the landlord business for a long while.

Office Equipment

Nearly half of all assets used by businesses today are leased. Dental practices lease equipment at a lower rate than general businesses. The decision whether to lease or buy is obviously one that astute business owners need to understand. There are both financial and nonfinancial reasons that a person might choose to lease or to buy assets for the practice.

There are several types of leases, depending on what is being leased. A property lease occurs when a property owner allows a tenant to use a property for a defined rent payment for a defined time. This does not occur often in dentistry (except office space leases). The entire lease payment is tax deductible, if the property is used for business purposes. An operating, or true lease, is similar to a property lease (the equipment is rented), except the person has an option to purchase the equipment at the end of the lease. (The minimum is 10 percent of the initial value and it must be a true option, not a requirement.) In operating leases, a person can deduct the full value of the lease payments but because he or she does not own the asset, he or she cannot claim depreciation on the asset. Maintenance, upkeep, and often taxes on the equipment must still be paid, although the asset is not owned. A financing, or capital lease is really a method of paying for an asset that is more closely akin to gaining a bank loan. In this arrangement, a leasing company buys the asset a person wants and

Table 10.12 Advantages and Disadvantages of Leasing Equipment Versus Purchasing Equipment

Option	Advantages	Disadvantages
Purchase		
	You own the asset	Asset may decrease in value
	Less expensive (long run)	Uses up free money
	Depreciation and interest expense	Uses up borrowing ability
	Shows on B/S	
Buy with cash	No finance charges	Lose alternative use of money
Borrow and buy	Uses leverage (other people's money)	Interest expense (finance charge)
		May require down payment
Lease		
	Lower monthly expense	More total expense
	No down payment	
Property lease	Occurs on P&L (not B/S)	You do not own the asset
	Less initial expense	You make leasehold improvements
Operating lease	Payment is deductible	You do not own the asset
	Occurs on P&L (not B/S)	
	Option to purchase (often)	
Capital lease	Appears on B/S (not P&L)	
	Depreciation and interest expense	
	May have favorable terms	

B/S, balance sheet; P&L, profit-and-loss statement

then leases it to him or her. Because the person owns the property, he or she can not claim the entire lease payment amount (only the interest portion) as a tax deduction. However, because he or she owns the asset, he or she gets to claim depreciation. There is no buy out option at the end of the lease because he or she already owns the asset. There are usually stiff prepayment penalties and even larger penalties if the person wants to break either of these leases.

Most equipment leases in dental practices are operating leases for specific pieces of equipment. Dental suppliers often have purchase or lease "deals" for the clients. They may offer no down payments, favorable interest rates, or other inducements for the dentist to purchase or lease the equipment. Dentists should look at the terms and conditions of any purchase or lease deal carefully. The suppliers recognize that few dentists go bankrupt. Still, remember that their business is to sell dental equipment.

Why should a person consider leasing equipment? He or she might already be deeply in debt and banks are not willing to lend that person more money. Leasing companies will often offer more flexible terms (e.g., graduated payments) than banks. Although lease contracts are more flexible, they are also more complex, so there can be more hidden pitfalls. A person may not have money for a down payment (often 20 percent or more of the price) required by a bank. Or he or she may have the money but want to hold it as a cushion in case it is needed in the future. A lease does not show up on a credit report or balance sheet as a loan does. The payment is taken from operating capital, so if a person is profitable but highly in debt, a lease may be a good option. Finally, some aggressive tax strategies involving putting business property (real estate or equipment) in family partnerships and then leasing it back to shift income into family members' lower tax brackets (Table 10.12).

Business Taxes and Tax Planning

Over and over again courts have said that there is nothing sinister in so arranging one's affairs so as to keep taxes as low as possible. Everybody does it, rich or poor, and all do right, for nobody owes any public duty to pay more than the law demands; taxes are enforced exactions, not voluntary contributions. To demand more in the name of morals is mere can't.

Justice Learned Hand
U.S. Supreme Court, 1947

Objectives

At the completion of this chapter, the student will be able to:
1. Differentiate between a tax deduction and a tax credit.
2. Describe depreciation as applied to a practice.
3. Differentiate between deductible and nondeductible expenses for operating a dental practice.
4. Discuss business taxes that impact a dental practice.
5. Apply the basic principles of tax planning to the dental practice.
6. Discuss the effect of the business entity on tax obligations.

Key Terms

ad valorem taxes
amortization
automobile expenses
barter
capital asset
capital gain
capital loss
cash basis accounting
casual labor
Circular E
commission
deductible expenses
depreciation
depreciation recapture rules
disposable asset
employee benefit programs
Employer Identification Number (EIN)
federal income taxes
Federal Insurance

Contributions Act (FICA; Social Security)
Federal Unemployment Insurance Act (FUTA)
flow-through entity
Form 1120: The Corporate Income Tax Form
Form W-2: Wage and Tax Statement
Form W-4: Employees Withholding Allowance Certification
governmental mandates
gross receipts
I-9: Employment Eligibility Verification
income
interest/dividend income
land
legal and professional

expenses
local income (occupational) taxes
marginal tax rates
meals and entertainment
office expenses
ordinary income
pension plan contributions
returns and allowances
Schedule "C"
state income taxes
state sales and usage taxes
State Unemployment Insurance Act (SUTA)
unwithheld expenses
unwithheld expenses for the employer
workers' compensation insurance

Business Basics for Dentists, First Edition. David O. Willis.
© 2013 John Wiley & Sons, Inc. Published 2013 by John Wiley & Sons, Inc.

Goal

This chapter will cover tax obligations of the business owner. The methods and timing of tax compliance will be discussed, as well as the various methods that the business owner can use to minimize the tax burden and potential problems with taxing agencies.

This chapter presents the common taxes that businesses pay. Depending on the type of business entity that established, it will be reported to the government differently. The basic tax principles remain the same, regardless the entity. Income and deduction are reported, equipment depreciated, and employer-related taxes are paid. An accountant will complete forms and do other paperwork for the business owner. However, the business owner should understand the principles so that he or she can communicate effectively with an accountant and other advisors.

In this chapter only federal taxes are discussed. Many states and municipalities have similar, additional taxes if a person practices in their jurisdiction. These taxes also follow the same principles outlined here. The specific implementation of those principles and rules may differ. An accountant will help with these taxes as well.

Principles of Business Taxation

The principles of business tax planning remain the same from year to year. Specific rules, amounts, and thresholds change constantly. Some are pegged to the inflation rate. Congress changes others as they attempt to affect social policy and the economy. If the principles are understood, changes in specifics will make much more sense and will be easier for a person to use to his or her advantage.

Income

The IRS has a simple rule concerning whether money made is "income" or not for tax purposes. They consider any money made to be taxable income unless they have made a specific waiver for that specific type of income in the tax codes. By this definition, almost any income gained by the dental practice is taxable. This includes collections from patient payments, money paid by insurance companies, capitation payments, interest or dividends earned, the gain from sale of assets owned by the practice, the value of trade or barter, and rebates. (This does not include money that the practice borrows.)

Some business entities (C corporations) pay income tax on any profits in the business at the end of the tax year. Others (proprietorships, partnerships, S Corps, and limited liability companies [LLCs]) do not pay income tax, but let income and deductions flow through to the individual owners. These flow-through entities report to the IRS who received the profits for the year. The IRS then checks to be sure that the individual has claimed the right amount of income on his or her individual tax return.

After the practice pays for the costs of doing business, the money goes to the owner or employee of the business. The owner or employee then pays individual income tax on it. This includes profit from a proprietorship or partnership (self-employment income), wages paid from an employer (proprietor or corporation), bonuses paid, profit sharing, and sometimes excessive employee benefits. An individual must decide the type of income that is paid because the IRS taxes it all differently. Ordinary income is the same as earned income. This money is made by working. Income and self-employment (SETA) taxes are paid on earned income. Investment income (e.g., capital gains, interest, or dividends) are called unearned income. The IRS taxes it at a lower rate. Because it was not earned, Social Security or Medicare (or SETA) tax is not owed on this type of income. Tax laws and rates change frequently at the whim of Congress, specific rates will not be detailed in this text. Dentists should check with an accountant for the current tax rates.

Most dental practices fall under the cash basis accounting rules. This means that a person realizes income when he or she takes constructive receipt of it. Therefore, a person only pays tax when he or she has control of income and can use it for whatever purpose desired. For example, assume a patient has a bill for $1200. They pay $800 on December 31 of the year X1, and the remainder ($400) on January 2 of year X2. The dentist pays tax on $800 of income in year X1 and pays tax on $400 in the year X2, the year it was constructively received. By this definition, a person pays no income taxes on accounts receivable because they are not income to until patients pay them. (It is not income until the check crosses the receptionist's desk.) A few large practices use accrual-based accounting rules. However, these rules cause income and expense recognition problems that do not favor the practice.

If a person sells a practice, or a component of the practice (such as dental operatory equipment), he or she receives money for the asset(s). The IRS calls this money either a capital gain or ordinary income, depending on the circumstances. The difference is important because different tax is paid on the two types of income. This leads to some obvious tax-planning issues. These are covered in different chapters of this text.

Business Deductions

A deduction is an expense that is a cost of operating or maintaining the practice. A person may need to prove the amount and necessity of this business expense to the IRS, so he or she should keep a receipt and canceled check for the item. The IRS may also require that the person prove the other criteria listed previously, so he or she should be sure to keep excellent records. Canceled checks, by themselves, are not enough documentation.

The IRS considers no expense to be deductible unless they have specifically granted deductibility in the tax codes. For a business expense to be deductible, it must meet *all* of the following criteria:

1. It must be "**ordinary**," which means that it is common to other taxpayers in similar situations.
2. It must be "**necessary**," which means that it is helpful in the conduct of a trade or business.
3. It must be "**reasonable in amount**," which means that any other taxpayer would pay a similar amount for a similar good or service.
4. It is *not* a **personal** expense (separate business from personal expenses).
5. It is *not* a **capital** expenditure (accounted for as depreciation.)
6. It does *not* relate to **tax-exempt income**.

The IRS expects everyone to follow these rules for deductions when they file their income tax for the year. However, the only way the IRS knows for sure that a person has followed th rules is if the IRS audits that person and finds a problem. Therefore, many taxpayers take a risk, get away with breaking the tax rules, and do not get caught. This is a risky practice. If the IRS catches that person, there are substantial fines, penalties, and interest payments. He or she might even receive a prison sentence for gross or willful tax cheating. The IRS recently increased the audit rate on high income individuals (such as dentists) decreasing the chance of getting away with breaking the law.

There are several points to consider about deductions:

- Expenses in getting to be a practicing dentist (or any other *new* occupation) are not deductible. Therefore, expenses for dental education and first state board exam are not deductible. The IRS considers a specialty to be a new occupation, so those expenses are not deductible. (Dentists frequently challenge this point in the tax courts.) The costs associated with setting up a practice are deductible.
- Expenses incurred for maintaining an occupation or profession are a required expense of doing business and are, therefore deductible. Relicensure fees, continuing

Table 11.1 Assets and their Lifetime

Useful Lifetime	Asset
Dental building	39 years
Leasehold construction	15 years
Office equipment	7 years
Office computers	5 years
Professional books	7 years
Office furniture	7 years
Automobiles	5 years
Any intangible asset	15 years

education expenses, dues, professional books, and publications are all deductible, once a person is a practicing dentist. He or she may deduct the costs of taking another licensing exam, after an initial license is earned.
- Business loan payments are not directly deductible. The interest paid on a business loan is a cost of business and therefore deductible. The principal portion of the loan payment represents a long-term asset. The value of the asset itself is deducted indirectly through depreciation.
- It never pays to incur an expense simply to "get a deduction." If it is an expense a person would take anyway, then that expense should be structured so it is deductible.
- The first step in maximizing deductions is to learn which items are deductible, so as not to miss one or more authorized deductions. Examples of deductible and nondeductible expenses for the dental office are given in Table 11.1.
- The marginal tax rate influences the value of a deduction. A $1,000 deduction in the 15-percent marginal tax bracket translates into a $150 tax savings. Conversely, the expense only "costs" a person $850 (1,000 − 150) instead of the full $1,000. That same deduction in a 28-percent marginal tax bracket translates into a $280 savings.
- When establishing a checkbook register, a person should be sure to establish categories that are the same as appear on Schedule C. This makes tax time much easier in that he or she does not need to go back over all receipts and categorize them for tax purposes. They have already been allocated to proper categories and the year-end totals are used.

Capital Assets and Depreciation

Some business purchases are assets that last for several years. These are considered "capital" assets of the business. As an example, a dental chair should last for several years, and a building for many years. Tax law says that because those capital assets have a lifetime greater than 1 year, the deduction for the expense of that item must be spread out over the estimated "useful lifetime" of the asset. (The IRS has a list that tells what the useful lifetime of most assets is.) If the IRS says that a dental chair should last 7 years, then logically one-seventh of the value of the dental chair should be deducted each year. Another way to think of depreciation is wear and tear on long-term assets. By this definition, the dental chair "wears out" over its useful lifetime of 7 years. It is written off over the same period.

Depreciation is the term used for hard, tangible assets. Intangible assets may also have a useful lifetime or wear out over time. A restrictive covenant that lasts for 3 years has a 3-year lifetime. *Amortization* refers to depreciation of these intangible assets. The idea is the same as depreciation. *Depletion* is similarly used for natural resources, such as timber or coal deposits.

Some points to consider about depreciation:

- Depreciation Form 4562 is the form by which the cost of assets that have a life span is deducted. This deduction starts the tax year the asset is placed into business service and occurs each year after that according to the depreciation law in effect in the first year. The IRS allows several accounting methods to set depreciation (wear and tear) on an asset. These methods include:
  1. Straight line
  2. Double (200%) declining balance
  3. Modified accelerated cost recovery system (MACRS)
- As a rule, the alternative methods (2 and 3) speed up the deduction for depreciation over the straight-line method (1). A person gets a larger portion of the depreciation in early years, less in later years with these accelerated methods. A person does not need to know how to calculate these amounts, just that several methods exist that generally speed up the deduction.
- A person should discuss with his or her accountant whether or not to speed up depreciation deductions. The MACRS method loads the deductions much more heavily on the front end. That is fine if a person estimates that his or her income will be steady over the next several years. That person will gain more of the tax saving immediately. However, if income will be significantly higher in the future (as, for example with practice growth), he or she may want to defer those depreciation deductions until he or she is in a higher tax bracket, thereby getting more "bang" for the depreciation expense. In the straight-line method, the person is trading off the certainty of an immediate deduction for the possible higher value of a future deduction. That person might find that later in the asset's life, he or

she has a cash flow problem. He or she is still paying for the loan for the asset (primarily principal) although he or she has used all of the depreciation deduction for the asset.

- When a person puts an asset into service during the year affects how much depreciation that can be deducted in the first year. If an asset is bought in January, he or she gets to claim much more of a full deduction than if it is bought in December. The IRS also has several methods for calculating this amount. An accountant will do that. A business owner needs to be aware that he or she may not receive the entire deduction the first year when buying a large asset.
- Disposable assets (those used up within 1 year, such as dental supplies) are a deduction in the year purchased.
- Land does not "wear out" over time, so it can not be depreciated. Buildings do wear out over time. If a building and land are purchased, the appropriate percentages of the cost to each must be allocated, depreciating the building but not the land.
- A person may depreciate any piece of equipment that is purchased, even if it is used and someone else has already depreciated it. It is essentially "new" to that person and has a new useful lifetime for him or her. An asset may be depreciated as often as it is bought. The sale price determines how much depreciation can be claimed. The previous owner is subject to capital gain or loss, and recapture.
- If a person sells an asset that he or she has previously depreciated, he or she might be subject to "recapture" rules, which means that the person must recapture as income any previously reported depreciation. For example, if a dentist bought a dental chair for $7,000, then depreciated it (straight line) for 3 years of its 7-year life, he or she is telling the IRS that the chair is now worth $4,000 ($7,000 − 3 years × 1/7 × $7,000). If that person sells that same chair for $5,000, he or she has made a book profit, or "capital gain" of $1,000 ($5,000 − $4,000). This person *must* "recapture" this depreciation expense and claim the gain on a capital investment as ordinary income, which is a higher tax rate than a capital gain. This happens frequently in practice sales, where the seller has fully depreciated the assets of the practice.
- As a rule, any "high-tech" equipment for the dental office (computers, lasers, etc.) are 5-year properties. Other dental equipment (chair, compressor, etc.) are 7-year properties. There is some capital equipment that does not fall neatly into these categories (Box 11.1).
- Congress has enacted special tax rules to encourage small businesses to purchase assets. These rules allow a small business to immediately expense (take the value in year 1) the value of assets instead of claiming the value over several years through normal depreciation. (This is the "179 Election" because it

Box 11.1 Examples of Deductible and Nondeductible Expenses

Deductible Expenses	Nondeductible Expenses

Deductible Expenses
1. Lease payments
2. Professional supplies
3. Office supplies
4. Stamps
5. Stationary
6. Printing costs
7. Advertising
8. Phone bills (utilities)
9. Lab bills
10. Malpractice insurance
11. All employee wages, taxes, workmen's compensation, and unemployment insurance
12. Office insurance policy
13. Continuing education
    a. Registration
    b. Travel
    c. Room and board
14. Office taxes
15. Mileage from office to lab, office to post office, office to buy office supplies and back.
16. Interest on office loan
17. Depreciation
18. Collection costs
19. Relicensure fees
20. Magazine subscriptions

Nondeductible Expenses
1. Loan payments
2. Mileage to office from home
3. Cost of land
4. Disability insurance premiums paid
5. Amounts you fail to collect from patients
6. Personal draw

refers to that section of the tax code.) According to these rules, a person may elect to expense (take in year 1) the deduction for up to $100,000 worth of depreciable assets. This election can be an advantage for the small business person if he or she wants to increase current deductions, at the expense of future ones. That person may elect to deduct 0 to 100 percent of the allowable amount in year 1 of the asset and depreciate the balance. However, early in your practice life, a person may find it more advantageous to push those depreciation deductions into later years, when a larger dollar deduction is claimed. Congress changes the rules on this deduction annually.

- Depreciation is a "noncash" write-off. This means that a person never writes a check that lists "depreciation" as the payee. Yet the expense for depreciation is claimed on an income statement. The person has taken the expense write-off, but not paid any cash. This leads to differences in the income statement and cash flow statement.
- If a person uses an asset for both personal and business use (such as an automobile), he or she must allocate the proportion that it is used for business. A person may then take as depreciation the portion that it is used for business.

Tax Credits

Tax credits are similar to deductions, but they are even more valuable. A deduction lowers income, and by that, lowers tax. A tax credit is a dollar for dollar reduction in tax.

For dental practitioners, presently the biggest potential tax credit is for installation of equipment that allows a business to comply with the Americans with Disabilities Act. The law does not apply to new building and requires that the equipment purchased be "reasonable and necessary" to comply. The credit amount is currently 50 percent of eligible expenses that are more than $250 and less than $10,250. This works out to a $5,000 maximum credit. The IRS is still debating what is necessary for compliance and what is for the benefit of the dentist. Widening hallways and making restrooms wheelchair accessible clearly qualify. Buying a new digital radiography unit so that visually impaired patients can see radiographs better is more problematic. Tax credits change constantly as the profession and the IRS work out definitions. A pass-through entity allows the tax credits to flow through to the individual tax return. This is usually an advantage because the credit is not as valuable at the entity level.

Nonincome Taxes (Mandates)

Governmental agencies also require business owners to comply with regulations written and enforced by the governing body. These mandates result in a hidden tax in that a business person must respond to. A common present example is the Occupational Safety and Health Administration (OSHA), which requires that dentists (and other businesses) meet certain safety standards regarding the operation of the workplace. The business owner must finance the cost of these mandates, although no true "tax" has been levied or paid. The cost of these mandates can be significant.

The Basic Business Income Tax Formula

The general business formula for determining profit or loss is the basis for Schedule C, partnership, or corporate income tax returns (Box 11.2). The prototype, Schedule C, is the tax form that the individual proprietor uses to report profit or loss from operating a business, such as a dental practice. If a person practices as a partnership or a corporation, this information is reported on a different form, but it contains similar information. Only income and expenses relating to this particular business should appear on this schedule. If a person has more than one business, he or she will file a different form for each of them. (Multiple dental office locations are generally considered one business.)

1. **Gross Receipts**   This is the actual amount of money collected by the practice because most dentists use a cash basis accounting. (If a dentist uses an accrual basis, this number must be adjusted.) This is not how much dentistry a person produced, but how much was collected as cash, patient checks, insurance checks, and capitation payments.
2. **Returns and Allowances**   If a person refunds money to an individual or third-party payer (for an overpayment), it should be recorded as a "Return." He or she has already received this money and accounted for it as a gross receipt. In this section, it is taken back off, if the situation warrants.

Box 11.2 Income Tax Formula

Gross Receipts
 – Returns and Allowances
 – Cost of Goods Sold and/or Operations
Gross Income
 – Deductions
Profit or (Loss)

---

3. **Cost of Goods Sold**   This section is for businesses that have an inventory base (such as a dress shop). Most dentists do not have a significant inventory or work in process, so they do not worry about this section. If a dentist sells a significant amount of a product, such as toothbrushes or nutritional supplements, he or she probably qualifies and must include this section. Some accountants will include dental laboratory costs or dental supplies in this category, calling a dental prosthesis a product as opposed to a service. Others will record these costs under the "Other Costs" section of the form. It really does not matter where they are placed, as long as they are somewhere in the expense list.
4. **Gross Income**   Gross income is gross receipts adjusted for any returns and cost of goods sold.
5. **Deductions**   Deductions are costs of doing business. (Definitions of valid deductions are given later in this chapter.) Deductions are expenses for supplies and equipment that a person will use up within a year. If the items will last longer than that, they are depreciated.
6. **Profit or (Loss)**   This is simply how much is left after a person collects fees and then pays the costs of running the business this year. If collections are greater than expenses, the result is a profit. If expenses are greater than collection, then the result is a loss. The IRS has rules to be sure that a person is trying to make a successful business, not merely using a hobby to take tax-deductible expenses. These "hobby loss rules" presume an enterprise is for profit if it makes a profit in at least 3 of the last 5 tax years, including the current year. There is some latitude for start-ups and other business conditions.

Employer Taxes

A business owner will probably hire employees. (In fact, 98 percent of practicing dentists have one or more employees.) If a person hires employees, he or she has another area of tax with which to be concerned. These are the employer taxes. An employer must withhold tax from each employee's check, report the amount to the employee, and then send this withheld amount to the appropriate agency. The chapter on staff compensation details these taxes. The responsibilities as an employer are listed here (Box 11.3). As before, an accountant or bookkeeper will help a business owner establish systems to pay and account for these taxes.

Obtain and Use Employer Identification Number

If a person has employees, he or she must obtain, by application, an Employer Identification Numbers (EIN). There is one for federal and others for state and local

---

Box 11.3 Responsibilities as an Employer

1. Use Employer Identification Number (EIN)
2. Verify that the employee can legally work in the United States
3. Withhold income taxes from employee paychecks
4. Withhold FICA (Social Security and Medicare) taxes from employee paychecks
5. Match FICA (Social Security and Medicare) taxes
6. Report wage and withholding information to employee
7. Report and pay withheld amounts to government

tax reporting. (A federal number is usually allowed to be used for all. Check the rules in each locality.) Once a person has an EIN, the taxing agency will automatically send yearly instructions, rates, forms, and tables. This number is used when paying and reporting employer taxes.

Verify Employee Eligibility to Work

An employer can not hire individuals who are not authorized to work in the United States. So he or she must verify an employee's immigration status. An IRS form (I-9) that the employer and the employee complete verifies the employee's status. This must be done after the person is employed.

Withhold Income Taxes from Employees' Paychecks

A business owner must withhold a certain portion of income from each employee's check. This money is then sent to the government monthly. At the end of the year, each employee computes their actual tax liability and compares it to the amount withheld along the way. If an employer withheld too much, the employee gets a refund. If an employer did not withhold enough, the employee has to pay the difference. The IRS has charts to use when calculating withholdings. If state or local government imposes income taxes, they also provide tables and forms to use.

Withhold FICA Tax from Employees' Paychecks

Social Security and Medicare taxes are employment taxes (tax on earned income) to fund these federal programs. This tax is also withheld from employees' pay,

similarly to the income tax. Presently, the tax is a flat amount (7.65 percent).

Match FICA Taxes

An employer must match the tax withheld with an equal amount from the practice. Presently, the total tax is about 15.3 percent (7.65 percent from the employee and 7.65 percent from the employer) for most employees.

Report Wage and Withholding Information to Employee

Employers must report earnings and the amount of tax they withheld to each employee (or former employee) by February 1 of the following year. This report (Form W-2) details the employee's earnings and the amounts withheld for the previous year so that he or she can accurately complete personal tax returns. The employer sends a copy to the government so the government can check to be sure the employee claims the proper amount. State and local taxing agencies have similar forms.

Report and Pay Withheld Amounts to Governmental Agencies

The employer pays the federal government the income taxes that he or she withheld from employees' paychecks. The payment frequency depends on size of withholding (federal+FICA). Most dentists make these payments monthly online at a special federal tax payment Web site. The IRS electronically debits (takes) this money from a business checking account. The IRS levies significant penalties if an employer misses a payment or filing date, even by 1 day. State and local governments have their own procedures for reporting and paying employee withholdings, so check with an accountant about setting up these payment mechanisms.

Unwithheld Expenses for the Employer

Four items cost the employer money beyond wages for each employee. Legally, an employer may not withhold money from employees' check to pay for these costs. Therefore, they are called "unwithheld."

Workers' Compensation Insurance

An employer must have this insurance before any employees are hired. The employer gets the insurance policy from a private carrier, paying an annual premium.

These insurers must register with the state. The insurance covers job-related accidents and illnesses.

State Unemployment Insurance (SUTA)

SUTA is the state unemployment insurance program. This is a really a tax, although it also has some characteristics of insurance. Unemployment insurance is a federal program, but it is run by the state. So SUTA and FUTA are coordinated programs. The state portion of this program requires quarterly reporting and payment. Typical rates are 1.7 to 2.7 percent of gross wages (first $8,000 per employee).

Federal Unemployment Insurance (FUTA)

An employer reports and pays FUTA taxes separately from FICA, Medicare, and withheld income taxes. An employer must pay FUTA from the practice and may not withhold it from employees' pay. This program requires annual reporting and payment or quarterly when the amount exceeds $1,000. The typical amount is 0.8 percent of first $7,000 per employee, although it depends, to a degree on how much an employer pays in the state program.

Matching Portion of Social Security and Medicare Tax

As described previously, an employer withholds a portion (currently 7.65 percent) from employees' pay for Social Security and Medicare tax. An employer must also match that with an equal amount. The matching portion is unwithheld.

Miscellaneous Hiring Issues

There are several miscellaneous issues regarding hiring and employee taxes.

Commission

An employer may use a commission as a basis for pay but only with dentists and hygienists (professional staff). If the dentist is an independent contractor, report to the IRS income paid by the employer to them. This special form (1099-MISC) is sent to both the IRS and the independent contractor. The payee must file a Schedule C or otherwise account for income and self-employment taxes. If the employee has "employee" status, then the

dentist withholds and reports commission employees as other pay methods.

Temporary Services

People contract temporary services through a temporary placement agency. The temporary worker is under contract to the temporary agency, not the employer. As such, no one requires an employer to withhold taxes, match FICA, retirement plan participation, or be responsible for any of the other unwithheld expense normally associated with employees. If an employer uses someone long term (i.e., staff leasing), then the IRS views that person as a bona fide employee and the rules change.

Hiring a Spouse or Child

An employer can hire a spouse or child to work in the office. The employer gains certain tax advantages by doing this. The rules are different for spouses and children. To deduct the expenses for hiring a close relative (spouse or child), the employer must meet the following four tests:

1. The service must be ordinary and necessary for the business operation.
2. The fee charges must be reasonable, or similar, to what other dentists would pay for comparable services.
3. The payment must be for services actually performed. If the services were not done, or were done by someone else, the employer may not deduct the payment.
4. The money must be paid. That means that the employer must write a check and the relative must cash it.

If an employer hires a spouse, he or she can deduct the full cost of reasonable wages. These wages are subject to FICA taxes (if the employer is a corporation or partnership), which makes the spouse eligible for Social Security benefits for which they might otherwise not qualify. (Unincorporated doctors do not pay FICA taxes on spouse or children.) The spouse is also eligible for employee benefit plans offered through the office. This way, an employer may take the full deduction for medical insurance premiums paid for the family. These wages are subject to all applicable income taxes. So an employer must do full withholding, just as if the relative were a normal employee.

If an employer hires a child, the employer gain more tax advantage. The salary or wage paid to a child is earned income and therefore not subject to the rules that apply to children younger than age 14 (the "Kiddie

Tax.") For earned income, the maximum standard deduction available to a child is currently about $5,000. Therefore, if an employer pays a child $5,000 in compensation, the standard deduction eliminates all tax on the income. The child is also eligible for benefit plans and retirement plans offered through the office. The child may also make a contribution to an IRA of the lesser of $5,000 or earned income. Combining the IRA and standard deduction allows the child to earn up to $10,000 and pay no tax.

It does still pay to employ family members in certain cases. The employer can shift some income from taxable income to the children's (presumably lower) taxable income, savings significant amounts of taxes. Depending on the employment status of the spouse and the office retirement fund, an employer might shelter additional income in a tax-deferred retirement fund by hiring his or her spouse.

Other Business Taxes

Some areas have a couple of other business taxes.

State Sales and Usage Tax (Sales Tax)

This is a sales tax. Some states require vendors to charge sales tax on all services (including dentistry). Others require that an employer pays this type of tax on any items purchased from out-of-state vendors. Because in-state purchases have already had sales taxes paid, they include only purchases from out-of-state vendors. Examples of items that are taxable if purchased from an out-of-state vendor include dental supplies, lab bills (materials only), printing services, and magazine subscriptions.

Ad Valorem Taxes

These are property taxes on the assets of the business. Generally local taxing agencies levy them. As a rule, these are paid yearly. Depending on the particular jurisdiction, assets may include financial items such as accounts receivable, and "hard" assets of the practice such as dental equipment.

Effect of Business Entity

Depending on the business entity, an employer will pay and account for taxes differently. The total tax liability is generally the same. The difference is in whose name they are paid.

Proprietorship

If a person is a proprietorship, he or she is the business. He or she pays all employee taxes under his or her name and EIN. He or she pays any property or other taxes under his or her name as well. Because the employer is not an employee, the proprietorship does not withhold income taxes. Instead, the owner estimates his or her tax liability and prepays it quarterly to the IRS. A Schedule C is filed with personal Form 1040 to report profit from the practice as income. He or she pays SETA on earned income. Losses pass down to the owner personally and offset other forms of income.

Partnership

If an owner is a partnership, he or she reports and pays employee taxes under the partnership's EIN. Like a proprietorship, the person estimates and prepays personal income taxes. The partnership will provide an information return to the IRS that details how much each partners should report for income and expenses related to the business. The owner pays SETA on earned income and losses flow through to his or her personal return.

Corporation

A corporation is a separate tax entity. Employee taxes are reported and paid under the corporation's EIN. The person is an employee of the corporation. Therefore, the corporation withholds tax from his or her paycheck according to Circular E, similarly to all other employees of the practice. The corporation withholds Social Security and Medicare taxes and matches them, like other employees. The corporation then issues a W-2 at the end of the year that details how much was earned. If a person is an owner of the corporation, he or she may receive dividends from the profit of the corporation. This is unearned income (not subject to Social Security and Medicare taxes), but the C corporation pays it from after-tax profit of the corporation. If the C corporation has a loss or tax credit, it does not pass down to shareholders. Instead, it stays at the corporation level.

Pass-through Entity (S Corporation, LLC)

S corporations and LLCs are separate entities that have elected to be taxed as a partnership. Pass-through entities do not pay income taxes. Instead, they divide profit or loss among the shareholders (members) who report these on their individual tax returns. (The term *pass through* refers to the portion of the corporation's income, losses, deductions, or credits that passes through to the shareholder.) If income is a wage, then the corporation withholds and matches FICA (Social Security and Medicare) taxes. If income is a dividend, then it is unearned and not subject to FICA. (The IRS requires that a person take a "reasonable" salary for work done.) Single owner LLCs report taxes as a proprietorship (on Schedule C). Multiple member LLCs report income as a partnership.

Business Tax Planning

Record Keeping

An employer must keep excellent financial records for many reasons. Tax compliance is only one. Box 11.4 gives several other reasons for keeping good records.

An employer can (and should) keep records himself or herself. He or she can train a receptionist or business office manager to take care of most financial issues in the office. The employer can (and should) verify those records. (The chapter on accounting discusses specific procedures.) If a person has good financial records, accounting fees will be much less and he or she can use an accountant's knowledge to best advantage.

Timing Issues: Recognizing Income and Expenses

Most dentists use the cash basis of accounting. This means that he or she recognizes income when it is received (check in hand) and recognizes expenses when they are paid (write the check or sign the credit card slip). An employer can accelerate some deductions by paying or prepaying before the end of the year. For example, if a dentist receives his or her dental association dues statement at the end of December, he or she can pay it December 31 (receiving the deduction this year) or pay it January 1 (receiving the deduction next year). As a rule, the employer should speed up deductions as much as possible. The owner should count any money

as income that is in hand this year. If he or she does not and the staff members do not go to the office and process the mail, any checks in the mail will not be counted as income until the following year. As a rule, the employer should slow recognition of income as much as possible.

Specific Techniques for Owner–Dentists

There are several specific techniques that dental practitioners who own their own practices might use to take best advantage of tax laws.

Using a Professional Corporation to Advantage

The biggest advantage of incorporation (from a tax perspective) is the tax deductibility of employee benefits. A person is an employee of the corporation. Medical insurance premiums are completely deductible for self and family and tax deductible to the corporation. A person may indirectly deduct disability insurance premiums. In this technique, the owner pays the disability premium personally. At the close of the policy year, the corporation reimburses the dentist the cost of the policy premium if he or she was not disabled. The corporation gets the cost of the deduction. If the owner was disabled and collected benefits, then the corporation does not reimburse the dentist. The benefits are tax free. As an employee of the corporation, the owner can use a medical reimbursement plan. This can be set up so that an insured medical reimbursement plan can be deductible to the corporation but not income to the owner.

Any business can establish a cafeteria benefit plan. In a C corporation, the dentist is an employee, not just the owner. As an employee, they can participate in the cafeteria plan. In these plans, the doctor and employees carefully choose among various benefit options. Money that goes into the plan comes from the individual, not the practice. Employees buy $1 of benefits for 60 to 65 percent of after-tax cost. The business withholds no payroll or income taxes.

A employee can do business with a separate entity, such as a corporation. He or she might own his or her office building in a separate entity, then pay the highest reasonable rent for the space. This makes that expense rental (unearned) income not subject to FICA or SETA tax.

There are monetary costs associated with a corporation. An accountant or advisor should "run the numbers" both ways to decide if incorporating is worthwhile. Tax law changes are making it less advantageous, from a tax perspective, to incorporate the practice.

Box 11.4 Reasons for Keeping Good Records

1. Identify sources of income
2. Track deductible expenses
3. Determine depreciation expenses
4. Determine proof of payment
5. Support items on tax return
6. Aid in tax-planning process
7. Minimize the possibility of embezzlement

Maximizing Business Write-Offs

All deductions that are legitimate business expenses should be taken through the practice. In that way, they are fully deductible. If they are taken as a personal deduction, the owner must take them as a "Miscellaneous Deduction" on Schedule A, where there is a 2 percent adjusted gross income (AGI) floor for these deductions. No such floor exists on Schedule C or the corporate return. This amount can be reduced even further for many high-income practitioners. The IRS has special rules that reduce total miscellaneous deductions for taxpayers whose income levels exceed a threshold amount (currently about $125,000). That leads to a double hit on business-related expenses claimed on the personal tax form. A person can deduct the cost (e.g., luggage and travel) for continuing education and assets bought for the business.

Using a Tax-Sheltered Retirement Plan

This technique works for most dental practitioners. Dentists should have the right type of plan to reduce staff contributions and administrative costs and should establish the plan as early in career as possible and fund the plan as early in year as possible.

Maximizing Business Automobile Write-Offs

Typical dental practitioners take about 60 percent of their automobile costs as a tax-deductible business expense. A person should write off his or her most expensive car. If a dentist is incorporated, the corporation should own the car. If unincorporated, the dentist should leave it in the practice's name. The dentist should pay for all operating costs out of practice to maximize deduction. Record keeping is critical. The dentist should prove business usage for 1 month of the year and then annualize for the year.

Using 179 Expense Election, as Appropriate

Congress intends this deduction for small business owners. Rules change frequently, but business owners should be sure to investigate if this election saves money. If a business owner expects income and tax bracket to increase significantly in the near future, he or she should put off depreciation expenses into the future by using a slower depreciation method.

Putting Family Members on the Payroll

If a person hires a spouse, he or she qualifies for Social Security benefits, child care credit, deductibility of travel expenses, and retirement plan income sheltering as well.

A business owner can save up to $5,000 per year (maximum tax free earnings) when a child is hired. This can be used to fund college educational costs. An accountant will know the latest rules for hiring a spouse or family member.

Specific Techniques for Employee Dentists

If a dentist is an employee of a practice (rather than the owner), he or she has special problems when it comes to tax savings. These stem from the fact that he or she does not make decisions concerning the practice; the dentist loses several advantages written into the tax laws that are an advantage to owners, and he or she files different returns than owners. However, dental practitioners who are employees might use take best advantage of tax laws by using several techniques.

Taking Advantage of Employee Status

If a dentist is an employee, he or she should participate in employee benefit plans and retirement plans. These are valuable benefits; these should be maximized. If the owner has a cafeteria style benefit plan, he or she should use it.

Having the Employer Pay for Professional Expenses

A dentist can pay for his or her professional expenses and deduct them on Schedule A as "Employee Related Business Expenses" under "Miscellaneous Deductions." The problem here is that there is a 2 percent of AGI floor before any miscellaneous expense can be deducted. In essence, the person loses 2 percent of AGI in deductions. Instead, the dentist should have the employer pay the expense and then reduce compensation by an equal amount. This makes the expense 100 percent deductible for the employee and saves the employer the cost of FICA and Medicare taxes on the difference.

Establishing a Schedule C

As an alternative, a dentist can do some consulting or outside independent contact dentistry. This way, he or she ca develop a Schedule C and deduct all expenses on that schedule. (No profit has to be shown.)

Maximizing Retirement Plan Contributions

Depending on whether a dentist participates in the employer's retirement plan, he or she can establish an IRA. If an employee does participate in a plan, he or she should maximize the contribution.

Using Business Car Write-Offs

An employee can still take a tax deduction for valid business use of a car. He or she should keep good records. Like other professional expenses, the dentist should have the employer pay these costs and deduct them from compensation.

Looking at the Home Office Deduction

Tax laws allow dentists to deduct part of their home as a "principal place of business" to include situations in which the home office is used for administrative or management activities, if there is no other fixed location where he or she can conduct these activities. Although this will not affect most dentists, a few can take advantage of the provision. If, for example, a dentist consults with an insurance company or does other nonpractice professional activities, he or she can probably use this provision. An accountant will know the rules to the home office deduction because the deduction frequently triggers an audit.

Management Principles

chapter 12

Lots of people confuse bad management with destiny.
Kin Hubbard

Objectives

At the completion of this chapter, the student will be able to:
1. Define the functions involved in managing a dental practice.
2. Describe the common types of decisions.
3. Describe the roles that the dentist–manager plays.
4. Differentiate between a business and a profession, and describe how a dental practice incorporates elements of both.
5. Differentiate between an entrepreneur and a small business owner.
6. Define the management competencies required by practicing dentists and describe why each is needed.
7. Describe the types of behaviors commonly found in small groups.
8. Describe assets and liabilities in group problem solving.

Key Terms

controlling
dental practice management
entrepreneur
financial resources
human resources
information resources

leading
organizing
physical resources
planning
practice philosophy
preferred future

profession
roles of an owner–dentist
small business owner
vision

Goal

This chapter acquaints the student with the meaning and importance of the concepts of practice management and the roles that the dentist plays as a professional and a business person.

Business Basics for Dentists, First Edition. David O. Willis.
© 2013 John Wiley & Sons, Inc. Published 2013 by John Wiley & Sons, Inc.

Most people that choose dentistry as a career have weighed their perceptions of various careers. The length of time in preparation, cost of training, qualifications for entrance, expected income, and expected lifestyle all contribute to their career choice. Most applicants to dental school understand that dentistry involves caring for people, technical and artistic expertise, and scientific and technical knowledge. Most profess loyalty to the notions of being independent (their own boss) and a member of a learned profession. However, few applicants pause to consider that they will be operating a small business. If they do consider it, they probably do not understand all that it entails. Most have the belief on entering dental school that they will have friendly patients, work on some teeth, make good money, and play golf or go fishing on Wednesdays. That vision is only partly accurate. They have loans to secure, taxes to pay, payrolls to meet, meet with suppliers, staff disagreements, and patients who have unreasonable expectations. If a person properly handles these business problems, then dentistry becomes a richly rewarding career and satisfying daily experience.

Success in dental practice comes from a combination of clinical, behavioral, and managerial skills. Each of those domains has a rich history and large body of knowledge. Each can be taught and learned. Learning business principles is no different than learning the principles of operative dentistry. Once a dentist understands the fundamental concepts, he or she can apply them to each particular circumstance. Lacking the concepts, that dentist can search for a new solution to each problem. If he or she understands the principles of business management and uses them to develop a modern business model, then the dentist can run a practice and it fulfills all of his or her personal expectations. If he or she does not understand and practice sound business management, then the practice runs the dentist, leaving him or her a victim of the needs of the practice.

Characteristics of Dental Practice

Dental Practice as a Business and a Profession

Dental practice has many characteristics of both a profession and a business, although dentistry and management come form entirely different mind-sets (Box 12.1). Dentistry (and therefore dental education) is scientific, procedural, and dogmatic. Most procedures have a right and wrong way to do them. Management is much less dogmatic. In fact, management teachers praise students and practitioners who do things differently than everyone else as innovators. They are encouraged to try something different, even if it does not work. (Imagine the opinion of dentists to another practitioner who tries a new way of cutting an alloy cavity

---

> **Box 12.1** Characteristics of Businesses and Professions
>
> *Characteristics of a Business*
> 1. Distribute goods or services for a profit
> 2. Provide an economic good or service
> 3. Profit motive
> 4. Treat customers fairly and honestly
>
> *Characteristics of a Profession*
> 1. Members possess special knowledge
> 2. Long training requirements
> 3. Self-regulation
> 4. Free from lay control
> 5. Necessary for society
> 6. Members place the good of society above personal interest
> 7. Members do what is best for patients

preparation?) Dentistry teaches conformity; business management teaches to be different. Dentistry teaches the safe, proven, tried, and true methods; management teaches innovation and experimentation.

Dental practice is a business. A business is an individual or group effort to distribute goods or services for a profit. This is done by providing an economic good or service that the public wants and needs. A business tries to make a profit. In fact, this profit motive separates businesses from public organizations that are often only held to the standards of accountability and not losing money. Society expects business owners to treat customers fairly and honestly but not necessarily to look out for the best interest of the customer. In fact, there is always some tension between the business and customer as each tries to gain in a transaction. Dental practices are businesses in that society expects them to generate income, pay bills, and follow regulations the same as any other business.

Dental practitioners are also professionals. Society has created the professions and granted them certain privileges. To be considered a profession, members must possess special knowledge that the public does not have. Gaining this knowledge often involves long training requirements that are not necessary in other vocations. Because the professions hold this advanced knowledge, society allows them to regulate themselves through licensure, education standards, and disciplinary actions. They are then relatively free form lay control. The knowledge that professionals hold and apply is necessary for the ongoing functioning of society as a whole, not something from which only few benefit. Because society grants so much authority in the professions, they also expect members to place the good of society above personal interest. That is not to say that society expects a vow of poverty from the members of professions, but they expect professionals to do what is best for patients, not just their own pocketbooks. If professionals abuse this power, then society can unilaterally change the rules through legislative actions.

A dental practitioner can satisfy both views in his or her practices when these differences are understood. In interactions with patients, concern for the patient must drive suggestions for treatment, and the treatment itself must be given as a professional. Business interest must not dictate or even influence patient interactions and the delivery of the care. The structure in which a professional delivers *is* the business of dentistry. Here, systems and methods are established that allow a dental practitioner to profit from the dental care that provided. The hazy line that separates the two often leads to tension for the practitioner. Which side "wins" if a given insurance plan's reimbursement for a procedure is too low to allow for adequate profit, but it is in the patient's best interest? Such problems lead professional to continually rebalance business and professional interactions.

To add to the problem, the dentistry that is done in the practice is technically based. That is to say, dentists need to know the science and have the technical ability to do excellent dentistry. However, this is only a starting point for a successful practitioner. When this technical discipline is applied, it is done on people who bring their own set of wants, needs, preferences, and desires to the practice. These behaviorally based factors form the basis of the doctor–patient and business–customer relationships. Dentists want to be the most proficient technical dentist with hand skills that amaze colleagues, but without a behavioral skill set that allows them to apply those technical skills, they can not be successful.

To accomplish all of this, dentists must not only practice the art and science of dentistry properly, but they must also practice the art and science of management. Practice management is based on a huge body of science and history in the business world. It is founded in mathematics, psychology, sociology, and logic. Each individual manager applies management information differently, depending on his or her own situation, needs, personal style, and frame of reference. So although management has a large scientific basis, its application, like dentistry, is more of an art as applied to the science on an individual, day-to-day basis. As a practice owner and manager, a person's job is to learn and understand the basic principles of management and then to apply them to meet a practice needs best.

Dentists as Entrepreneurs or Small Business Owners

Many people believe that entrepreneurs and small business people are one in the same. In fact, studies have shown that the two types of people (and their resulting businesses) have a different set of goals, strategies, and needs from the business. Neither is right nor wrong. There are many obvious examples of dentists who fit into either type. People's view of themselves, the dental profession, and the practice's objectives will help someone understand where he or she "fits in."

Entrepreneurs are builders. They try to gain market share and to make the business grow rapidly. The purpose is to take over or acquire other businesses or sell the existing business to someone else. This means that the entrepreneur must use aggressive business practices, both externally and inside the business to gain the speed of growth required by outside venture investors and initial public offerings. They may "mortgage the farm" or family fortune to finance the start-up phase of the business. They have a river boat gambler's sense of calculated risk; they do not play the game without knowing the rules, the odds, and how to use them to their advantage. They investigate possibilities, estimate the chances of success and failure, and calculate the expected return from each possibility. Only then do they decide if a venture has an adequate financial return to pursue. They are maximizers. Adequate is not enough. If they can make a million dollars this year, they will try for $2 million next year. Every city has dental entrepreneurs, those who accumulate offices, grow and sell practices, or build networks. Their vision is different from the individual lifetime practitioner.

However, most dental practitioners approach their practice like a small business owner (Table 12.1). Few dental practices fail as business ventures. People enter dentistry to be safe, not to take risks. Dentists understand that their income is limited by their personal skill and ability and by how much time that they devote to their practice. Many could make more money if they worked longer hours, but they choose family and personal time instead. Most aspiring dentists do not plan to be rich, but they do plan never to worry about money. Because most dental services require that the practitioner personally deliver the service, the size of most practices is limited. Growth involves adding highly trained (and compensated) professionals. Most dentists want to satisfy themselves and others they contact. Once they have established an adequate income, they take Wednesdays

Table 12.1 Characteristics of a Small Business Owner versus Entrepreneur

Small Business Owner	Entrepreneur
Low risk, low return	High risk, high return
Personal profit	Growth of business value
Informal systems	Formal systems
Social orientation	Commercial orientation
Personal (family) staff	Impersonal staff relations
Personal satisfaction	Financial return

off and play golf. So although they take some financial risk when establishing a practice, most dentists do not continue to grow the practice once it reaches a certain size and style.

Characteristics of Successful Business Owners

Successful small business owners and entrepreneurs share several important characteristics, as well (Box 12.2). First, they have a vision of what they want the business to be. This type of dream is not a nebulous notion or a conglomeration of possibilities. Instead, it is a specific and concrete idea of what the business owner wants or this specific business to be. This vision of a preferred future looks 5 hours, 5 days, 5 months, and 5 years into the future at once. Every action taken then supports the achievement of the preferred vision. Secondly, successful business owners show persistence. Nearly all businesses have difficult periods as a result excessive growth, lack of business, staffing problems, or any of hundreds of business problems. Successful business people take set backs in stride. They retain their preferred vision and continue to work toward its achievement. Finally, successful business people are willing to manage. Management is not pie in the sky dreaming, it is "roll up your shirt sleeves" day-to-day work. Good management means that a person is involved in every aspect of the business daily. Successful business people do not leave the details to others. Instead they dig into the details of the business to make it run most efficiently.

For most of this book, it will be assumed that the reader is the owner, manager, and producer of a dental practice. That owner may have partners or associates in the office, but the essence of the ownership issue is that the reader is responsible for more than just doing dentistry. He or she is responsible for seeing that the office runs smoothly as a business, that it is compliant with all laws regarding businesses, that staff (and an owner) feel that each are fairly rewarded and productive members of the practice, that the owner presents the proper professional image that he or she wants to promote to the public, and that he or she is involved in professional activities to improve the profession and access to health care services by the community. Sounds like a huge task, and it is.

Box 12.2 Characteristics of Successful Small Business Owners

1. Vision of a "preferred" future
2. Persistence
3. Willingness to manage

Definition of Dental Practice Management

The definition of dental practice management is "to plan, organize, lead, and control the human, physical, financial, and information resources of the business of delivering dental care." Notice that this definition is composed of four functions and four resource areas. If this is thought of as a matrix, then there are sixteen different functional problems to manage in the practice.

Functions of Dentist–Manager

Function 1: Planning

Planning is the process of determining courses of action, direction, goals, and objectives for the practice. Plans may cover long periods or be much more immediate (days or weeks). Plans start with the practice philosophy, which is the overall guiding vision of what a dentist wants the practice to be. They are supported by goals that define an expected outcome or desired future situation. Once a dentist knows where he or she wants the practice to be, he or she develops strategies to for getting there. The owner should also identify likely barriers to overcome and a time for completion. Finally, objectives give concreteness to the planning process. Objectives define what the expected outcomes are. They should be both measurable and specific to decide if the practice has met them.

When a dentist decides to expand the office or move to a new location, he or she is planning. For major initiatives, such as these, the dentist will probably use advisers, such as accountants, equipment representatives, and bankers. For many smaller initiatives, such as hiring an additional staff member or changing recall systems, the dentist will plan what to do with little outside help. In all these planning instances, a preferred future is desired and changes are made to try to reach that goal.

Function 2: Organizing

Organizing means coordinating resources and activities by designing the physical facility and by structuring tasks and authority. The organizing function involves setting up the physical space and systems in the office, deciding information needs and solutions, deciding what types and numbers of staff to hire, and how the office will operate on a daily basis.

Many dental practitioners develop office manuals that contain policies, rules, procedures, and standard operational methods. They find instrument set ups and sterilization methods that work effectively. They develop equipment maintenance and repair schedules, supply vendors, office cleaning and redecorating schedules, and hundreds of other routine organizational policies that allow the office to function smoothly.

Function 3: Leading

Leading is selecting, motivating, and directing staff members to work at the peak of their abilities. Most dental offices have employees. The planning and organizing functions describe the types and numbers of staff members that will be needed. Many new dentists believe that all a dentist needs to do is to plug people into the various slots. In fact, at this point a dentist must engage in what many people believe is the most difficult piece of the management puzzle: leading and motivating those employees.

Employees each bring their own set of wants, needs, family histories, backgrounds, and personalities to the workplace. The astute manager works to understand people so that they can stimulate high performance from them, both as individuals and as groups. As the owner of the practice, the dentist sets the office environment. That environment consists of the compensation package (pay and benefits), the communication process, group interactions, and job duties. The way the office environment is set up can either support or discourage motivated workers from doing their best on the job.

Function 4: Controlling

Controlling means monitoring and evaluating activities to ensure that the operational and performance outcomes resulted as planned. As the practice moves toward its goals, the owner must monitor its progress. If it is not acting in a way that will allow it to reach its "target," then the owner needs to either change processes or change the target.

In fact, controlling is an ongoing function in the office. At the end of each day, the dentist examines the office daily production and collection numbers, looking for problems. The dentist gives immediate and constructive feedback to members of the dental team, so that they know what they are doing correctly and incorrectly. The dentist examines work that was previously done and changes materials or procedures if problems are found. These are included in office control. Some are more formal than others, but all these (and more) feed back to help the dentist make better practice decisions.

Resources of the Practice

The definition of practice management is to plan, organize, lead, and control the resources of the practice. But what are the major resource groups of the practice?

Resource 1: Human Resources

Most dentists in practice in the United States employ staff. Yet staffing the practice continues to be one of the practitioner's greatest problems. Staff typically is the single greatest area of expense for a practitioner and the most important limit to practice growth. Dentists want long-term, committed individuals to be employees, yet generally do not know how to establish pay, compensation, and reward systems that optimize staff performance. Dentists and staff members work closely together in a physically confined space. They often become genuine friends, making employee discipline and rewards difficult to administer fairly. The variety of staff job duties and legal requirements of job classifications can lead to petty jealousies and interpersonal conflicts that the manger–dentist must arbitrate.

Resource 2: Physical Resources

The physical resources include the office space itself and the equipment and supplies required to do dentistry. Dentists typically rent office space, although many own their own building and space. Maintenance, upkeep, and decoration all add expense to the basic office cost. New equipment, especially high technology equipment, has a short useful lifetime. (Most computers are obsolete within a few years of purchase.) Yet new techniques and materials are coming to the dental marketplace continually. This means that a dentist must plan for the continual change and upgrade in the physical plant and equipment of the office.

Resource 3: Financial Resources

Dentists must properly manage the finances of the office to be profitable. Initial (start-up or buy-in) loans significantly affect cash flow. The dentist's plans and decisions regarding payment plan and credit policies, personal financial planning, retirement plans for self and staff, staff pay schedules, and even bill paying schedules affect the practice's profitability.

Resource 4: Information Resources

Dentistry is presently becoming more of an information service and less of a product or personal service-based industry. Patients want information on their dental and general health conditions. Insurance carriers and other third parties want information on services provided and the costs associated with them. Dentists need patient information for legal and ethical reasons, and for mailing and other appropriate marketing services. Dentists need information about the profession, evaluations of new materials, descriptions of new techniques, and responses from third-party carriers. Information drives the practice. Modern dentists understand and manage the information needs of the practice.

Roles of an Owner–Dentist

Private dental practice is both the long-term goal and result of most graduating dental students. The vast majority of these are solo practices. Most of the rest are two practitioner offices. Because there are few practitioners in most offices, most dentists must play many different managerial roles. In larger organizations, one person can be responsible for staffing, another for supplies, and yet another for accounting. The small dental office is different in that the owner–dentist must wear many different hats during the day (Box 12.3). The dentist must produce dentistry. Legally, the dentist is the only person in the office who can do many daily dental procedures. As owner, the dentist must be a decision maker. These decisions deal both with the dentistry produced and with the management in the office. The dentist possesses the primary storehouse of information for patients and staff. He or she is the technical expert in dentistry, the chief of accounting for the office, personnel manager, production supervisor, vice-president for marketing, and the ceremonial head of the practice.

Box 12.3 Roles of an Owner–Dentist

Producer
Decision maker
Information provider
   Mentor
   Teacher
Technical expert
Interpersonal facilitator
   Figurehead
Accounting, operations

Add to this the many roles played outside the office (e.g., parent, spouse, church member, little league coach), it is little wonder that some dentists are victims of personal and professional burn out.

The dentist who is a student of management is better able to control the problems that occur on a daily basis in the practice. In that sense, to do management properly in the office means that the study of management is an ongoing concern, just like the study of dental techniques and materials. It is not an end in and of itself, but a road, path, or Tao. If a person understands basic management principles and applies them appropriately, he or she will take the first steps toward a lifelong career that is satisfying and rewarding in both a personal and financial context.

Planning the Dental Practice

It was the best of times, it was the worst of times, it was the age of wisdom, it was the age of foolishness, it was the epoch of belief, it was the epoch of incredulity, it was the season of Light, it was the season of Darkness, it was the spring of hope, it was the winter of despair, we had everything before us, we had nothing before us, we were all going direct to heaven, we were all going direct the other way—in short, the period was so far like the present period, that some of its noisiest authorities insisted on its being received, for good or for evil, in the superlative degree of comparison only.

Charles Dickens
A Tale of Two Cities

Objectives

At the completion of this chapter, the student will be able to:
1. Describe external environmental factors that affect dental practices.
2. Describe internal environmental factors that affect dental practices.
3. Describe the amount of control the practitioner has over the various factors.
4. Describe an environmental analysis.
5. Describe how a SWOT analysis can be applied to a dental practice.
6. Describe several environmental trends that are important for planning in dentistry.

Key Terms

allies
competitors
economic domain
environmental analysis
environmental planning
process
ethical and professional
domain
external environment
general environment
influence groups

internal environment
internal management
legal and regulatory domain
opportunities
patients
personal position
personal style of the dentist
professional strengths and
weaknesses
risk aversion
sociocultural domain

strategic issues
strengths
suppliers
SWOT analysis
technological domain
the operating environment
threats
views of dentistry
weaknesses

Goal

The purpose of this chapter is to acquaint the student with the internal and external factors that affect the planning and operation of a dental practice.

Business Basics for Dentists, First Edition. David O. Willis.
© 2013 John Wiley & Sons, Inc. Published 2013 by John Wiley & Sons, Inc.

Starting a practice is much like having a child. A practice must be birthed, allowed to grow, and helped through problems before it becomes a fully functioning mature practice. The problems and opportunities faced by a child are different from those faced by an adolescent. Similarly, a start-up practice faces different challenges from a mature practice. With both children and dental practices, a well-articulated plan must be in place to move to the next level of development. In both instances, change happens regardless whether there is a plan. Nevertheless, having a plan helps to guide the process and maximize opportunities that occur.

Practice Stages

Dental practices typically develop through several stages. Depending on where a dentist is in the practice development stage, planning needs and practice profile will be different.

There are four stages in a practice's growth (Table 13.1). During the first phase (start-up), the practitioner is concerned with getting warm bodies in the door. Marketing efforts become critical. Practitioners often use managed care, welfare patients, emergency call, or other methods to increase the number of patient visits. Efficiency is not as much of a problem as in later stages because there is often slack time. The growth phase sees an acceleration in patient visits. Schedules begin to fill, and the practitioner begins to "weed out" managed care and other less profitable patients. The maturity phase sees practitioners concerned with making the practice efficient from a production, cost, and revenue basis. Finally, during the development phase of practice, the dentist readjusts the practice to meet long-term personal and professional life goals. The practice is concerned with different problems in each phase of its development. Different problems and solutions will then be more important at different phases as well.

Stage 1: Practice Establishment

This initial stage begins with the set-up, buy out, or buy-in of the practice. The practitioner's main concern is to increase the patient base and to acquaint those

Table 13.1 Stages of a Dental Practice

Stage	Major Concern
Establishment	Warm bodies
Growth	The right warm bodies
Maturity	Becoming efficient
Redevelopment	Personal goal attainment

patients with the style and personality of the practice. To this end, he or she will see virtually anybody, any time. Marketing and advertising are important to attract people into the practice so that they may be won over as regular patients. Profits are low or nonexistent because revenue is low and slow to be collected whereas debts and start-up costs are high. Operational efficiency is not a big problem because there are often extra appointments available and the practitioner is increasing his or her clinical and management skills. During this time, the practitioner develops operational systems and management skills that will be the basis of later practice efficiencies.

Stage 2: Practice Growth

The growth stage occurs when the practitioner continues to acquaint the patient base with his or her individual practice style. Because of the unique style, patients begin to self-select for or against the practice. This leads to patients leaving the practice to find a dentist who is more compatible with their needs and wants or patients who enjoy the style of practice and refer patients with similar wants and desires. This internal referral process allows the practice to approach a "critical mass" of patients that will help the practice to sustain itself from internal referrals.

Many marketing efforts begin to pay off as well. There is often so much new and previously deferred work that the practice begins to run the practitioner, rather than vice versa. This can leave the practitioner with little time for personal growth or family interests. Although a large amount of money comes into the practice, there is low profit because overhead is still high because of loan pay offs and personal debt associated with typical family start-up expenses. This often leads to a "cash crunch" in which the practitioner has trouble paying the bills each month, though production reaches an all-time high. Operational efficiency becomes a large problem as the number of patients increases. The practitioner needs to assess carefully when to add additional staff, change hours, or make other critical operational management decisions.

Stage 3: Practice Maturity (Realization)

The practitioner reaches his or her intended level of practice busyness during the maturity stage. Referrals increase as the dentist concentrates on the types of work that are of greater interest to him or her for personal, professional, or financial reasons. The dentist takes control of the time spent with the practice and balances this commitment with personal and family time uses. Involvement with professional societies and organizations increases as the practitioner gains professional and personal stature. Profits increase as fixed costs decrease from loan payoffs. Production peaks and fees increase so that this stage becomes the most profitable. The dentist's time is the limiting factor to production, so office operational efficiency is vital to maximum profitability. Many dentists' goal is to maintain a mature type practice for many years.

Stage 4: Practice Redevelopment

This stage of practice can take two different paths. One group of practitioners is content to continue the existing practice pattern. The patient pool begins to contract as patients move away, die, or have decreased need for dental care. If the practitioner has not encouraged children into the practice, the patients age with the practitioner as the patients' families grow and move away. Often the treatment scope is fairly limited, especially if the practitioner has not incorporated the newer techniques, methods, and materials. The practitioner takes more time off for outside pursuits. Profits continue to be high because the overhead is low, although profits and revenues are decreasing as a result of the shrinking patient pool. Operational efficiency is not important if the practitioner is satisfied with the profit and workload of the practice.

The second group of practitioners wants to maximize the value of the practice. To do this, they take in associate dentists, sell part to a new partner, or merge their practice with another. They find ways to continue to develop and grow the practice so that the practice becomes more of the focal point, instead of them. As the practice grows, they often require additional, specialized staff to run the practice. Office manager, sterilization clerks, and insurance management staff members do tasks shared in smaller practices. Operational efficiency is paramount to these larger practices maintaining profitability in the face of this increased bureaucracy needed to run the practice.

The Environment of Dental Practice

A dental practice does not exist in a vacuum. It exists in an environment that affects the practice either directly or by influencing the climate in which the practice operates. These environmental forces may be external to the practice or may exist internally as management-related concerns or as personal positions taken by the owner–dentist. But each of these factors may profoundly affect the way a dentist structures the practice. The individual practitioner should identify these forces, anticipate their effects, and use this information to plan practice growth in the most advantageous manner. An "environmental analysis" assesses the practice's environment so that the dentist can anticipate problems and make changes in the practice's direction to increase the his or her chance for success. This becomes the framework for planning the successful practice.

External Environment

The external environment, by definition, lies outside the practice itself and is composed of both specific individuals and general groups. It includes those people who influence the practice and those whom its actions affect. This is obviously a large, diverse, and complex group of factors. For that reason, external environmental factors generally fall into two categories, general environment and operating environment.

The General Environment

The general environment includes the business, regulatory, legal, technological, cultural, and social factors that affect the climate in which dental practices operate (Box 13.1). It includes factors that affect both the number and types of patients and the number and types of inputs into the practice (labor, supplies, etc.). The general environment is divided into several domains.

Sociocultural Domain
The sociocultural domain consists of the demographics (e.g., age, education level, income level, etc.), values, customs, and historical interests of the people within the society served. Because dental practices exist to serve the needs of the population base, it is no wonder that these cultural factors should influence the organization and operation of the dental practice. The people whom the practice employs bring many of those cultural factors with them as background knowledge on the job. Social and cultural roots, for example, may in part determine an individual's "work ethic" on the job or affect their personal interactions with the clients of the practice.

Dental practices face a host of sociocultural influences. Demographic changes in the population will affect the practice's future productivity. The US population, overall, is aging, becoming more affluent and better educated. Twenty percent of the population moves their home in any given year. People value preventive health care and practice more "self-help" than ever before. Ethnic and racial composition of communities and the population at large are rapidly changing. The myriad ways, both positive and negative, that these factors might affect the dental profession overall (and a specific dental practice) are considered the sociocultural factors of the external environment.

Box 13.1 General Environmental Factors

Sociocultural
- The graying of the United States
- Social attitudes toward health behaviors
- Rise of consumerism
- Changing character of dental needs
- Quality of life issues
- Decline of the traditional family

Economic
- Inflationary trends
- Interest rate changes
- Specific local employer changes
- The decrease of unionization of workers

Technological
- Nonsurgical periodontal techniques
- Caries "vaccine"
- New materials and techniques

Legal and Regulatory
- Changing governmental spending for health care
- The tax status of health benefits
- Ethical/Professional

Economic Domain

The application of sociocultural factors requires an exchange by both the dentist and the population. This process results in the economic domain. On a macro level, general economic conditions such as inflation, unemployment levels, and benefit packages negotiated by workers affect the number and type of dental services demanded by patients. Interest rates, resource prices (e.g., gold, silver, computers, and dental instruments), and alternative employment possibilities all affect the general atmosphere that in part determines practice costs. Although the individual practitioner has little control over economic environmental factors, understanding how these factors can affect the practice is still important. In this way, a dentist may anticipate future effects and react appropriately to developing trends by anticipating the outcome and planning accordingly.

Technological Domain

Technology is the third major general external environmental domain that affects dentistry. Technology is the means, knowledge, training, and systems used in the delivery of dental services. Just as robotics has revolutionized the manufacturing sector, research and technological changes have as dramatically influenced dental practices. A few of the new dental technologies from the past 25 years that have dramatically influenced dental practice include community water supply fluoridation, the high speed handpiece, four-handed auxiliary skills, fiber optics, lingual braces, castable ceramics, desktop computers and supporting software, light cured composite restorations, spherical cut alloys, implant materials and techniques, CAD/CAM restoration formation, laser cutting, electronic insurance filing, improved nonsurgical and pharmacological periodontal treatments, and newer filling and cementing agents. The rate of change of technology is accelerating rapidly. Future dental practices will be vastly different from today's in materials, techniques, and information processing. This will affect the nature and character of dental practice. A dental practitioner must constantly monitor the technological domain of the external environment for developments. He or she then decides how those developments might affect dental practice and to incorporate those developments into the growth plan when appropriate.

Legal and Regulatory Domain

The sociocultural environment strongly influences the legal and regulatory domain. In a sense, they are outgrowths of our cultural norms. They define what is acceptable and unacceptable behavior by members of the society and translate into laws and regulations aimed at controlling them. In this country, laws are formed by the legislature, enforced by the executive, and interpreted and judged by the judicial branch. As such, they are closely tied to the will of the society. The legal and regulatory environment has obvious and profound impact on the dental practice. Every dentist remembers the state board ("trial by fire") clinical exam required for licensure. State Dental Practice Acts define limits of auxiliary duty delegation and practice ownership. Through legislation and regulation, Congress affects how much money is spent on indigent care, workers' health benefits (and tax deductibility of those benefits), and inclusion or exclusion of dental care in health policies. The Occupational Safety and Health Administration (OSHA) and the courts are presently redefining the dentist's responsibilities to employees and patients while handling potentially infectious materials. The litigious nature of today's US society has caused many dentists to change the way they practice dentistry. The individual practitioner should monitor the political and regulatory system closely to anticipate shifts in ideology and priorities among regulators.

Ethical and Professional Domain

The profession of dentistry is relatively autonomous, in that dentists decide the prevailing entrance and educational requirements of its members, set the practice and technological norms, define behavioral expectations, and discipline members who do not adhere to their norms. Society grants the profession this autonomy with the understanding that the professional abuse the power and that they look out for the best interest of the public and individual patients under their control. So individual practitioners must respond to and follow a set of socially and professionally determined ethical norms. These ethical expectations change slowly over time as new influences in the other environments change public and professional expectations and opinions.

The Operating Environment

The operating environment is the direct influence that the general environment makes on the dental practice (Box 13.2). It is the environment in which the dental practice actually operates. In a sense, it is the concrete embodiment of the abstract general environment. As such, these are factors that the practitioner contacts and can exert some influence over. For example, the general demographic trend is that, because of fluoridation and the end of the "baby boom," there are fewer young people with significant dental caries. The periodontist may feel the direct influence of this trend in the changing character of the service mix of the practice. Conversely, the local environment may not mirror the overall trend. Several new subdivisions in the area may bring an influx

of new families, lowering the age of the patient base. Focusing efforts to cope with changes in the operating environment (e.g., inclusion of orthodontics or adolescent marketing) is more productive than trying to fight or influence the underlying general trend. The operating environment is divided into several components.

Suppliers

Suppliers provide the resources needed for the dental practice to operate and consist of much more than simply dental supplies. They also include personnel or labor (assistants and hygienists), financial capital (banker), subcontracted work (laboratory), and information (accountants, lawyers, continuing education courses, practice consultants). A dentist, for example, competes for labor with other local businesses that offer alternative forms of employment, such as grocery stores and manufacturing plants. If local employers are offering high wage and benefit packages, the dentist must compete for the suppliers of labor by offering comparable compensation packages for comparable level jobs.

Patients

Patients (customers) are the second major component of the operating environment. Every dental practice serves a defined and segmented portion of the population. Marketing attempts to match the service provided to the wants and needs of a lager population segment. Developing profiles of whom actively uses the practice's services is the first step toward developing a plan to increase the number of people who would be patients. Customers have different amounts of bargaining power with the service provider. Preferred provider organizations (PPOs) are an example of the power a group may exert when bargaining for services. Plant openings or closings in the geographic area will increase or decrease the buying power and the number of potential customers, and therefore exert indirect bargaining power with local dentists and other business people.

Influence Groups

Influence groups become a real part of the operational environment every time a regulation is enforced. Zoning commissions can profoundly influence the growth plans for a dental practice by allowing or not allowing a favorable zoning change. Professional associations and organizations (such as the American Dental Association [ADA] or the various specialty groups) act as information exchange centers and may propose policy or laws that affect the general environment of the practice. Interest groups (such as parent–teacher organizations.) may influence the immediate environment through concerted effort (e.g., boycotts) or through informing and influencing its members and the public to its position.

Box 13.2 Operating Environment Factors

Suppliers
- Unionization of dental auxiliaries
- New laboratory procedures

Patients
- Increasing number of people with insurance
- Changing affluence of the population
- Changes in insurance coverage

Regulators and Influence Groups
- State laws regarding delegation of duties
- Changing nature of third-party organizations (capitation plans, preferred provider organizations, etc.)

Competitors
- Efficiency of large competitors
- Changing character of established practices
- Competition from new practitioners
- Corporate practices

Allies
- Group purchase plans
- Advertising and marketing networks
- Independent practice associations

Competitors

Competitors influence the operating environment of the practice. If a patient is not satisfied with the service provided, he or she may find another practice that does satisfy those wants and needs. Desired growth opportunities may be shut off because of existing competition in the area. New forms of dental service payment plans (e.g., capitation plans) may alter the traditional competitive environment and cause patients to choose dental practices based on reasons that an individual dentist cannot control.

Allies

Allies are groups or individuals that develop an inter-dependent relationship with the practice. In this function, they share resources or information to the mutual benefits of both parties. Individual dentists may have well-established referral patterns, study clubs, group purchase plans, or kindred spirits with whom they share a special bond. More formal groups of allies may also develop, such as independent practice associations (IPAs), that seek to influence the marketplace though group action.

Internal Environment

The internal environment consists of the elements of the practice when viewed as a business (Box 13.3). Personnel, marketing, financial, organizational, and production-related functions all fall within the practice's internal environment. The owner–dentist can control the quality and quantity of internal factors easily (when compared with external factors). In fact, until and unless the practice is operating with excellent efficiency and effectiveness, it probably cannot take advantage of external environmental opportunities.

Internal Management

Internal management issues are the focus of many practice management texts, lectures, continuing education courses, and consultants. Internal management includes the marketing, staffing, the efficient provision of services, and office financial management. The dental practitioner has almost unlimited control over the internal manner in which his or her office will operate. It is important that the practitioner adapt his or her internal management philosophy and techniques to fit other internal and external environmental considerations.

Personal Style of the Dentist

Practice growth is a notion similar to "motherhood" or "the American way." People profess to believe in it, but each person would come up with a different definition and method of carrying out his or her plan for achieving

---

Box 13.3 Internal Issues

Organizational Concerns
- Office communications
- Policies and procedures manual
- Management skills and interest of the owner
- History of the practice

Personnel Concerns
- Worker relations
- Recruitment of employees
- Performance appraisal system
- Incentive system
- Training and certification of employees
- Doctor's management style–staff relations
- Employee turnover

Marketing Concerns
- Internal marketing efforts
- Community visibility activities
- Recall system effectiveness
- Patient satisfaction
- Patient education programs

Production Concerns
- Service mix provided
- Facility design and expansion potential
- Inventory control
- Scheduling
- Delegation of tasks
- Quality control and assessment program
- Procedures referred
- Staff and doctor continuing education course taken

Financial Concerns
- Liquidity of the practice
- Profitability to the owner
- Investments
- Personal lifestyle desired

---

it. This is because everyone approaches personal and professional decisions with a unique history, set of values, abilities, and beliefs.

The first step in analyzing the internal environment is to appraise individual circumstance, as to wants, needs, desires, and abilities. The result is that a appropriate and realistic strategies will be formulated that fit a unique style. The four primary areas of self-appraisal are views of the profession of dentistry, personal risk aversion or attraction, personal position, and professional strengths and weaknesses (Box 13.4).

Views of Dentistry

Some dentists believe that dentistry is a cottage industry; others that it is a multibillion dollar-a-year service industry.

Box 13.4 Personal issues

Views of Dentistry
- Dentistry as a profession and a business
- Professional image in the community

Risk Aversion
- Amount of personal wealth accumulated
- Time until retirement
- Ability and desire to incur additional debt

Personal Position
- Standing in the community
- Desire and ability to work closely with other dentists
- Professional autonomy desired
- Work and leisure time trade-off
- Personal and family time desired
- Outside interests, businesses, and hobbies
- Religious, social, and civic commitments
- Tolerance for ambiguity and change

Professional Strengths and Weakness
- Business management and patient treatment skills
- Technical and behavioral competencies
- Professional treatment strengths and weaknesses

Every dentist has a different view of dentistry and the dental profession and, therefore, has a different answer to the question. Many aggressive growth strategies (such as opening a satellite location or participating in a managed care program) require that the participants have a business-oriented view of the profession that would be anathema to a cottage industry dentist. Conversely, a conservative strategy of internal referrals and community education may appear stifling and unimaginative to a dentist with a true entrepreneurial spirit.

Risk Aversion

Everyone has a unique tolerance for and aversions to both risk and debt. The US hero is a swashbuckling daredevil entrepreneur who risks the family savings and mortgages the ranch on a new idea and wins. Few have the river boat gambler's tolerance for risk. In fact, most people avoid risk whenever they can, especially as they progress through their professional lives and accumulate assets that represent goal attainment or that make their lives more comfortable. People must decide how much risk and uncertainty they can tolerate.

Any growth action involves taking some risk. That may take the form of placing personal or professional assets at risk as collateral (financial risk) or may take the form of possible loss of professional standing, bearing, or reputation (professional risk). The inclusion

of an associate dentist may lead to a decrease in income as a result of increased expenses or a decrease in professional bearing in the community if the associate is not carefully chosen or acts unprofessionally. Use of novel treatment approaches may lead to either new opportunities for patient satisfaction or poor clinical results and the concomitant loss of reputation. The success of a satellite office may paradoxically risk a decrease in personal and family time that the practitioner cherishes.

Every growth strategy or action has some attendant risk. The higher the risk associated with a growth strategy, the higher the pay off should be. Otherwise, the dentist would choose a strategy that has the same potential pay off but involves less risk. The pay off may be in financial or entirely nonfinancial currencies. A feeling of success, service to people in need, religious goodwill, and other "good feelings" are adequate pay for many dentists in certain situations. Depending on how much risk aversion is identified through self-assessment, (see Fig. 13.1). the dentist will pick a growth strategy that adequately compensates him or her for the associated risk taken. If the dentist is only willing to accept limited risk despite the potential returns, the acceptable strategies may similarly be limited to those that have a limited return.

Personal Position

Each person has a set of personal issues that act as profound factors in the growth decision. Families grow accustomed to certain income levels and time commitments from family members. Individuals need different amounts of personal time for such activities as hobbies, outside interests, and personal development efforts. Most professionals require time for personal health-related activities and spiritual and religious devotional efforts. Many require time and efforts for political, environmental, community, or social causes. It is essential, that each dentist constantly explores and recognizes those personal factors that are critical for his or her spiritual, mental, and social well-being. Practice growth cannot take place until the personal position is identified, developed, and reconciled with professional opportunities.

Professional Strengths and Weaknesses

A critical self-appraisal is also necessary in the professional arena. Every clinical dentist has areas of technical, behavioral, and managerial strength and weakness. Dentists are often unaware of them either through lack of introspection or through the inability or unwillingness to gain an honest appraisal from selves, patients, staff, or peers. An honest appraisal is difficult because it involves personal risk. A person might find out something that he or she does not want to know, or the person might gain confirmation for something suspected but wishes were not so. Yet an appraisal is critical to successful growth.

A successful growth strategy uses an individual's strengths and reduces his or her weaknesses. Without an honest appraisal of professional strengths and weaknesses, the dentist cannot intelligently choose an appropriate and successful growth strategy. For example, suppose a person identifies the need for a periodontal maintenance program. If the dentist does not have adequate skills or knowledge in this area, it would be foolish, destructive, and unethical to pursue this strategy without continuing education in the field. Or if the staff reports that the dentist is particularly adept at interpersonal communication with apprehensive patients, the dentist could initiate a "Dental Phobic" program and expand office revenues by referral and program development in this area. Without an honest appraisal, the dentist might have been unaware of this staff-perceived strength and lost the opportunity for practice growth and patient service.

Environmental Analysis and Planning

Planning is the primary management function. A dental practice can change or influence many elements in its environment. The practice cannot change but must respond to others. Planning allows the dentist to affect rather than simply accept the future. The purpose of planning and goal setting is to guide the practice to excellent performance. By establishing a practice mission, goals, and strategies, the dentist guides the practice and makes it happen rather than simply responding to whatever the marketplace offers. The practice becomes more efficient and more profitable as practice goals are achieved. The practitioner is more satisfied with his or her personal and professional lives. Finally, the mental exercise involved in planning for various options helps the dentist to understand the operational and financial foundations of the practice and to make him or her a better practice manager. The purpose of the environmental planning process is to provide a direction and concrete steps that the dentist can use to decide where the practice is going in the future. Rather than simply letting the environment dictate the future of the practice, the planning process assesses the environment and adapts the practice to take advantage of the environment. The framework for developing a strategic plan involves looking at both the internal and external environments in a logical and systematic way. These assessments are then use as the basis for developing a plan (Fig. 13.1).

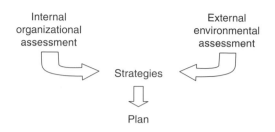

Figure 13.1 Strategic planning framework

The relationships between the components of the operating environment are dynamic; they change over time and with different circumstance. They are founded on the trends seen in the general environment and so may be predicted with more or less accuracy, depending on the circumstance. Dentists should assess the factors that are at work in the operating environment and attempt to influence the environment rather than simply allow the operating environment to control the practice. The method used for this assessment is called an *environmental analysis*.

An environmental analysis attempts to assess the internal and external environmental factors that are important to the growth process. Constantly scanning the environment is useful for identifying trends and developments that may affect the practice. These ongoing scans may use many sources of information but should be done continually. Factors that are important should be sorted from the ones that are less important to the immediate operating environment. Any individual tends selectively to filter and discard information that may be vital to the practice's growth. The more people involved, the less likely this is and the better the information becomes.

Finally, the dentist must honestly appraise and compare the strengths and weaknesses of the practice and attempt to find a growth opportunity that enhances the practices capabilities. This is, after all, the whole purpose of environmental analysis, to assess the organization's internal and external environmental factors so that the practice can anticipate and react to them in a way that enhances success.

The Practice Planning Process

When planning for a practice, the dentist first decides what is important for him or her professionally. Those core values then drive the practice mission. An analysis of the environment helps determine the problems and opportunities for success. Strategies say how a dentist will satisfy that mission. He or she then further defines the strategy as goals and objectives for the practice that measure the effectiveness of the methods in meeting goals and the mission.

Step 1: Develop Core Values

A statement of core values is a summary of the beliefs and values that a person holds to be important. These core values are a set of beliefs about the practice and the philosophy about how a person wants to practice dentistry. The include personal values, beliefs, concerns, and attitudes. Businesses often develop them as a set of bullet items. The core value statements concern the approach to patient care, the work environment, the organizational culture, and personal responsibilities. If a dentist does not understand and follow core values, he or she will never be satisfied in practice. Box 13.5 lists areas that might fit with a dentist's core values and gives examples of specific value statements.

Step 2: Establish a Practice Mission

Whereas the core values describe what a dentist believes, a practice mission is a set of active statements that describes what a dentists want the practice to accomplish on a daily and a long-term basis. (Some people call this the practice philosophy because it puts in writing how the practice is run.) The mission is a set of action verbs. It puts core values into actions. Like core values, the mission includes how a dentist manages the practice's business and the types and levels of treatment that he or she does for patients. The practice's mission is not a secret document. A dentist should proudly share it with patients, staff members, and suppliers so that everyone knows goals and expectations.

A written practice mission is essential if team members are to work together in a way that reinforces this philosophy with patients. To have an idea of a mission is only a beginning. Putting those ideas on paper is the challenge that forces a dentist to come to grips with the elements that he or she thinks are important. No single mission statement is appropriate for all dentists because dentists have individual attitudes, backgrounds, wants, and needs. However, at least one item in the practice mission should be included for each core belief.

Box 13.6 gives examples of practice mission statements. These are intended to give dentists ideas about how to develop a practice mission. These should be rewritten as action verbs to reflect core values. Like the core value statements, this is not an exhaustive list.

Step 3: Assess the Environment

The first step in the planning process is to assess the environment of the practice. This process is often called a SWOT analysis. SWOT analysis attempts to define the organization's *Strengths* and *Weaknesses* and to identify

environmental *Opportunities* and *Threats* that may occur (Box 13.7). Strengths and weaknesses are environmental factors that come from inside the practice. They are issues that are under the control of the dentists. Opportunities and threats come from outside the practice. They are issues that the dentists can not control but must respond to. Something can be both a threat and an opportunity at the same time. Managed care may be viewed as a threat for many dentists in the potential financial impact on the practice but may also be an opportunity to generate additional patients for the practice.

Box 13.5 Example Core Value Statements

Patient Care Objectives
- The optimal care for patients is first concern.
- Patients are engaged in their treatment decisions.

Quality of Care
- The highest quality technical care is essential to success.
- Behaviorally sophisticated patient management is necessary for a practice to prosper.

Work Environment
- The practice should be a fun place to work.
- A team-centered work environment is important for doctors, staff, and patients.

Management Style or Structure
- A strong, participative, management style is valued.
- The doctor is the primary decision maker in the dental practice.

Team Members' Responsibility
- All members share in organizational responsibilities.
- Team members are expected to work hard and to be well compensated for their work.

Team Members' Professional Growth
- Individual team member's continual professional growth is encouraged.

Reward Structure
- A competitive wage will be paid and a benefit package will be offered for team members.
- Rewards for all team members depend on the profitability of the practice.

Relationship to the Community
- All members of the team participate in community health missions.
- A portion of practice time is devoted to serving less fortunate members of community.

Box 13.6 Elements of Practice Mission

Approach to Patient Care
- Patients are involved in the choice of their treatment options.
- Patients are served in a modern facility with the most modern equipment and materials.
- Poor treatment choices by patients will not be enabled.

Financing Dental Care
- Patients are served who can comfortably afford care.
- The practice participates in all major dental insurance plans.

Personal and Staff Preparation
- Each member of the team will participate in annual continuing education.
- Staff members will provide care to the best of their abilities each day.

Community Responsibilities
- The practice provides care for all members of the community.
- The practice annually will donate a portion of profits to worthy community causes.

Box 13.7 SWOT Analysis for a Dental Practitioner

What are the practice's STRENGTHS?
1. _____
2. _____
3. _____
4. _____
5. _____

What are the practice's WEAKNESSES?
1. _____
2. _____
3. _____
4. _____
5. _____

What are the greatest environmental OPPORTUNITIES for the practice?
1. _____
2. _____
3. _____
4. _____
5. _____

What are the greatest environmental THREATS to the practice?
1. _____
2. _____
3. _____
4. _____
5. _____

When a SWOT analysis is done, a dentist should remember to think of all of the stakeholders of the practice. A stakeholder is any person, group, or organization that can place a claim on the practice's resources or output or is affected by the organization. Stakeholders then become everyone that the practice has an effect on. This includes staff, patients, suppliers, landlords, special patient groups, and other dentists in the area, to name a few. If all the stakeholders are identified when doing a SWOT analysis, the dentist has less of a chance of inadvertently missing an important element to be included in the plan.

SWOT analysis may be as formal or as informal as needed, however, it must be complete so that no important factors are overlooked. In fact, the quality of the SWOT analysis generally rests with the accuracy of the environmental assessment. SWOT analysis is a brainstorming technique, in which participants identify strengths, weaknesses, threats, and opportunities. After these are identified, participants then "make sense" of the listings by analysis and planning actions to take advantage of opportunities while minimizing threats.

SWOT analysis does not identify a course of action, but points out areas that should be addressed in a strategy. It involves a certain amount of "guestimation" and is only as valid as the information gathered in the analysis of the environment. If done honestly and as accurately as possible, SWOT analysis can be used to identify areas for growth and to avoid possibilities that, at first blush, appear enticing.

An important point is to look for confluences of weaknesses with threats, and opportunities with strengths. Real problems are identified where there is a threat in an area in which something is weak. Conversely, real potential exists where an external opportunity occurs in an area in which something is strong.

Step 4: Determine Strategies

Strategies are the long-term plans a dentist has to implement his or her mission. It may not be realistic to have an insurance-free practice from the start, but it may be possible to develop that style practice over several years. The strategy then is to decrease the amount of insurance each year. This becomes a long-term plan, a road map to achieving this mission while fulfilling core values. Every practice must grow and evolve over time. Developing a strategic view of the practice allows a person to control where he or she wants the practice to be, instead of merely reacting to where it is.

Box 13.8 Example Strategies

The following are examples of strategies to achieve the practice mission. Like the core value statements, this is not an exhaustive list. A person might have other areas or values that are not included here.

Third-Party Plans
- The practice will participate in managed care plans in the start-up phase of practice to generate patient base.
- The practice will end managed care participation when a sufficient patient base is built up.
- The practice will participate in Medicaid throughout the practice to fulfill community responsibilities.

Credit and Collection Policy
- The practice will start with an easy credit and collection policy to build patient pool.
- The practice will keep a strict credit and collection policy to keep accounts receivable and uncollectibles low.

Fees
- The practice will keep fees low to penetrate the market.
- The practice will be a high-end dental provider, keeping fees at the upper end for the area.

Operatories
- The practice will build operatories as patient demand dictate.
- The practice will build operatories and drive patient visits to fill them.

Hours
- The practice will keep only weekday business hours.
- The practice will work extended hours to increase patient base.
- The practice will not work more than 40 hours per week to avoid overtime pay.

Continuing Education
- The practice will only take the amount of continuing education that is needed for license renewal.
- The practice will take more than the required amount of continuing education to improve service offerings to patients.

Staff Compensation
- The practice will pay above average pay and benefits to attract and keep the best staff members.
- The practice will pay above average pay but below average benefits to keep staff members who are motivated by money.

Practice Style
- The practice will keep a general practice style so that the target population is maximized.
- The practice will develop a niche style practice so that there is more freedom with fees and credit policy.

Advertising
- The practice will gain patients through other marketing efforts, not advertising.
- The practice will advertise heavily to generate patient base.

Loan
- The practice will pay off start-up loans as soon as possible to be debt free.
- The practice will pay off loans as needed to free cash for other uses.

Step 5: Set Goals and Objectives

Goals put a strategy into action. Objectives are specific elements of goals. For example, a dentist may have a goal to increase the patient base of the practice. A related specific objective might be to increase new patient visits to one per day. Box 13.9 describes five areas in which a dentist should want to establish goals and objectives. If appropriate goals in each of these areas are satisfied, then the dentist will have a successful practice. These goals and objectives should be measurable or quantifiable, specific, and time related. Measuring goals over a given period is the only way to know if they have been met. The goal "to provide an adequate income" leaves too much discretion to be an adequate goal. What is adequate for one practitioner may be inadequate for another. "To provide an income of $200,000 per year" is measurable and allows the person to decide whether the practice has achieved the goal for a particular period. Any individual goal

---

Box 13.9 Areas for Practice Goals

1. To have a profitable practice
   Productivity
   Collections
   Profitability

2. To have a reasonable workload
   Patient visits
   Hours worked
   Recall effectiveness

3. To have adequate financial and personal rewards
   for the staff and doctor
   Financial rewards
   Personal satisfaction rewards
   Personal and professional growth
   Staff recruitment and development

4. To have patients that are satisfied with the care
   that they receive
   Treatment completion rates
   Posttreatment surveys

5. To be a good and responsible citizen in the office
   and in the greater community
   Indigent care
   Philanthropic giving
   Responsible advertising
   Legal and proactive staff relations

Box 13.10 Some Methods to Achieve Goals

- Increase advertising
- Increasing evening or weekend hours
- Accepting insurance plans
- Hiring (terminating) staff
- Adding operatories
- Lowering or raising fees
- Tightening or easing the credit policy
- Raising pay for employees
- Lowering benefits for employees
- Borrowing additional money

---

may be inappropriate for a specific practice. If a goal is unattainable, it becomes disruptive for the practice. People may give up or view the entire goal process as a sham. If goals are inconsistent with the practice's philosophy, they are disruptive as well. An inappropriate reward system may subvert goal attainment as employees try to achieve the wrong ends. Finally, poorly stated or contradictory goals leave employees unsure of which direction they should follow.

In this discussion, only practice-related goals have been discussed. To be a truly complete and actualized professional, the dentist must also establish personal goals that are congruent with the practice goals. Many people advocate setting personal goals in the four areas of work, love, play and worship to find personal satisfaction; however, this discussion is limited to work, understanding that it affects the other areas of personal happiness.

Step 6: Develop Methods

Methods describe how a person will meet his or her goals. They are things that a person does to accomplish

a purpose. Therefore, although goals tell what a person what he or she is trying to do, methods tell how he or she is trying to do it. Depending on personal philosophy, different methods will be appropriate for different practices. For example, if the goal is "to generate at least one comprehensive new patient per day," then dentist might use a combination of advertising, managed care participation, rewarding existing patients for referrals, or keeping extended office hours. The methods should be consistent with the philosophy of the practice. If a dentist disdains advertising in the professional practice setting, then a different method would be more appropriate.

Each of the decisions that a dentist makes for the practice is a potential method and affects the outcomes of the practice. Box 13.10 gives several possible methods that can be used in this simulation to achieve goals. There are many others. Part of a dentist's job is to put these methods together into a coherent plan that leads to the fulfillment of his or her philosophy. Each method has consequences in several different areas. A dentist might increase evening hours to generate additional patients, but staff members may become dissatisfied working those hours. Dissatisfied staff members are not as productive and are more likely to leave.

Step 7: Measure Outcomes and Follow-up

Outcome measures are the numbers that a person examines to decide whether he or she has met goals. When a person measures the attainment of his or her goals, he or she is really measuring the effectiveness of the used strategy to meet that goal. (This assumes that the goal was appropriate and attainable.) If a person is not meeting established goals, then he or she should use a different approach (strategy). The section of this book on "Financial Analysis and Control" helps to establish outcome measures in critical areas of the practice.

Section 3

Dental Office Success Factors

Success is simply a matter of luck. Ask any failure.
Earl Wilson

Successful dental practices do not just happen. They are managed by an owner who has a clearly defined vision of where he or she wants the practice to be and works each day to guide the practice to that vision. That is the same thing that managers, from CEOs of Fortune 500 companies to start-up entrepreneurs, do every day. For people who have no training or background in business management that can seem like an overwhelming task. However, the philosophies, methods, and techniques that successful business managers use in other large and small companies can be learned. If those techniques are applied to the business operation of a dental practice, the dental practice can be like any other well run business.

The first step is to examine the business and decide what factors lead to its success or failure. Then try to measure whether those factors are being met, and if not, what can be done to improve operations to be more successful. Financial ratio analysis helps to show areas that need to be improved.

Major Goals of the Dental Office Success Factors Section

Business foundations relate to three major goals:

1. **Understand What Makes a Practice Profitable** Several factors lead to the success of a dental practice. Financial ratio analysis is a technique that business managers use to gauge the financial health of their firm. Just as someone's blood pressure is an indicator of his or her cardiac health, financial measures can show the financial health of a practice. When a dentist looks at the "numbers" of the practice, he or she measures whether those success factors are being met.

2. **Understand How to Manage an Efficient and Effective Operation** The daily operations in a dental practice must be managed to develop successful practice.

3. **Know and Manage the Sources of Risk in the Dental Office** Every business faces risk. Some of this is common to all businesses. Some risk is specific to the industry or individual firm. Regardless, a dentist needs to understand the risk so that he or she can reduce its effect on practice profitability.

Objectives of the Dental Office Success Factors Section

Given these three main goals, the objectives of the success factors for a dental practice are given here. These success factors are the indicators of a well-run dental business.

Chapter 14: Financial Analysis and Control in the Dental Office Dentists need to know the factors that lead to success in a dental practice and how they can measure whether they are achieving those factors.

Chapter 15: Maintaining Production Production is the key to practice health. Unless a dentist is generating an adequate production (and therefore dollars), then no amount of management skill can gain profitability. **Part 1: Duty Delegation** If dentists can legally have staff members do tasks in the office that the dentist would have done, dentists have time to do other, more profitable procedures. This improves production. **Part 2: Scheduling Patients** Dentists need to keep an orderly flow of patients to use their practice

Business Basics for Dentists, First Edition. David O. Willis.
© 2013 John Wiley & Sons, Inc. Published 2013 by John Wiley & Sons, Inc.

resources effectively. This keeps patient visits, and therefore production, at healthy levels. **Part 3: Dental Fee Policy**   The fees that dentists charge, along with the number of patient visits, are the basis of office production.

Chapter 16: Maintaining Collections   Once dentists do the dentistry, they must collect a fee from patients and insurance companies. **Part 1: Patient Financial Policies**   Dentists need to establish payment policies that encourage patients to have the needed work done and to pay for it. **Part 2: Office Collection Policies**   If patients do not pay for services as they had agreed, dentists need to have methods that encourage patients to fulfill their financial obligation.

Chapter 17: Generating Patients for the Practice   Patient visits are the basis of all income generated in the practice. Dentists need to be sure that they generate enough patients to meet their financial goals. **Part 1: Generating New Patients**   New patients increase how much work dentists do in the practice. They often result in large, expensive cases that directly improve profitability of the practice. **Part 2: Managing Continuing Care**   Existing patients of the practice have improved oral health outcomes when dentists see them regularly for periodic maintenance of dental conditions. They also improve the financial outcome of the practice.

Chapter 18: Gaining Case Acceptance   Any patient who comes to the office may have additional dental work to be done. However, the patient does not automatically accept treatment recommendations. Dentists must properly communicate patient needs to them and help the patient to understand how the treatment will improve their health and life. **Part 1: Communications in the Office**   All human interactions involve some form of communication. If dentists understand how they transfer information, they can improve communication in the office. **Part 2, Case Presentation and Acceptance**   Dentists must turn a patient who has dental needs into a patient who wants treatment for those needs by using proper case presentation techniques.

Chapter 19: Controlling Costs in the Practice   Profit is gained by keeping cost less than revenue. Dentists can not eliminate costs in the dental office, but they can manage and control the costs. Understanding the nature of the various office costs helps dentists to manage cost in the most effective way.

Chapter 20: Promoting Staff Effectiveness   Successful practices have effective staff members. Effective staffs do not just happen. The owner–dentist creates them by hiring the right people, compensating them well, and motivating them to high levels of performance. **Part 1: Selecting and Hiring Staff**   Dentists need to find people with the right skills to do tasks and the right attitude to fit into the staff team in the office. **Part 2: Compensating Staff**   Everyone works, to some degree, for compensation. Dentists need to develop a competitive pay and benefit package to attract and retain the best employees. **Part 3: Leading and Motivating Staff**   People work, to some degree, for reasons other than pay. If dentists understand what motivates people in the workplace, they can develop a system and atmosphere that promote employee performance. **Part 4: Assessing Employee Performance**   Employees want to perform well on the job. As employers, dentists need to let employees know what is expected, reward them when they do well, and discourage inappropriate behaviors.

Chapter 21: Maintaining Daily Operations   Dentists need to manage daily work in the office. They need to ensure that supplies are ordered, laboratory cases are completed, instruments are sterilized, and payments are properly accounted. **Part 1: Office Operations**   The most profitable practices are those are those that use their resources effectively and efficiently. **Part 2: Office Accounting Systems**   Dentists need to establish proper accounting systems to use in the office. **Part 3: Instrument Management**   Each office needs to establish methods to clean, disinfect, or sterilize instruments and equipment used in the dental office. **Part 4: Lab and Supply Management**   Each office needs to establish methods to ensure that there are enough supplies for procedures and that lab work is properly prepared and returned in time for delivery to the patient. **Part 5: Dental Insurance Management**   Dental insurance is a reality for most practitioners. Dentists need to understand how dental insurance programs work so that they can manage the programs in the office.

Chapter 22: Managing Risk in the Office   Practices face many types of risk. Dentists need to identify and mange those risks so that they do not face a financially devastating incident. **Part 1: Office Risk Management**   Risk management identifies and decreases the sources of risk in the office. These may develop from the dentist's role as a practicing dentist or as the owner of the business. **Part 2: Compliance**   Dentists must comply with regulatory agencies' requirements. **Part 3: Quality Assurance**   Many third-party providers require that dentists prove quality assurance activities.

Financial Analysis and Control in the Dental Office

chapter 14

Put all your eggs in one basket and WATCH THAT BASKET!
Mark Twain

Objectives

At the completion of this chapter, the student will be able to:

1. Discuss the steps in the financial control process.
2. Describe the common stages in the practice development cycle.
3. Describe the six critical factors that lead to dental practice success.
4. Compute typical office analysis in the areas of:
   Office production
   Office collections
   Practice costs
   Patient generation
   Case acceptance
   Staff effectiveness
5. Discuss the importance of and give common normal values for the following dental office financial ratios:
   Overhead ratio
   Office monthly production
   Service mix
   AR amount
   Collection ratio
   AR over 60 days
   Managed care percentage
   Managed care efficiency
   Total staff percentage
   Variable cost ratio
   New patients per month
   Recall effectiveness
   Marketing dollars per new patient
   Case acceptance ratio

Key Terms

AR amount over 60 days	managed care percentage	ratios
basic profitability formula	mix of devices	staff efficiency ratios
collection ratio	lab-to-labor ratio	standards
fee profile	overhead	variable cost ratio
managed care efficiency	overhead percentage	

Business Basics for Dentists, First Edition. David O. Willis.
© 2013 John Wiley & Sons, Inc. Published 2013 by John Wiley & Sons, Inc.

Goal

This chapter examines the financial control process for use in the dental practice. It discusses the factors that lead to dental office success and gives common financial ratios that are used to assess attainment of those success factors.

Financial control looks at the "numbers" of the practice in an attempt to maximize profit from the practice. Dentists can make the financial control process as simple or as complex as they want. The possibilities for gathering data are endless. If dentists have an in-office computer system, the problem is often deciding which of the many reports and analyses they truly need. Dentists should not inundate themselves with information and should look for major problem areas first. They should start with some basic ratios (production, profitability, and collection ratios) and look for problems in these areas. If dentists find no major problems, they probably do not need to do any in-depth analysis. Conversely, a practice may be having problems in one certain area that needs particular, additional attention. Other areas may be functioning well and only require periodic monitoring.

Most people only think of costs when they look at financial control. The revenue side is equally important. For example, costs may be under control, but low production leads to low profitability. Many also think that business owners should reduce overhead wherever possible; however, there is "good" overhead and "bad" overhead. Good overhead is money that dentists spend that makes them more money. Bad overhead does not contribute to making more money; it is, therefore, wasted. For example, suppose a dentist hires a new staff member with pay of $15 an hour. That staff member allows the dentist to produce an additional $50 per hour. That is money well spent (a good piece of overhead). However, if the office does not increase production enough to make up for the additional costs, the additional money spent on the staff member would be bad overhead. This is simple in idea. The problem is trying to decide which costs cause waste and which contribute to the practice's profitability. That is what financial analysis is about.

Many dentists want to leave the numbers to an accountant. Such a policy is OK if the accountant is familiar with dental practices and understands a dentist's personal philosophy, goals, and where the dentist wants the office to be. The problem is that most accountants do not know these things. They are more interested in tax numbers. If a dentist finds an accountant who is knowledgeable about dental practice numbers, he or she should use that accountant to his or her advantage. If not, then a dentist will need to be his or her own financial analyst.

Steps in the Financial Control Process

Understanding the financial control process is important. Otherwise, a dentist might apply a simple rule that is not appropriate for the given situation. The previous chapter on office finance presents the fundamental information on finances in the office. This chapter continues the analysis by looking at how those concepts should be interpreted.

Step 1: Setting Standards

The first step is for a dentist to establish a target against which he or she will measure subsequent practice activity. The standard serves as the mechanism to monitor practice performance and should meet the needs of a particular practice. For example, a dentist may set a standard of wanting to see 200 recall patients per month. A slight deviation from this standard (180–220 patients per month) is expected, but a major shortage of recall patients (50 patients per month) would suggest a more serious problem.

Dentists often use national or regional averages as the basis of setting a standard. For example, an average overhead ratio may be 65 percent. Does that mean that a dentist's practice *should* have a 65 percent overhead ratio? Not necessarily. If a dentist hits this mark, then half of the practices will have a higher mark and half will have a lower percentage. A dentist's practice may be a start-up practice in which he or she is not fully scheduled. So any time a dentist compares his or her practice to others as a standard, that dentist must be sure that the analysis is adjusted appropriately.

The key is to decide the appropriate standard—what is it that a dentist wants to measure? He or she should look for measures that relate to the changes made or suspected problems rather than trying to measure everything. In this way a dentist can make a higher impact by concentrating on specific target areas rather than trying a "shotgun" approach to measuring his or her practice.

Step 2: Measuring Performance

Although standards set forth "what should be," measuring performance examines what has happened in a practice. This reality measure is crucial to successful and effective practice management control. Dentists may make these measurements daily, monthly, or annually depending on the variable. Practice policy may define them such as "all patients receive a survey questionnaire when they complete treatment and are placed on recall status," or dentists may gather them from ongoing practice record systems (day sheets, time records, etc.). The measures may be formal or informal, simple or elaborate. Whatever system is used, it should relate directly to the standard a dentist wishes to measure. It should also represent the entire dental practice and be reliable (consistent) and valid (measure what is intended). Reliable measures require, for example, that a dentist uses the same survey questionnaire for the exit interview of patients who have completed treatment. Dentists cannot expect to gain useful information if they ask different questions each time the questionnaire is given. Valid standards measure what they are supposed to measure. "Percent of recall patients seen by the hygienist," for example, may be a measure of scheduling rather than hygienist performance.

Historical practice data will serve as a good starting point for determining future standards. Previous costs, revenues, or intangible measures should all be considered. A dentist may also find comparative standards from other dental practices useful. One excellent source of this data is from the American Dental Association's (ADA) periodic "Survey of Dental Practice." Other sources include the popular dental press (e.g., *Dental Economics*), an accountant, and national organizations, such as the ADA.

Step 3: Comparing Performance to Standards

In this step, dentists compare actual performance with what should have happened. This comparison is easy if there are established standards and measured information. The actual results and the desired outcomes will rarely match exactly. A dentist should set acceptable ranges for performance, evaluate the performance outcomes within these ranges, and then look for exceptions. Management by exception permits a dentist to concentrate on the significant problems that may arise in the practice without becoming overburdened with the minutia of all the standards. For example, as stated previously, if a dentist has a standard of wanting to see 200 recall patients per month but only sees 180 in a month and 197 the next month, he or she may not be too concerned about the 2-month average of 188 recalls a month. However, if he or she saw only 55 recalls 1 month and 127 the next month, the dentist would want to explore more fully the reasons for much lower-than-expected recall patient visits.

Dentists should be sure to pick an appropriate period for their analysis. Many numbers and ratios may fluctuate widely over a given time range. If so, a dentist would want to lengthen the period being reviewed. Dentists should track some numbers daily. Some offices set daily production goals. Other offices feel that daily production is too unsteady and prefer, instead to use monthly numbers. If a dentist examines a month in which he or she took 2 weeks of vacation, unrepresentative numbers will be the result. A quarterly analysis might be more appropriate. Most aggressive dentists look at their numbers monthly. Many others look quarterly, believing that this smoothes out the monthly variations. Still other dentists only look at numbers when accountants prepare their taxes. The final group never looks at them. They simply believe that things are going OK, and they are making an adequate living, so why bother? All are perfectly acceptable.

Step 4: Correcting Deviations

This is the essence of control. It is during this step that dentists take actions to adjust the plan or operation of the dental practice. For example, if the office did not meet the standard of "95 percent of recall patients due are appointed each month," the dentist would take corrective actions to meet the standard in the future.

Correcting deviations from planned standards requires astute problem-solving skills. Knowledge of dental practice management helps a dentist decide when to modify standards, replace personnel, restructure office policies, set up new staff development programs, and so forth. The key to setting up an effective control system is taking corrective action. Failure to act when a dentist detects a substantial deviation in a planned standard undermines the purpose of this evaluation system.

The plans that a dentist started may be inappropriate for the actual conditions that develop. Then, he or she needs to correct the plan itself. If a dentist assumes a steady economic climate and plans to expand the dental practice by finding additional office space, equipment, or staff and the general economy declines instead, he or she will need to alter the plan. If a dentist only finds slight deviations, he or she may decide simply to monitor these changes and take action when they reach a certain point. For example, if a patient satisfaction survey reveals slight displeasure with the receptionist from one or two patients, a dentist would probably choose to monitor this situation rather than discuss it with the receptionist. If other patients also reported dissatisfaction over a period, then the dentist may decide to speak to the receptionist.

Profitability Analysis

The basic statement that shows profitability is profit-and-loss (P&L) statement (Fig. 14.1). What dentists want to do is to maximize the "bottom line" and

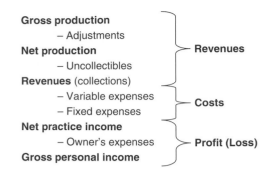

Figure 14.1 Profit-and-loss statement

makc practices as profitable as possible, given certain constraints. (Dentists could increase income by working 80 hours per week, but most are not willing to do that.) There is no magic formula. To increase profit, dentists can only increase revenues, decrease costs, or make some combination of the two. So dentists need to examine the components of the income formula (both revenues and costs) when planning an office analysis.

Dental Practice Revenues

Total collections (gross practice revenues) are the result of the number and type of procedures that dentists do, the fee that they charge for each of those procedures, any adjustments granted from full fee, and the collection ratio shown by the office. If collections are low, any of the four factors may be at fault. The following formulas describe these relationships:

Gross Production = Number of Procedures × Fee

Gross Production − Adjustments = Net Production

Net Production × Collection Ratio = Revenues

Gross production is the total amount of dentistry produced by the office for the period, before any discounts or adjustments. Production levels vary with the number and types of procedures done and the fee charged for those procedures. It is the combination of all individual procedures and fees. Production is obviously the cornerstone of practice profitability in a dental practice because without production, no money flows through the office.

Adjustments are the amounts of money that the office "wrote off" for discounts because of payment plan (such as Medicaid) requirements, marketing efforts, or professional courtesies. Dentists may decide to track particular types of adjustments to detect the impact of that plan has on the office finances. For example, a dentist may wish to track how much Medicaid and capitation plan payment that the office adjusts each month.

Net production is mathematically, production less adjustments. It is the amount of money that dentists want to collect. Because dentists do not expect to collect the money that has been adjusted, they should exclude those amounts from many analyses.

The *collection ratio* is the percentage of net production that the office collects from patients and insurance companies. *Uncollectibles* are the monies that dentists have given up trying to collect. Mathematically, it (collection ratio) is multiplied by net production.

Revenues (collections) are the amounts of money (i.e., cash, checks, and credit cards) that crossed the receptionist's desk for the period. Some of this may be from production for this month, whereas the rest of it may be for dentistry done several months ago but is now being paid. Individuals, insurance companies, or government programs may make payments.

Dental Practice Costs

Cost for a dental practice fall into two conceptual categories, fixed and variable.

Fixed costs do not change with production. Rent, for example, remains the same regardless if 10 or 100 patients are seen in a month.

Variable costs change directly with the level of gross production. These are supplies and laboratory charges. If a dentist produces twice as much dentistry in a month, he or she would logically expect to have twice the lab and supply bill from the increased amount of work.

Profit

Profit is the money that is available for the owner of the practice to take from the practice accounts and use for personal benefit and enjoyment.

Net practice income is the amount that is available to the owner as profit from operating the practice.

Owner's expenses are expenses that the owner has chosen to take from the practice that they could have taken as profit. Examples include personal automobile expenses, personal retirement plan contributions, and many continuing education expenses. Because taking these costs is discretionary, they are included in the practice profit.

Gross personal income is the amount that the practice owner claims for initial personal tax computations.

Critical Success Factors

There are six factors that lead to business success of the dental practice. Dentists should aim their practice assessment at these factors, judging whether they are meeting the factors. Box 14.1 lists the success factors. The rest of Section 2 gives much more detail on each of these items, showing how dentists can change the practice to improve these indicators.

Factor 1: Maintaining Production

Production is the key to practice health (Box 14.2). Unless dentists are generating an adequate production (and therefore dollars), no amount of management skill can gain profitability. Production is a result of both the number of procedures done and the fee charges for each procedure. The number of procedures completed is the result of all the management functions in the office. The front office influences this through scheduling. A dentist's abilities and wants and the efficiency of the production personnel also affect production.

Office production per month tracks the total amount of dentistry done by the entire office for the month. Assuming an individual practitioner, production should remain steady or rise each month. (Obviously, if a dentist takes a week off, then production may be down for

that month.) Many dentists set production goals for the office. This then becomes the production measure. To do production, the office must adequately schedule patients. "Adequately scheduled" does not just mean being busy. Instead a dentist needs a good mix of highly productive procedures (such as crown and bridge) and preparatory procedures (such as restorations).

Some practitioners like to track gross production, others, net production. Gross production describes how hard a dentist is working because it is before any insurance adjustments. It is a gauge of patient visits. Net production (after adjustments) shows how much money the office generates. It is a more accurate gauge of practice finances and insurance plan participation. Net production defines income, whereas gross production determines costs. Either is an appropriate indicator, depending on what a dentist wants to measure.

The *procedure mix* examines the types of services done in the office. As a rule, a general practice should have about one-third of the revenue generated from hygiene procedures, one-third from non-lab production, and the final one-third from high-margin lab-related procedures. This shows enough patients in the pipeline for diagnostic, basic, and complex procedures. If a practice mix is significantly different from this, then a dentist might look at new scheduling priorities.

A *fee profile* compares fees to the average fees in a certain area. Most dentists want to position themselves so that they are in the upper half of fees in the area. More aggressive practitioners prefer to be above the upper 75th percentile. Dentists must be sure to keep fees current for the area in which they practice. Even a small increase can have a dramatic influence on production numbers. Fee level is the single biggest determinant of production levels in the mature dental practice. Monitor fees regularly.

Box 14.1 Six Factors that Lead to Business Success

1. Maintaining production
2. Maintaining adequate collections
3. Controlling costs
4. Generating patients for the practice
5. Gaining high case acceptance
6. Promoting staff effectiveness

Box 14.2 Maintaining Production

Office Production per Month
 Not decrease
Mix of Services
 One-third hygiene
 One-third lab-related production
 One-third nonlab–related production
Fee Profile
 Fiftieth to 75th percentile

Factor 2: Maintaining Collections

Once the dentistry is done, dentists need to be sure to collect from the patients for the work done (Box 14.3).

The *accounts receivable (AR) amount* shows the proportion of production that dentists are not collecting. A raw amount for AR (e.g., $30,000) is meaningless. Was that from a practice that grosses $25,000 per month or one that grosses $80,000 per month? (AR will be larger for larger practices, all other things being equal.) This indicator says that for any practice, about 1/2 to 1 times the average month's net production is acceptable as an AR amount. Credit and collection policies will have an obvious impact on this indicator. Easy credit policies will generate higher AR; stricter

---

Box 14.3 Maintaining Collections

Accounts Receivable Amount
   Half- to 1 month's net production
Collection Ratio
   >98 percent
   One-third counter, one-third insurance, one-third billed
Accounts Receivable Amount over 60 Days
   One-fourth to one-third month's production
Managed Care Percentage
   <50 percent total production
   <25 percent in any one plan

Box 14.4 Managed Care Programs

Managed Care Percentage
   Total managed care <50 percent production OR managed care adjustments <20 percent production
   <25 percent production in any one plan
Managed Care Efficiency
   Total plan collections
   Full fee value of services

---

policies lower. Practices that process a large amount of insurance (greater than 60 to 70 percent of patients) will also have a larger AR as they wait for insurance companies to process forms and mail checks. Immediate fee-for-service practices on the low end of this range. This also assumes that the office processes insurance electronically, rather than through paper and mail. These latter practices will have higher AR (up to 1 and 1 1/2 months' production) because of the slower insurance processing.

The total *collection ratio* should be at or more than 97 percent of net production. Ideally, everyone should pay. Most dental offices collect between 95 and 99 percent of the billable amount. (Because dentists do not really expect to collect adjustments, they are not included in this ratio.) A lower collection ratio may suggest problems with collection procedures or a temporary surge in production, resulting in an increase in AR and potential cash flow problems. A high collection number may suggest a credit policy that is too strict, discouraging patients from accepting large treatment plans. This may be a particular problem in younger, growing practices. Established practices with an excess patient base have more freedom to set stricter financial policies.

The *AR amount over 60 days* tells a dentist how well the front office is collecting the money from patients that the office has billed. Sixty-day-old accounts are becoming problem accounts. Any insurance payments should have cleared on these accounts. They are becoming difficult to collect, and the dentist has lost the use of the money for that time. Dentists should see, at most, one-fourth to one-third of 1 month's production in this number. If this number is high, then either credit policies are too loose or collection efforts are not strong enough.

Managed care programs (preferred provider organizations, dental maintenance organizations, etc.) significantly affect the analysis of a dental practice. For example, using gross production will give an unrealistic result in determining collection ratios. If dentists discount 20 percent of the work done, then the highest that can be expected to be collect is 80 percent of gross production. This is a seemingly abysmal amount that may be excellent for the circumstance. Using net production as a basis finds a more accurate collection efficiency. Few dentists in the United States want to deal with any managed care plans. However, most dentists do. If a dentist does, then he or she needs to track how well he or she is controlling the managed care in the office.

Managed care percentage looks at the portion of a practice's gross production represented by managed care insurance plans. This measure has two options. First, if total managed care production exceeds 50 percent of total gross practice production, then managed care is simply too great a part of the practice. Not only is a dentist losing a lot of money, he or she is also losing control of the schedule because managed care patients replace full fee-for-service patients. The practice may be in a "risky" position if the programs change reimbursement schedules or cancel provider contracts. A second measure is to look at managed care adjustments. These adjustments should represent no more than 20 percent of the total office production. This takes into account the efficiency of all of the plans (in total) a dentist is working with but does not assess an individual plan. Both measures give similar results. The first is a bit easier; the second is more accurate. Finally, no plan should account for more than 25 percent of gross production (Box 14.4). In this way, if the employer changes insurance plans, closes temporarily, or goes bankrupt, the change does not devastate the practice. This may be difficult to accomplish in areas that have only one major employer and the practice depends on that employer for a large portion of the patient pool. It also encourages locating a practice in an economically diverse area.

Dentists also need to track how well each plan is reimbursing the practice. *Managed care efficiency* looks at each individual plan. It asks the percentage returned compared to a similar, full-fee patient. This way, dentists know how much of a discount is implied with each plan. To calculate this measure, take the total collections from each plan (including any capitation payments) and divide by the full-fee value. Dentists need to track this regularly because plan administrators change their reimbursements and rules, often without telling providers. This is discussed in the chapter on dental insurance.

Factor 3: Controlling Costs

Because both output (revenues) and input (costs) contribute to productivity, dentists obviously must control both to be productive. There is a cost of doing business. For example, dentists can not practice without spending money on space or supplies. Any cost that adds to profitability is a good cost; any cost that decreases profitability is a bad cost. The key is to decide which is which. To accomplish this, most management experts compare a practice to norms, or "average" practices of a similar type. For example, every dentist has a cost associated with rental (or purchase) of office space. If the "average" dentist pays 9 percent of his or her production for rent and another dentist is paying 12 percent, then some rent may be decreasing the profit of the latter's practice.

The *overhead ratio* rearranges the information contained in the income statement. Rather than showing how much profit was made, the profitability formula shows overhead, or how much it costs for a given amount of work. The profitability formula answers the question "What percentage of my production went to pay the bills?" (It also answers the converse, "What percentage of my production was left as profit?") The traditional overhead percentage is the total cost of doing business divided by the total collections. This shows, in a rough way, the percent of

every dollar generated that pays the costs of the practice. The inverse (1 – overhead percentage) represents the profitability of the practice. (If the overhead is 70 percent, then the profitability of the practice is 30 percent.) Production or net production is often used instead of collections in the profitability formula. This gives a more accurate picture of costs, especially in practices that participate with highly discounted insurance plans. However, most national reference numbers still use collections as the base. This can lead to confusing practice comparisons.

In general dental practices, overhead (and the overhead ratio) falls into ranges: more than 65 percent is high; less than 55 percent is good; and 55 to 65 percent is about average. This ratio balances for different parts of the country. High-fee areas are also generally high-cost areas. If overhead falls into the "good" range, a dentist may be satisfied, realizing that the trouble of additional analysis and control may not produce enough return to worry about. Conversely, a dentist may want to maximize the potential profit from the practice and continue the analysis to detect areas to increase profitability further. If the overhead percentage is out of line compared with other practices, a dentist needs to look at his or her numbers more carefully. Generally the problem is that the overhead ratio is too high, but the overhead ratio may also be too low. This happens when dentists unrealistically staff the office, do not account for all costs (such as working spouses), if collections surge because of anomalies in the collection pattern, or if they do not purchase adequate supplies, equipment, and material to keep up to date. Specialty practices have different acceptable ranges because of the different character of those practices. This also assumes that a dentist is not doing any fancy tax avoidance strategies (e.g., renting space from self or hiring family members at an unusually high price) that can skew results.

When a dentist looks at his overhead ratio compared with others, he or she is comparing his or her practice with other dental practices. When making this comparison, the dentist makes two implicit assumptions: that the dental practice is similar to other practices and that dentists are rational businesspeople making similar, rational business decisions. These assumptions can both be challenged; however, given a broad mix of practice types and styles, a dentist can use these comparisons as a beginning point in understanding his or her practice's financial structure.

The overhead ratio is dependent on the point a dentist is at in the practice cycle. If a dentist is in a start-up phase, with few patients and high debts and expenses, then overhead will obviously be very high. New practitioners are often paying off the buy-out or start-up loans.

Box 14.5 Controlling Costs	
Overhead Ratio	55–65 percent
Staff Efficiency Ratios	
Clinical efficiency	10–12 percent
Front office efficiency	7–9 percent
Hygiene efficiency	33–42 percent
Specific Cost Ratios	
Staff ratio	22–30 percent
Variable cost ratio	13–20 percent
Office space ratio	8–10 percent

Table 14.1 Specific cost control

Category	Percentage of Collections
Staff Costs Wages, Benefits, Taxes, Insurance	25–30%
Variable Costs/Supplies Lab, Dental Supplies, Office Supplies	13–20%
Facilities Rent, Utilities, Depreciation	8–10%
Miscellaneous Legal, Accounting, Advertising, Taxes, Insurance, Interest	9–14%
Owner's Expenses Dues, subscription, automobile, continuing education, retirement	8–10%
Profit	35–45%

The interest and depreciation expenses represented by this outlay are additional costs that established practitioners generally do not have. New practitioners in a buy-out situation often must replace or update equipment, supplies, and materials at an additional cost. Finally, many new practitioners simply cannot do the volume of dentistry that established practitioners do. This may be from the need to increase patient pool or the new practitioner's clinical inexperience. Regardless, if production is less than a comparable established practitioner, then the overhead, and most other ratios, will appear to be out of line. New practitioners can expect an additional 5 percent overhead for debt service while paying off loans. They may even run at a loss (more than 100 percent overhead) while building patient pool.

Dentists' personal and professional wants, needs and desires will modify what they consider to be acceptable range in all these analyses. For example, a dentist may be considering two practice options. Practice one produces $600,000 with a 70-percent overhead on 5 days per week ($180,000 net). Practice two produces $400,000 with a 60-percent overhead on 4 days per week ($160,000 net). A dentist must decide if the added management problems and time commitments are worth the additional net income.

Specific Cost Control

This really looks at the same thing as the overhead percentage but begins to break it into specific units, using typical ranges of costs for each area of cost allocation. These standards attach values to various components of the expenses of operating a dental practice. Most are related as a percentage of collections.

(Some, such as variable costs, may more logically relate to gross production, but industry norms use collections as the basis of comparison.) When using these numbers, a dentist is comparing his or her practice to the "norm" or other similar practices. A dentist can compare every cost if he or she wants, but that is not a good use of time. He or she should concentrate on the areas where a change can make the most impact.

Total staff costs involve all of the expenses of hiring and retaining staff members. This includes gross wages paid (including withholdings), FICA matching, unemployment and workers' compensation insurances, retirement plan contributions, and any other benefits (such as health insurance) paid by the practice. The acceptable number is a range. Practice without a hygienist should be at the low end of the range. Practices that employ a hygienist (or multiple hygienists) should expect to be at the upper end of the range. Staff is the single largest area of cost in the dental office. A little savings here can make a large difference on the bottom line.

Variable Cost Ratio

Variable costs change directly with production. The more dentistry produced, the greater these costs should be. Variable cost ratios run 13 to 20 percent for most general dental practices. Breaking these costs down further, dental supplies run 7 to 10 percent, office supplies 1 to 3 percent, and dental lab costs from 6 to 12 percent.

Office Space (Facilities) Ratio

Dentists should hold total cost for office facility to the range of 5 to 10 percent of collections. (The average is about 7 percent). This is true whether a dentist owns or rents space or whether the facility is freestanding or part of a larger facility.

Proper Staffing Configuration

Because staff costs are such an important part of the cost equation for dental practitioners, a series of ratios has been developed to assess whether they have properly staffed the office. These are "negative" ratios. That means the lower the percentage, the better the ratio.

Clerical Efficiency

Clerical efficiency looks at total clerical compensation as a percentage of office collections. Typical practices run 8 to 10 percent for this number. Higher than that, either a dentist is overstaffed or his or her production or fees are too low. Less, a dentist may be understaffed or the existing staff may be underpaid. If a dentist is understaffed, front office personnel probably cannot do billing, make appointments, or make collection calls in a timely manner. Problems with general office productivity may result. Remember to include all costs of employment (e.g., wages, benefits, insurances, FICA, retirement plans, etc.) when calculating total compensation.

Clinical Staff Efficiency

This ratio compares nonhygiene clinical labor costs and revenues. Ideally, clinical labor should run 7 to 10 percent of the doctor's collections. (Hygiene labor and collections are excluded and calculated later.) The doctor's productive capacity and the state's expanded function laws will obviously influence this number.

Hygiene Efficiency

Hygiene efficiency examines the relationship between the hygienists' total compensation (including taxes and benefits) with the revenue produced by the hygiene area. The "exam" portion of the periodic visit is generally included in the doctor's production because that is the person who does that service. This is probably a better ratio than production per hour for looking at hygiene productivity because areas with higher fees also usually have higher salary levels. (They balance each other out.) Hygienists should be producing 2 1/2 to 3 times their compensation. That is to say, compensation should be 33 to 42 percent of hygiene revenue (not production).

Factor 4: Generating Patients for the Practice

Without patients, dentists have no practice. Patients are either existing (recall) patients of the practice or patients that are new to the practice, generated either from internal referrals or outside marketing efforts

(Box 14.6). Patient satisfaction with a dentist's care leads to internal referrals. Money that dentists spend for marketing programs leads to outside new patient generation. All are important sources of patients. Dentists should monitor all regularly. Established practitioners can often live off internal referrals without the need or expense for marketing programs. New and growing practitioners often need a planned marketing effort to generate the patient pool needed for success.

Because new patients present with most of the large cases in an office, *new patients per month* keeps tracks of this statistic. Each practitioner should see at a minimum 20 new patients per month (or about one per day) to keep the practice adequately busy. "New" patients imply comprehensive care patients, not emergent or episodic care patients.

Recall effectiveness measures the percentage of patients due for recall in a given year that dentists saw for recall visits. This ratio examines how effective the practice is in encouraging patients to return for periodic maintenance visits. In established urban practices, production resulting from the recall visit and subsequent findings account for 60 to 75 percent of the total production. Managing the recall program is obviously an important component of overall practice management. Dentists expect some patient attrition as people move from the area or find different reasons to switch dentists or forego dental treatment. However, dentists should try to reduce these two latter reasons through effective recall planning. Dentists should strive to see 90 to 95 percent of the patients who are due for the month. If they fall short, the front office person or hygienist (whoever is responsible for recall management) should begin procedures to increase recall acceptance. (This is also, in part, a scheduling issue.) Normal monthly variations may suggest that an annual recall effectiveness ratio is better than the shorter, more volatile monthly analysis.

Marketing Dollars Spent Compared to New Patients

This ratio examines how much it costs to generate each new patient, compared with the production each new patient represents. If a dentist is spending $10 to generate a patient who has a typical treatment plan of $800, the marketing program is obviously effective. Most in-office computer accounting programs will track patient referral sources and dollars generated from the referral source. This is particularly important in assessing the cost–benefit ratio of specific marketing plans. Dentists should generate at least $5 of production

---

Box 14.6 Generating patients

New Patients per Month
   Twenty per practitioner per month
Recall Effectiveness
   >90 percent of recalls due
Marketing Dollars per New Patient
   Treatment = 5 × marketing dollars
Patient Satisfaction
   >95 percent satisfied

> **Box 14.7** Gain High Case Acceptance
>
> **Proper Case Presentation**
>   Case acceptance ratio >75 percent
> **Appropriate Sales Technique**
>   Case completion ratio >95 percent

> **Box 14.8** Promoting Staff Effectiveness
>
> **Compensation System**
>   Compare to published averages
> **Motivating and Team Building**
>   Performance appraisals
> **Selecting Staff**
>   Probationary appraisals and retention

for every dollar spent in marketing. Less than that may still be profitable but only marginally. Another measure is that dentists should not spend more than $100 to generate each patient unless the patients are highly profitable.

Patient Satisfaction

These standards include patient attitudes about the practice, quality of care, staff interaction, public relations, and promotional activities of the practice. Qualitative (intangible) items are more difficult to measure than other standards. Patient surveys, questionnaires, or interviews are effective techniques to measure these variables to set standards. These questionnaires ask how patients "feel" about certain aspects of a practice, staff, or promotional activities. Satisfied patients tell other potential patients about the office; so do dissatisfied patients (in unkind terms). Strive for the highest satisfaction that is realistically possible.

Factor 5: Gain High Case Acceptance

Generating patients for the practice is only one step in generating income. A person who comes to a dentist for an examination is only a potential patient (source of revenue). Dentists must turn each of those potential patients into patients who accept recommended treatment, becoming comprehensive patients of the practice (Box 14.7). How many accept the recommended treatment is determined, largely, by how the dentists present the case and how the office completes the "sales" of dental services. The case acceptance ratios judge how well dentists can convince patients to complete recommended treatment.

A dentist's *case presentation technique* is what turns a prospective patient into a comprehensive patient. It involves patient psychology, patient education, selling techniques, and ethical behavior. During the presentation, a dentist should establish what the patient wants and provide solutions to those wants. Everyone will have objections to treatment proposed. This is a healthy skepticism that, if properly answered, leads to a commitment to act. Despite presentation

techniques, not everyone will immediately accept the total proposed treatment. However, dentists should aim for at least a 75 percent acceptance of complete treatment plans.

The *appropriate sales technique* involves all of the office systems that help a potential patient commit to the treatment recommendations that dentists give. These include a flexible payment plan, proper collection techniques, appointment availability, follow up of missed or broken appointments, and reminders of upcoming appointments. If any of these fail, the patient may not initiate or complete the proposed treatment. The case completion ratio compares all of the cases completed with those initiated (accepted). Dentists should complete at least 95 percent of the cases to which patients commit.

Factor 6: Promoting Staff Effectiveness

Successful practices have effective staff members (Box 14.8). Effective staffs do not just happen. The owner–dentist creates them by hiring the right people, compensating them well, and motivating them to high levels of performance. Analysis items that examine staff effectiveness do not have standard numbers associated with them. They are specific to an individual practice. However, some general guidelines are provided.

The *compensation system* must reward individuals and the team for high performance. Compensation includes both wages and benefits. Staff members compare these with other, similar jobs in the area. They then decide if they believe they are fairly compensated for the work they do. Dentists should compare their compensation to published averages for the area. The total compensation package should be at or above average for the area. Although simply paying a high wage will not guarantee loyal, hardworking employees, paying an inadequate wage will almost guarantee an unmotivated workforce.

People work for many reasons besides pay. Social interactions found on the job, personal growth, and a belief they are contributing to improve people's lives all play a part. As the practice leader, it is the dentist's job to tap into all these emotional reasons for working and to use them to build a cohesive and productive team that meets the philosophy and goals of the practice. That is the essence of motivation and team building. Dentists should check how well they are doing through their staff performance appraisals. Staff members should be meeting or exceeding a dentist's expectations.

To have excellent staff members, a dentist first must select staff. This is done through the recruitment, application, and interview processes. Dentists should asses their performance by looking at the probationary period appraisals and retention. If the selection process is effective, most of the dentist's probationary appraisals should be positive. Dentists should also have few staff leaving their employment.

Tracking the Factors

Table 14.2 guides dentists in tracking these important factors. It gives expected ranges. Table 14.3 can be used to assess the operation of a practice. The table can be photocopied and completed once per quarter. (It can be completed once per month but often normal fluctuations that confuse are seen the analysis.) When the numbers are completed, dentists should look for areas of improvement and then set goals for the upcoming quarter and reassess to look for progress.

Table 14.2 Critical Factors in Practice Success and their Measures

Success Factor	Measure of Factor	Value of Measure
Maintaining Production		
Scheduling	Office production per month	Level or increasing
Proper Mix of Services	Procedure mix ratio	1/3, 1/3, 1/3
Fee Profile for Services	Fee comparison with norms	50th to 90th percentile
Maintaining Adequate Collections		
Collection Effectiveness	AR amount	1/2 to 1 month's production
Collection Efficiency	Collection ratio	98% of billable amount
Managing Accounts Receivable	AR over 60 days	1/4 to 1/3 month's production
Managed Care Contribution	Managed care percentage	<50% total gross production
	Managed plan size	<25% production in any one plan
Generating Patients		
Adequate New Patients	New patient ratio	One new patient to practitioner per day
Effective Recall System	Recall effectiveness ratio	>90%
Marketing Effectiveness	Marketing expenses compared to new patients	Five times the marketing expenses divided by new patients
Patient Satisfaction	Patient surveys	95% patient satisfaction
Gaining High Case Acceptance		
Proper Case Presentation	Case acceptance ratio	>75%
Appropriate Sales Technique	Case completion ratio	>95%
Controlling Costs		
General Cost Control	Overhead ratio	<60%
Specific Costs Control	Specific cost ratios	Staff ratio 25 to 30%
		Variable cost ratio 13 to 20%
		Office space ratio 8 to 10%
Proper Staffing Configuration	Staff efficiency ratios	Front office <9%
		Clinical <12%
		Hygiene 33 to 42%
Promoting Staff Effectiveness		
Appropriate Compensation Systems	Comparison with norms	Low staff turnover
Motivating and Team Building	Performance appraisal	Acceptable appraisal
Selecting Staff Members	Probationary appraisal	Acceptable appraisal and retention

AR, accounts receivable

Table 14.3 Practice Analysis Form

Practice Analysis		Quarter: _____		Year: _____	
		Quarter		Year to Date	
Dr. _____		Planned	Actual	Planned	Actual
Production Measures					
Office Production, Total					
Hygiene production	33%				
Lab-Related production	33%				
Nonlab production	33%				
Collection Measures					
Accounts receivable (EOM)	½–1 month				
Collection ratio	98%				
AR over 60 days	33%				
Managed care percentage	<50%				
Managed plan size	<25%				
Patient-Generation Measures					
New patients	1/day				
Recall effectiveness ratio	90%				
Marketing $$/new patient	5 ×				
Case Acceptance Measures					
Case acceptance ratio	75%				
Case completion ratio	95%				
Cost Control Measures					
Overhead ratio	60%				
Staff ratio	25%				
Front office efficiency	<9%				
Clinical staff efficiency	<12%				
Hygiene efficiency	33–42%				
Variable cost ratio	15–25%				
Office space ratio	8–10%				
Staff Effectiveness					
Compensation system					
Staff motivation					
Staff selection					

AR, accounts receivable

Maintaining Production

chapter 15

Part 1: Duty Delegation

When a man tells you that he got rich through hard work,
ask him: "Whose?"
Don Marquis

Objectives

At the completion of this part, the student will be able to:
1. Describe the types of dental staff and their duties.
2. Differentiate between the types of supervision in the dental office.
3. Describe the methods of labor substitution.
4. Describe how state dental practice acts affect duty delegation in the dental office.
5. Describe typical extraoral tasks that dentists delegate.
6. Describe typical intraoral tasks that dentists delegate.
7. Describe the principles of duty delegation.
8. Describe the steps in proper duty delegation.
9. Describe the benefits of cross-training.
10. Describe arguments for and against using expanded function auxiliaries.

Key Terms

authority
bookkeeper
capital
chairside assistant
cross-training
dental hygienist
differential pay rate
direct supervision
dentist time
efficiency

effectiveness
expanded duty dental
assistant (EDDA)
expanded function dental
assistant (EFDA)
flexible staff time
general supervision
indirect supervision
insurance clerk
job sharing

labor substitution
laboratory technician
marginal jobs
midlevel practitioners
office manager
outsourcing
receptionist
responsibility

Goal

The goal of this part is to make students aware of principles of delegating tasks to dental auxiliaries.

Business Basics for Dentists, First Edition. David O. Willis.
© 2013 John Wiley & Sons, Inc. Published 2013 by John Wiley & Sons, Inc.

To schedule patient visits in the office effectively, dentists must decide which procedures various staff members in the office will do. Dentists must schedule not only each staff members' time, but also their own time. Each staff member has a cost and allowable duties associated with their position. Duty delegation means time management. It fits procedures to the appropriate staff position. Dentists are trying to maximize the use of their time by having other people in the office do some procedures or tasks that the dentist could do. However, dentists choose to delegate these tasks for any of several reasons, including:

1. Dentists have other, more profitable tasks that they could be doing.
2. Dentists do not enjoy the tasks and want someone else to do them.
3. A staff member is better at the task or procedure than the dentist is.

Everyone in the office (including the dentist) should be busy throughout the day. If not, the office is probably overstaffed, incurring an additional, unneeded expense that decreases profit. To be efficient, dentists need to manage both their own time in the office and their staff members' time. The principles of duty delegation are based on the idea dentists have additional patients to see or additional work to do in the office. If not, the key problem is to increase patient visits and decrease costs. Principles of duty delegation, therefore, become important for cost-effective operation of a dental practice.

Types of Dental Staff Members

Several types of dental staff members are found in a dental practice. The use of these auxiliary personnel depends largely on the individual state's laws regarding what dentists can and cannot delegate to nondentist personnel. Their pay rate depends on local market factors (supply and demand of workers), the skill and training necessary for the job, and certification that dentists may require. Often one person may serve several functions in the office. Their overlapping roles often evolve as the practice grows and hires additional staff members. Larger offices usually have more personnel doing more specialized tasks.

Dentists traditionally delegate many tasks in the dental office. They often think only of intraoral tasks when they think about duty delegation. In fact, there is a broad range of duties that dentists can direct staff to do that frees their time for other, more lucrative procedures (Box 15.2). Dentists must be sure that the staff member knows how to accomplish the duty and that he or she is given proper support.

Box 15.1 Tasks Dentists can Delegate

- Front office tasks
- Bookkeeping
- Office cleaning
- Equipment maintenance
- Dental laboratory work
- Instrument management (sterilization)
- Supply management
- Chairside assisting
- *Some* intraoral procedures

Box 15.2 Types of Dental Staff

Clinical Staff
  Midlevel practitioner
  Dental hygienist
  Expanded duty dental assistant (EDDA)
  Expanded function dental assistant (EFDA)
  Dental assistant (certification)
  Sterilization clerk
Clerical Staff
  Receptionist
  Office manager
  Insurance clerk
  Bookkeeper
Other Staff
  Laboratory technician

Clinical Staff

Midlevel practitioners have the highest independence. They function between a licensed dentist and a hygienist or other auxiliary who is present in the office. These people may operate independently (without a dentist present). They may do restorative work, prophylaxes, basic extractions, and other common dental procedures independently. Training requirements and allowed procedures are not standard but are evolving. Often a dentist must be available for consultation or follow-up care if needed. Some dentists may use these staff members in the office, freeing the dentist to do more complex restorative procedures. Proponents tout them as a solution to the problem of lack of dentists in underserved areas, particularly rural and impoverished areas. State laws do not commonly allow this type of dental auxiliary, but they are becoming more frequent. This is currently a hot political issue for the dental profession.

State dental law usually allows dental hygienists to do prophylaxis, polishing, and deep scaling on patients, besides taking radiographs. Many states allow hygienists to administer local anesthetic or nitrous oxide conscious sedation, if the hygienists have adequate prescribed training and certification. State law describes whether a dental hygienist is subject to general or direct supervision. Most states do not allow hygienists to diagnose intraoral disease, so they generally require some supervision. (A few states allow independent practice for dental hygienists.) They then refer to a licensed dentist for evaluation and treatment any dental needs that are beyond the scope of their treatment.

Expanded duty dental assistants (EDDAs) are the same as *expanded function dental assistants (EFDAs)*. Each state is specific regarding what intraoral functions dentists may delegate to EDDAs. EDDAs generally can expose and process radiographs, place amalgam and composite restorations, fabricate temporary crown or bridge restorations, take preliminary or final impressions, and cement restorations. Although some states allow auxiliaries to perform all these tasks, others allow them to do few or none. Some states require formal training and certification for EDDAs, whereas others do not. So depending on the state in which a dentist practices, he or she might delegate a significant part of many routine procedures to these trained auxiliary staff.

Traditional *chairside assistants* operate chairside, mixing materials and medicaments, passing instruments, and keeping the operating area clean and dry through rinsing and suction. Most states allow chairside assistants to expose and process radiographs, if they have had formal training and certification. Formal programs often offer a certificate as a Certified Dental Assistants (CDA) through the Dental Assistants National Board (DNAB). The Commission on Dental Accreditation of the American Dental Association (ADA) accredits dental assisting programs. This shows a higher level of formal training, passing knowledge examinations, and annual continuing education requirement for recertification. Some states require certification, but others do not require this certification to act in the role as a traditional dental assistant.

Many larger dental offices hire a person as a *sterilization clerk*. Their job is to clean, package, and process instruments for the rest of the team to use while seeing patients. Smaller offices require the dental assistant and often the hygienist to process instruments between patients and during designated times during the day. Although this job is critical to the office functioning, it is a low skill, low training, entry-level job.

Business Office Staff

The number and type of business office staff members depend on the size of the office. As the office sees more patients, then it needs more front office (business) staff members (Box 15.3). In some offices, these additional

> **Box 15.3** Business Office Functions
>
> - Initial patient contact
> - Meeting, greeting, and dismissing patients
> - Answering and routing telephone calls
> - Entering information into computer system
> - Developing financial plans for patients
> - Collecting insurance information
> - Collecting payments
> - Sending statements
> - Writing and sending checks as payments
> - Processing office payroll

staff members share all duties among themselves. More commonly, they begin to specialize and are responsible for specific duties, such as insurance management, account collections, or patient scheduling. This allows staff members who are more skilled at specific function to do those functions and decreases training needs because their jobs become narrower but deeper.

The office *receptionist* is responsible for running the business office in smaller dental practices. In larger offices, he or she is often only responsible for patient interactions, telephone communications, scheduling, and computer entry.

Managing the insurance for patients has become one of the largest jobs in many dental offices. Even medium-sized offices will often assign one person to be an *insurance clerk*. This person verifies eligibility, finds benefits schedules, and benefits used for the year. Although it may not be the dental office's job, it is often in their best interest to try to maximize a patient's insurance benefits.

A *bookkeeper* is responsible for paying bills and verifying income from the office computer system.

A true *office manager* runs the business office. One to several business office staff members report to the office manager. The office manager has authority to hire and fire staff, to make office policy, and to develop operational procedures. There is a continuum of responsibility from an office receptionist to a true office manager.

Dental lab technicians are responsible for fabricating crowns, bridges, removable appliances, and other complex appliances that the dentist cannot easily delegate to clinical staff members. Most dentists have found it easier and more cost effective to outsource this function to external laboratories.

Levels of Supervision

Each state has laws that govern the procedures that a staff member may do while in the dental office. Additionally, some states require certain education or certification of different classes of employees. Dentists must know the dental laws of the specific state in which they practice because some states even interpret these definitions differently. (Most state dental boards have a Web site that describes these duties.) However, some general concepts throughout the nation can be applied.

Levels of supervision are important because they define how much work dentists can have staff members do, freeing them to do other high-skill duties in the office. For example, if a state allows expanded functions, dentists can delegate placing and carving restorations and many other procedures. If a dentist has an adequate patient base, he or she can have more operatories and more staff than a more restrictive state. Hygienists can gain anesthesia in many states, freeing dentists from this task. Some states allow hygienists to operate under general supervision, allowing them to see patients while the dentist is not present in the office. Many states are now considering allowing some form of midlevel practitioner or dental therapist. Depending on the laws regarding supervision of these paraprofessionals, the dental practice may take a different size and form.

Direct supervision means the dentist is in the dental office personally diagnoses the condition, personally authorizes the procedure, remains in the dental office while the staff member completes the procedure, and examines the patient before his or her dismissal. The dentist takes full responsibility for the work done. For example, many states allow EFDAs to place and carve restorations, if the dentist exercises direct supervision. So the dentist may inject and cut a cavity preparation. The assistant then would place the restoration while the dentist does other procedures in the office. When the assistant is finished, the dentist evaluates the final product.

Indirect supervision means the dentist is in the dental office personally diagnoses the condition, personally authorizes the procedures, and remains in the dental office while the dental auxiliary does the procedure, although he or she may not evaluate the final product or procedure. As an example, the dentist may authorize a prophylaxis by a hygienist or a lab procedure by a technician. The dentist may remain in the office for the procedure, although he or she does not evaluate the final product or service.

General supervision means the dentist has authorized the procedures (often in writing) and the dental auxiliary carries them out according to the dentist's diagnosis and treatment plan. The dentist does not have to be physically present for the staff member to do the work assigned. For example, a dentist may make rounds at a nursing home and write a prescription that certain patients should have their teeth cleaned by a licensed hygienist. The hygienist may then come to the facility later to do the prophylaxes. Some states allow the hygienist to see patients in the office without the dentist

---

Box 15.4 Methods of Labor Substitution

Capital (machinery, computers)
Outsourcing
Eliminating marginal jobs
Using lower-paid employees
Flexible staff time
   Part-time employees
      Time
      Duties
Job sharing

---

being present. Often this also requires a written prescription. The states' requirements for general supervision vary considerably.

Labor Substitution

In dental practice, the cost of labor (i.e., wages and benefits paid to employees) is the largest single item of expense. Typically, a individual practicing dentist spends from 25 to 30 percent of collections to pay staff members. If dentists can decrease this cost, then they will see the difference (after substitution expenses) as profit. Two major ways to decrease those costs are to control the number of staff members and the wage rate paid and to substitute other methods for labor. The cost of replacing the labor (over time) must be less than the cost of the labor itself. This results in either decreasing costs or allows an employee to become more efficient (doing more work), thereby decreasing the cost of hiring an additional employee. Businesses use several common methods to substitute for expensive labor, as listed in Box 15.4 and detailed in this section.

Capital (Machinery, Computers)

Dentists commonly see this method in large manufacturing plants, where machines and robotics have replaced many workers. This involves a higher initial cost, but a lower long-term expense. It is also common in dental practices. For example, buying digital radiographic equipment involves a large initial cost but saves staff costs involved in processing and maintenance of radiographic facilities. A new office management computer system (or software upgrade) may allow the existing person to do additional work rather than hiring an additional front office person. Other dental examples include purchasing instrument cleaning systems, voice-activated charting systems, or CAD/CAM restorations.

Outsourcing

Outsourcing means that instead of hiring an employee, dentists pay another outside company to do the work that the employee would have done. This is especially effective if the work is not a full-time job for someone in a highly skilled position. For example, dentists may hire a laboratory technician to make crowns and bridges in the office, but if the dentist does not do enough crown and bridge cases to keep the person fully employed, then it is more efficient and effective to outsource the laboratory work by sending it to an outside lab. Similarly, the payroll and bookkeeping functions in large offices are often outsourced.

Eliminating Marginal Jobs (Reduction in Workforce)

A common method of labor substitution is to eliminate a staff line (through firings or though attrition). The dentist then assigns that person's job duties to other people in the office. The work continues to be done but at no additional cost. The down side of this method is that the remaining employees may resent having to do additional work. If the remaining employees were fully busy before, then some part of their job will not be done. So this becomes an appropriate efficiency method if the remaining employees were not fully busy.

Using Lower-Paid Employees

A related technique is to use lower-skilled, lower-paid employees to do the job that higher-paid employees do. This frees the higher-paid (more skilled) employee to do higher margin, more profitable procedures. This is the basis of substituting for dentist time, but it is also applicable to other dental office staff. If two different people in the office can do a job, the lower-paid employee should generally do the job, if the higher-paid employee has other duties that he or she can be doing during the substituted time. Dentists may need to hire a lower-paid employee to do the job. For example, a hygienist can clean instruments and trays. However, if there are enough patients, he or she should see the additional patient, and a lower-paid employee (such as a sterilization clerk) should clean the trays. If there are not enough patients for the hygienist to see an additional patient, then a dentist should not hire the sterilization clerk but should have the hygienist clean trays instead of doing nothing. Likewise, dentists should not hire a hygienist if they will routinely be sitting in their office working the crossword puzzle while the hygienist does the prophylaxis. Many dentists hire high school workers part-time to file

Table 15.1 Labor Substitution in the Dental Office

Type	Hourly Wage	Substitution
Dentist	$100	100%
Hygienist	$40	90%
EDDA	$25	65%
Assistant	$15	30%
Sterilization clerk	$10	10%

EDDA, expanded duty dental assistant

charts and do other routine, low-skill jobs, freeing the receptionist or office manager to call insurance companies, make collection calls, or arrange financing for patients. Table 15.1 estimates the percent of the dentist's time that a trained and competent staff member could substitute for those procedures in which they are involved.

Flexible Staff Time

Using flexible staff time also controls staff costs. Hiring part-time employees instead of full-time employees saves in several ways. Part-time employees may not qualify for employee benefits. Dentists can have them work only peak hours, so that the part-time employees are not "sitting around doing nothing" when the office is not busy. These peak times may occur during the week (Tuesday evenings) or at special times during the year (school holidays or local plant shutdowns). Part-time employees can be hired based on time (e.g., Monday mornings) or based on job duties (e.g., collecting accounts). If more than one employee wants to work part-time, dentists can often allow them to share a job. Job sharing allows the individuals flexibility in taking time off for vacations and family issues such as day care. If one employee is present when dentists need them, job sharing can keep excellent employees engaged at the office while meeting their individual time needs.

Principles of Duty Delegation

Before delegating duties and procedures to staff members, dentists need to understand the principles of delegation.

Know What the Expected Results Are

Both dentists and the subordinate should have a clear understanding of the expected outcome. This may involve a technical procedure, self-assessment, or interpersonal skills of the auxiliary. There is a line to walk between being a "control freak" who manages every decision and a pushover who does not care the outcome of the decision. With proper training, dentists can let go of the authority to act and follow-up where needed.

Delegate the Authority to Act

Dentists must allow the subordinate to act independently. That implies that the subordinate can decide and act on those decisions without asking the dentist. The dentist sets the boundaries within which the subordinate has the authority to act. However, the dentist must allow and encourage the subordinate to act independently within those boundaries or the delegation will be worthless. For example, assume that a dentist wants to delegate to the receptionist the responsibility for scheduling emergency patients. First the dentist must decide what constitutes an "emergency" patient (e.g., pain, swelling, hemorrhage). Developing a script for the receptionist to use in determining if a patient is a true emergency helps this. Then the dentist defines rules for how and when to appoint these patients. The dentist must also decide what the receptionist should do when a case does not fit the rules. Finally, the dentist should follow-up with the receptionist to ensure that he or she is acting appropriately within the established boundaries. If the dentist does not let the receptionist act independently in this area, then he or she should schedule all emergency patients.

Dentists Retain Responsibility

Delegating does not mean that dentists are free from responsibility or that the auxiliary has all (or no) responsibility for a bad outcome. Both dentist and the auxiliary share that responsibility. However, because the dentist is the employer and directs the employee to do the task, the dentist is ultimately responsible for the actions or (inactions) of the employee. Therefore, dentists must be sure to delegate appropriately to the right person (who has training, abilities, certification, etc.). Dentists must ensure that the work is done properly. This means both from a technical standpoint (the procedure is clinically acceptable) and a behavioral standpoint (the auxiliary behaved appropriately while doing the procedure). Whether a dentist delegates an oral prophylaxis on a nursing home patient to a hygienist under general supervision or delegates preliminary impressions to the chairside dental assistant, he or she retains responsibility for correctness of actions of the subordinate.

> **Box 15.5** Bases of Pay Rates
>
> Marketplace determined based on:
>   Certification
>   Training
>   Abilities

Use Differential Pay Rates

Different classes of employees earn different rates of pay in the office. This is based on the supply-and-demand considerations of how difficult replacing someone is. This, in turn, is based on the employee's abilities, training, and certification (Box 15.5). Hygienists earn more than assistants because hygienists have additional training and licenses that assistants do not have. This allows the hygienists to do certain functions in the office (dental prophylaxis) that assistants can not. The hygienist carries a higher financial value. Likewise, an EDDA demands a higher wage in the marketplace than a traditional assistant because they can do more functions. As a rule, dentists should hire at the lowest pay level first, then hire higher pay-level employees as the demand for their service increases.

Delegate to the Lowest Pay Level

For maximum efficiency, dentists should delegate tasks to the lowest level possible. Three factors dictate this. The state dental practice act defines what is legally permissible. For example, dentists may not delegate deep scaling to someone who does not hold a license as a dental hygienist. Dentists must delegate commensurately with abilities of the staff member. Although delegating placing a composite restoration to an assistant may be legal, if no one has trained them or they cannot do the restoration, then the dentist should not delegate the procedure. Finally, dentists must keep the higher paid employee busy doing higher level tasks. Dentists should not delegate dental prophylaxes to a dental hygienist if the dentist does not have other (more lucrative) procedures that can be doing during the same time. For example, assume that a dentists' staff members consists of a hygienist (paid $35 per hour), an expanded duty dental assistant (paid $22 per hour), and a chairside assistant (paid $12 per hour). The dentist needs instruments sterilized. Legally, any of the staff can do the procedure. Why pay the hygienist or EDDA to do the procedure, when it can be done less expensively by the assistant? (This assumes that the other staff members are doing other, more lucrative procedures.) If a patient needs a scaling procedure, then the dentist can do it or he

Box 15.6 Benefits of Cross-Training

- Avoid overtime and temporary employees
- Avoid being "held hostage" by key employees
- Promote teamwork
- Handle peak demand more easily
- Uncover hidden talent
- Prevent embezzlement

Box 15.7 Patient Tasks to Delegate

Extraoral Procedures
  Patient education
  Oral hygiene instruction
  Patient financial counseling
  Medical history
  Chairside assisting
  Passing instruments
  Mixing materials
  Workspace management
    Evacuation, etc.
    Operatory set-up and break-down

Intraoral Procedures
  Scaling
  Prophy or polish
  Examination
    Existing conditions: charting
    Periodontal charting
    Radiographs or photographs
  Placing and carving restorations
  Diagnostic impressions
  Temporary restorations

or she can delegate it legally to the hygienist. It is more efficient to delegate, if the dentist have other, higher-value procedures to do while the hygienist is doing the scaling.

Cross-Train When Possible

Cross-training means that a dentist trains a person who holds one job to do the tasks normally done by someone in another job (Box 15.6). Often the replacement will not do as good a job as the original person (because of lack of experience), but he or she can more than adequately substitute for a short time. This is especially useful if a staff member becomes ill or needs to leave work for a time for other reasons. (If the dental assistant can process instruments and the sterilization clerk must leave early, the assistant may fill in.) This helps to avoid paying overtime or using temporary employees, both adding to cost in the office. This also promotes teamwork in the office because each employee understands and appreciates other employees' jobs. A dentist might also find an employee who has hidden talents. For example, the dental assistant may have excellent telephone skills and would be interested in expanding his or her duties to include confirming and scheduling patients.

Steps in Delegating in the Dental Office

Dentists should use the following steps to delegate procedures in the dental office. Table 15.2 gives an example of a procedure (a two-surface amalgam) and the decisions dentists must make to delegate properly.

1. **Determine the State Law** Each state has a dental practice act that details which procedures dentists can delegate to auxiliaries and which they cannot. It also describes the training and certification requirements for each type of employee. Some laws are negative laws; that is to say, they describe the procedures that dentists may not delegate to a particular type of employee. Other states have positive laws, which describe the procedures that dentists may delegate to staff. Both types of laws will describe the

level of supervision that dentists must exercise for the procedure. (Some states have different definitions for the levels of supervision from the ones given here; so each dentist should be sure to read his or her state's laws carefully.)

2. **Decide Which Procedures to Delegate** Depending on the state law, dentists should then decide which procedures that they want to delegate to staff. Dentists may need to hire or train staff before they can legally delegate those procedures. Most extraoral and management procedures (except laboratory work) have few training requirements. Most intraoral procedures have significant rules to follow. Dentists should remember the rules of delegation and determine the lowest level to which they can delegate. Box 15.7 gives several intraoral and extraoral tasks that dentists might delegate, depending on state laws.

3. **Break Procedures into Steps** Each procedure is really a combination of many procedural steps. Some procedures, dentists can delegate entirely to staff members. For other procedures, dentists may delegate some steps but not others.

4. **Determine Which Steps Dentists Can Delegate and to Whom** After dentists have decided what the steps are, they should decide which of the steps they can delegate and to whom.

5. **Estimate the Time Needed** Each step requires a certain amount of time. Although each procedure is unique,

Table 15.2 Time Estimation

Procedural Step	Delegate?	Time (min)	
1. Seat patient	Yes	3	
2. Review med Hx	Yes	3	
3. Apply topical anesthetic	Yes	2	13 Minutes
4. Anesthetize (inject)	No	2	
5. Apply rubber dam	Yes	3	
6. Cut cavity preparation	No	15	15 Minutes
7. Apply bases and lines	Yes	5	
8. Apply matrix band	Yes	3	
9. Place restoration	Yes	5	
10. Contour and finish	Yes	5	
11. Remove rubber dam	Yes	2	
12. Check occlusion	Yes	1	33 Minutes
13. Evaluate restoration	No	1	
14. Postoperative instructions	Yes	2	
15. Complete record	Yes	3	
16. Dismiss patient	Yes	1	
17. Disinfect operatory	Yes	5	

dentists can begin to estimate the time required for each step of a "generic" procedure of the type.

Table 15.2 shows the time breakdown for a hypothetical two-surface amalgam. The state law allows trained staff to place and carve restorations but not to inject anesthesia. These are done under direct supervision.

The procedure's steps are in the first column. Steps 4, 6, and 13 are those that the dentist must *personally* do (may not delegate as in column 2). The time estimate is for a generic two-surface restoration. (Personal times may vary.)

From this breakdown the total *chair time* for the procedure is 61 minutes (13 + 15 + 33). Of that, the dentist is needed for 18 of those minutes, and he or she can delegate the rest. The first and last times for the dentist are so small (1 or 2 minutes) that they are impractical to schedule. The only block of *dentist time* that needs to be scheduled is the 15-minute block for the cavity preparation. The dentist will need to find time among other activities to inject anesthesia and evaluate the completed restoration.

6. **Plan Appointments** When dentists have decided who will do each step and how much time they need for that step, the dentist can plan the appointment, scheduling the patient for the correct amount of time. (The chapter on scheduling describes how to use this information to construct daily patient schedules.)

7. **Schedule Appropriately** The next part on patient scheduling describes how to use these planned appointments in a comprehensive office scheduling system.

Using Delegation in the Dental Practice

Every office delegates some procedures to auxiliary personnel. The question usually focuses on the delegation of intraoral procedures, using expanded-function auxiliaries.

Advantages of Using Expanded-Function Auxiliaries

Using expanded functions develops a more efficient practice. This allows the dentist to see more patients in a given time. The office can participate with more insurance plans because dentists require a lower income to be profitable in the additional chair. This provides more care to people at a lower (insurance mandated) fee. Although advocates have claimed that this would lead to lower fees, in fact, most dentists keep their fees and the resulting higher income. Patients benefit from more appointment availability and the previously mentioned expanded insurance plan participation. Staff members have a higher job satisfaction because of the increased responsibility and job enrichment that accompanies expanded functions.

Disadvantages of Using Expanded-Function Auxiliaries

The biggest downside to using expanded functions is the additional management required. Dentists have more staff members to manage, which leads to more interpersonal interactions that can sour. Preplanning the appointments takes additional time. A larger operation is riskier and more expensive. If a dentist is away from the office, the higher costs of a larger office continue in his or her absence. Some patients do not want auxiliaries to do technical intraoral procedures. (Studies have shown that dentists can decrease, but not elim-

inate this, with proper patient education.) Depending on state laws, finding certified, competent staff members may be difficult. In these cases, the certified staff generally demands a premium wage. This concerns some practitioners who worry that auxiliaries may "take over" the profession or demand independent practices.

Part 2: Scheduling Patients

This is the earliest I've ever been late.
Yogi Berra

Objectives

At the completion of this part, the student will be able to:
1. Define the prerequisites for proper appointment control.
2. Differentiate between a treatment plan and an appointment plan.
3. Describe an appointment plan, its use, and construction.
4. Describe the proper use of the appointment book.
5. Describe treatment time codes and how they are used to plan dental appointments.
6. Make appointments in a multioperatory office.

Key Terms

appointment book
appointment control
appointment plan
confirming appointments
delegation of duties
direct supervision
emergency patients
indirect supervision
look sees
new patient appointments
"outlining" the appointment book

prime time appointments
priority column
procedure column
quick call list
series appointments
treatment plan
treatment time codes
　EFDA time units
　hygienist time units
　traditional time units

Goal

The goal of this part is to demonstrate an appointment control system for the office.

Traditionally, dentists have approached appointment control in a dental practice simply. They schedule patients one after another usually for a standard amount of time such as one half-hour. The appointment may specify the

type of treatment to be done, for example, alloys. When a staff member seats a patient, the dentist will quickly review the patient's record and select those teeth that he or she will try to restore in that half-hour appointment. With the constant pressure to "produce," the dentist often works over the half-hour, rather than select an amount of work that he or she may finish early. Thus, what occurs is that the dentist gets off schedule with the first patient. He or she then either must do little work on patients at the end of the day or work over at lunch and at closing. This results in the practice in which everyone rushes all day, overtime is common, everyone is nervous, work satisfaction is low, and auxiliary turnover is high.

Purposes

Appointment control is a system carried out for the convenience of the dental office. A treatment plan is a listing of the procedures that will be done for a given patient. The appointment plan organizes those procedures so that the office staff can schedule more efficiently, prepare for, and execute those treatment procedures. Appointment control systems are valuable for several reasons.

An effective appointment scheduling system helps to promote smooth operation of the office. It does this first through ensuring that dentist and staff members use their time to maximum efficiency and effectiveness. Second, it encourages dentists to see patients on time for their dental procedures. Finally, an effective appointment system helps to balance the patient treatment load and service procedure mix. Simply stated, a properly operated appointment system increases patient satisfaction and staff productivity.

A proper appointment control system is versatile. The dentist and staff should constantly observe and receive responses from the practice. Dentists can adjust the appointment control system to meet the changing needs of the practice easily. This system is to small or large offices. The appointment system that is described here works in large, expanded-function practices or in the small individual practice. The important principles that underlie the system are that dentists:

1. Schedule the appointment for time needed, not for a standard amount of time for all visits. All appointments do not take 1 hour. Some take considerably less, others more.
2. Schedule procedures with the appropriate staff person. Dentists should schedule dental prophylaxes with the hygienist and basic restorative procedures with the EDDA, as permitted by law.
3. Schedule dentist time separately from chair time. A patient's total visit may take an hour. Of that, the dentist may only spend 30 minutes with the patient. If dentists schedule correctly, the dentist can see another patient while the staff completes procedures on the first patient.

Prerequisites

Before starting an effective scheduling system, the office (dentist and staff) must meet several prerequisites.

Written Treatment Plan

The first requirement of any effective appointment control system is a formally written treatment plan. This treatment plan is the basis for the entire scheduling system. The office schedule will reflect the accuracy of the treatment plan. Without a formal treatment plan, the practitioner must rediagnose each time the patient is seen.

Proper Delegation of Responsibility and Authority

The keys to appointment schedule control in any type of practice are duty delegation and preplanning. To delegate effectively, the dentist must know the laws in the state in which he or she practices regarding delegation of duties to auxiliaries. As described in the previous part on duty delegation, dentists want to delegate any procedure to the lowest level legally possible.

For effective schedule delegation to take place, dentists must give the receptionist enough information to schedule patients efficiently. Only the dentist can provide this information. If the dentist supplies this information each time he or she appoints the patient, the dentist might as well make the appointments himself or herself because it would be so time consuming. What the dentist needs is a means of preplanning for each patient visit. That is called *process appointment planning* (and it is discussed later).

The practitioner must delegate to a staff member the authority for keeping the appointment book. In the traditional system, the dentist essentially does the scheduling, either by escorting the patient to the front office and telling the receptionist how long and when the next appointment should be or by giving the receptionist standard appointment lengths (such as 30 minutes for a restorative visit) without regard for the actual time anticipated for the procedure. Either of these approaches is inefficient and inappropriate because the dentist, and not a staff member, is doing the clerical duties of scheduling patient appointments.

Appropriate Appointment Book

The third requirement of the system is that the appointment book itself accurately represents the scheduling needs of the office. If a dentist is using a computer system, he or she should be sure that the system adapts to the needs of the office, rather than requiring that the office adapt to the needs of the computer system. Before dentists can use the scheduling module of a computer system, they must set the preferences to meet their office needs. Setting the computer program includes:

1. The dentist should "outline" the appointment book before making any appointments. Outlining sets up the appointment book "matrix" so that staff knows what times are available for appointments. The dentist should mark off the times the office is closed; mark off holidays and note the time the office is closed for staff meetings and other administrative functions; and show "buffer periods," if they are used (e.g., emergency patients, new patients). Professional meetings and other professional obligations should also be noted. The dentist should be sure to note local school holidays because many teachers and parents want to find appointments on those days.
2. There should be one (and only one) column for each operatory. (There can only be one patient in the chair at a time.) It is assumed that the auxiliary stays with the chair. So if there is an EDDA chair, the EDDA stays in that operatory.
3. Proper time increments should be set. Dentists should be sure that the time increments in the schedule are the same as in the appointment planning process. These must reflect the smallest increments of time for which a dentist is comfortable scheduling patient visits. Initially, a dentist will probably use a 15-minute interval. As he or she becomes more familiar with how long it takes to do the various steps of the procedures, it may be shortened to 10-minute intervals to schedule more efficiently. Some experienced offices use 5-minute intervals.
4. The dentist should schedule dentist time separately from patient chair time. Dentists must schedule both

the time that the patient is in the chair and the time that the dentist is captive with that patient.

Appointment Plan

The last prerequisite is that the dentist takes an extra few minutes at the time of preparing the treatment plan to organize and sequence the treatment procedures into a plan for the appointments. This requirement is fulfilled through the use of a work sheet, called an appointment plan. The appointment plan is completed just after the dentist formalizes the treatment plan. This plan is the mechanism by which dentists preplan the treatment to be done at each visit, duty delegation (if appropriate), and length of time required to complete each appointment. Using this method, dentists indirectly control the receptionist's appointment choice.

Appointment plans are useful for grouping procedures together. Dentists can combine several different procedures or parts of procedures to reduce the number of patient appointments. Quadrant dentistry is much more efficient than single-tooth operations. The appointment book should reflect this.

Dentist can schedule appointments for the time needed. A simple occlusal alloy and a difficult pin-retained build up obviously will take different amounts of time. The appointment plan allows the receptionist to schedule appropriately for those procedures.

Appointment plans help to organize multiple visit procedures into discrete units. This helps staff to have proper instrumentation, materials, and other needed items ready for the procedure. Staff members can schedule specific patients or procedures for specific operatories. If, for example, radiologic facilities are only available in one operatory, the receptionist can, through proper appointment control systems, ensure that they schedule procedures involving radiographs for that particular chair.

Treatment Time Codes

A time code is always written as three digits separated by two dashes (e.g., 1-1-1). This is a three-digit time code. The time code designates:

a. who the primary operators are,
b. their sequence of operation,
c. how much time each operator needs, and
d. total chair time. In any time code, both the first and third digit positions refer to an auxiliary.

The middle or second digit always refers to the dentist. Thus, in a three-digit time code containing no zeros, the auxiliary operates first, the dentist second, and the auxiliary again operates at the end.

Set Time Increments

Dentists must have a consistent increment of time. It is recommended that one increment or unit is equal to 10 minutes of time for the experienced practitioner and one unit is equal to 15 minutes of time for the less experienced practitioner. In this discussion and example, one unit is equal to 15 minutes. Thus, the digit "2" equals 30 minutes of time. Consequently, the time code 1-2-3 would mean the following:

a. First operator is an auxiliary needing 15 minutes (one 15-minute time unit)
b. Second operator is the dentist needing 30 minutes (two 15-minute time units)
c. Third operator is the auxiliary needing 45 minutes (three 15-minute time units)
d. Total chair time is 90 minutes.

When the first operator is the dentist, use a zero in the first digit position (e.g., 0-1-2). A single 10-minute block is required for operatory set up, breakdown, and disinfection, even if the designated auxiliary is not required during the visit.

Develop Standard Time Codes

To schedule dentist, assistant, and total chair time, a dentist must have a notion of how long typical procedure will take to complete. A copy of this should be given to the receptionist. Unless the receptionist is instructed otherwise for a particular procedure, he or she should use these time codes to schedule appointments. For example, if Mrs. Jones has a particularly difficult alloy or a quadrant of composites to complete, note on the appointment plan the three-digit time code needed for this appointment.

Table 15.3 should be completed with numbers from a practice. Table 15.4 is given as an example only. A dentist's frequent procedures and time requirements for each procedure will be different from this example. These time codes will also change over the practice life as skills, abilities, staff, and physical office change.

- *Code* is an abbreviation for the step in the procedure. For example, "E2M" means "Endo, 2nd visit, Molar." A dentist can decide which procedures the office commonly uses and an appropriate abbreviation for each. If dentists generally take twelve visits to complete a denture, then develop twelve procedure steps for

Table 15.3 Time Codes

	Treatment Time Codes				
Code	Treatment	Delay (Days)	Units (Traditional)	Units (EFDA)	Units (Hygienist)
Initial Exam					
IA	Adult		___	___	___
IC	Child		___	___	___
EM	Emergency		___	___	___
Recare Exam/Prophy					
RA	Adult		___	___	___
RC	Child		___	___	___
Amalgam					
AM1	1 Surface		___	___	___
AM2	2 Surface		___	___	___
AM3	3 Surface		___	___	___
AM4	4+ Surface		___	___	___
Pol	Polishing		___	___	___
Composites					
CM1	1 Surface		___	___	___
CM2	2 Surface		___	___	___
CM3	3+ Surface		___	___	___
Complete Denture Construction					
CD1	Initial Impression	___	___	___	___
CD2	Final Impression	___	___	___	___
CD3	Jaw Relations	___	___	___	___
CD4	Try-In	___	___	___	___
	Delivery				
CD5	Nonimmediate	___	___	___	___
CD5	Immediate	___	___	___	___
CD6	Adjustment	___	___	___	___
Endodontics					
E1	Initiate	___	___	___	___
E2M	File (Molar)	___	___	___	___
E2A	(Anterior)	___	___	___	___
E3M	Fill (Molar)	___	___	___	___
E3A	(Anterior)	___	___	___	___
Extractions					
EXT	Simple Extraction		___	___	___
	Multiple Simple Extractions		___	___	___
EXTQ	Quadrant Extract, Alveoloplasty		___	___	___
SUT	Suture Removal	___	___	___	___
Crown and Bridge					
CR1	Crown: Preparation, Temporary, Impression		___	___	___
CR2	Crown: Seat	___	___	___	___
BR1	Bridge: Preparation, Temporary, Impression		___	___	___
BR2	Bridge: Seat	___	___	___	___

dentures. If the office commonly does other procedures, add them to the list.

- *Treatment* is a word description of the step code.
- *Delay* is the number of days between the previous visit and this visit. If, for example, the office routinely needs 10 days to get lab work back on crowns, a "10" is put in this column for the second crown visit.

Constructing Appointment Plans

The appointment plan has columns that consist of the procedures, time code, and date completed. The first step is to make a diagnosis and construct a treatment plan as usual. Then complete the appointment plan.

Table 15.4 Example Time Codes

Code	Treatment	Delay (Days)	Units (Traditional)	Units (EFDA)	Units (Hygienist)
Initial Exam					
IA	Adult	2-3-1	2-3-1	2-1-3	
IC	Child	2-1-1	2-1-1	2-1-1	
EM	Emergency	1-2-1	2-1-1	2-1-1	
Recare Exam/Prophy					
RA	Adult	1-3-1	1-3-1	2-1-2	
RC	Child	1-1-1	1-1-1	2-1-0	
Amalgam					
AM1	1 Surface	1-1-1	1-1-1	1-1-1	
AM2	2 Surface	1-2-1	1-1-2	1-2-1	
AM3	3 Surface	1-3-1	1-2-3	1-3-1	
AM4	4+ Surface		1-3-1	1-2-3	
Pol	Polishing	0-1-0	1-0-0		
Composites					
CM1	1 Surface	1-2-1	1-1-2		
CM2	2 Surface	1-3-1	1-1-3		
CM3	3+ Surface	1-3-1	1-2-3		
Complete Denture Construction					
CD1	Initial Impression				
CD2	Final Impression		3	1-3-1	4-0-0
CD3	Jaw relations		5	1-2-1	3-0-0
CD4	Try-In		5	1-2-1	3-0-0
	Delivery				
CD5	Nonimmediate		5	1-2-1	2-2-1
CD5	Immediate		5	1-4-1	2-3-1
CD6	Adjustment		1-1-0	2-0-0	
Endodontics					
E1	Initiate		1-3-1	1-2-2	
E2M	File (Molar)	3	1-4-1	1-3-2	
E2A	(Anterior)	3	1-3-1	1-2-2	
E3M	Fill (Molar)	3	1-4-1	2-2-2	
E3A	(Anterior)	3	1-3-1	3-1-2	
Extractions					
EXT	Simple Extraction	1-2-1	1-2-1	1-2-1	
	Multiple Simple Extractions	1-3-1	1-3-1	1-3-1	
EXTQ	Quadrant Extraction, Alveoplasty	1-4-1	1-4-1	1-4-1	
SUT	Suture Removal	0-1-0	1-0-0	0-1-0	
Crown and Bridge					
CR1	Crown: Preparation, Temporary, Impression			1-4-1	2-2-2
CR2	Crown: Seat		8	1-3-1	2-1-2
BR1	Bridge: Preparation, Temporary, Impression			1-6-1	3-2-3
BR2	Bridge: Seat		8	1-4-1	2-3-2

Decide Appropriate Operatory (Staff Person)

The dentist needs to decide which operatory the procedure will be done in. This is really an indication of which auxiliary type will see the patient. If, for example, the office employs an EDDA who is trained and capable, then dentists schedule the patient in the EDDA chairs, freeing themselves the time required to place and carve the restoration.

The dentist should estimate how long each of these common procedures takes to complete, filling a time code for each type of staff and each procedure. Each time unit should be the same as the appointment book (5-, 10-, and 15-minute intervals). The three-digit time code reflects how long:

1. the staff member has to set up the operatory, and for patient meeting, greeting, and seating, and time for

initial treatment procedures, such as removing temporaries;

2. how long the dentist will have with the patient; and
3. the staff member has alone with the patient for completing work, patient dismissal, and operatory break down and clean up.

- *Units (Traditional)* is the three-digit time code that the office uses for this procedure if it is done with a traditional chairside dental assistant.
- *Units (EFDA)* is the three-digit time code that the office uses for this procedure if it is done with an EFDA. If the state practice act does not allow these auxiliaries in the office, then dentists should not bother with this column.
- *Units (Hygienist)* is the three-digit time code that the office uses for this procedure if a dental hygienist does it.

Group or Split Procedure Steps into Appointment Blocks

The treatment plan lists all of the dental procedures that a dentist will do for a patient. Some of those procedures require several visits to complete. Dentists need to break them into their individual steps for treatment visits. Others are quickly accomplished and can be combined with other procedures in a single appointment. The appointment plan then groups those procedures, and procedural steps, together so that the dentist knows what will be done at each appointment.

In Table 15.5, the patient, Susan Smith, will have the procedures listed in the treatment plan done. The appointment plan shows that it will be done in seven appointments. The first appointment, for 30 minutes, will be with the hygienist for scaling and root planing. The next appointment is to initiate endodontics on tooth 3 in the chairside assistant's chair. The next visit is also with the assistant for filling the endodontic preparation. The patient then will be in the EDDA chair for completion of a core on tooth 3, then again with the EDDA for preparation, impression, and temporization of crowns on teeth numbers 7 and 3. The final visit is in the assistant's chair for cementation of the crowns.

Group the treatment steps for each appointment based on efficient delivery. For example, if several teeth in a quadrant require restorations, restoring the entire quadrant at one visit is more efficient than restoring each tooth at a separate visit. (There is less operatory set up and break down time, less time for anesthesia, etc.) It should be noted that in grouping procedures, there are no restrictions on grouping

Table 15.5 Comparing a Treatment Plan with an Appointment Plan

Treatment Plan: Pt Name: Susan Smith	
Tooth #	Procedure
All	SRP&P
3	Endo
3	Core
3	FGCrown
7	PMCrown
19	MOD Alloy
20	DO Alloy

Appointment Plan: Patient Name: Susan Smith		
Procedure	Time Code	Chair
1. SRP&P	3-0-0	Hyg
2. E - 1 #3	1-3-1	Asst
3. E - 2 #3	1-3-2	Asst
4. Core # 3	1-1-2	EDDA
5. R # 19, 20	1-1-3	EDDA
6. CR ! #3, #7	1-4-2	EDDA
7. CR 2 #3, #7	2-2-2	Asst

Asst, assistant; EDDA, expanded duty dental assistant; hyg, hygienist. See text for description of procedures.

different types of treatment such as preventive and restorative at the same visit. In fact, combining different types of treatment often results in better scheduling.

Notice several additional guidelines for allotting time. First, no time is allotted for an auxiliary to assist the dentist; the assistant is always at the chair. Second, no time is allotted for local anesthesia. Because this procedure generally takes such a small amount of time, it is not worth scheduling even the shortest appointment (e.g., 10 minutes) for that procedure. Third, no time is allotted for evaluating procedures that have been delegated, for the same reason. The quantity of time allotted in each digit is based on the number of procedures to be done, the difficulty of the procedure, the experience and speed of the operator, and individual patient management factors.

Making Patient Appointments

Proper planning greatly simplifies the task of making appointments for the receptionist or other front office person. Computer scheduling modules have evolved to become effective, if the staff members set them up properly. However, most programs do not have effective appointment planning modules. A dentist may need to develop paper systems (such as the ones in this chapter) to communicate the appointment planning needs. The process for making appointment includes several steps:

The scheduler uses the appointment plan for each patient to schedule the next visit. As the appointments are completed, the receptionist schedules the time code for the next appointment in the priority column. If the dentist has no appointment plan (e.g., for a new patient visit), then the receptionist uses standard time codes to decide how much time to schedule.

One person, usually the receptionist, should be in charge of making appointments. If a dentist finds problems, or if changes are required, then the dentist can deal with them by involving only one person. (Obviously, other office staff members should know how to make appointments in the case that the primary person is out of the office.) If the hygienist is in charge of preappointing periodic (recall) visits, then he or she is in charge of that component of scheduling.

The computer scheduling program should enforce the following guidelines when making appointments:

1. Do not overlap patients in a chair. (Only one patient can be in a chair at a time.)
2. Show dentist time and chair time.
3. Do not overlap dentist time horizontally across chairs. (The dentist can only be at one chair at a time.)
4. Include the patient's name, phone number, and abbreviated procedural listing for the appointment.
5. Schedule appointments as determined on the appointment plan or standard time codes.

Example Schedule

An example daily schedule is given in Figure 15.1. This is a conceptual appointment calendar that shows the principles of proper patient scheduling. This conceptual schedule uses an arrow to represent the time that the operatory is dedicated to the patient, either direct patient time or breakdown and setup time. The barbells represent doctor time, when the doctor is directly tending to the patient. Office management software systems use color codes that replace the arrows and barbells, hot links that show patient contact information and alerts, and other features that enhance the scheduling function. Nevertheless, the software *must* support the basic idea of scheduling chair time and dentist time as separate functions.

It is assumed that an auxiliary is associated with each chair. The first two chairs are dedicated for traditional dental assistants, the third chair for an EDDA, and the fourth chair for a hygienist. (In the example, state law allows an EDDA to place and carve final restorative materials.)

The dentist has previously determined the appointment increments when he or she developed the appointment plan and associated time codes for each visit. An example of determining these delegated time increments was given in Table 15.2. (Fifteen-minute increments for both schedule and time codes are used in this example.) In the schedule, Pat Greene has an appointment in chair 2 at 9:00 for the second visit for a crown on tooth 4 (Cr 2 #4). The dentist set a time code of 2-2-1 for this visit. This means that the patient is with the auxiliary for 30 minutes (i.e., operatory set up, anesthesia, and temporary removal), with the doctor for 30 minutes (i.e., try-in, adjustment, and cementation), followed by 15 minutes with the auxiliary (i.e., clean up, patient dismissal, operatory breakdown and disinfection). Remember, there is no time block assigned for anesthesia or checking completed work.

In the schedule, the lines with arrows (patient appointment time) cannot be overlapped vertically or two patients would be in the chair at the same time. So it can be seen that Anne Woods will occupy chair 2 from 8:00 until 9:00, Pat Greene from 9:00 until 10:15, Kevin Ross from 10:30 until 11:00, and Bob Hoffman from 11:15 until 12:00. There are two 15-minute intervals when chair 2 is not scheduled this morning.

The barbells show the time that the dentist is with the patient in the indicated chair. Dentist time cannot be overlapped horizontally, or the dentist would need to be in two places simultaneously. The dentist is with the patient in chair 3 at 8:00 for 15 minutes, then in chair 2 to initiate endodontics on tooth 9 for 30 minutes. He or she then moves to chair 1 for 30 minutes for extractions and then to chair 3 to prepare amalgam restorations on teeth 3 and 4. (The EDDA will fill these latter preparations.) The dentist then moves to chair 2, chair 3, and so forth throughout the morning. As previously mentioned, no dentist time is scheduled for anesthesia or final evaluations. At some point during the first 15 minutes, the dentist will stop by chair 1 to administer anesthesia, and during the first hour will attend chair 4 (the hygiene chair) to check the adult recall on Connie Judd.

Appointment Issues

Several additional notes about appointments:

Patient Communication

The receptionist should offer the patient appointment options. He or she should not simply ask the patient "When do you want to come in again?" (The patient may not want to come again!) He or she should offer

⟷ = Chair Time •—• = Doctor Time

Date: _____

Time	Chair #1 – Assistant Patient and Service	Chair #2 - Assistant Patient and Service	Chair #3 EDDA Patient and Service	Chair #4 - Hygiene Patient and Service
8:00				
8:15		Anne Woods	Mary Adams	Connie Judd
8:30	Eva Sands	E-1 #9	New Patient	Adult Recall
8:45		Confirmed		Left Message
9:00	Ext 1,32		John Smith	Bobby Franklin
9:15	Confirmed	Pat Greene	Am 3,4	Child Rec Confirmed
9:30		Cr2 #4	Left Message	
9:45		Confirmed		Mary Worth
10:00	Joe Morgan		Ted Ford	Quad Scale UR
10:15	Brl 4 X 6		Comp #3	Left Message
10:30	Left Message	Kevin Ross	Left Message	
10:45		Suture Rem - Confirmed		Hank Studer R Adult
11:00			Amy Hand	Confirmed
11:15		Bob Hoffman	Am # 19, 20, 21	Jenny Combs
11:30		CD3	Left Message	R Child
11:45		Left Message		
12:00	Lunch	Lunch	Lunch	Lunch
12:15	Lunch	Lunch	Lunch	Lunch
12:30	Lunch	Lunch	Lunch	Lunch
12:45	Lunch	Lunch	Lunch	Lunch
1:00				
1:15				
1:30				

Figure 15.1 Example schedule

188

the patient "Tuesday at 10:00 or 1:30." This allows the receptionist to fill 1 day before moving to another. The receptionist should also avoid the mind trap of just "filling holes" in the schedule. Instead, he or she should consider the procedure, the patient, and other procedures scheduled near and opposite this procedure.

Series Appointments

Many patients prefer a series of appointments (every Tuesday morning at 8:30). For patients with long treatment plans, the advantage is that they provide a consistent time for the patient. However, patients may feel freer to cancel series appointments, knowing that they have another already scheduled. Dentists should be sure to allow time between appointments for lab turn-around and that treatment does not go too far ahead of a patient's payment plan.

Vary the Day

A variety of procedures should be scheduled during a typical day. Long, productive appointments should be scheduled during the dentist's best time (Some of dentists are morning people, some are afternoon people.) At least one "big-ticket" item (bridge, partial, or other large-fee procedure) should be scheduled per every morning or afternoon session.

"Prime Time" Appointments

Evening hours and Saturdays are high-demand times. Many dentists restrict these appointments to private pay or traditional indemnity plan patients. Others charge an additional fee for evening hours, not so much for the income as to make patients aware of how valuable those time slots are. Many dentists have especially strict cancellations and "no-show" policies for these prime hours.

"Look Sees"

A look see is a quick evaluation of a small problem. The dentist does not plan to do anything, just look at the problem and see what should be done about it. These visits may be for follow-up of previous treatment or as a triage method for emergent problems. The minimum time allotment should be used for these quick appointments. Some dentists have an extra operatory for such use.

New Patient Appointments

New patients should be scheduled as soon as possible. A maximum wait of 2 to 3 days is suggested. New patients are the lifeblood of a practice. They may have waited for months, building their courage to call. They may have just won the lottery. Whatever the reason, they are ready *now*. Dentists should get the new patients an appointment quickly. They may schedule "buffer time," which is an hour allotted for new patients, and is kept open for new patients only until the day before the appointment. The new patient should be told of the fee required and the need for insurance forms and plan information (if any).

Children

Children should be scheduled in the morning if possible. They are less tired, and therefore better acting that way. Their parent may want the appointment after school, but the scheduler does not have to schedule the appointment at that time.

Elderly Patients

Many elderly patients do best in the mid- to late morning slots. They can get up and dress, take their daily medicine, and get out before lunch or getting tired in the afternoon.

Emergency Patients

The dentist should have standard list of questions for the receptionist to use in determining if the caller has a true dental emergency. Depending on the availability of time and the practice philosophy, the dentist can then set parameters for whom he or she should see and

---

Box 15.8 Questions to Ask an Emergency Patient

1. Where is the pain?
2. When did it begin?
3. Is it constant or intermittent?
4. Is there fever or swelling?
5. Does anything trigger the pain (e.g., hot, cold, sweets, or chewing)?
6. Is there any recent treatment or injury to the area?

how quickly. As with all transactions in the office, the dentist should have a written script for the receptionist to follow in assessing and appointing emergency patients.

Confirming Appointments

Dentists should confirm appointments daily for the following day. If a dentist is unable to talk with the person at home, he or she should leave a message. The patient should be asked before they are called at work. Many people (and their employers) do not want to be bothered while working.

Problem Patients

All offices have "problem" patients. These are the patients who are habitually late, consistently break appointments, or fail to show for scheduled appointments. What a dentist does with these people is a matter of personal preference and where he or she is in the practice cycle. If a dentist has a young practice he or she is trying to build, he or she will tolerate more of this behavior than if the dentist has a well-established, "full" practice. Some practitioners charge patients for broken appointments. The purpose is to try to instill the importance of the visit rather than try to generate any income. If the purpose is to anger people who break appointments and drive them away, then the dentist should use this technique. It works well for that.

"Quick Call" List

Most dentists maintain a "quick call" list. These are patients who live or work nearby and can come in with short notice to have work done. Most computer management programs have these lists built into the program. (Actually, either a 3-in × 5-in file card box or a simple list on a legal pad is sufficient.) If a patient expresses a desire to be seen sooner than the office schedule otherwise permits, write their name, phone number, procedure, time code and present appointment on the list. Whenever a cancellation occurs, the receptionist checks the list for an appointment code that will fit into the newly vacated time slot. As the dentist completes a patient's appointment plan, the receptionist can easily update the code for the next visit.

Quick call lists have several uses. The most obvious is filling a time slot when a patient cancels their appointment. This lets us use of the office's valuable (and expensive) time the best. It is also used when confirming appointments (usually 1 to 2 days ahead). If a patient cannot keep their scheduled date, staff members can fill it with the quick call list. Finally, many practitioners keep new patient slots open until the day before the appointment slot. (This allows the office to see valuable new patients quickly.) If the dentist has scheduled no new patients for the day, the receptionist can use the quick call list to fill those time slots as well.

"Tickler" List

Dentists should keep a list of patients who have missed appointments and need to be rescheduled. Some patients will miss an appointment and forget to call back for another appointment. Others do not have their schedule with them or need to check conflicting appointments. Whatever the reason, keep a list of those missed appointments and call them back to make the appointment.

Production Goals

Some offices set daily production goals for the scheduler. This can work if there are adequate patients to pick the procedures. (Other offices are more concerned with filling the appointments for the rest of the week.) As a rule, these scheduling philosophies stress scheduling high margin (i.e., lab-related visits) first, then filling around these more profitable procedures with the other, less profitable procedures (i.e., restorations). The idea is that this keeps a steady flow of the more profitable procedures. If a potential appointment is lost, losing a lower margin procedure is better than the more profitable ones.

Part 3: Dental Fee Policy

It is a socialist idea that making profits is a vice;
I consider the real vice is making losses.
Winston Churchill

Objectives

At the completion of this part, the student will be able to:

1. Describe fee-setting objectives, giving an example from both the general business and dental practice environments:
   Market skimming
   Satisfying
   Market penetration
2. Describe fee-setting methods, giving an example of each from both the general business and dental practice environments:
   Cost based
   Demand based
   Competition based
3. Discuss the effect that managed care programs have on dental fees.
4. Discuss consumer or patient sensitivity to fees.
5. Describe how to raise fees.
6. Discuss the effect of fees on practice profitability.
7. Define "elasticity of demand," and relate it to dental fees.
8. Calculate a procedure's cost-based fee.
9. Describe the consumer price index and its use in dental fee determination.

Key Terms

apparent fee
competition-based fee setting
consumer or patient fee
sensitivity
cost-based fee setting
cost shifting
demand-based fee setting

consumer price index (CPI)
elasticity of demand
fee objectives
market penetration
market skimming
satisfying
practice profitability

Goal

This part presents the basis of fee determination for the dental practitioner. The nature of dental fees and the behavior of the buying public regarding dental fees will be explored.

Fees dramatically affect practice profitability and patient perception. A profitable practice can only be attained by careful attention to the financial details of both income generation and management of practice cost. A dentist's self-esteem is closely tied to fees, both as a cause of low fees (the dentist must believe that the fee is fair and valuable) and in the resulting practice profitability. The fees that the practice sets have obvious and important implications for income generation. Principles from the marketing and economics can help the dentist in setting practice fees.

Professional Fee Objectives

As a practitioner, a dentist should initially determine what he or she expects to accomplish with practice fees. Those objectives may include, depending on the type and style of the practice, market skimming, satisfying, and market penetration. Various strategies accomplish these alternative profit objectives.

Market Skimming

Skim pricing occurs when a business prices goods or services so high that only a few consumers can afford them. In the automotive world, they sell Porsche and Bentley automobiles on this basis. Dental practices that make large profits from a few patients by charging high fees employ skim pricing.

A paradoxical value of high fees is that consumers may use them as an indicator of quality. A patient who perceives the quality of dental care as high is not as concerned about the cost of that care. For these patients, treatment decisions are based on nonfee considerations, such as aesthetics, image, treatment outcome, or personal interaction with the dentist and office staff. Often then, high fees may lead to higher patient satisfaction.

Market skimming also has limitations for use in a dental practice. The number of patients who will buy dental services without regard to the price is not large. So only a few practices in an area can use this skim pricing. Each of those practices must offer something unique for which the patient is willing to pay a premium price. Practitioners must be sure to differentiate themselves from other dentists in the area. In that way, a patient who becomes dissatisfied with the fee will be less likely to leave because they have no (or few) other substitute or comparable providers. Patients with dental insurance may question a procedure fee when their insurance carrier notifies them that the charged fee exceeds the carrier's usual, customary, and reasonable (UCR) fee schedule. When other practices in the area discover these higher fees, they may provide similar services, market the service similarly, and charge fees similar to the practice that originally adopted a market skimming strategy.

Satisfying

Many dental practices may not emphasize extreme profitability, either in the short or long run. These practitioners may exhibit behavior that produces satisfactory, rather than maximum, profit. Satisfying behavior is an economic notion that emphasizes attainment of a desired level of something without maximization of anything. Ford Motor Company "satisfies" in its mid-sized line of automobiles. They produce adequate numbers of automobiles, charging a reasonable price, paying their workers a satisfactory wage, and earning a satisfactory profit. They could maximize profits in the short run by charging more, but in return might lose satisfied customers or workers. A dental practice that uses the satisfying strategy structures its fees so that everyone is "fairly happy." The practice meets current expenses and allows the dentist to live comfortably and to reward the staff adequately (*comfortable* and *adequate* obviously have different meanings for different people.)

Creating this perception of satisfying behavior helps the practitioner to earn a reputation of being fair and equitable. Studies on dental consumer satisfaction suggest that the attributes of professionalism, quality, and reputation are significant determinants for consumer selection and retention of a dentist. Patients who perceive that their dentist is satisfying rather than maximizing may assume a higher level of satisfaction in the dentist–patient relationship. The cost of care alone does not lead to satisfaction but can be significant in exacerbating patient dissatisfaction. (Patients will not become more satisfied if they believe the fee is fair but will become dissatisfied if they believe that the fee charged is too high.) Therefore, a satisfying fee strategy is a helpful component in developing patient satisfaction.

Market Penetration

Fees may be set at a low level to attract new customers or "penetrate" into a new market. Many stores have grand opening sales to develop markets for new outlets. Ford Motor Company also uses this strategy in pricing its entry-level line of automobiles. The hope is that the low price will lure initial Ford buyers who will then, in later years, upgrade to larger, more expensive (and more profitable) automobiles in the line. In dentistry, the price or fee may be set below that of similar services offered by other dental practices to attract potential patients based on lower fees and, hopefully, keep them in the practice. It is often used for such services as initial exams, cleanings, economy dentures, or even orthodontics.

Many high-volume retail dental operations use this pricing objective. Their goal is to attract patients based on a lower price for a common service, such as an initial exam. By doing this, they hope to attract enough patients to penetrate the market. Once they establish a patient load, the retailer may adjust fees upward to approximate those of other dentists in the area.

Advertising dentists who offer initial price reductions in their advertisements or coupons use a similar strategy. A free or reduced price examination, prophylaxis, or radiograph is an attempt to penetrate a market and generate new patients for the practice. This strategy is especially effective for cost-conscious dental consumers. It is much less effective for consumers for whom cost is not a significant decision factor. These groups include families with higher discretionary income and managed care participants.

Managed care dental plans often use a similar strategy to become established in the dental benefits market. Their goal is to price the managed care plan at a low-entry level price compared with conventional dental reimbursement plans. By doing this, the dental plans hope to attract companies or organizations as clients rapidly and, so, build a market share. Once they build this share, they may eliminate the introductory offer, and prices may rise. Profitability to the participating dentist under this objective is small or may not exist at all during the plan's growth phase.

The use of a low-price, market penetration strategy is only advisable under certain circumstances. The markets in which this strategy is most effectively used include markets that are highly sensitive to fee levels (demand for a service increases as the fee declines), in which a lower fee would discourage competition, and those in which a lower fee does not equate with poor quality. It is debatable whether the traditional dental practice marketplace meets any of these criteria. Many patients may use price as an indication of quality, particularly for intangible services, such as health care. Dentists must also inform potential patients of the price, which means that they may incur expensive advertising costs to inform the potential patients. However, advertisements rank low as an important dental consumer decision factor. Therefore, undue emphasis on advertising of dental services may be counterproductive to the effective marketing of dental services. A market penetration strategy may be used by independent practice associations (IPAs), preferred provider organizations (PPOs), or other groups who are competing based on price and are willing to accept low profits to build a presence in a particular market.

Fee-Setting Methods

Once a dentist has established an objective and strategy for setting fees, he or she should select a method to use in determining those fees. The methods of setting professional fees can include casual conversation at a professional meeting, "gut-level" estimates, or analytical business techniques. These fee-setting methods can be grouped into three broad categories: cost-based, demand-based, and competition-based methods.

Cost-Based Method

One common method that dentists use to set fees (price) is based on the practice's cost structure. The dentist determines total office cost per hour, determines the time required to do each procedure, and then computes the required fee for each procedure based on the time needed to complete the procedure and any additional costs (e.g., lab). A normal or desired profit (personal income) can be added to the overhead cost to decide the fee. For example, assume that a dentist knows that the practice must generate an average of $200.00/hour to meet the operating costs and he or she wants $100 per hour in profit. If the dentist also knows how long it takes, on average, to do a given procedure, then he or she can calculate the amount required to "break-even" on that procedure. If he or she can do the "average" two-surface alloy in 20 minutes, then he or she should charge $100 ($200 per hour overhead + $100 profit divided by three procedures per hour) to meet this projection. These numbers are given as examples only. Individual practice numbers will, of course, vary.

This type of fee planning is particularly important if a dentist participates in managed care or contract dental plans. In this instance, dentists must know how much a given procedure will "cost" the practice to produce. Because the practice receives a predetermined fee for any given procedure, dentists must know the cost structure of the practice to figure out if they will be making or losing money by participation in the program. A capitation plan may decrease the fixed costs of a practice (by supplying a monthly fixed revenue amount) but not pay a high enough fee to recover variable practice expenses. If the managed care plan fee will not cover at least variable expenses, then it literally costs dentists money to participate in the plan and treat patients covered by the plan. There may be reasons other than simple profit for participating in a plan. The marketing and practice growth implications of gaining additional patients for the practice may, in fact, outweigh the strict financial justifications.

Cost-based fee determination has its shortcomings. It leads to a satisfying fee strategy. Its intent is to be "fair" to all parties involved, and it accomplishes that end. However, it is not an aggressive fee strategy and does not lead to the maximum profit or income for the practitioner. Most practitioners want to be viewed as

fair and not overly concerned with money. This strategy reduces dissatisfaction of involved parties. It involves considerable calculation work. Dentists must have excellent time records, which either involves considerable time with a stopwatch, consistent schedule records, or a good guess. This can also lead to the dentist who is clinically faster being compensated less than the slower dentist.

Demand-Based Method

A second method used to set a fee is based on consumer demand for a service or product. This method is represented by the adage, "charge what the market will bear." This infers that the firm or dentist will charge the highest fee at which enough people will buy the product or service. It is important to note that there is no price at which everyone will buy dental services; nor is there a price at which no one will buy services. Demand-based pricing says that some people will be dissatisfied with the price or fee and go elsewhere to purchase their services or simply *not* purchase the service at all. However, demand-based pricing also says that the other people who value the good or service will pay the price. Demand-based pricing is a technique used for specialty and image-based goods and services. Luxury automobiles, designer clothing, and gourmet restaurants set price on a demand basis. The business could sell more products or service at a lower price but not enough more to make up for the income lost from lowering the price. Thus, these firms optimize profit, rather than the amount of goods or services produced.

As an example, assume that a dentist could "sell" 30 gold crowns a month at a fee of $900 each. If the fee of a gold crown was raised to $1200, some people would not buy a gold crown that would have previously purchased crowns at $900. Assume that the dentist could now sell only 20 crowns at this higher fee. Which fee would result in a higher income for the dentist? If one assumes a $150 laboratory fee for each crown, then selling 30 crowns at $900 results in an income of $ 22, 500 per month (30 × [$900 − $150]). Selling fewer crowns at the higher price results in a higher income of $ 26, 250 (20 × [$1200 − $150]). Here, the dentist has increased income by selling fewer crowns at a higher price.

The obvious problem is to figure out how many people will purchase various services at the various prices. Economists determine this by estimating the elasticity of demand for a product or service. *Elasticity* is a term that describes how much "give" or "flex" will occur in purchase amounts because of a change in price. Demand is elastic if a large change (either increase or decrease) in the amount purchased results from a price change. An example is the purchase of soda drinks. If a person's favorite brand of cola raises its price, many consumers will switch to a competitor's brand. Demand is inelastic if there is not a large change in the amount purchased because of a price change. An example of inelastic demand is the purchase of pharmaceuticals. If a particular drug gives relief of symptoms, a person will purchase the drug at virtually any price. Dental services appear to fall in a mid-range of elasticity. That is, patients are not sensitive to changes in price (fee). Increasing dental fees causes some (but not all) potential patients not to purchase the service. Elasticity of demand for dental services varies considerably with socioeconomic and demographic factors. People who have higher disposable incomes are less sensitive to changes in prices or economic conditions.

Dentist can use the consumer price index (CPI) along with estimates of disposable income as indicators of how much change in demand there may be in response to dental fee adjustments. If the CPI is increasing, then the public is generally aware of higher prices and will accept increases in dental fees as a matter of course. If, on the other hand, prices (i.e., the CPI) are stable, then the public will expect a smaller increase in dental fees. Whether or not people can pay these higher fees will be influenced more by their disposable incomes than the CPI. If income is going up faster than prices, people will have more money to spend on discretionary or optional services, such as routine dental care. They will be less sensitive to increases in fees. If the price index is rising faster than incomes, then people will have less money to spend on such services and will be much more sensitive to increases in dental fees.

Traditional dental indemnity insurance plans tacitly encourage demand-based fee determination. The insurance portion of the total fee will largely absorb any fee increase. Capitation dental plans, on the other hand, virtually eliminate demand-based pricing because the fee is contractually determined. Interestingly, the sponsoring organization then is using demand-based pricing (in reverse) to set fee reimbursement levels. If enough dentists presently are willing to provide the needed quantity of services at the given contract price, the price will hold. However, if the market of dental providers is unwilling or unable to provide the services at the prescribed fee level, the contract plan would have to raise the reimbursement level until enough dentists would be willing to participate to provide the required number of services.

Demand-based fee determination is an aggressive strategy. It leads to maximum profit for the practitioner, although many patients may be dissatisfied with the high fees and leave the practice. This is acceptable if a practice is mature and has a backlog of patient demand. If one patient becomes dissatisfied, another will take its place. New practitioners who are growing the practice and practitioners in competitive markets find it difficult to use this aggressive strategy. Managed care plans are irrelevant to the demand-based fee practice. Because fees are high, managed care is not involved.

Competition-Based Method

The third major method that dentists can use to set dental fees is based on what the competition charges. This is the method that dentists traditionally use when they "casually discuss" fees. With the addition of third-party payers, competition-based pricing becomes more complex. The basic problem with this system of fee determination is in verifying the source of information about other dentists' fees.

The most common source of information is to ask other dentists in a geographical area what their fees are for given procedures. This method has several shortcomings. Besides being possibly illegal (because of price fixing), the other dentist may not accurately represent his or her fees. The inquiring dentist often asks friends and contemporaries about dental fees and, therefore, does not get a true cross-sectional sample of the dental community.

A second, and more accurate, source of information concerning competing dentists' fees is the data published regularly in the dental literature. These data are often broken down by region of the country, city size, and dental specialty to make the comparisons more meaningful.

The third source is for the dentist to establish a system in the office to track insurance and other third-party reimbursements. Dental insurance carriers will generally keep fees for a specific area or region, often to the point of establishing UCR fees for part of a metropolitan area or even an individual zip code. By gradually raising fees, the dental office can determine when the "cutoff" occurs for a particular plan. For example, if a plan will pay the UCR fee up to the 80th percentile, a dentist can learn when his or her fee for that procedure reaches the 80th percentile for the area; the insurance carrier will no longer reimburse the full amount. Because most offices see several different plans with different payment schedules, a dentist can develop an accurate notion of prevailing fee levels through this method. A dentist must have a detailed knowledge of each plan's limitations and constant monitoring to make this system work.

Once a dentist has a range of fees for his or her geographical area and type of practice, he or she must decide how to position fees compared with other practitioners in his or her reference group. Many practitioners want to establish fees at the mean or average level. Others are more aggressive and prefer to be at the 75th or even 90th percentile. (That is, their fees are higher than 75 or 90 percent of the practitioners in the area.) If a dentist's fees are too high, patients will notice that dentist like the sore thumb. If a dentist takes this approach, he or she should have a "name" in the community. Also, be aware that if his or her fees are above the 80th percentile, third-party carriers may not reimburse the full amount. In this case, patients may require extra education to understand how their relationship with the third-party carrier.

Implications for Dental Practice

Price is a factor in almost every purchase decision that consumers make, although it is only one decision factor. Everyone has some price that will cause them to switch to a different brand, a different style or model, or a different health care provider. For dental consumers, that switching behavior is a result of the uniqueness of the practice, consumer discretionary income, third-party involvement, and consumer attitudes about dental health care.

Effects on Practice Profitability

The fees that dentists charge affect practice profitability tremendously because the greatest part of a dental practice's costs is fixed. Once this fixed cost component has been met, then additional revenue becomes almost pure profit. (For more explanation, see the chapter on break-even analysis.) Table 15.6 illustrates this point. Assume that there are three equal dental practices, Drs. Red, White, and Blue. Their practices are in the same building, employ similar staff members, and have the same exact cost structures. Dr. White charges the average fees for the area, in this example $100 for a procedure. Dr. Red's fees are 10 percent below the average for the area ($90); Dr. Blue's are 10 percent above ($110). They all do identical numbers and types of procedures for the year. The table shows the financial results from this scenario.

Dr. Red made 25 percent less than Dr. White and 40 percent less than Dr. Blue, although they had essentially identical practices. The actual difference in fees for a given procedure was small (in the example, $90, $100, and $110), but the outcome was quite dramatic. The

overhead ratio changes considerably as well. Because costs are the same among the three practices, increased revenues affect the overhead ratio. Because fee level makes such an impact on productivity, it seems that all dentists would simply raise fees and become more profitable. Several constraints keep dentists from charging whatever fee they want to charge. The greatest constraints are patients' sensitivity to fees and the effect of insurance plans.

Consumer or Patient Fee Sensitivity

Most people shop for certain goods based solely on price. This is the basis of selling many commodity type goods, such as generic soap, paper products, or canned tomatoes. Some people also buy dental services solely based on the professional fee. The patient who calls the dental office and asks as to the price of an extraction or denture is "shopping" for services and will buy primarily based on price. Some dentists are concerned about attracting these people and desire to use a low-fee or penetration fee strategy to make them "regular customers." Dentists should be aware that people who shop on price are often looking for specific, not comprehensive, dental care. Therefore, these patients may not represent a large potential source of income. Because the patient was originally won on price, the dentist can just as easily lose them because of price. If he or she finds a dentist who will do dental services more cheaply, the patient might leave the practice and patronize the new dentist. Therefore, the use of a low fee strategy often does not result in the establishment of a stable patient pool for the dental practice. It may, however, generate an initial patient pool that can be a referral base. Additionally, dentists can convert some of those people whom they initially won on price to buy dental services based on factors other than price. These patients may become loyal patients. However, many dentists are too sensitive to these "price shoppers."

Dental consumers are concerned with the apparent, or out-of-pocket, cost for a service. The third-party payer decreases out-of-pocket expense. If a patient has

Table 15.6 The Effect of Fees on Practice Profitability

	Dr. Red	Dr. White	Dr. Blue
Fee Level	10% below = $90	Average = $100	10% above = $110
Gross Collections	$450,000	$500,000	$550,000
Practice Costs	$300,000	$300,000	$300,000
Practice Profits	$150,000	$200,000	$250,000
Profit Difference	25% below	Average	25% above
Overhead Ratio	67%	60%	55%

dental insurance that reimburses 50 percent of a procedure that costs $800, the apparent cost to the patient is $400. Patients are not particularly sensitive to the price of dental services, but they are sensitive to payment options and other forms of credit. (See the chapter on credit and collection policies.) A patient will balk at an $8,000 treatment plan the same as at a $9,000 treatment plan. Using the same principle as automobile leasing, if a person can make the monthly payments affordable, the cash flow price for the consumer becomes tolerable. Dental consumers are also more concerned with and knowledgeable of frequently "bought" procedures. Many patients know when a dentist raises the prices of a "recall" exam by $1 but are oblivious to a $25 increase in the price of a crown because they have never bought a crown.

Effects of Dental Insurance Plans

Managed care is any plan that the dentist provides services for a contractually reduced fee. Managed care plans change the traditional relationships between the dentist and the patient. They do this by upsetting the familiar methods of reimbursement for services. Managed care plans take much of the power to influence the purchase behavior of clients from the dentist. It is now vested in the payment plan administrators through their choice of participating dental offices. This changes the "rules" that have governed the competition between dentists. The nonparticipating dentist finds it difficult or impossible to compete based on demand or price criteria. The participating dentists find their traditional cost structures changed and their traditional pricing decisions eliminated. The public finds their dental shopping choice severely limited. (Judging from the continuing growth of these plans, this may not be as significant an issue to the public as dental practitioners would hope that it would be.)

Closed panel, capitation, and PPO plans remove the elasticity of demand as a criterion from the dental purchase decision. Fees become irrelevant to the consumer except in a yes–no participation criterion. If a dentist is a plan participant, then his or her fees (and, therefore, the patient's monetary costs) are both fixed and inelastic. The nonparticipating dentist's fees are prohibitively high by comparison. The purchase decision is then governed by elasticity. Patients will purchase few services at this higher (nonparticipant) price. This also negates the possibility of competition-based pricing by nonparticipants because the fees that the competition sets are irrelevant to the demand for the service.

Managed care plans severely limit the dentist's ability to raise fees. If the patient is a participant in the plan, then the dentist has signed a contract that stipulates what the fee for the procedure will be. It does not matter what the office charges enrolled patients for the service, the dentist only will collect what the plan allows. The plan may raise or lower the fee schedule. The dentist than must decide whether to continue to participate in the plan. Practitioners can negotiate fee schedules with insurance plans. Individual practices or practice networks that see many plan patients have more negotiating leverage than a smaller plan participant. The chapter on dental insurance discusses these issues more completely.

Managed care plans also affect the participating dentists' cost structure and therefore affect cost-based pricing. If a PPO or capitation plan reimburses at a 65-percent level and the office costs or overhead is 65-percent, then the dentist or participant just cover costs. (For a more detailed explanation, see the chapter on practice costs and control.) The practice's full-pay patients provide the profit. Here, either the dentist must accept a lower income, or he or she must charge the full-pay patients more to make up the difference. This is called price differential "cost shifting." It occurs when the practice shifts the profit lost on the managed care patient to the traditional insurance and private payment patients in a hidden way. The notion of using different prices for different patients may seem unethical or at least unsavory to many health care providers. However, this is a common practice in the business world. Hotels charge different rates, depending on a particular convention or group. Senior citizen discounts, volume discounts, buying cooperatives, and preferred customer plans are all examples of charging different customers different prices for identical goods or services.

Raising Fees

Most management experts agree that dentists should adjust dental fees, at a minimum, annually. January 1 and July 1 are the most common dates, with the first of the calendar year being the most prevalent. Many practitioners time staff members' raises to follow fee increases closely. This has several advantages. It helps staff members remember that practice revenues dictate their pay. If patients question fees, the staff member will have more interest in justifying the fee charged. Staff members will look forward to fee increases because they know their salaries will soon increase as well.

Many dentists use the CPI to set changes in their practice fees. The CPI is an index that measures the change in prices of a hypothetical "basket" of goods and services that the "average" consumer might purchase. It is a statistical index computed by the US government based on selected urban standard metropolitan statistical areas and a few sample cities. The CPI includes payments made for housing, food, transportation, and health care costs. Dentists assume that their cost of doing business will generally rise in proportion to the CPI. When dental practice costs are rising, it is logical to assume that dental fees should rise in relation to that change in cost. Dentists have a much better measure of their practice costs than the CPI. They have the actual costs. The CPI is valuable in determining changes in compensation levels for employees because their costs of living are reflected in the index's basket of goods and services. The CPI is not as useful for cost-based pricing decisions. It is, however, more useful in assessing the public's demand for services.

Some fees, such as the fee for a routine periodic oral exam or prophylaxis, are visible to the dental consumer. Because these services are the most commonly performed, many patients can use these as benchmarks or comparison figures, either between practitioners or over time. One strategy to cope with this problem is to list every procedure done on the maintenance visit. Rather than simply list "Recall exam, Prophy" on the patient's statement, a dentist should list everything to be done. This should include a medical history update, oral cancer exam, blood pressure check, home care instructions, radiographs, toothbrush, floss, hard- and soft-tissue exams, and any other education or services that are routinely provided at the maintenance visit.

Other procedures, such as cast posts and periodontal surgeries, are less frequent. Patients have a much more difficult time comparing the costs of these procedures. Dentists may have more discretion when setting fees for these procedures. Routine patients become accustomed to fees for routine procedures. Often problems arise when dentists confront patients with procedures that are uncommon or which they have not seen in many years. A form of "sticker shock" sets in. Like an automobile consumer who has not priced cars for several years, these patients are amazed (and appalled) at the total price for the package of services. ("Why, the last crown I got in 1948 cost me $30 and it was all gold!") A dentist's patient education skills become important at this point.

Maintaining Collections

chapter 16

Part 1: Patient Financial Policies

Every tooth in a man's head is more valuable than a diamond.
Miguel de Cervantes, *Don Quixote*, 1605

Objectives

At the completion of this part, the student will be able to:
1. Define the elements of a patient financial policy.
2. Describe the common methods of payment in a dental office.
3. Establish a credit policy for a dental practice.
4. Establish payment plan alternatives for patients.
5. Describe typical methods for presenting financial plans to patients.
6. Describe the effects of financial policies on office operations.

Key Terms

account guarantor
bank plan
cash
cash discounts
credit
credit bureau
credit cards
  recourse

health care credit cards
credit check
down payment
financial policies
interest on unpaid amounts
marketing incentives
payment methods
payment plan

payment plan policy
personal checks
  returned checks
practice production and profitability
professional courtesies
third-party payers
truth-in-lending laws

Goal

This part presents guidelines for formulating credit and collection policies.

Business Basics for Dentists, First Edition. David O. Willis.
© 2013 John Wiley & Sons, Inc. Published 2013 by John Wiley & Sons, Inc.

Every dentist and every business has a financial policy, whether they know it or not. The consumer is well aware of the policy. When a person goes to a fast-food restaurant, he or she knows their credit policy: cash at time of purchase. Yet many patients continue to believe that they can (and should) get a bill from the dentist at the end of the month, let it set for another 20 days, then write a check for part of what is owed, without worrying about late charges or accrued interest. It is the dentist's job to inform the patient if this is not the case.

Dentists must decide before the fact what their policy is regarding payment for services. Patients need to have this information to make informed treatment acceptance decisions. They will also become angry if dentists spring a financial surprise on them without informing them ahead of time. Having a written policy improves patient compliance, increases collections, decreases uncollectible accounts, improves scheduling (by decreasing broken appointments), and makes more appreciative patients. Although they may not like a dentist's policy, at least they know and understand it!

Elements of A Financial Policy

Dental office financial policies commonly contain several elements (Box 16.1).

What Patient Information a Dentist Collects

Every person that dentists agree to allow to pay them over time is essentially applying for an interest-free loan. If the dentist offers extended payment plans, he or she wants to have some indicators of the credit worthiness of the account guarantor or applicant for the loan. If someone does not pass the test, the dentist does not have to offer the patient credit. The patient must pay for services as the dentist provides them or the dentist does not offer the patient another appointment.

The dentist (or office staff) needs to gather certain information to ensure payment for services from patients who do not pay in full at time of service. The account

---

Box 16.1 Elements of a Financial Policy

- Patient information collected
- Qualifications for credit
- Payment methods accepted
- Payment conditions accepted
- Charges for late payments
- Rules regarding dental insurance plans
- Marketing incentives in place

---

guarantor is the person who is responsible for paying the bills. They "guarantee" the patient's account. The guarantor may be the person themselves, a spouse, or the parent of a minor child. An adult child may be a guarantor for a marginally capable elderly adult. A divorced parent, who lives in another city may be the guarantor for a child who comes to the dentist with their custodial parent. A trustee or guardian may have financial control for an incapable adult. The account guarantor may or may not be a patient of the practice. Regardless, the dentist's job is to ensure that he or she knows who the guarantor is and to let the guarantor know the financial policies of the practice. (The guarantor, not the custodial parent or anyone else who does not have payment responsibility, should sign financial agreements.) Dentists also must send any bills to the guarantor; so dentists need to keep a current address and telephone number for the guarantor. A Social Security number is important to have to track people down or check on credit histories, but they are becoming more difficult to obtain. Driver license numbers are also valuable for tracking people down.

Dentists can legally make a credit check (order a credit report) on any patient who makes a financial commitment to them. In practice, dentists will use this only for large amounts. What is a "large" amount? That is up to the dentist to decide. A $1000 treatment for one dentist may be appropriate; another will not bother with amounts less than $10,000. Dentists can join a credit bureau. The cost is several hundred dollars per year. Individual credit histories may still cost an additional fee. The report does not give the dentist a yes–no reply, but instead describes the person's history of payments on credit cards, loans, and mortgages. It is up to the dentist to interpret that information and decide if he or she wants to extend credit. To run a credit check on someone, the dentist must have the patient's Social Security number. If the patient will not give it, the dentist can refuse to offer credit.

Who Does Not Have to Pay at Time of Service?

Credit occurs when a person buys a good or service but does not entirely pay for it until sometime in the future. A dentist's credit policy dictates the conditions under which he or she allows patrons to pay in the future for dentistry done today. It describes to whom the dentist is willing to extend credit. In a sense, a dentist is lending patients money when he or she agrees to send a bill at the end of the month. Dentists should qualify ahead of time to whom they are willing to lend, to whom they are not, and under what terms they will lend it to the patients.

Dentists do not have to extend credit to anyone. They may require full cash payment at the time the service is rendered, no exceptions. The problem is that a credit policy that is too strict may discourage people from proceeding with treatment plans (i.e., "buying the dentistry") who might otherwise go on with treatment. Patients are not particularly sensitive to fees, but they are sensitive to credit and collection policies. Think about a patient who has $8,000 of dentistry to be done. They are interested in having the work done. They can not really discriminate between a total price tag of $8,000 or $9,000. One price over the other will not make their decision. However, the difference between 100 percent immediate payment and a payment plan of $1,000 per month can help decide whether to have the treatment at all. The real issue becomes how they fit the payment into their monthly family budget, rather than the simple cost.

Remember, not everyone that dentists treat deserves credit. Dentists may think of the public's creditworthiness as a continuum, from very credit worthy (will always pay as agreed) to not credit worthy (will never pay) and everything between. A dentist's job is to decide how far he or she is willing to go on the continuum to go to generate the production he or she wants. Dentists should be aware that only 30 percent of Americans qualify for a VISA or MasterCard with more than a $500 limit. If these companies will not extend credit to someone, the dentist should seriously consider if he or she will.

What Payment Methods a Dentist Accepts

Dentists may or may not accept any of several methods of payment for their services. Each has advantages and disadvantages and may be part of a financial policy.

Cash

A patient may make a payment in cash. If dentists often have patients who pay with cash, they must have extra cash on hand to make change. Dentists know that cash will not "bounce" like a personal check might, but dentists also must be careful to account for all cash in the office accurately. Cash can be a problem in the office. Cash is difficult to track, and therefore easy to steal. In the unlikely event of a robbery, cash can be easily spent, while checks and credit card slips can not.

Personal Checks

Dentists may refuse to take a personal check anytime. From their perspective, they want to ensure that a person's check is "good." In other words, dentists want to ensure that they have enough money in their account to cover the check. From the consumer's perspective, they need to be sure dentists protect their personal

information. If dentists put personal information on a check, that information is open not only to their office staff, but throughout the paper trail that the check travels. As a result, states have passed laws governing what dentists can and can not do regarding check verification. Each state is different, but the general rules are:

- Dentists can not require a consumer to show a credit card as a condition of accepting a check.
- Dentists can not condition accepting a check on a consumer's authorizing charges to a credit card if the check is return from the bank (i.e., it bounces).
- Dentists can require and record a person's name, address, and phone number on a check.
- Dentists can require a driver's license or other form of photo identification.

If the bank returns a check, the dentist has a problem. The first thing to do is for the dentist to call the patient and determine what the problem is. The dentist may, and should, charge the consumer a "reasonable" fee for reprocessing the check. (Often the bank charges the dentist to reprocess the check.) It should be added onto the patient's ledger as a separate code. (This is a charge adjustment, but not part of a dentist's production numbers.)

When the bank returns a check from a patient, it will be stamped with one of four reasons:

- *Insufficient funds* means that the patient did not have enough money in the account; the check bounced. This is the most common reason for returned checks. It might not be a big problem. The receptionist should call the patient when this is discovered. The patient may have a reasonable explanation of the problem ("My pay check was late"). In this case, the dentist should tell the patient that he or she will be sending the check through a second time. If it clears, then great, the dentist has payment. If it bounces again, the dentist will need to take legal action. A dentist should give it to a lawyer or collection agency for immediate action.
- *Payment stopped* means that the patient has stopped payment on a check. The dentist should call patient immediately to find out the problem. More often than not, the patient is dissatisfied with work the dentist has done. (Hopefully, the dentist will know about this before the bank returns the check.) The dentist should discuss how he or she can correct the problem.
- *Closed account* means that the account has been closed. Often this shows intentional fraud by the patient. Sometimes, it may be an honest mistake, if a patient closed an account and "forgot" that he or she wrote the check or their spouse wrote the check. In these cases, the dentist may let the patient immediately make payment (generally in cash) rather than sending the check for prosecution.

- *No account* usually shows fraud because the bank has no record of any such account. The dentist should try to call the patient (but they may not be found). Unless they have some unusually inventive excuse, the dentist will probably need to turn this type of check over to a lawyer or call the local sheriff or police department to prosecute the patient for intentionally writing a bad check.

Box 16.2 Example Health Credit Cards

Care Credit: www.carecredit.com
Dent-a-Med: www.helpcard.com
PFS Patient Financing: www.p-f-s.com

Credit and Debit Cards

Many practitioners accept bank cards (e.g., VISA, MasterCard) for payment of dental services. Dentists will have a bank that establishes a deposit account in their name, often the bank in which a dentist has his or her office checking account. The bank then deposits any charges that patients make to that account. The dentist then can withdraw money from that account whenever he or she chooses. The upside of this process is to speed cash flow through the practice and encourage patient payment. The down side is that the issuing bank retains approximately 2 to 4 percent of the amount charged as their fee for processing the account. The bank calls this a "discount." In the end, this probably saves the dentist money if he or she sends these people bills at the end of the month. If the dentist collects well in the office at time of service, it is more costly.

Bank Plan or Health Card

Another common payment mechanism is a bank line of credit for the patient. In rural areas, banks offer these more often. In urban areas, finance companies offer them more frequently. Either way, the method is the same. In this arrangement, the dentist tells the bank the estimated amount for treatment. The bank then qualifies the patient (checking credit history) and makes a loan to the patient for the amount of service. The bank pays the dentist for the dental services. The patient then pays the bank over time as an installment loan. These arrangements have the advantage of keeping the dentist out of the money-lending business, speeding payment, and decreasing billing costs. The bank generally charges the patient the costs of originating the loans.

Several national companies offer this service calling themselves "health credit cards" or other similar names. They often have Web sites and can qualify a patient for payment for services while they are in the office (Box 16.2). A dentist will need to sign up for these services as the practitioner. (This is generally at small charge.) The patient then pays the finance company over time, with interest included for the finance company. (Depending on the size of the case and the payment history, the loan may be interest free to the patient.) The finance company pays the dentist as the work is completed, or sometimes when the work is scheduled. Each

has different rules, so a dentist should check them out to find the one that best suits his or her needs. These plans take the dentis out of the finance business. They do not approve everyone for credit. (Currently, they approve about 60 percent of the applicants.) If an independent credit agency refuses to extend credit to a person, the dentist should seriously consider whether he or she can offer them any credit as well.

Special Cards

Patients may have flexible spending accounts or other employer-sponsored payment methods. The tax advantage of these plans encourages many people to participate. This becomes a significant stimulus for demand. The plan may require patients to bring a receipt for reimbursement of services, or the sponsoring organization may issue a special debit card for the person to use in health care offices. Dentists process these cards like others.

What Payment Conditions a Dentist Accepts

If a dentist decides to extend credit to patients by sending a bill, he or she must decide the conditions of repayment in his or her financial policy. Will the dentist allow people to send $50 per month to pay off a $5,000 treatment plan? Will the dentist require 50 percent down, before starting any treatment or a specific procedure (e.g., a bridge)? Does the dentist's payment plan policy differentiate between cash (fee-for-service accounts), traditional insurance accounts, and managed care accounts?

There are several points to consider when developing a payment plan policy. (Remember. This is for the patient portion of the total charge.)

Complete Plan

Dentists should develop a payment plan for a complete treatment plan. If they develop separate requirements for individual procedures, the patient may become easily confused.

Written Plan

Dentists should have a definite plan of repayment for every patient to whom they extend credit. This arrangement should be written, not verbal. (An example agreement at the end of this part.) Require the account guarantor to sign it. This does not make the debt more legally binding. (The patient owes the dentist for the service whether or not he or she signed a piece of paper.) It does place in the patient's mind the idea that he or she has signed an agreement to pay the dentist for the service. The patient *thinks* that it is more binding to see it in black and white.

Down Payment

The size of the required down payment affects treatment acceptance. A lower down payment is a means of easing the dentist's credit policy. A requirement for a higher down payment tightens the dentist's credit policy. The dentist should get an initial payment large enough to cover any lab bills. That way, at the least the dentist will not lose money if someone does not pay his or her bill. Many dentists require half the fee for the procedure as a down payment to begin treatment. Require a down payment of 33 to 50 percent, even if there is no laboratory work.

Length of Payment

Billing should not be extended beyond 3 months after treatment has been completed. If the payment period extends further out than this, patients often "forget" to complete their scheduled payments.

Amount of Plan

The total amount of the payment affects the options the dentist offers. A dentist might say, for example, that patients must pay all amounts less than $200 at time of service. Amounts more than $200, but less than $1,000 may be paid in three monthly installments (with an acceptable credit check). For amounts more than $1,000, the patients must gain financing through a health credit card.

Charges for Late Payments

Dentists may charge interest for any unpaid amounts. If a dentist does charge interest, he or she must be sure to meet the truth-in-lending laws. These laws state that dentists must make complete disclosure of all financing costs to the borrower; dentists must calculate the annual percentage rate; and the borrower must sign a statement containing this information. Dentists really need a computer system and software designed for this task. (Most of the major dental management software contains this option.) If a dentist wants to charge interest, feel free. Dentists should know and abide by all of the laws. Many dentists find it easier to charge a nominal "billing charge"

(such as $5 per month) to all accounts that have aged more than 60 or 90 days. No one intends this monthly charge to make money but rather to induce patients to pay. Because a dentist does not charge interest, he or she is free of the requirements of truth-in-lending laws. Good dental office management software allows dentists to set up various payment plans for patients. Most will also print out a set of payment coupons for the dentist to give the patient as a reminder of the payment due. The software may also have truth-in-lending forms, interest calculators, and other requirements if a dentist charges interest.

Rules Regarding Dental Insurance Plans

Third-party payers are insurance companies, managed care companies, and others who write a check to reimburse the cost of care for a patient. A traditional indemnity dental insurance plan is a contract between the patient and the insurer. The dentist has no legal responsibility in the contract, although most practitioners help patients by completing insurance forms and often allowing the benefits (payments) to be assigned or paid directly to the dentist. Managed care contracts are different in that the contract does involve the dentist who has legal obligations fulfill. This topic is covered in more detail later in other chapters of this book.

Whether or not a dentist accepts assignment of benefits for insurance payments is an important part of their payment policy. If a dentist does not accept assignment of benefits, patients must pay the full amount and then receive reimbursement from their insurer. This means that the patient must come up with more money up front, and it results in a stricter credit policy. Patients have been known to take their insurance reimbursement check and buy other desired goods or services, putting off payments to the dentist. If the dentist does accept assignment of benefits, he or she should have the front office estimate the patient portion of the bill, charging them for their portion when the service is done. When the insurance "clears," the office reconciles any difference and charges or refunds the patient the difference between the estimated amount and the actual amount. This speeds cash flow through the office. If the office keeps accurate computer insurance information and uses pretreatment estimates appropriately, there will be few differences. If the dentist waits for the insurance to clear, then cash flow slows considerably. Dentists must wait several weeks for the insurance process to complete, and then send a statement of the remainder to the patient. This may be at the next billing cycle, which may be several weeks in the future. If the patient is late or makes a partial payment, many weeks may elapse before the dentist records complete payment.

Marketing Incentives

Many practitioners offer cash discounts, either as part of a marketing plan or as a payment incentive. If patients make a cash payment ahead of service, some practitioners offer a 3- to 10-percent discount. (Five percent is probably the norm.) This obviously speeds collections and cash flowing through the practice. It also saves the dentist money through decreased billing costs. Marketing discounts are those that dentists offer to encourage patients to come to their office. Dentists might offer a 10-percent senior citizen discount to those seniors who pay cash (or check) at the time a service is initiated for patient portion more than $500. (Dentists may offer similar discounts to members of their church, temple, or mosque or employees at a spouse's place of employment.) Other dentists offer professional courtesies, or discounts to other professionals, such as physicians and optometrists, and they return services similarly. Managed care plans may require dentists to offer discounts to their members as a condition of being a provider. If dentists offer any of these discounts, it is a good idea to require payment in full at the time of service for the remaining portion. After all, the dentist has already reduced his or her return by offering the discount. To require the patient to pay the remainder in full is both reasonable and appropriate.

Dentists may have different financial arrangements for the type of patient visit. Communication is especially important for patients who are making their initial office visits. This is a fine balancing act. Dentists need to let patients know their financial obligations without appearing to be only concerned with money. It is a good idea to send a "welcome to the practice" letter, which describes financial policies. The receptionist should remind new patients on the phone to bring any insurance information and payment for the initial visit. Emergency patients require a similar type of arrangement. If the emergency patient is a regular patient of the practice, then he or she should be aware of the payment policy. Emergency patients who are not regular patients of the practice are another matter. Here, dentists want to be sure to collect the fee for any work they do, but they also (probably) want to encourage the patient to become a regular patient of the practice. Dentists should be sure that the receptionist informs the patient professionally what the estimated fee is and that the dentist expects payment at the time of the visit. Patients who are making routine office visits should know the policies. One type who may not be fully aware is the long-term patient who has not had significant work done. He or she has had routine prophylaxes, recalls, and occasional filling completed. Now he or she breaks a tooth, requiring root canal therapy, core, and crown. The receptionist should be sure to review payment options with this patient rather than assuming that he or she knows the policy.

Presenting Financial Plans

Dentists should be sure that their office presents financial plans at the time treatment plan is presented. Then they will have an accurate estimate of costs and length of treatment time. Dentists will also have the patient's commitment to go on with the treatment. Part of that commitment is an understanding of how the patient will handle the financial arrangements. Dentists should make financial arrangements in a quiet area of the office that is away from other patients. Many people view financial discussions as a private issue and do not want other people listening to their private conversations. Dentists do not want other patients in the office overhearing treatment plan amounts. The patients may worry that their treatment may be as costly.

Who presents the financial arrangements is a matter of personal preference. Some dentists make all the financial arrangements for their patients. They quote amounts based on treatment plans and know the financial policies thoroughly so that they can define payment amounts and conditions. These conditions may encourage patients to go on with their planned care.

Other dentists gain treatment acceptance from the patient, with a general understanding of the cost. After that, they turn over the patient to the office financial coordinator (receptionist or business manager) to arrange specific amounts and conditions for payments. Then, the financial coordinator provides truth-in-lending forms, payment coupons, contracts, or other financial forms. An advantage of this approach is that the dentist presents themselves as looking out for the patient's oral health interest. It is the financial coordinator that insists on payment conditions. Through this method, the office sets up a "good cop, bad cop" scenario in which the patient understands that the dentist is looking out for his or her needs, rather than "selling" a service that he or she may not believe that he or she needs.

Effect of Financial Policies

A dentist's financial policies affect practice production and profitability. The policies are one of the most important methods of increasing case acceptance, and therefore, productivity. Obviously, dentists cannot please all patients (unless they give away the dentistry or allow people unlimited time to pay). Dentists need to design their policies so that they get the best balance of money flowing through the practice and patient acceptance of treatment plans. To a degree, what is customary in the community in which a dentist practices will dictate his or her financial policies. If the community norms are that patients pay the full amount at time of service and then the insurance company reimburses them, then develop a policy that has

Your Name, DMD
1000 Main Street
Anytown, USA
Phone (502) 459-9999

EXTENDED PAYMENT CONTRACT

For Professional Services:

Rendered to: _____

Name of Responsible Party: _____

Address: _____

City: _____ State: ____ ZIP: _____ Phone: _____

Description of Services Rendered:

_____

_____

_____

Approximate Number of Appointments: _____

Financial Considerations:

1. Total Fee for Services: _____

2. Estimated Insurance Benefit: _____

3. Estimated Patient Portion of Cost: _____

4. Down Payment: _____

5. Balance Due (Extended payment): _____

The amount listed as "**Balance Due**" is payable in ____ monthly payments of $ _____. The first payment is due on _____, 201__, and each following payment is due on the same day of each consecutive month until full payment is received. A $10 Service Charge will be added to the account for any month in which the payment is received in this office after the due date.

Occasionally, problems may arise that prevent you from making payments as scheduled. To avoid misunderstanding, if this happens, please notify us immediately so that we may make adjustments to your plan.

_____

Date   Signature of Patient or Guardian

Figure 16.1 Example payment contract

similar parameters. That same policy would not be as effective at generating patients in an area where dentists customarily accept assignment of benefits and offer credit through extended payment plans. Does that mean that that a dentist is simply a sheep and must follow community dictates? No, but the dentist must be aware of community norms, especially as a beginning practitioner. As he or she builds the patient pool, the dentist can tighten the credit and collection policy. His or her financial policies will probably change over time as the character of the practice changes. A credit policy can be too strict, decreasing the

portion of patients who would have work done with a more generous policy. However, a plan can be too generous as well. If a dentist extends credit to everyone (even those who do not need credit), he or she is hampering the cash flow of the practice, resulting in large accounts receivable and uncollectible amounts.

Payment plans are important in stimulating demand for dental services. A patient generally will not know if a fee of $8000 for a set of procedures is too high or not. He or she often will not let that be the deciding factor in whether or not to have the procedures done. However, the patient

Your Name, DMD
1000 Main Street
Anytown, USA
Phone (502) 459-9999

We believe that it is in out patient's best interest to have a definite understanding about payment of fees for dental services. We offer the following payment options for your convenience:

1. We will gladly accept MasterCard and VISA for payment of professional services. We accept personal checks if you provide acceptable picture identification.

2. Without exception, for any treatment which involves the services of a dental laboratory, you must pay at least one half of the total fee as a down payment. The remainder may be financed as listed below.

3. For routine services (patient portion less than $200) you must make full paymentat the time of service.

4. For services which involve $200 to $1,000 of patient expense, we may arrange three equal monthly payments on a 30-, 60-, 90-day schedule. We will arrange definite payment dates and amounts.

5. For services which involve more than $1,000 of patient expense, we require the involvement of an outside lending agency if not paid in full. We will help you to arrange financing for these services through the First Union Bank of Anytown.

4. We offer a 5% courtesy for cash or check pre-payment of the patient portion of professional fees.

5. We offer our Senior Citizen (65 and older) patients a courtesy of 5% for all professional services in excess of $100 (patient portion). The cash prepayment courtesy of 5% may be applied by seniors as well. (Total courtesy of 10% is possible for seniors.)

6. Due to the substantially discounted nature of contacted dental plans, we require that the patient portion of these services be paid in full at the time of service.

We will complete and process all insurance and other third-party forms without any additional charge. Your insurance companies may provide some reimbursement for certain professional services. However, each patient must realize that they are responsible for payment of their account, regardless the level of insurance reimbursement. We will assist you in any way possible to see that you receive the entire insurancebenefit to which you are legally entitled. We ask that you help us by providing us with claim and authorization forms, as well as a current copy of your insurance policy, so that we can more accurately estimate your benefits from the plan. To avoid disappointments, we will request a pre-treatment estimate of benefits from an insurer for any treatment over $200. If you desire, we will accept assignment of benefits, which means that the insurance company will send any reimbursements directly to this office to decrease your portion of the total bill. You are responsible for the estimated patient portion of the treatment cost at the time the services is provided, as well as any services which are unpaid by the insurance company at the completion of treatment.

Occasionally, problems may arise that prevent you from making payments as scheduled. To avoid misunderstanding, if this happens, please notify us immediately so that we may make adjustments to your plan.

Figure 16.1 *Continued*

will know if they can afford a monthly payment of $800 and will often make that a deciding factor in whether to have the work done. In this sense, payment options are more important then the actual fee in influencing patient acceptance of treatment recommendations.

Poorly designed financial policies cost dentists money in several ways. A dentist may lose the patronage and goodwill of a patient and all their future referrals to the office because of misunderstood financial policies. The patient may never pay the dentist the amount that is owed. The longer a bill is outstanding, the less likely a dentist is to collect it. The older a bill, the more it costs the dentist to collect it. Dentists must pay billing expenses, postage, and staff time to prepare the bills. The money that the dentist receives becomes "less valuable" over time as inflation eats away at its value. Finally, a dentist has lost the interest that he or she could have made on the money if he or she had it to invest, instead of the patient.

Part 2: Office Collection Policies

It is the wise dentist who collects his fee while the tooth is still hurting.
Chinese Proverb

Objectives

At the completion of this part, the student will be able to:
1. Describe the elements of a collection policy.
2. Determine accounts receivable and properly age patient accounts.
3. Establish a collection policy for the dental office.
4. Describe common office collection techniques.
5. Describe common outside collection methods.

Key Terms

account aging
accounts receivable (AR)
collection agency
collection calls
collection policy
collection techniques
delinquent accounts

dunning messages
factoring service
in-house collections
Small Claims Court
statements
writing off accounts

Goal

This part presents guidelines for developing an office collection policy.

A dentist's office collection policies describe how he or she plans to collect payment from people who owe money. These people represent failures of the dentist's financial policies because if the financial policies qualified people properly and established timely payment procedures, nobody would fail to pay on time. This, of course, only happens in the ideal world. In the real world, people intentionally abuse kindness with no plan ever to pay their bill. Others may have life circumstances change (a death in the family or loss of a job) that makes it difficult for them to make payment as agreed. Still others may fully intend to pay what they owe but decide to use their current limited financial resources elsewhere.

A dentist's collection policies should integrate with patient financial policies. Patient financial policies describe how patients normally pay for services. The collection policy describes what happens when they do not (Table 16.1).

Table 16.1 Percentage of Dentists Collecting Payment

Net Production Collected	Dentists
99–100%	18%
97–98%	34%
95–96%	23%
93–94%	14%
92% and less	11%

An issue health care providers face that nonhealth business people do not is whether to continue treatment on patients who have not paid for past or current treatments. The dentist–patient relationship demands that a patient not be abandoned or harmed by failure to pay. This means that if a patient has treatment partially completed, a dentist should not stop in the middle of treatment because the patient might be harmed. So if a patient that has several teeth prepared for crowns, a dentist is obligated to complete those treatments because the patient might be harmed by the dentist's failure to complete treatment. However, if a patient has had several quadrants of restorations, needing several more, the dentist could halt treatment until payment is up to date. Patients also have an obligation in the relationship to pay for the service. With large-ticket items, be sure that the financial policy calls for adequate down payment and that the office staff follows the policy.

Accounts Receivable

Accounts receivable (AR) are the amounts that patients owe. This is a running tally. It changes each time a dentist bills a procedure or opens the mail and posts a payment. There is no absolute acceptable level for AR. That depends on a dentist's production level, amounts of insurance, practice philosophy, and even time during the year. (Patients are notoriously slow paying just after the holidays.) As a rule, a dentist's practice is healthy if the AR value is about 1/2 to 1 month's collections. This amount may be higher in practices with significant (greater than 80 percent) insurance patients, especially those that do not process claims electronically. It may be lower in practices that accept no assignment of benefits and have other, strict credit policies. AR will change over time. If a dentist has a particularly good month (from a production standpoint) it may take several months to see all of those payments come across the receptionist's desk as payment.

Billing Systems

Most dental offices that have computer management systems process and send their own bills to patients. The sequence of sending bills to patients is important. Most

---

Box 16.3 True Collection Ratio

One-third front desk	100 percent
One-third insurance	100 percent
One-third statements	91 percent
Total	**97 percent**

3 percent uncollectible = 9 percent uncollectible ratio

33 percent billed

Box 16.4 Elements of a Collection Policy

Collection techniques
Delinquent accounts
Outside collection aethods

---

offices send bills once per month. Dentists should be sure to use a consistent date so that patient does not forget the bill. Larger offices may need to send bills several times per month. This helps smooth the work load and cash flowing through the office. For example, an office may send accounts with last names beginning with letters A to M on the first of the month and N to Z on the fifteenth. Other offices send a second bill 2 weeks after the primary with a special dunning message to all accounts more than 60 days old. This is an attempt to encourage the older accounts to pay.

Billing is expensive. It involves staff time to process entries, staff time to review and print bills, mailing charges, stationery and other paper products, and lost implied interest earned. Some estimates have put the total cost of sending a single bill at $16.00. If it requires two statements to collect, the cost rises to $32.00 for each patient, essentially eating away the profit on smaller cases. It obviously pays to collect fees as soon as possible. As Box 16.3 shows, in a typical dental practice, dentists collect about a third of the fees at the front desk. The collection ratio on these accounts is 100 percent. Dentists send about a third of the fees to insurance carriers. The insurance also pays these at virtually 100 percent. The fees that dentists send by way of statements (the last third) account for almost all of the uncollectible amounts. So if the total collection ratio is 97 percent, the actual collection ratio (on the billed amount) is much less, perhaps 91 percent. The uncollectible ratio is then actually 9 percent. Not many dentists would be happy with a 91 percent collection ratio, although that number is the more accurate reflection of the real collection percentage in this practice. The obvious solution is to move more of the collections to the front desk, leaving less in AR. Dentists do this by asking for payment, making payments easy, and accurate estimate of insurance payments.

Collection Policy

If a dentist's credit policy has failed to screen bad credit risks adequately, he or she will have a problem collecting money owed by patients. A dentist's collection policy determines the rules that he or she and staff use in collecting that money. It establishes collection techniques, defines what a delinquent account is, and decides methods outside the office that the dentist uses for collecting problem accounts (Box 16.4). Dentists can use any or all of several different collection methods.

Collection Techniques

Collection techniques describe the methods that the dental office uses to collect money from patients.

In-House Collections

By far, the best way to collect money that patients owe is to collect it at the time of service. By using this "in-house" method of collecting, dentists do not worry about sending a bill, uncollectible amounts, or AR. Patients are free of worrying about paying later. However, many dentists are reluctant to have their staff members ask for payment. Staff members should remind every patient, as they leave the operatory and pass by the receptionist's desk, what their new current balance is and ask for payment. If a patient comes for treatment and owes money before they receive any treatment for the day, staff members should try to collect all that is owed, not just the day's amount. Dentists should develop scripts for staff members to use with patients who do not to make a payment at this time. These might include patients who say "I forgot my checkbook" or "Just send me the bill."

Statements

A statement is a printed report sent to the patient that details the status of his or her financial account. Computerized accounting systems allow dentists to customize the process, choosing who to send statements, when to send them, add special messages, and account charges. Often the program will allow any of several types of statements, depending on how the dentist wants the statement to look. A dentist should be sure that his or her statement contains a return envelope to make it easy for people to pay. Most offices set a minimum amount to bill. If a patient owes less than $5, it is probably not worth the trouble or expense to send the bill.

Most offices place "dunning messages" on statements. A "dun" is a repeated or insistent request for payment.

Table 16.2 Example "Dunning Messages"

Age	Message
30 Days	We have not received your payment. Please send it as soon as possible. Thanks!
60 Days	We have not received a payment from you in more than 60 days. Please pay your bill immediately to keep your account current.
90 Days	Your account is seriously past due. Please send payment immediately to avoid collection action.
120 Days	We have not received a payment from you in more than 120 days. If we do not receive payment in full within three working days, your account will be turned over to a collection agency for further action.

Box 16.5 Things to Keep in Mind When Making Collection Calls

1. Be accurate.
2. Be truthful.
3. Show concern and understanding.
4. Be persistent.

Computer programs allow dentists to place ever-more insistent messages on statements, depending on the age of the account. Accounts that are 30 days old receive a polite reminder for payment. Accounts that are 60 days old receive a not so gentle reminder. These messages are marginally effective for people who have simply forgotten to pay their bill. They are not effective for people who have intentionally not paid.

Letters

Personalized letters are more effective than messages on monthly statements. With the use of in-office microcomputers, the receptionist can generate word-processed letters personalized with the individual patient's personal information and payment history.

Telephone Calls

Telephone call from the office staff is the most effective method of collection. Unfortunately, they are also the least enjoyable and least liked by the staff members. They will find all sorts of other tasks to be done first and come up with many valid excuses for not having made collection calls.

There are several things to keep in mind when making collection calls. Have the staff member find an area away from the patients to make collection calls. Patients in the reception area or those waiting to make an appointment do not need to hear a collection call in progress. Dentists should be to have accurate records and that the caller reviews the chart and account before contacting the patient. A collection call is worthless and destructive if the patient has sent payment as required, but the caller discovered this fact too late. A dentist should not say he or she will do something if he or she will not. For example, if a dentist that says he or she will send an account to a collection agency if the payment is not received by this Friday, then he or she should do it. Idle threats are illegal and unwise. The dentist should show concern and understanding for the patient. Sometimes people lose jobs or have illness or other personal life difficulty. New payment schedules can be arranged if the patient truly needs one. Dentists should be persistent. It is an unpleasant job, but they should keep it up. If patients know that a dentist will give up, the patients will expect it. Any required follow-up should be noted on the financial record. For example, if a patient has promised and not completed payment, the dentist should call on the day payment was promised. The dentist should let the patient know that he or she has not forgotten. Finally, laws (such as the Fair Debt Collection Practices Act) govern how dentists can conduct telephone collection calls. These are described in the section on legal considerations.

When the staff member makes the collection call, most responses fall into one of four categories. The most commonly given excuses are:

- **It was an oversight** The most frequent response is "The check's in the mail." Often, in fact, the patient quickly writes a check and the payment comes in the mail in several days. If it does not, follow-up immediately.
- **The patient has a temporary financial problem** This happens from seasonal jobs, illness, or other reasons that limit their cash flow. People often will not call to tell the dentist that they are not making payment. They just do not make it. A new payment schedule can be worked out, if required.
- **The patient wants their insurance to pay for the procedure** Patients often believe (erroneously) that their insurance will cover all, or most, of the cost of a procedure. They then want to put the dentist in the position of being their advocate with the insurer to get them a higher reimbursement. Dentists should be sure that patients understand their portion of the fee before beginning treatment. Patients must also understand that if the insurance changes or changes reimbursement, they are responsible for the bill. As insurance contracts become more complex, more patients are confused by their contracts and need help in understanding their benefits.
- **The patient is unwilling to pay** Often this is because the patient is dissatisfied with the work a dentist has done. At this point, the dentist should try to satisfy the patient by making the work right. He or she can then continue to press for payment or pursue payment less

aggressively. The decision rests on how sure the dentist is that the work is proper and how willing he or she is to face a potential malpractice suit. (The single largest cause of malpractice claims is continued collection effort.) Some states have a 1-year statute of limitations. This means that the patient has 1 year, from the date of discovery of a problem, to initiate a lawsuit. If a dentist waits 366 days to initiate aggressive collection efforts in these states, a dentist should be safe. Dentists should check with a lawyer to find the statute of limitations in the practice state.

Delinquent Accounts

Delinquent accounts are the next level of the collection process. The first step at this point is to define a delinquent account. This means that dentists must have a system to "age" the accounts. When accounts are aged, they are categorized by how long it has been since the patient made the unpaid charge. (Some people use the time since the last payment made on the account. Either system works.)

Aging Accounts Receivable

Keeping track of the age of accounts is important because the older the account, the less valuable it is to the dentist. The dentist may have already spent a lot of money sending statements in an effort to collect the account. He or she has a lower chance of collecting the account, additional staff time, postage and supplies to spend trying to collect it, and the dentist has gone longer without the money. Because of these problems, the value of the account decreases significantly as it ages. Figure 16.2 shows the estimated value of an account as it gets older. As it shows, an account that is 6 months old is only worth 50 percent of its original value.

An account that has a charge made less than 30 days previously is considered "current." Account aging classifications generally run in 30-day increments, up to 120- or 150-day-old accounts. A "30-day" account is one in which no payment has been made in at least 30, but not more than 60 days. A "60-day" is one in which no payment has been made a payment in at least 60, but not more than 90 days, and so forth. That means that the patient (or the account guarantor) has not made a payment in at least that amount of time. The account will be older than the listed amount. If, for an example, a patient made a payment the first day of the month and the office aged the accounts on the last day of the month, that patient would be listed as current because they had made a payment within the 30-day window. (Even though there has been actually 29 days since the last payment.)

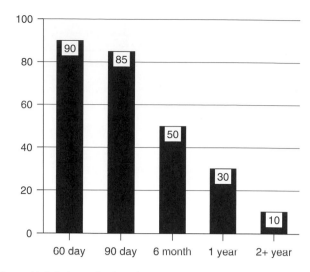

Figure 16.2 Estimated value of an account as it ages

The account aging report gives a listing of all the patient accounts that owe money, categorized by the time since the last payment (Table 16.3). A dental office management system will easily generate this report. The front office staff should use this report to make follow-up telephone calls and letters to patients who are late in their payments. Often the 30-day accounts are waiting for insurance to clear before making the final payment. The 30- to 60-day accounts are the ones that staff should aggressively pursue so that they do not become older, harder-to-collect accounts. Any account more than 60 days old is becoming a problem account. A dentist should pursue it aggressively.

Purpose of Pursuing Delinquent Accounts

Dentists really have two purposes in collecting delinquent accounts. First, they want to get the money owed. After all, they did the work, the patient should pay for it. If possible, the dentist also wants to retain the patronage and goodwill of the patient. That patient may have future work to be done; he or she may refer patients to the practice; or he or she may have friends or family members who are patients of the practice. If a dentist is too aggressive, he or she risks angry or embarrassed patients, counter-claims, suits, malpractice suits, and adverse publicity. Again, dentists should be sure their work is above reproach before aggressively pursuing a delinquent account.

Outside Collection Methods

Just as collection efforts represent failures of a dentist's patient financial policies, outside collection methods represent failures of his or her in-office collection policy.

Table 16.3 Aged Accounts Receivable Report

							Date: June 30, 2012 Page: 1
Pt No.	Acct Name	Balance	Current	30+ Days	60+ Days	90+ Days	120+ Days
12568	Abel, John Last Pay: 50.00	235.25	0.00 Pay Date: 04-22-12	0.00	100.00 Phone: 502-589-8942	135.25	0.00
10064	Edgers, Ann Last Pay: 36.00	1,674.00	0.00 Pay Date: 04-15-12	0.00	1,200 Phone: 502-783-8945	474.00	0.00
7682	Haas, Timothy Last Pay: 25.00	956.50	0.00 Pay Date: 03-06-12	0.00	0.00 Phone: 502-378-1267	135.25	956.50
9847	Nante, George Last Pay: 00.00	197.00	0.00 Pay Date: 05-18-12	197.00	0.00 Phone: 812-854-3852	0.00	0.00
11234	Powell, Dawn Last Pay: 100.00	65.00	0.00 Pay Date: 01-20-12	0.00	0.00 Phone: 502-378-9567		65.00
16548	Smith, Roy Last Pay: 250.00	1,274.00	0.00 Pay Date: 03-18-12	0.00	0.00 Phone: 502-378-4223	400.00	874.00

When a dentist has decided that an account is delinquent, he or she has several avenues to continue collection efforts. By this point, the dentist's costs will probably equal any money that he or she gains from continued efforts. Often the dentist will pursue collection efforts just to feel vindicated.

Collection Agency

The most common method dentists use to collect delinquent accounts is a collection agency. A collection agency really can not do anything to collect an account that a dentist can not do in his or her office. The collection agency should not be a major source of income, if the dentist and staff are doing their jobs correctly. They collection agents do know the system and have access to credit reports that the dentist may not. Collection agencies take a percentage (generally from 33 to 50 percent) of the amount they collect from patients as their fee. (Some also have membership or retainer fees.) Therefore, it is not worth much of their time to work a $50 account. The collection agent usually spends time with larger accounts so that their return is better. The dentist has the satisfaction of knowing that the delinquent patient knows they are subject to a collection action. The collection agency should put a notice in the delinquent patient's credit report, so the next time he or she tries to buy something on credit, he or she will at least have a problem.

In selecting a collection agency, the dentist should be sure that the agency has the proper credentials and that the state has licensed and bonded the agency. The dentist should ask for a list of dentists and other health professionals in the area who use the agency's service. Several of the dentists should be contacted to see if they are satisfied with the results. The dentist should have the agent explain the exact sequence or steps that he or she uses when attempting to collect and should note what the agent does with accounts that are not paid. Poorly handled, collection efforts reflect badly on the dentist's practice.

Small Claims Court

Every county has a Small Claims Court. The purpose of these courts is to adjudicate civil claims that are of low value (generally $1,500 or less). The court is informal; it has some initial basic paperwork to be completed. Anyone can sue or defend themselves or bring an attorney. Small Claims Court uses no juries. A judge listens to both sides of the story, views evidence brought by the parties, and renders a decision.

Some dentists use Small Claims Court to try to collect money that patients fail to pay. If the dentist has evidence that he or she rendered the service appropriately and that the patient owes the bill, he or she will probably receive a judgment in his or her favor. However, the dentist may also not get paid then. A judgment is a legally enforceable court order, but the dentist is still responsible for collecting the money (which is why the dentist is there in the first place). The dentist may need to return to court to get a garnishment of the patient's wages (if he or she is employed) or an attachment of personal property. Postjudgment collections can be difficult, time consuming, and tricky. A dentist might even need an attorney to collect his or her judgment.

Some dentists are true advocates of using the Small Claims Court as a collection method. Others find that their time is better spent in the office doing dentistry or on the golf course relaxing. A dentist can send staff in his or her place to present his or her case in court, but then the dentist has the added expense of the staff salary, with still no guarantee of collection.

Lawyers

Another common method of collecting overdue accounts is to have a lawyer write a letter to the nonpaying patient. Letters from lawyers usually get action. A dentist has to be willing to pay the lawyer to write the letter (usually a small fee) and then continue with the case if a patient refuses (potentially a large fee).

Selling Accounts Receivable (Factoring Service)

Some dentists sell their AR to a bank to collect. These are also called factoring services. They generally pay dentists about 80 percent of the face value of the accounts. The problem here is that they generally only buy accounts less than 90 days old because the banks realize the problem in collecting the older accounts.) So essentially, they collect the easy-to-collect accounts, leaving the dentist with the difficult, older accounts. The primary use for these services is during practice sales or transfers, when other arrangements do not work out.

Writing Off Accounts

Dentists should write off uncollectible accounts regularly and periodically (usually annually). When a dentist "writes off" an account, he or she is declaring doubt that he or she will ever collect the money owed by that guarantor. The dentist then removes it from his or her AR total, resets the account balance to zero, and removes the account from his or her files. If the patient ever returns and pays the account, the dentist reactivates the account and all unpaid balances. Dentists should write off accounts when they are turned over to collection agency or other third-party collector. Write back any money that is received from the collector to a reactivated account.

Periodically writing off accounts lets the dentist keep an accurate running tally of the AR total. This is important so that the dentist knows if there are problems with normal collection efforts. If the dentist values his or her practice for any reason (e.g., bank requirements, practice sales), he or she also needs an accurate AR figure.

Keys for Effective Collections in the Office

Dentists should be honest and upfront about fees. They should let patients know what the patient's estimated portion of the fee will be. Dentists should believe in what they are doing and in what they are charging. If a dentist believes the service is overvalued, he or she cannot effectively convince patients that it is properly valued. Dentists should practice telling people how much the service is going to cost. Some dentists go as far as to practice in front of a mirror until they are comfortable with the idea of "selling" a service. Dentists should never assume a patient does not want or can not afford the best dentistry that they can offer. Dentists should be sure patients understand, up front, what their portion of the fee will be and what portion they can expect for their third-party carrier to cover. Dentists should always remind patients that the bill is the *patient's* obligation, no matter what the third-party carrier will pay. Dentists should have a written policy and should give it to all patients; they will appreciate that the dentist informs them before beginning treatment. Dentists should have a definite plan with everybody. They should train staff and delegate to them because they can arrange payment plans as easily as a dentist can, if given the proper direction.

Box 16.6 Keys for Effective Collection

- Dentists should be honest about their fees.
- Dentists should believe in what they are doing and what they are charging.
- Dentists should practice telling people how much the service is going to cost.
- Dentists should never assume a patient does not want or can not afford the best dentistry that they can offer.
- Dentists should be sure that patients understand, up front, what their portion of the fee will be.
- Dentists should have a written policy and should give it to all patients.
- Dentists should train staff and delegate to them.

Generating Patients for the Practice

chapter 17

Part 1: Generating New Patients

So you think that advertising doesn't pay? We understand there are 25 mountains in Colorado higher than Pike's Peak. Can you name one of them?
The American Salesman

Objectives

At the completion of this part, the student will be able to:
1. Describe the evolution of marketing of professional services.
2. Discuss the relationship of professional ethics and marketing.
3. Define what marketing is and is not.
4. Compare the nature of services with products, and discuss how this affects their marketing.
5. Describe the stages of the growth of a dental practice and its relation to the marketing effort.
6. Define the "four P's" of marketing and relate them to marketing dental services.
7. Describe why people purchase dental services.
8. Describe ways to segment the dental marketplace.
9. Describe how common internal marketing efforts generate patients for the practice.
10. Describe how common external marketing efforts generate patients for the practice.
11. Describe the market planning process.
12. Describe some common problems in marketing professional services.

Key Terms

0-2-10 rule
40-40 rule
advertising
benefits
bundle of services
consumerism
external marketing
  media use
  professional relations
  public relations
  signage
fees
"four P's" of marketing dental

services
inseparability
intangibility
internal marketing efforts
  branding
  performance
  facility
intestability
marketing
perishability
place
price
problem-solving purchases

product
promotion
routine purchase decisions
segmenting the market
  behavioristic
  demographic
  geographic
  psychographic
service vs product
target market
top-of-the-mind awareness
variability

Business Basics for Dentists, First Edition. David O. Willis.
© 2013 John Wiley & Sons, Inc. Published 2013 by John Wiley & Sons, Inc.

Goal

This part presents the basis of marketing of professional services. The nature of dental services and the behavior of the buying public will be explored.

Dentists use many methods to help attract new patients to the practice, retain existing patients, and convince patients to purchase services. Actually, every management decision that dentists make in the practice has implications for patient generation. These efforts are called *marketing*. External marketing looks at generating new patients to the practice, whereas internal marketing aims to retain existing patients. Both are necessary for a successful practice. The hours that dentists keep, the fees dentists charge, insurance plan participation, and the types of services that dentist do all affect patient generation and retention. Together, these are marketing efforts.

Depending on the competitiveness of the practice area, dentists will need to put more effort into marketing. If the practice is as busy as it wants to be (or busier) with the right kind and mix of patients, there is less need for marketing expenditures. Even practices that have a full complement of patients and do not advertise continue to market the practice through their communications and management of the office.

What is Marketing?

Marketing is a managerial process that focuses a practice's activities on the benefits sought by a target group of clients, thereby satisfying their needs and desires more effectively. Notice that marketing looks to satisfy the needs of a group of patients. The major task is to learn clients' needs, wants, and preferences, and then to develop services and products that satisfy those needs. This affects how dentists deliver the service, and even how they organize the practice. It means listening to people and providing goods and services that they demand (or want). Marketing means that dentists view the practice through the patients' eyes, thereby generating and retaining patients in the practice (at a profit).

It is almost as instructive to say what marketing is not, as to start by defining marketing. Marketing is not advertising, although advertising can be a part of marketing. Marketing is not the sales technique of a used car salesperson, although sales technique is a component of marketing. Marketing does not mean high-pressure techniques, convincing people to buy what they do not need, or slick four-color ads.

Marketing looks at dental consumers' desires (not dentists' professional assessment of their need). Those desires fall into three broad categories:

a. To avoid something, such as pain, disfigurement, noise, odors, X-rays or cost.
b. To gain something, such as health, a pretty smile, or relief from pain.
c. To prevent something, such as pain, disfigurement, or embarrassment.

Notice that consumers do not want amalgams, partials, or bridges. Instead, from their perspective, they are avoiding, gaining, or preventing something happening to them. Dentists can probably provide a service that helps the patient achieve their goal. That service may be a prophylaxis, tooth whitening, or orthodontics. If it solves the patient's wants, then the dentist has acted with a marketing orientation. Part of the marketing orientation is to provide information to patients so that they know the procedures and techniques that are available. This education process makes consumers more aware of their needs, raising their level of wants, and, therefore, their desire for dental services.

Why do Dentists Market?

Dentists market to gain patients for the practice. Dentists have marketed their services since the first dental practice was created. In recent years, dental marketing has become much more sophisticated as dentists have brought business techniques to bear on the world of professional practices. Several factors have brought this on.

The increased competition among dentists for the available patient pool has stimulated marketing. As described in the economics section, this is really a question of relative supply of practitioners and relative demand of patients. Factors such as the number and age of dentists, auxiliary use patterns, technology, and practice patterns influence the supply of practitioners. The number of patients, usage patterns, disease patterns, third-party reimbursement, and efficiency of preventive measures influence the demand for service. When dentists see holes in their appointment book, the first thing they try to do is encourage more patients to come to the office. In other words, they market their services.

Dentists have two kinds of competition. The first is to gain the attention of the potential patient and to have the patient patronize them, instead of another nearby dentist. In this sense, dentists compete against each other for their share of the available patient pool. A dentist's internal operational policies (such as the hours that the office is open) and the external marketing strategies (such as advertising campaigns) help to attract new patients. Once the patient comes to the office, then the dentist faces a second, equally important marketing problem. That is to educate and convince the patient that their dental needs are important enough to spend (often large amounts of) money to repair. Because most dental procedures are considered discretionary services, then dentists compete against other forms of spending for the consumer's dollar. In this sense, dentists do not compete against other dentists but compete against travel agents, home remodelers, big-screen television sales agents, and fine-dining restaurants. Convincing the patient to come to a dentist involves external marketing plans. Once the patient is in the chair, then the internal marketing and sales techniques become more important.

The changing nature of third-party contracts has encouraged many dentists to market their services. Various contract organizations (capitation plans and referral plans) may limit where patients can go for reimbursed dental care. The act of deciding whether to participate in one of these plans is a marketing decision because it addresses the patients' desires for reimbursed dental care. Beyond that, a practitioner may see patients who sign up with a given plan leave the practice. The dentists then feels that they need to generate additional traditional fee-for-service patients to compensate for the managed care patients who have left. A dentist's insurance plan participation becomes one of the most important marketing decisions that he or she makes.

The rise of consumerism and a revised legal and ethical climate in the profession have increased marketing in dentistry. In years past, the profession considered any advertising to be unethical. The American Dental Association (ADA) Code of Ethics and many state dental practice acts described advertising to be an illegal act. In 1977, a court decision (*Bates and O'Steen v. Arizona*) effectively ended professional prohibitions against advertising. This case stated that a professional must be allowed to advertise the services that he or she provides, if the advertisements were not false or misleading. Simultaneously, consumerism was beginning to be felt as an underlying trend in the United States. This trend advocates for more information for consumers to use while making informed decisions. According to this tenet, a consumer should differentiate among dentists. Dentists must tell the public how they are different from others. Some professionals have a problem with this notion. The public agrees with it.

Changing technologies have brought many new services to the arsenals of practicing dentists. These address consumer desires by fulfilling the benefits sought. Patients want to know about these services. Dentists who provide them want patients to know about them. Marketing answers both desires.

What do Dentists Market?

Before a dentist begins a marketing policy, he or she needs to understand the characteristics of dental services, so that appropriate marketing strategies can be used.

Dentists Market a Service, not a Product

A product is a tangible object. Services, on the other hand, are intangible. Consumers can see the results of the service, feel, or hear the service. However, they cannot pick it up and examine it. So services are, by nature, different from products. These differences lead to significant difference in the ways that dentists market products and services, as well.

Inseparable from the Provider of the Service

Retailers or other third-parties can buy, repackage and resell a product. They can put a different label on a product, move it across the country or the world, but the product remains unchanged. Services, on the other hand, cannot be separated from the provider of the service. The delivery of service is the service. If someone else delivers the service, it really becomes a new service.

Variability

Because services show low standardization, the providers of the service and the service itself are inseparable. Food preparation is a tremendously variable service. Virtually every restaurant prepares food differently. Fast-food franchises have decreased variability through strict standard operating procedures. A person knows that a "quarter-pound burger" from a favorite fast-food franchise will be the same whether it is bought in New York, Atlanta, or San Francisco. This standardization essentially turns a service into a product.

Perishability

A service is perishable. It can not be put into a warehouse or put it into inventory as a product can. This means that timing is critical. Because there are only a given number of hours in a day, one person can only provide a given amount of service. Once time is lost (through a "no show" or cancellation) it is lost forever. Production can not be increased to make up for the lost time.

Intangibility

Services are intangible. A maxim of marketing is to "tangibilize the intangible, and intangibilize the tangible." This means that dentists should try to provide an intangible service as a reminder of a tangible product and give a tangible reminder for an intangible service. Whether it is a little sign in a yard from the lawn service company, a mint on a motel bed pillow, or a toothbrush after a dental prophylaxis appointment, tangible gifts serve as reminders that someone provided an intangible service.

Intestability

Consumers are unable to test services before they purchase the service. They can not pick them up, examine them, take them for a test drive, or kick their tires to check for soundness. Instead, they use surrogates to test the service before they purchase it. Patients are similarly unable to test dental services before they purchase them. Instead they use surrogate measures for testing quality of health services. Those surrogates include reputation, recommendations from trusted others, cost (as a reverse measure), and familiarity. The inability to test the service beforehand leads to more postpurchase testing and dissonance.

Dentists Market Based on the "Four P's" of Marketing

Marketers often speak of the four P's of marketing. That is to say, nearly all marketing efforts involve four major concerns. Those concerns are:

1. *Product* is the good or service that is being provided. It involves both the core product and all extensions of the product itself in the bundled of services purchased.
2. *Price* is the money that the consumer pays for the good or service. It includes not only the price for the core product but also all extensions. For example, the total price of a veneer includes the fee charged, how much work time the patient missed, the payment plan offered, and how much the insurance pays.
3. *Place* is where the good or service is sold or delivered. Generally, for dentists, the core is the dental office. The extended place includes parking and public transportation availability, disabled accessibility, office decor, and cleanliness.
4. *Promotion* involves all the efforts that a person does to make people aware about his or her good or service. For the dentist, it includes the core advertising efforts and extended promotions such as signs, community service, and health promotion efforts by the dentist and members of the office staff.

Why Consumers Buy

The consumer wants to buy. That is a huge conceptual difference. People want their purchase to solve a problem for them. In that sense, they buy benefits, not features of the good or service. The expected outcome is generally not simply to own the good or service but instead to use it for some end. Consumers do not really purchase aspirin. They purchase relief from a headache. If another product (acetaminophen or ibuprofen) offers a better benefit at a reasonable cost, then they will purchase the other product. They do not really care about how they make the product or deliver the service.

Definition of Features

A feature is a characteristic of the good or service that is sold. Need to know the type of metal, the characteristics of the material, and the method of making the product. That is vitally important when fabricating a dental restoration or appliance. However, consumers do not care about the features of the product. An implant has the features that it is made of titanium and osseointegrates with the bone, and a porcelain crown is placed on top of the implant (Box 17.1).

Definition of Advantages

Advantages are the characteristics of one feature over another that makes a product or service different. They help the consumer to differentiate among choices, but advantages do not cause the consumer to buy. An implant has the advantages that there are no clasps or wires that look unnatural, and dentists do not have to cut on adjacent teeth to replace a missing tooth. This simply compares the features of one solution with the features of another.

Definition of Benefits

A benefit is the expected outcome of a purchase. Consumers do not purchase a filling, a partial, or cosmetic bleaching. They purchase the benefit of a more attractive, more youthful smile or the ability to chew food effectively. The more that consumers see the benefit

---

Box 17.1 Why a Consumer Would Buy Implant Service

Features
    Titanium
    Osseointegration
Advantages
    No clasps or wires
    Do not cut down adjacent teeth
Benefits
    Looks great
    Functions like natural teeth

as solving their problem, the more they are willing to pay for the solution (Box 17.2).

Most dentists sell services based on their features, not the benefits that the consumer wants. When dentists talk "to" patients about their proposed treatment plan, they discuss the features of the bridge (what materials it contains, what steps the procedure requires) rather than the benefit that the patient can expect (a better smile, improved chewing). Any given patient will weigh the alternative solutions (partial versus bridge versus implant versus no treatment) and determine, in their mind and for their case, the best solution to their problem. Patient education plays an obviously vital role in helping people understand their problem and the benefits of the various treatment choices. In the end, it is the patient's perception of a solution to their problem that is important.

Patients Buy a "Bundle of Services"

People do not buy a simple good or service. Instead, they buy a bundle of goods and services that all combine to make the purchase decision. When a person buys a car, he or she buys the core product, which is the automobile. However, he or she also buys the reputation and location of the service facility, the delivery date of the car, and financing options. These all make up the extended product that is purchased. Likewise, patients buy more than the core dental service. They purchase not only a veneer, but the time that the office is open, the date they can have the procedure completed, payment plans, and reputation of the dentist. So the simple price of the service often will not be the only determining purchase factor.

Marketing Plan Development

When dentists are ready to begin marketing their practice, they need to develop a marketing plan. Developing this plan makes the dentist look at the people he or she

will be serving to meet their needs. It also makes the dentist look at what he or she is doing well and what he or she needs to improve, what competitors are doing, and how he or she will tell his or her story. It should fit with the dentist's strategic plan and vision for the practice. The marketing outputs that are desired (e.g., additional new patients) are a function of these marketing inputs. The marketing plan consists of several discrete steps.

Defining the Market

The first step is to define who the patient base will be. This defines the market. The location of a practice is one of the most important marketing decisions a dentist makes because it is crucial in defining the market. Most patients live within 5 miles of the dental practice (in urban areas). If a dentist intends to develop an upper-class "white collar" practice, but his or her practice is in a "blue collar" side of town, the dentist needs to make an honest appraisal of goals and possibilities.

Segmenting and Targeting the Market

Segmentation of the market refers to dividing the population into smaller groups of similar individuals. Dentists may assign these groups on several bases. Geographic segmentation groups people by where they live or work. If a dentist uses any direct mail, he or she will probably look at zip codes to decide where to send mailings. Demographic segmentation groups people by some outward characteristic, such as age, sex, race, or income level. Many dentists aim marketing efforts at people who subscribe to a particular insurance plan. When a dentist advertises in a senior citizen's newsletter, he or she is employing demographic segmentation in the marketing effort. Psychographic segmentation does not care about a person's outward characteristics. Instead, this form of segmentation groups people by how they think or feel about a particular issue. If a dentist develops a fear reduction program with the hope of attracting fearful dental patients, he or she has used psychographic market segmentation. Behavioristic segmentation groups people by how they act. It is well known that people who display high general preventive health behaviors also have higher dental usage rates. When a dentist places flyers in the local fitness center or health foods store, he or she is employing behavioristic market segmentation.

Market segmentation is the true art in successful marketing. Segmentation tries to group people so that a particular group is more effectively appealed to, with less wasted advertising effort and money. This is called *target marketing* (as opposed to *mass marketing*). The

Box 17.3 Example Dental Market Segments

1. Fearful patients (dental phobics)
2. Smile seekers (esthetic conscious)
3. Status seekers (perfect smiles)
4. Utilitarians (basic care that works)

target marketer is much more efficient because more of the marketing message reaches the person for whom it is intended. There are no fixed rules about market segmentation. A dentist can set and develop his or her own target groups (Box 17.3).

Developing the Marketing Mix

Dental office marketing consists of a mix of procedures and techniques for getting the word out about an office. The key is to decide who the target market is and then develop strategies that appeal to that target group. A dentist will probably find that he or she needs several strategies to deliver the message. Even a well-defined target group uses several channels to find information.

Tracking the Effectiveness of Marketing Efforts

Marketing efforts are expensive and time consuming for the practice. Therefore, it is important to track how many patients each marketing effort generates so that a dentist can decide if the marketing effort has been worth the cost and time spent. The best way to find out how a patient found out about the office is obvious, ask. When the patient first calls the office, the receptionist who takes the call should ask, "And how did you hear about our office?" The patient may respond with one specific method ("I was referred by Doris Smith") or may mention several methods ("I saw your ad in the Yellow Pages and looked up your Web page online"). All modern dental management computer software has fields for entering this information. At the end of the month (or quarter), a dentist then generates a report that lists all of the patients who listed each marketing source (e.g., Yellow Pages) and the amount of dentistry treatment planned and completed for the source. By comparing the cost with the amount generated, a dentist can establish if a program is worth continuing.

When looking at this relationship in more depth, the cost to generate a patient needs to be allocated by type. For example, assume a dentist spent $1,500 per month on yellow page ads, generating 3 patients, each with $400 worth of dentistry. He or she also spent $3,000 per month for direct-mail program, generating 15 patients with an average of $400 per month. The yellow page ad patients "cost" $500 each, losing $100 each. The direct mail patients cost $200 each, earning the dentist $200 each per patient. Given these numbers, the direct-mail campaign, although more expensive, is more profitable.

Marketing Strategies

Marketing strategies are the methods that dentists use to get their message to their target group. These efforts can be grouped into two types, internal and external. Internal efforts focus the attention on the existing patients of the practice, whereas external efforts focus the effort on people who are not present patients of the practice.

Internal Marketing Strategies

Internal marketing efforts are those that dentists have traditionally called "professionalism." These efforts cater to the existing patients, with the hope that they will stay with the practice and bring in additional new patients.

Branding

Branding is an internal function with large external implications. A dentist's brand is the image of his or her product in the marketplace. It is how consumers perceive the dentist to be different from other similar providers in the area. Their information and expectations about their dental experience should be the same as their actual experience. If so, they will see a particular as both relevant to solving their problem and unique in that ability. Branding involves all of the intangibles that drive consumer perception of a business. These include logo, stationery, advertising, office décor and ambience, staff training and attire, and Web site. These should all be consistent and offer consistent messages about the value of the service provided. If a dentist can establish a strong brand image, then he or she has more freedom in pricing and other management decisions that lead to increased profitability.

Table 17.1 Types of Marketing Strategies

Internal	External
Existing patients	New patients into practice
Current patients of record	Target group
Traditional "professional"	Nontraditional methods
Existing resources within office	External resources, media
Less costly	More costly

Performance

The single most important trait of a dentist (according to public opinion surveys) is quality of care delivered. Quality care is the basis of the "product" that a dentist provides. Quality dentistry is necessary for a successful practice. But quality dentistry alone is insufficient to guarantee a successful practice. A dentist's performance of the technical side of dentistry is an assumed trait by the public. If a dentist violates that assumption, the patient will be dissatisfied and probably leave the practice. It is not even the dentist's actual performance that the patient judges but rather the patient's perception of the performance compared to the patient expectation of the performance. Patient expectations then become crucial to their satisfaction. If the dentist did not meet the patient's expectations, the patient will be dissatisfied with the service, even if their expectations were unrealistic in the first place. (To his or her mind, the expectations were realistic!) Even if a dentist does the most technically perfect procedure, if the patient does not like it (or the way it was delivered), he or she will be dissatisfied. If a dentist builds patients' expectations with slogans such as "special care," "painless," "low fees," or "cowards welcome," then he or she better deliver what is promised. The worst thing a dentist can do is to gain someone's trust to come to the office and then not deliver promised services. Patients are concerned with the total time of treatment. From the dentist's perspective, the time is the chair time in treatment. From the patient's perspective, time is the total time involved in the dental visit: travel time, waiting time, return-to-work time, and additional time to go to the baby sitter, school, or other places. Other examples of influencing patients' expectations include promptness, pain control, availability, and amount of health information provided.

Insurance Plan Participation

Whether or not a dentist participates in a given insurance plan has a large impact on generating patients for the practice. People generally gain their dental benefit through their work, often with little input into which plan to choose, or the specifics of the plan. The plan administrator then gives them a list of dentists who are providers for the plan. They then choose a dental provider based on which ones are providers for the plan. The insurance carrier then steers hundreds or thousands of patients to participating providers. From the perspective of a practitioner, he or she may gain many patients if he or she is a participating provider. (The dentist must also offer the patients substantial discounts from normal fees.) If the dentist is not a participating provider, then he or she may lose patients as their insurance package at work changes. Because of this, a dentist will need to compare insurance plans and decide with which, if any, he or she wishes to participate. This is currently one of the greatest marketing issues faced by dental practitioners.

Fees

Depending on the objective, a dentist will have a different fee strategy. Those strategies and their uses are described in the chapter on fee determination, and the various methods of determining fees (cost, demand, and competition based) are also in that chapter.

If a dentist wins a patient today based on price, the dentist can also lose them tomorrow based on price. When patients call asking the fee for a particular service (e.g., a denture), try to deflect the answer (e.g., "the dentist will need to do a complete exam and determine a best course of treatment for your particular case"). However, the dentist should not worry about giving the fee because he or she may have chased the patient away, but was that patient worth having in the first place?

If a dentist is different, price is less important. If he or she offers a unique service or offers a service uniquely, then the patient will find it more difficult to go to another dentist to have the service done. As patients bond to the dentist and the staff, the personal relationship becomes unique as well. The value attached to a product or service is proportional to the ability to solve the problem for the consumer. The patient is seeking a benefit or solution to a problem. The better the service solves the patient's problem, the more they are willing to pay for the service.

Customers (patients) buy clusters of values for a multiplicity of reasons. Those reasons may not always be obvious to the dentists. Patients buy based on their values, not the dentist's. Dentists should be careful of *should* statements. These statements imply the dentist's values, not the patient's. It is the process of being sold, not just the product or service that sells. How the dentist delivers the service is as important as the service itself. A particular dentist might make the most esthetic crowns in town, but if he or she can not convince the patient of the value, the dentist will not be making any of them.

Box 17.4 Performance Affects Patient Referrals

- If someone has simply the experience expected, he or she will tell no one.
- If someone had a better experience than expected, he or she will tell 2 people.
- If someone had a worse experience than expected, he or she will tell 10 people.

Credit Policy

Every practice has credit and collection policies, whether they know it or not. (A separate chapter discusses this in detail.) The public and all patients become aware of that policy every time they say, "Just send me the bill." An easy credit policy encourages people to have work done and continue with treatment plans. A stricter plan requires patients to have more money upfront and discourages some from accepting planned treatment. Dentists want to establish a policy that is consistent with the clientele they are serving in their practice. If a dentist is too lenient when extending credit, his or her production will grow along with the accounts receivable and bad debts (uncollectibles) as people take advantage of his or her kindly nature. On the other hand, accounts receivable may be too low, suggesting that the dentist may be losing some "sales" and production as a result of an excessively restrictive credit policy.

The credit policy interacts with fees to be a powerful marketing influence. Patients refer other patients based on how they perceive they are treated in the office, including payment plans. Patients look more at the monthly cost of a payment plan than the total cost of the procedure. The credit policy therefore, has a huge impact on how much dentistry a dentist can "sell."

Facility

A facility is the "place" in marketing dentistry. As a health care facility, the public absolutely expects cleanliness. (Cleanliness includes dust, cob webs, and finger prints.) Dentists should match decor to the desired clientele. Decor includes color, lighting, furniture, and open or closed operatory arrangement. Accessibility for disabled and geriatric patients is important for those groups. Dentists should try to isolate the reception area isolated from the noise and odors of treatment area. Labs are usually messy. The lab should be hidden from view by either placing it the back of the office or keeping the door closed. Try to have diversions in the reception area. Most practitioners have reading material that is appropriate for their patients. Many others have an aquarium or a "kid's corner" to use as a diversion for their patients.

A facility-related marketing strategy is the hours that a dentist keeps the office open to see patients. A dental practice is a business that "sells" dental services to the public. Successful practices make those services available at times that are convenient to the clients or patients. Many dentists have as a goal to work only traditional hours during the day. However, new practitioners may find a wealth of patients by providing services during nontraditional hours. Changing demographics in this country point to a continued decline in the "traditional" family unit (wage earner father, nonworking mother, and two school-aged children). Patients may be single parents or two wage-earner couples who find it difficult to take off work for dental appointments. These people often have either dental insurance (or dual coverage) or have the discretionary money to spend on sophisticated dental care. As a result, many dentists find their nontraditional hours (evenings and Saturdays) to be most productive. On the down side, neither the owner–dentist nor the employees may want to work during these hours. The providers want time with their own family or for outside, personal interests. Depending on family situations, some people may not be able or willing to arrange schedules, day care services, or other obligations to work these hours. Some dentists have hired part-time workers to fill times when other staff members can not work. Most state laws require that any employee is paid "time and a half" for working more than 40 hours per week, for each additional hour. (A few states base overtime on 8 hours per day.) The additional patient revenues may be worth the added cost of overtime and staff turnover.

Communication

Communication is the "advertising" of dental office internal marketing. The dental office communicates in several different ways. Verbal communication is the most obvious form. A dentist's (and staffs') choice of words is important. A word that has common and innocuous meaning to the dentist may strike fear into the heart of an apprehensive patient. (Does *operatory* mean that the dentist is going to do an operation?)

Nonverbal communication is as important as the conversation itself. The tone of voice, by the provider or person on the telephone, tells more than the words themselves. Kinesics "body language" and proxemics "personal space" are understood by patients on an intuitive level. A dentist should be aware of how he or she and staff use these techniques.

Written communications should all convey the sense of professionalism that a dentist wants the office to project. It is a good idea to have a logo or other style of stationery used on all office communications. These include letters, brochures and information, postoperative instructions, and payment options and plans.

Recall (Recare) Systems

A dentist's recare system is one of the most visible internal marketing efforts that the office makes. (*Recall* implies defective care, as in a product recall. *Recare* or "periodic maintenance" implies ongoing care.) Dentists should aim all of their efforts in this area to help patients achieve an optimum level of oral health. All communication should support this idea. Specific techniques are given in a separate chapter.

Information for Patients

Dental patients want information to make health care decisions. They want information both about dental issues and general health concerns, so many dentists provide brochures about these topics. (For example, "What is a root canal?" or "How can I stop smoking?") Many dentists also have video or DVD presentation about dental care topics that they can show to patients. This helps in educating patients about complex procedures, helps in the informed consent conversation, and decreases the time that the dentist spends in direct patient conversation.

People who use dental services preventively usually have a preventive health lifestyle that shows as other healthy lifestyle habits and procedures. They also exercise more, smoke less, eat healthier foods, and use seatbelts more than those who do not use dental services preventively. This preventive lifestyle group especially values health information. They appreciate and recommend the dentist because of it.

Asking for Referrals

One of the best ways to encourage patients to send additional patients is simply to ask them. Often patients do not know that dentists are looking for new and additional patients. Many dentists have developed reward systems for thanking patients for referring their friends or coworkers as patients of the practice. After a referral, the office may send a nice note of thanks. After several referrals, the office may send a note with a gift card or other more tangible method of thanking the referral source. Box 17.5 gives a simple formula method of verbally asking a patient for additional referrals.

External Marketing Strategies

External marketing efforts are those that dentists have not traditionally used. These efforts are to bring new patients into the practice. The hope here is that they will stay with the practice and bring in even more additional new patients. Most external marketing involves advertising and promotional efforts because dentists are trying to reach a new group of patients.

Public Relations

This strategy often involves speaking to groups. It is important that dentists identify whom they will be speaking to and what they want the outcome to be. Is the desired outcome a better-educated group? Or does the dentist want to generate three patient referrals from the presentation? Depending on the desired outcome, the talk will have a different orientation.

Public relations efforts often involve brochures or newsletters. Dentists may write these, or they can purchase them already written (prefabricated or off the shelf). (Making a newsletter involves a significant amount of time that might be spent more productively doing other tasks.) Dentists can purchase prefabricated newsletters from many dental form and stationery companies. They can then have the dentist's name printed on them to customize the look.

Professional Relations

Interacting with other professionals is the second important part of the external marketing effort. Dentists need to let other professionals in the area know where they are and what they can do for the other professionals regarding patient referrals. This usually takes the form of announcements to physicians and other area dentists when a dentist opens a practice. Dentists should join local study clubs to learn and share special procedures and agree to take emergency calls for local established dentists, being sure that their patients return to the dentist of record for follow-up treatment. Specialists appreciate referrals from generalists and often refer different patients to the generalist. A dentist should not be afraid to get on the phone and ask for help if he or she runs into a particularly difficult problem. If a dentist refers regularly, the specialist will usually be glad to help out. Many dentists give a bonus to their own staff who refer patients and send gifts to the staff of their referring dentists.

Signage

Office visibility is crucial for a dentist's success. The public needs to know that he or she exists and where he or she practices. Where a dentist places the office is important in this regard. The most visible location is on a busy arterial feeder street where thousands of cars pass every day. If a dentist has a visible sign on such a busy road, thousands of people will see the location each day. Keep the sign simple. The "40–40 rule" says that a person should be able to read a sign from 40 yards away at 40 miles per hour as they drive past. This

Box 17.5 How to Ask a Patient for Referrals	
Thank the patient by name	Mrs. Jones, Thank you for coming to see us.
What you want	If you know anyone who is looking for dental care,
Ask them to send	Please have them call us.
Confirm their care	We would love to see them and will take excellent care of them.

does not mean that they will all come to see that dentist, but when they decide to see a dentist, he or she will be one of the dentists that they consider. The dentist should "cut through the clutter" of other signs in the area. If all businesses have 20-foot wide neon signs, the passersby will not see the 1-foot black-and-white sign. Internal lighting makes it viewable at night. If the office is located in a site that is not easily visible, then the dentist will need other forms of marketing to make up for the problem location.

Advertising and Promotions

Advertising and promotion bring a service to the attention of potential and current patients (customers) to increase patient visits. Advertising uses the media to inform potential patients of the services that are offered. That media can be the Yellow Pages, direct mail, radio or television advertising, or a Web site. Advertising intends to inform the public of the services offered.

A promotion is a planned effort to increase sales over a short period. Promotions add something of value to the service offered. It helps to stimulate sales for reasons other than the face value of the service's benefit. For example, if a dentist sends a direct mailing to the households in the zip code that surrounds his or her office, that dentist has engaged in advertising. If he or she includes a coupon for a free whitening tray, then that dentist has included a promotion with the advertising. Promotions are effective in stimulating potential patients to action. The advertising informs them of the services that offered, but the promotion gives then a reason to come and see that dentist.

Depending on the target market, a dentist will use different types of advertising and promotional efforts. Direct mail is more effective in blue-collar neighborhoods than in white-collar ones. Web sites are more important if a dentist is targeting a younger, more affluent group. Senior citizen newsletters, high school sport brochures, and new mother publications are effective media for their target audiences. A dentist is only trying to get the potential patient to come in to see him or her, not complete the treatment decision in the ad.

Network and franchise practices have an advantage over individual practitioners when using advertising and promotions in the mass media. Radio and television ads are effective, but also expensive. When someone places an ad in these venues, the ad goes to everyone. It is not targeted by geography or other demographic variables. Most of patients come from near practices. So, using mass media wastes many contacts because of too large a reach for the individual practice. If the franchise or network has practices throughout the media market, then each of those outlets shares in the benefits of the

marketing effort, drastically reducing the cost of acquiring each patient. This means that an individual practitioner often takes a more focused marketing strategy that targets patients that are more likely to come to the practice.

Professional advertising differs from advertising many other goods and services. It must be more factual (office hours, services offered, location, etc.) with no "puffery" or other claims of superiority. What is customary for the area influences professional advertising. Using a radio ad in one area may be mainstream for the dental market but may label a dentist as a pariah in a more traditional marketplace. Although a dentist may be legally able to use such advertising, the dental community may be small and close-knit. The dentist still needs to interact with fellow practitioners, so be aware of local customs in this area.

Good advertisements draw someone's attention, generate interest and desire for the product, and result in an action by the person (called AIDA in marketing). Professionals often accomplish these goals by developing a list of potential problems that someone can identify with (e.g., dry mouth, floppy dentures). They may show examples of their work (such as before and after photos) or have people give testimonials of the excellent care they have received. Most have a call to action ("Good for the next week," or "for a limited time"). Incentives are often use to evoke action by the patient (Box 17.6).

Web Sites

Web sites are becoming a more important source of information for consumers. This depends largely on the type of clientele sought. For example, if a dentist has an orthodontic practice that seeks young affluent families, then a Web presence is important. If a dentist has a prosthetic practice that seeks elderly patients with prosthetic needs, then a Web site is less valuable as a marketing

---

Box 17.6 Example Advertising Incentives

Bonus
   Call within 3 days, receive free X-rays
Discount
   Bring this coupon before September 1 and get 50 percent off new patient exam
Motivation
   Come in today and begin your life with a beautiful new smile
Consequences
   Do *not* wait. Dental problems only get worse without treatment

tool. Other forms of distributing a message (such as senior newsletters or yellow page advertising) are more important for this group. A Web site can introduce services, introduce the dentist and staff members, inform prospective patients of hours and policies, and provide health information. Forms (such as health history or Health Insurance Portability and Accountability Act [HIPAA]) that patients can download and complete before they come to the office can also be posted. Other forms of Web presence (Facebook, LinkedIn, etc.) can be valuable if the target market includes people who regularly use these media.

Mailings

Direct mailings can reach potential patients in an inexpensive way. These can target the zip codes or areas near the office or other target groups. Dentists can purchase brochures and mailing packages from marketing firms or develop their own. Direct mailings are especially effective for a working class neighborhood, especially when they include a coupon or other saving enticement. If using these direct mailings, the dentist should use them for at least 3 to 4 months to imprint his or her name on the minds of those who receive the mailings. Another form of direct mailing is to send current patients of the practice newsletters or other information about the practice. When a dentist purchases a practice, the outgoing practitioner often has a bank of patients that have not been active (seen in the practice) for one to several years. Sending a letter to these people is a cost-effective way to generate additional patients for the practice.

Yellow Pages

Many people will use the Yellow Pages to screen possible choices in dentists. They may use location in a large city or services offered as a screening criterion. (Dentists should include a map of the general location so that people can easily find the office.) A yellow page ad can be expensive, especially as the size is increased or placement of the ad is moved to be more easily noticed. If it generates enough patients, then it can more than pay for itself. As mentioned previously, older clientele use yellow page searches more than younger people. Dentists should identify and target the market to set the most effective use of their advertising budget.

The Financial Impacts of Marketing

Given the high cost of marketing efforts, dentists need to understand how marketing and patient generation affect the finances of the practice.

Marketing Is Necessary for Success

Marketing brings patients, both new and repeat, to the practice for treatment. Without patients, there is not practice. Many dentists claim that their office budgets do not allow them to spend money on marketing ("I can't afford to spend money on marketing."). This view assumes that marketing is an optional practice activity. The correct view should be "What do I need to spend on marketing to drive the number of patient visits that I need to meet my financial projections?" This second view says that marketing is the engine of practice growth. If a dentist wants to grow the practice, he or she needs additional patients. Marketing expenditures bring these patients to the practice. To the extent that a dentist limits marketing expenditures, he or she limits practice growth.

Value of a New Patient

Each new patient is worth a certain dollar value to the practice. That value is the average amount of dentistry that is done on new patients. Dentists can find it by adding the total collections for dentistry done on all new patients divided by the total number of new patients. Compare that dollar value to the average amount spent on marketing per new patient. On a basic level, if the dollar value of the patient is higher than the amount spent to generate the patient, the marketing program was worthwhile. If not, it was not.

Marginal Cost of Production

Taking this analysis one step further, the cost of doing the dentistry should also be allocated to the new patient to decide profitability. The issue here is whether the dentist has "slack resources" or empty chair time. If a dentist has no slack resources (chairs are all completely booked) then all of the costs of the office should be divided and allocated to all patients. If, on the other hand, a dentist has empty chair time, then the cost of seeing an additional patient is only the variable costs associated with production (dental supplies, dental lab, and office supplies). The dentist has already paid the rent and utilities, the staff (they are sitting around filing their nails), and he or she is doing the crossword puzzle in the morning newspaper. The dentist's only costs for seeing another patient—the marginal costs of production—are small (the additional costs associated with lab and material for doing the dentistry).

Repetition

Marketing means repetition. Dentists, who are used to the scientific method, believe that if something works once, then it will work always for all similar circumstances. When sending a message to people, dentists have to tell them over and over again. People hear the message when they are ready to listen, not simply when a dentist is ready to tell them. Someone may drive past the office every working day for 5 years, but it is only when they decide they need to find a dentist will they notice a dentist's sign. For the same reason, Proctor and Gamble constantly advertises Tide laundry soap, so that when a person is ready to buy laundry soap, he or she will think "Tide." This "top-of-the-mind" awareness means that a dentist may not see an effect of his or her marketing efforts in the first week, month, or even several months. Repetition is required of even a good marketing message. Although this appears to increase the cost of the marketing effort, it also increases its effectiveness and therefore its value.

Part 2: Managing Continuing Care

Remember that credit is money.
Benjamin Franklin

Objectives

At the completion of this part, the student will be able to:
1. Describe the patient care reasons to develop the continuing care function in the office.
2. Describe the economic reasons to develop the continuing care function in the office.
3. Describe common methods of setting continuing care appointments.
4. Describe the effect of retention rate on continuing care production.
5. Compare the cost of acquiring a new patient with a continuing care patient.

Key Terms

check up
periodic maintenance
preappointing

preheating
recall
recare

Goal

This part presents guidelines for developing the continuing care function in the dental office.

Internal marketing aims to generate patients from within the practice and to encourage existing patients to remain with the practice for their continuing care. This is healthy from two perspectives. It improves patient care and therefore his or her oral health and makes good financial sense for the practice. Supporting continuing care is truly a mutually beneficial situation.

Different offices have different names for the continuing care function. Although at first this seems a trivial exercise in semantics, how dentists convey to patients what they do has a tremendous impact on the patient's perception of them. Words do matter, and patients form opinions based on the words they hear. Although different patients may have different wants and needs that dentists cannot control, dentists can control how they communicate services to the patients.

The most common name is the recall system. This is an office-centric view of the function. Dentists are recalling the patient for their purpose and their procedures. In the patients' minds, this is similar to a defective product recall, where the manufacturer must repair or replace a defective part. (Is the gas tank going to explode? Did a filling go bad?) Because all dental services have a lifetime that is often dependent, in part, on the care taken by the owner, moving from dentist responsibility to partnered responsibility for long-term function seems appropriate. Some offices call the function *recare*. This moves the focus toward the patient's health and away from the office procedure. It helps the patient and staff members realize that the purpose is to care for the patient's oral health needs. Many offices call the process *periodic maintenance* or *continuing care* to emphasize the ongoing nature of the procedure and relationship. By calling the process maintenance, patients understand that they have a part in ensuring that their dental health remains good and their dental work remains defect free. Part of the responsibility is to return regularly for a follow-up evaluation and treatments necessary. Finally, some offices call the process a *check up*. Although this infers the ongoing nature of the process, it also trivializes the important function that the process plays in the oral health of the individual.

Value of Preventative Services

Patient Care Perspective

Continuing care, properly applied, prevents additional restorative work for the patient (Box 17.7). Through a personal preventive orientation, patients can avoid recurrent caries and the replacements that result. This also decreases the severity of future work, as each time dentists replace a restoration, it necessarily becomes larger, and the tooth weaker. Regular prophylaxis and reinforcement improve periodontal health and decrease the severity of this disease. Other oral problems—caries, periodontal, or pathological in nature—can be found and treated at an earlier stage. This all improves the patient's oral health and decreases the total amount that he or she spends on personal dental care. Finally, ongoing care visits help the patient and doctor develop a more personal relationship, instead of simply a client–provider relationship. This trusting relationship helps communication and patient involvement in treatment decisions and personal health awareness and ownership. All are important outcomes from the personal and public health perspectives.

Financial Perspective

From the financial perspective, encouraging continuing care makes good sense for the practice (Box 17.8). Dentists charge for preventive services such as periodic exams, diagnostic radiographs, and prophylaxes. Although not enormously profitable, these services do generate revenue and profit when properly managed.

Box 17.7 Value of Preventive Services: Patient Care Perspective

- Prevents additional work
- Decreases severity of future work
- Improves periodontal health
- Develops relationships
- Improves oral health

Box 17.8 Value of Preventive Services: Financial Perspective

- The value of the work itself
- Additional work generated
- Higher margin work generated
- Preparing patients for needed work
- Improved treatment acceptance

At the periodic exam, dentists often identify dental problems that need treatment. This generates additional revenue and profit for the practice. Often this work is complex in nature, which generates higher margin procedures, adding to the practice profit. Routine visits help to "preheat" patients for future needed work. When dentists remind a patient of a given problem ("That tooth needs a crown to avoid breaking"), they prepare the patient so that if the problem happens, he or she is ready for treatment. Dentists do not have to convince the patients of the need for the procedure. Finally, patients need to trust that the dentist is looking out for their best interest, not merely the dentist's own pocketbook, before they commit to complex and expensive treatments. Periodic visits help build that rapport and resulting trust.

Economic Value of a Continuing Care Patient

The economic value of a continuing care patient comes from several sources: the periodic work, additional work generated, and referrals from the patient.

Each patient that remains in the practice adds to the total production and compounds the profit and value of the practice simply from the periodic visit work. As an example, assume that a single patient comes to the practice every 6 months for periodic maintenance visits and never has any other dental work done. The value of the visit is $100, inflation increases the price by 4 percent per year, and each patient makes two visits per year. As seen in Table 17.2, the pure cumulative financial value of the periodic visits for that patient after 10 years is more than $2,400.

Now assume that, beyond the periodic visit procedures, the patient needs one additional restoration per year. That restoration has a value of $150, also compounded at 4 percent per year. As seen in the table, the cumulative value of the restorations is approximately $1,800. The total cumulative value of that patient over the 10-year example period rises to more than $4,000. This is for a patient who has no complex or high-value procedures done. Higher margin items (such as crowns) increase the value. This example only shows 10 years. The value also increases quickly over longer time as the fee compounds.

If then each continuing care patient will refer one additional patient every 2 years, Table 17.3 shows that the value triples to more than $15,400. If each of those patients also refers an additional patient with similar habits and needs, the value compounds to more than $25,000.

These numbers represent one patient. The value when added for many patients becomes dramatic. As is seen in Table 17.4, if a dentist gains 20 new patients per month and each of those patients returns for a periodic visit

Table 17.2 Economic Value of a Continuing Care Patient

Year	Value of Periodic Visits	Cumulative Value of Periodic Visits	Value of Restoration	Cumulative Value of Restorations	Total Cumulative Value
1	$200	$200	$150	$150	$350
2	$208	$408	$156	$306	$714
3	$216	$624	$162	$468	$1,093
4	$225	$849	$169	$637	$1,486
5	$234	$1,083	$175	$812	$1,896
6	$243	$1,327	$182	$995	$2,322
7	$253	$1,580	$190	$1,185	$2,764
8	$263	$1,843	$197	$1,382	$3,225
9	$274	$2,117	$205	$1,587	$3,704
10	$285	$2,403	$213	$1,801	$4,202

Table 17.3 Value of Referrals

Year	Total Cumulative Value Original Patient	Total Cumulative Value Referral 1	Total Cumulative Value Referral 2	Total Cumulative Value Referral 3	Total Cumulative Value Referral 4	Total Cumulative Value Referral 5
1	$350					
2	$714	$364				
3	$1,093	$743				
4	$1,486	$1,136	$394			
5	$1,896	$1,546	$804			
6	$2,322	$1,972	$1,230	$425		
7	$2,764	$2,414	$1,673	$867		
8	$3,225	$2,875	$2,134	$1,327	$460	
9	$3,704	$3,354	$2,613	$1,805	$938	
10	$4,202	$3,852	$3,112	$2,302	$1,436	$498

Total Cumulative Value = $15,402

Table 17.4 Hygiene Visit Production[*]

Months	New Patients	Recall Patient Visits	Total Hygiene Patient Visits	Total Hygiene Production per Month	Total Hygiene Production per Year
1–6	20	0	20	$2,500	
7–12	20	20	40	$5,000	$45,000
13–18	20	40	60	$7,500	
19–24	20	60	80	$10,000	$105,000
25–30	20	80	100	$12,500	
31–36	20	100	120	$15,000	$165,000
37–42	20	120	140	$17,500	
43–48	20	140	160	$20,000	$225,000
49–54	20	160	180	$22,500	
55–60	20	180	200	$25,000	$285,000

[*]Assumptions: Start at zero patients; add 20 new patients per month (20 × 6 = 120/six months; and keep 100% of patients for 6-month periodic visits.
Total hygiene patient visits = periodic patients + new patients
Average hygiene periodic production = Exam + Prophy + BWs/2 + Pan every 5 years = $105

every 6 months, then the total value of the hygienist's functions alone is worth $285,000 per year after 5 years. This does not include any additional work generated from the new patient or periodic maintenance visits.

The rate of retention of patients for the periodic visits is also important. The previous analysis assumed that a dentist retained 100 percent of the periodic patients. Table 17.5 shows the effect of lower retention rates. As dentists retain a smaller proportion of patients, the effect decreases the hygiene production significantly. Every continuing care patient then is important for the economic health of a practice. The loss of even

Table 17.5 Effect of Retention Rate

Retention Rate	Hygiene Production
100%	$285,000
95%	$270,750
90%	$256,500
85%	$242,250
80%	$228,000
75%	$213,750

a single patient, especially early in the practice cycle when the compounding effect is greatest, can have a large impact on long-term office finances. The importance of actively managing the system should be obvious.

Cost of a Periodic Maintenance Patient

Marketing looks to generate patients for the practice, either through internal (existing patient) method or through external methods (new patients). Depending on the method used, a new patient may cost tens or hundreds of dollars to generate. Some of these new patients will come with large, complex cases. The cost of retaining existing patients is much less than generating new patients for the practice. An existing patient costs the practice a postage stamp or a few minute of staff time for a telephone call. Existing patients know the staff and doctor and have developed some level of trust with the practice. They are often participants in favored insurance plans, so the staff does not need to investigate benefits or insurance plan requirements as often. These are higher-volume, lower-cost patients. Both contribute to practice profitability.

Periodic Maintenance Management

Several issues are common to managing periodic maintenance systems.

Completion of Treatment

When a patient completes active treatment and is placed on maintenance status, staff members should be sure to show the date in the computer. Dentists can also code any special instructions (such as required premedication) in the appropriate area. Dentists should place an exact date for the next visit. Many insurance companies pay for prophylaxis every 6 months (to the day) since the last one. If a patient returns for a periodic exam 1 day early, the insurance company may deny benefits.

Setting Appointments

There are two common methods of setting appointments, preappointing and month of recall. Which method is used depends on trial and error and what is customary in the community in which a dentist practices. In fact, a dentist may use a combination of the two, depending on patients' needs and wants.

Many offices make periodic appointments for patients as they leave the office, preappointing the patient's next periodic visit. This requires that the office have a defined schedule at least 6 months in advance. If patients are on yearly frequency, office schedules must be determined at least that far ahead. This limits a dentist's ability to take time off for continuing education courses or personal enjoyment without significant rescheduling problems. Offices that use this method claim that they are first on a patient's schedule. The patient then works other schedule items around their dental appointment. If someone cancels, the appointment can generally be filled with another patient. It also allows the practice to decide the appropriate level of future hygiene staffing. Many dentists who use this system leave blocks of time available for new patient prophylaxes or patients who must reschedule an appointment. Staff members should still call patients before the appointment for confirmation. Using this method works particularly well in offices that have multiple practitioners because these offices can ensure that the office will be open and "covered" in the future.

The second method is to wait until the month before the maintenance visit to appoint. The office sends either computer-generated cards reminding patients to call to schedule a periodic visit, or they generate a computer list of patients due and call them to remind and appoint them. If a dentist uses this method, computer-generated reminder cards should be sent at least 2 weeks before the month due so that the office can schedule people appropriately early in the month. Otherwise, a 6-month maintenance visit turns into a 7- or 8-month maintenance visit, compromising both the patient's oral health and the office maintenance system. Offices that use this method claim that it gives more flexibility in scheduling vacations and other time off. They also claim that patients often change appointments when they make them 6 months ahead, so it is easier to schedule once, rather than adjust appointment books. Some patients do not want to commit to a specific time that far in the future.

Follow-Up

Contact patients who do not have an appointment during their scheduled month. Then appoint and place them on the appropriate monthly lists or place them on inactive status. Follow-up and constant monitoring of the system is crucial to effective periodic system management.

Responsibility

Responsibility for maintenance of the continuing care system varies from office to office. Often the receptionist or office manager is in charge of maintaining and updating all periodic information on patients, mailing reminder cards, and scheduling appointments. In offices where a hygienist is paid a commission, he or she is usually responsible for maintaining the system because his or her productivity and income depend on the effectiveness of the continuing care program. One person should be responsible for the system, whether business office personnel, hygienist, or clinical assistant. That way, if problems occur, then the responsible person can be identified and corrective action can be taken.

Scheduling Time Increments

Dentists should set a standard time code per periodic visits. Hygienists on salary will generally want to see one patient per hour; those on a commission basis will schedule one patient every 30 minutes. Accurate scheduling differs with the practice philosophy and skills of the practitioners. Hygienists can generally complete children's visits in 30 minutes. Adults with routine "prophy" needs can generally be completed in 45 minutes. Those adults who have significant calculus present or periodontal condition may require reappointment for definitive periodontal scaling and root planing.

If dentists schedule the hygienist to do only hygiene procedures and an assistant to do nonhygiene procedures (such as history updates, charting, and radiographs) then the dentist can almost double hygiene production for each hygienist. This substitutes the assistant's time for the hygienist's time for those procedures the state law allows the dentist to delegate to the clinical assistants. This frees the hygienist to do hygiene-only procedures on a second patient while the assistant begins or completes the patient in the first chair. Some hygienists feel that this becomes a "prophy mill" as they move from patient to patient without the personal interaction that many cherish.

Some offices have operatories specifically set up for hygienists, often using older or inferior equipment. Although older equipment saves money in the short run, it has negative consequences. Not only does it slow treatment, but it also sends a subliminal message to the patient and the hygienist about the importance of the continuing care system. The additional cost of fully equipping an operatory over minimally equipping a "hygiene" operatory is small. Full equipped operatories are more flexible and can be used for small procedures on maintenance visits or on a day that a hygienist is not working in them.

As the maintenance function becomes larger, some practices dedicate a day a week in which the entire office sees periodic maintenance patients ("hygiene Thursdays"). The office hires part-time hygienists to see patients in chairs that are normally scheduled for dentist visits. The dentist then spends the entire day assessing periodic maintenance patients and treatment. This allows the office to see large numbers of periodic patients without constantly interrupting dentist–patient procedures.

Denture Patient Maintenance

Many successful practices insist that all complete denture patients return to the office once per year for a denture check up. These visits consist of an oral cancer exam and a check of denture fit and function. These practices generally find the time and effort well spent.

Gaining Case Acceptance

chapter 18

Part 1: Communication in the Office

All great writers have a built in, infallible crap detector.
Ernest Hemingway

Objectives:

At the completion of this part, the student will be able to:
1. Describe the steps in the communication process.
2. Describe the common methods of communication in the dental office.
3. Describe the types of nonverbal communication.
4. Describe how proxemics affects patient interactions.
5. Describe how patient position affects patient interactions.
6. Describe the oral communication process.
7. Define common barriers to communication.
8. Describe the types of listening.
9. Describe how to deal with common "problem patient" communication issues in the dental practice.

KEY TERMS

active listening	message	self-disclosure
body language	noise	semantic problems
content listening	oral communication	sender
decoding	personal zone	social zone
effective feedback	proxemics	therapeutic listening
encoding	public zone	value judgments
feedback	receiver	verbal/nonverbal incongruity
interpretive listening	relationship listening	written communication
intimate zone	script	
medium	selective perception	

Goal

This part presents guidelines for communicating in the office.

Business Basics for Dentists, First Edition. David O. Willis.
© 2013 John Wiley & Sons, Inc. Published 2013 by John Wiley & Sons, Inc.

Communication is a key to successful dental practice. Dentists must communicate with staff members to be sure that the office operates effectively. They must communicate with vendors and other professionals to ensure excellent patient treatment. And dentists must communicate with patients to inform them of their needs and to gain acceptance for treatment options. A successful dentist has to be a great communicator. This part discusses the communication process and how dentists can improve their patient communication process and abilities.

Communication in its most basic form is simply the transfer of information from one person to another. This seems simple on the surface, however, digging more deeply into the process, communication involves speaking, writing, thinking, and a heavy dose of psychology. It involves transmitting not just facts but also ideas, opinions, emotions, and attitudes. It is the primary method of forming interpersonal relationships. For example, to formulate a treatment plan for a patient, we need to understand their frame of reference, their wants, needs and desires. The only way to find this out is through interpersonal communication. Although many forms of communication are used in the office, face-to-face communication is the most common. It is also the richest method for processing issues, especially those that have a high degree of uncertainty or a large emotional component to the decision. Other channels of communicating, such as letters, e-mail, or telephone calls, do not share the depth of understanding is gained from face-to-face communication.

The Communication Process

The communication process is a shared experience between two or more people with importance given to both sending and receiving information. Really, all interpersonal behavior involves communication, either intentional or not, because most actions convey some meaning. Communication involves eight key elements. All eight must work for there to be an effective sharing of ideas. The important point in understanding this process is that when communication fails, any of the eight steps may be the cause. If someone understands the steps, he or she can decrease problems in the process.

1. The *sender* is the person who wants to transmit the idea or information to another. A dentist may wish to offer an idea, or his or her patient may want to express an emotion, fact, or concern with the dentist. The role of the sender and receiver shifts back and forth as communication progresses.
2. *Encoding* happens when the sender translates the communication into a language that the receiver will (hopefully) understand. If dentists use too much dental jargon that the patients cannot comprehend, their failure to properly encode may harm the communication process.
3. The *message* is the result of the encoding process. It is the idea that the sender wants to send to the receiver. It may be information, a feeling, value, belief, or attitude.
4. The *medium* is how the message is carried. The most obvious is the meaning of the spoken words. Other examples include text massages, e-mails, tone of voice, or body language.
5. The *receiver* is the recipient of the message. Receivers decode and interpret messages developing their own meaning of the message. This may be different from the sender's meaning.
6. *Decoding* happens when the receiver translates the message into their "language." They must interpret the direct words plus any additional messages carried by the medium. Because some media, such as face-to-face oral communication, are much more rich (i.e., they contain more additional information), they also have more room for misinterpretation and error. The receiver's perception of what was said is a reality for them. Therefore, their values, attitudes, beliefs, and concerns all influence the receiver's perception of the message.
7. *Feedback* occurs when the receiver responds to the message. A direct response (verbal reply, facial expression) allows the sender to assess whether the message was received and if it had the intended result.
8. *Noises* are factors in the system that distort the intended message. The receiver may not accurately interpret the message if there is too much distortion. Examples include physical noise in the conversational space such as other people talking, and psychological noise, such as fear, different frames of reference, and preconceived notions by the communicators.

Methods of Communicating

People use several ways of communicating in face-to-face situations. Verbal communication (either written or oral) is the most obvious. However, how people present the verbal communication tells the receiver about their state of mind during the process. Perceptive people use these cues to come to a deeper understanding of what was meant to be said, as opposed to what was actually said. This means that people have both an intentional communication (e.g., the meaning of the words) and an unintentional communication (e.g., the unease exhibited by nervous fidgeting during the conversation). The best communication occurs when these two match, when people communicate effectively what they want to communicate. Although this sounds simple, the process becomes muddied by peoples' perceptions, cultural and family histories, state of mind, and current condition.

Nonverbal Communication

Communication is the transfer of information from one person to another. This is usually thought of as simply the spoken word. However, face-to-face communication carries much more information than simply the words. People can view the other's facial expression and hear the tone of the voice or the emphasis of words or points that are not present without a personal encounter (e.g., think of a simple e-mail message and how simply factual it is without embellishment). Psychologists estimate that as much as 85 percent of the information conveyed in face-to-face communication is nonverbal. People use these nonverbal cues to learn additional meaning and emotional background. By examining the context of the communication, people validate or refute what was said verbally. People examine the other's body language, or what the person has said beyond the simple spoken word, so that they have a richer communication encounter. People do this continually and subconsciously. Even a person who is inactive or silent may be sending an intended or unintended message: that he or she is bored, depressed, or angry.

People also must remember that the other person is assessing them in the same way. Therefore, people must be careful of the nonverbal messages that they send to others (patients and staff) and manage that part of the communication process as well.

Verbal and nonverbal information is related. Nonverbal are usually the more powerful of the two. When they are congruent, the nonverbal message reinforces the verbal message. When they are not congruent, there is a cognitive dissonance that indicates that something is wrong. (Think of the person who has anger in his or her words and voice but is calm and smiling in his face.) Cultural and gender differences play a role in nonverbal cues also.

Posture

A person's posture gives a strong statement on how he or she feels about himself or herself. An upright, but relaxed posture shows confidence and honesty. Slumping suggests lower self-esteem. Crossing arms may feel like a relaxed position, but to observers it can suggest that a person is shutting them out. Fidgeting (including twisting hair, drumming fingers, or examining fingernails) shows boredom or nervousness to patients.

Eye Contact

Direct eye contact suggests honestly and openness, especially when a person is speaking to someone else. A person looking down or away while speaking shows boredom. To be effective, people should try to make eye contact for the first and last 15 seconds of a conversation. It creates a feeling of concern and honesty that cannot be gained otherwise. However, a person should not overdo eye contact because if it is held too long, others will see it as hostile.

Physical Contact

People expect to be touched when they visit the dentist. However, they expect a "therapeutic" or "professional" touch, not an aggressive or sexual touch. So dentists still must respect a patient's personal zones, only entering the closer zone when invited. Hand-shaking is a ritualistic way to move from a social to a personal zone. (A person's emotional state can be indicated by their hand. Are they cold and clammy? Warm? Sweaty?) A pat on the shoulder is a less ritualistic way of making a symbolic connection with a person.

Facial Expression

Facial expressions give away a person's emotions. A pallor shows fear. Squinting shows aggression. People can read surprise, happiness, anger, or a host of other emotions by carefully watching a patient's facial expression.

Tone of Voice

The tone of someone's voice can also be a giveaway to his or her emotional state. People can show (or see) anger, fear, boredom, or happiness depending on how they emphasize words and the tone of their voice. Dentists see this when a patient talks with them, or when the dentist or a staff member talks with patients. For example, consider the children's game where the speaker emphasizes a different word in the same sentence; entirely different meanings result:

I love my job.
I *love* my job.
I love *my* job.
I love my *job*.

Because no one knows how he or she sounds outside to someone else, the dentist should record himself or herself talking with a patient. Then the dentist should listen to the tape private and honestly evaluate his or her own vocal delivery. Then the dentist should develop one or two specific things to work on. If a dentist has difficult time speaking with patients, he or she should consider getting a voice coach. The coach will help the dentist develop the tone and method of oral delivery.

Proxemics (Personal Space)

Proxemics is the study of space and how people relate to space. Understanding people's comfort zones can help a dentist influence communication and professional relationships with his or her patients.

Everyone has a personal space that surrounds them. The social relationship that someone has with the other person defines this space. Psychologists have proposed that the reasons may lie in people's evolutionary behavior. When unknown people are kept at a distance, they cannot surprise attack. As people are invited closer, it becomes easier to talk with them. When people are invited closer, intimacy or affection is invited. When people are acting, they may deliberately threaten another by invading their space without invitation. Anytime someone enters a personal zone without invitation, it creates anxiety for the person whose space is invaded. This is seen as a threatening action. Some people do this intentionally to signal that they are more powerful.

The public zone is generally more than 12 feet. When people are encountered in public, the tendency is to leave space between each other. When adequate space can not be left, people begin to feel uneasy. The next social zone allows a connection with other people. People can talk with others but still keep them at a distance. Friendly people in a social setting adopt this distance. The personal zone is one in which people who know each other may directly converse. When a person is close enough to touch the other, they are in the intimate zone. They can harm or touch each other in intimate ways. There must be significant trust for the two to be comfortable in this area.

The sizes of these zones vary by culture (Latin Americans and Middle Easterners have smaller personal spaces), by gender (women have smaller spaces), and by personality. People who come from different cultures may have different views of personal space. For example, males in some cultures find it unnerving to have a woman touch them or be proactive in invading their space.

In the dental office, dentists see each of these spaces. Patients sit as far from each other as possible in the reception room. In the operatory, they must be prepared for their intimate space to be invaded. Dentists then go further by touching them and invading their bodies, by putting their hands in the patients' mouths. This can be disconcerting, especially for someone who is not accustomed to dental visits. The dentist should reduce space gradually: meeting the patient, shaking hands, and gradually decreasing space before starting dental procedures. Patients who are lying in the supine position in the dental chair are in an exposed and vulnerable position. (Dogs roll on their backs, exposing their bellies to show submission.) When a dentist discusses treatment options with a patient, he or she should have the discussion with the patient in the upright position with eyes level or in a treatment conference room. This is a coequal position that promotes trust and open conversation.

Verbal Communication

Verbal communication is the most common form of professional–patient communication dental offices. Too often dentists assume that when they say something, the other person understands what is said, why it was said, and the nuances of what was said. It involves the two sides of speaking and listening. People use verbal communication to transmit or obtain information, share experiences, or bring about change in another person. Depending on the purpose of the conversation, people rely on different elements.

Word Choice

Particular words that people use may have different meaning to others. This occurs especially when people are discussing a familiar topic with a person who is unfamiliar, or has preconceived ideas, about the topic. For example, dentists are familiar and comfortable with endodontics, but many patients fear the dreaded "root canal." Patients may have heard stories or jokes that have given them preconceived ideas about how horrible the procedure is. So a dentist using the more technical terms *endodontic procedure* over the emotionally laden term *root canal* may avoid a negative reaction by a patient. Table 18.1 gives several other common dental office terms that may generate negative responses from nondental people. The more nondental terms dentists

---

Box 18.1 Personal Zones

Public zone more than 12 feet
Social zone is between 4 and 12 feet
Personal zone is between 1 1/2 and 4 feet
Intimate zone is less than 1 1/2 feet

Table 18.1 Word choice in the office

Dental Term	Nondental Term
Waiting room	Reception area
Operatory	Treatment area
Price	Fee
Investing	Paying
Oral exam	Check-up
Recall	Routine visit

and their staff can use, the less likely they are to generate negative emotional responses from patients.

Types of Listening

As busy professionals, dentists become accustomed to talking, but not listening to patients. However, listening is half the communication process. To be an effective listener, dentists have to stop talking and listen. (This can be difficult for some people!) Dentists also must listen for more than facts by keenly observing patients during the conversation.

Each of person uses several levels or types of listening in his or her role as a dentist. People shift between the types depending on the purpose of the conversation they are holding.

Listening for Content

The basic level of listening is to hear and comprehend the meaning of what was said. This requires that people have an appropriate vocabulary and understanding the rules of grammar and syntax so that they can understand what others are saying. Some words carry more importance than others. Understanding the content requires that people rank key facts from the long stream of words that make up many conversations. When a dentist listens to a patient's medical history, he or she must initially listen for the simple, factual content of what the patient said. Once a dentist gathers this information, he or she can move to higher levels of evaluation and interpretation.

Listening for Interpretation

The next level of listening is where a person makes judgments about what the other person says. People listen to decide if the other person is telling the truth, about how strongly they believe what they are saying, and if they have other, hidden agendas. When people interpret what is heard, they must also listen visually. Picking up on cues of body language helps people to assess if what another said verbally is congruent with what he or she said through actions and mannerisms. This type of listening is important as dentists interview patients about their wants, needs, and desires in dental treatment. If dentists try to persuade a patient to change their health behaviors, they will use interpretive listening as they weigh the pros and cons of the dentist's position to decide if it makes sense for them.

Relationship Listening

Sometimes the reason that people listen is to develop or maintain a relationship. (Lovers talk for hours about things that would bore them when listening to someone else.) In relationship listening, a person tries to learn more about the other person, how he or she thinks, what he or she enjoys, and what motivates him or er. This type of listening is important in developing both business and personal relationships. Before a patient will commit to a large treatment plan, he or she must believe that the dentist is looking out for his or her interests, not the dentist's. For a dentist to gain that level of trust takes time in building a relationship.

Therapeutic Listening

In therapeutic listening, people gain understanding of how others are feeling. The purpose is to use this personal relationship to help the other change or develop in some way. To get others to expose these deeper and more sensitive parts of themselves, people need to show understanding and empathy toward them, not just in words, but in the way that questions are asked. Dentists must be sensitive to the patient's unease in a way that encourages self-disclosure. A common example in the dental office is discussing treatment history with a patient who is dental phobic. These types of patients are often embarrassed about their dental condition and their behavior in the dental setting. Through therapeutic listening, dentists may find the root of the dental aversion and help the patient respond appropriately to it.

Active Listening

Active listening is the process that uses the different types of listening. This process intends to improve understanding between the speaker and listener. The listener frequently checks with the speaker to be sure that their interpretation of what the speaker said is what the speaker intended.

Active listening focuses our attention on the speaker. The listener must be sure to listen fully, not think of other things such as what he or she is going to ask next. The listener also observes the speaker's behavior and body language, incorporating them into the content and interpretation of the conversation. Having listened, the listener then paraphrases the speaker's words, not necessarily agreeing, but simply checking what the speaker said. In emotionally charged conversations, the listener should recognize those emotional bases. The active listener often describes his or her observation of the underlying emotion. ("You seem to feel angry" or "I sense that you feel frustrated. Why is that?"). This validates the speaker's emotional statement in a nonjudgmental way. It allows and encourages the speaker to discuss his or her emotions in a way that is positive for the conversation and leads effective therapy.

Effective Self-Disclosure

Self-disclosure occurs when a person intentionally gives information (verbally or nonverbally) to another about themselves. Self-disclosure is important because it conveys openness. Openness is one requirement for developing a trusting relationship. Trust is an element that is necessary for patient to communicate effectively and accept proposed treatment.

People can see self-disclosure in the response statements "Really? I've had a similar experience" or "I've often felt the same way." When a dentist shares that experience or feeling with the patient, the patient understands that the dentist's opinions may come from a similar reference and, therefore, be more valid.

Effective Feedback

The only way really to know if the patient received and processed the dentist's message with the same meaning that was meant is to ask. A simple question such as "Does that make sense?" or "Do you have any questions?" ask for a response that tells the dentist if the patient understands what was said. Several other techniques also test for understanding. Parroting is a simple repetition of what the person said, and paraphrasing does the same thing, only rephrasing what the person said in the listener's own words. Both are good ways to encourage additional discussion of an issue.

Verbal Communication Barriers

People have often heard someone say during an argument "What you heard is not what I said." This points to a breakdown in the communication process. Several common reasons that oral communications fail in the dental office (barriers to communication) include:

- *Different frames of reference* is when people have entirely different and valid views of similar issues. These come from different backgrounds, experiences, and values. For example, dentists value excellent oral health. Some of patients may not share that view. If dentists discuss treatment options based on their frame of reference, they may not "get through" to the patient because of this different frame of reference.
- *Selective perception* occurs when people hear what they want to hear, blocking out information that conflicts with their beliefs and values.
- *Value judgments* occur when the receiver decides the value of the message before he or she receives the entire message.
- *Semantic problems* occur when words and terms have one meaning to one person and a different (or no)

meaning to the other. If dentists use too much dental jargon or use words too casually (*root canal* can have a negative meaning for many), they may impede the communication process.

- *Poor listening skills* can occur especially under times of stress. Many find the dental office to be a stressful environment. Others may be in severe pain or worried about a diagnosis or cost of a procedure. This can make effective listening difficult.
- *Verbal–nonverbal incongruity* occurs when the verbal message does not match the nonverbal message sent. If a dentist shakes his or her head back and forth but verbally says "Yes," patients will become obviously confused. More subtle incongruities exist when a dentist fidgets while trying to sound confident or grinning when telling a patient bad news about the patient's dental condition.

Improving Verbal Communication

Dentists can improve interpersonal oral communication in the dental office by using the following techniques.

1. Follow-up on messages to be sure the listener received properly. The simplest way is for the dentist simply to ask the patient if he or she was clear. This verbal feedback assures the dentist that the patient received and properly interpreted the message.
2. The dentist should simplify language by being sure not to use many professional terms. The dentist should write down a list of dental terms and acceptable alternatives to use in daily communication.
3. The dentist should watch body language. He or she should be aware of the body language that he or she projects and take time to read the body language of patients. If a patient is sitting cross-armed with his or her lips pursed, he or she is probably not accepting the dentist's message, regardless of the verbal response.
4. The dentist should work on effective listening skills. These are skills that people can learn and improve, if they take the time and make the effort.
5. The dentist should make sure that his or her nonverbal messages support his or her verbal messages. If they are not congruent, the listener will hear the worse one.

Scripts

Most communication in the office is repetitive for the dentist and the dental staff members. Some staff members are more skilled at saying things in a way that elicits positive response from the patient. Others have a difficult time spontaneously talking in an effective way. To solve this problem, many offices have developed scripts for staff to use when talking with patients. For example, the assistants may not know the words that the receptionist uses when he or she answers the telephone. If the receptionist is sick or away from the desk, the fill-in may not know to answer the phone. A script that the replacement can read the first several times ensures that he or she answers the telephone correctly, gathering the correct information for patient care and scheduling.

A dentist can write scripts for every common interaction in the office. He or she can then use staff meetings to practice and refine the scripts. In that way, the dentist can be sure that all the staff members are saying what he or she wants said in a way that the dentist wants it said.

Written Communication

Written communication has become less common in professional settings. Because of this, their use can become a powerful communication tool. From a marketing perspective, the dentist should be sure that the stationery and other communication devices (Web sites, etc.) have a similar look and "feel," including logos, slogans, and other branding devices.

Treatment Plans

Dentists often think of a treatment plan as a technical exercise in procedure sequencing. However, the treatment plan is also an excellent form of communication. It allows the patient to see the procedures the dentist proposes, the cost associated with those procedures, and gains the consent for and acceptance of treatment. If the dentist provides different treatment options, then these can be the basis of a discussion about the advantages and disadvantages of each and open a discussion of patient wants and values. The patient's "chief complaint" is more than a line on a form. It is the reason the patient came to see the dentist. The plan must acknowledge and address this.

Payment Plans

Like a treatment plan, a payment plan is really a patient communication device. It allows the office personnel to discuss finance options and requirements with each patient. A verbal contract, such as patient agreement to pay, is a legal binding contract. When a patient signs a payment plan, it becomes more binding in the patient's mind. It also removes any "he said ... , she said ... " discussions if the patient misses a payment.

Treatment Letters

Many offices follow up treatment with a posttreatment letter. In this letter, they will include before and after photos, showing the improved esthetics. They will also thank the patient for their patronage and ask for referrals of friends or colleagues.

Communication Issues in the Dental Office

The Dentist Is the Leader

The dentist is the communication leader in the office. How he or she speaks, acts, responds, and relates sets the tone for everyone else in the office. Staff members will follow the dentist's lead, doing as he or she does. If a dentist finds someone with a different communication style, the dentist should use that person's strengths to the office's advantage.

Address the Patient in the Way He or She Wants

Patients come to a dental office with different backgrounds and value systems. Some, especially elderly patients, are more formal than others. The dentist should call the patient by title and last name "Mr. Jones," 'Mrs. Smith," "Dr. Brown" until the patient invites the dentist to do otherwise. ("Oh, honey, call me June.") The dentist should not assume that someone wants to be called by their informal name (Steve instead of Steven, Kate instead of Katherine). The simple way to find out is to ask. People enjoy hearing their name. It says that the dentist is recognizing him or her individually. The dentist should use his or her name often but correctly.

Identify Patient Wants, Needs, and Desires

Each patient comes to the office with a unique set of needs, wants, and desires regarding his or her dental condition and treatment. Not everyone feels free to discuss them with others, especially strangers. The dentist's job is to find out what the patient wants so that he or she can respond effectively. The best way to do this is to ask questions.

Use Communication Aids

Adults learn best in many different ways. Some use the spoken word, but most (about 80 percent) learn best visually, through pictures and video. A dentist should use all of the patient education tools that are available to help inform the patient of his or her condition and treatment choices. This is not only good salesmanship. It is also the ethical basis of true informed consent. The dentist should have a variety of good education material available.

Speak the Patient's Language

The dentist should speak with his or her patient based on his or her individual level of understanding. The dentist should avoid dental jargon or hot button words. He or she can usually find the fine line between talking down to a patient and talking over the patient's head.

Use Co-Diagnosis

A dentist should use a mouth mirror or intraoral camera to show patients problems that are found. When a dentist shows a patient a problem directly, the patient generally wants to know what to do to fix it. The patient will be actively involved in the diagnosis, asking for treatment options, rather than passively being told what he or she needs.

Watch Body Language

Dentists can easily send conflicting messages to a patient. He or she may discuss treatment options verbally. However, if the dentist does not maintain eye contact, or if he or she slouches or fidgets, the verbal message says the dentist cares, but the more powerful nonverbal says that the dentist is distracted or uncertain. Upright posture conveys confidence.

Watch the Patient's Body Language

Patients will send motions about their emotional and physical state through their body language. Just as the dentist must be careful of the messages he or she sends, the dentist can read the messages that patients send and respond appropriately. If the patient's hands are sweaty when shaking hands, he or she is probably nervous. A patient with his or her arms crossed usually says that he or she is shutting out the dentist's ideas. The more the dentist studies the subtle body signals patients give, the better he or she will be at interpreting the communication.

Special Patient Problems

Dentists see several common types of "problem" patients in the office. These are often the result of a communication breakdown. Sometimes, the dentist (or the staff) can help resolve the problem.

Angry Patients

When a patient is angry, the most important thing for the dentist to do is to listen to the problem. Often the angry patient believes that his or her issue has been ignored or brushed off by the dentist or the staff. The dentist should not try to rationalize or counter every point that the angry patient makes. He or she should give the patient time to talk and explain his or her side of the problem completely. (The dentist should allow the patient to "vent.") When the patient has finished, the dentist should use active listening methods and paraphrase one of the points the patient made without being defensive or hostile. The dentist should reflect back on the issues the patient brought up. (Often that is all that is needed. The patient just wanted a forum to explain his or her side!) The dentist should ask the patient what he or she wants to happen to resolve the problem. Sometimes it is simple ("I need an extra month to pay off my bill"). Sometimes the patient will ask for another action that the dentist cannot do immediately. The dentist should tell the patient what he or she plans to do ("I will call Dr. Smith and discuss the problem with her"). The dentist should tell the patient when he or she will be back in contact with the patient.

Noncompliant Patients

Patients who do not follow up with appointments, take medications as prescribed, or do recommended home care procedures risk additional problems developing. This can be both a treatment and legal problem for the dentist. Therefore, if a patient is routinely noncompliant, the dentist needs to address the noncompliance. The dentist should note any compliance in the patient chart in a nonjudgmental way. If a patient misses a follow-up visit, the dentist should note the miss and any attempts to call or reschedule. The dentist needs to find out why the patient is noncompliant (misses appointments or does not follow through with recommendations) so that he or she can address those specific concerns. The dentist may need to write a stern and factual letter to the noncompliant patient that describes the additional problems the patient may face if he or she does not follow through with recommendations ("If you do not complete the root canal procedure that we started, the tooth might abscess and spread infection throughout your body. It also might break resulting in significant pain and require the surgical removal of the pieces at a specialist."). If the patient remains noncompliant, the dentist should dismiss the patient from the practice as described in the chapter on office risk management.

Anxious Patients

Patients may be anxious in the dental office for many reasons. They may have experienced past pain or discomfort or may fear upcoming procedures because of stories they have heard from friends, family, or acquaintances. They may worry about the cost of treatment or feel guilty for failing to seek care sooner. Some fear that they will receive bad news or fear that the doctor will find out they are afraid (the "he-man" syndrome). Regardless, the best solution is to deal with the issue directly. The dentist should acknowledge to the patient that it is normal to have such feelings. Many people have similar feelings brought on by many reasons. An open discussion using effective disclosure and feedback will often help to find the "real" cause of the anxiety. The dentist can then try to address the cause of the anxiety instead of simply trying to reduce the anxiety itself.

Part 2: Case Presentation and Acceptance

I have never worked a day in my life without selling. If I believe in something, I sell it, and I sell it hard.
Estée Lauder

Objectives:

At the completion of this part, the student will be able to:
1. Describe the common types of consumer purchase and relate them to dental office treatment.
2. Define the common treatment acceptance decision points.
3. Define the steps in presenting a case to a patient.
4. Describe the common methods of gaining patient commitment.

Key Terms

adjournment close	patient needs
concession close	patient wants
direct close	problem-solving purchases
extended cost of service	routine purchases
objections	testimonial close
office atmosphere	trust
opportunity cost close	

Goal

This part presents guidelines for and presenting cases to patients.

A dentist's case presentation skills convert the patient's interest in dentistry into an action step: deciding to continue with treatment. Case presentation is analogous to "selling" in the business world. In the professional practice, dentists look out for patients' best interest, taking care not to "oversell" what they can do or what the patient needs to have done. However, if dentists truly believe that a particular course of dental care is in the patient's best interest, it becomes their duty fully to inform the patient of the options, presenting advantages and disadvantages of the options. In this way dentists develop a true informed consent before proceeding to treatment. The problem develops when dentists take the information presentation step and turn it into a coercive or manipulative process, either stressing or withholding information to make their point, which does not involve a free decision by a fully informed patient. However, dentists want the patient to accept the treatment. First, dentists really believe that it may improve the patient's life, and second, it improves their bottom line. If patients do not accept treatment, dentists have limited production, and therefore, limited profit.

Types of Consumer Purchases

Marketers say that consumers have two types of treatment decisions: routine and extended. Patients behave differently and use different purchase criteria in each type. A dentist should appeal to patients differently in each type as well.

Routine Purchase Decisions

Consumers buy many low-cost, frequently used goods and services. These are often called *low-involvement purchases* because they do not involve much thought or consideration by the consumer. These purchases do not involve much financial or psychological risk. (Examples include soap, fast food, and routine dental care). The buyer often has strong brand preference (or loyalty) that is strongly affected by "top-of-the-mind" awareness rather than conscious decision making. When a person goes to the store to purchase bath soap, he or she generally does not agonize over the decision, weighing the merits of each type of soap, and researching the values and consumers' preferences of each. Instead, most shoppers, without thinking much about it, pick up their usual brand. (This is brand loyalty.) Advertising keeps the brand at the top of the consumer's mind, so that when they are ready to make the purchase, the consumer remembers their brand.

In dentistry, regular dental patients make routine purchases every time they respond to a call for a "recall" or "periodic maintenance" visit. Most of the dental work at this visit is considered routine as well, for most patients. (This includes cleanings, fillings, and often basic crowns.) Patients, as dental consumers, do not really think about whether to purchase the service or not and from whom to purchase it. Like buying their usual deodorant at the store, they simply make the purchase based on familiarity and habit.

Routine purchase behavior works to a dentist's advantage when a patient returns for routine periodic maintenance without consideration of going to another dentist. It works to a dentist's disadvantage when consumers do not have brand loyalty to his or her office, but instead go to an office that is on their insurance panel. In this sense, consumers view dental care as a commodity, with no brand loyalty. They do not have much involvement in the purchase decision. They are simply looking for the most inexpensive care, which may be dictated by their insurance plan. In these cases, dentists should try to develop "brand loyalty" for their particular practice. Nevertheless, dentists should realize that they may lose some consumers (patients) to other "brands" (dentists) because of the insurance pricing inducements.

Problem-Solving Purchases

These purchases involve purchase of high involvement, generally expensive items that have a long lifetime. (Examples include new cars, stereos, and reconstructive dental care.) The buyer often must first learn the criteria for selection, then shop for the good or service based on those criteria. Many people, when they buy a new car, research the various makes and models, check *Consumer Reports* or other consumer guides, and agonize over the model, color, and options. This is all because automo-

biles are generally purchases that a person will live with for several (or many) years. They are expensive purchases, so there is a high desire to be satisfied with the decision. (Many people even justify a poor purchase, simply to reinforce their previous decision.) If a person finally admits that he or she made a poor choice, chances are that he or she will tell everyone the shortcomings of the item purchased.

In dentistry, dentists see problem-solving purchase decisions each time the patient worries about the treatment. This may be because of large cost, potential side effects, or excessive fear by the patient. (A simple alloy may be a major life-altering event for an extremely fearful patient.) Before a patient commits to spend many thousands of dollars for complex treatment, he or she may check with trusted friends or family members. The patient may research the expected treatment or even get a second professional opinion. The dentist should not see these efforts as distrust but instead as the consumer's search for information and an evaluation of alternatives before committing to treatment. In other words, this is healthy consumer behavior. Because patients evaluate the service after it is completed, dentists need to follow-up with the patient, ensuring that he or she is satisfied with the work and try to solve any problems identified. In this way, dentists encourage a positive postpurchase evaluation by the patient. This in turn encourages the patient to recommend the dentist to friends, family, and trusted others.

Patient Treatment Acceptance Decision Points

Patients base whether or not to accept a dentist's treatment recommendation on four major points. These are all patient perceptions, *not* facts. Patient perceptions are as real to the patient as concrete facts, so the dentist must address them as such. The dentist must address each of these points to gain treatment acceptance.

Office Atmosphere

Patients often make a conscious or subconscious decision about a dentist within the first minute they are at the dentist's office. They make this based on the feeling they get about the interpersonal relations and office atmosphere. If patients perceive a warm, trusting relationship between the dentist and the staff, they will assume that the same trusting relationship will develop with them. Likewise, they will perceive a rigid, formal, or controlling atmosphere as one that does not lead to trust. Many patients view office cleanliness as a surrogate measure for the dentist's attention to detail.

Trust

Patients must believe that the dentist is working in their best interest, not the dentist's own. This is especially true for large, complex treatments. Simply telling a patient, "Trust me, I'm a dentist" is usually not enough. The dentist must prove it through his or her actions and office personnel interactions. It may take a long time for some patients to develop that trust. That is why dentists may see patients for several years of routine maintenance visits before the patient feels comfortable enough to commit to a large, expensive treatment plan.

Extended Cost of Service

Money is always a consideration in the treatment decision. The absolute price is not as important as the conditions of payment. How long do patients have to pay, and how will the payment fit into their family budget? If payments are reasonable (a patient perception) then most patients accept this decision point.

Preventing Discomfort

The dentist must not cause pain before, during, or after treatment. This means that the dentist practices excellent injection technique, using sedation (nitrous oxide/oxygen or chemotherapeutic agents) when indicated, and halting treatment if the patient has pain. The dentist can ease discomfort with soothing atmosphere, music headsets, and other distractions. Nearly 15 percent of the US population are true dental phobics. They need special help (beyond that normally done for patients) to have a pain-free dental experience.

Steps In Case Presentation

The case presentation is a combination of patient education and sales technique. There are several steps to follow in gaining patient case acceptance.

Establish a Relationship

The dentist must establish a one-to-one personal relationship with the patient. Until that relationship is established, most people will not commit to large treatment plans. Patients may make smaller, routine purchases (such as a "cleaning" or basic fillings) but generally will not commit to a large, high-involvement purchase (such as an oral reconstruction) without a relationship and the trust that is inherent in the relationship.

Often, patients will not "buy" expensive treatment for many months or years, until they have developed the trust required for such a commitment. The patient comes to the dentist knowing that he or she is the expert. The patient needs to gain trust by finding out that the dentist is looking out for the patient's interests.

Learn Patient Wants

In this step, a dentist's listening skills become critical. The dentist should ask probing questions and listen to the answers. This allows the dentist to offer solutions that satisfy the patient's needs, not the dentist's technical solution to a dental problem. The dentist should listen to the emotional side of the patient. The part on communication gives several techniques to use, including feedback and self-disclosure. The patient may make an off-hand comment about how pretty someone's teeth look. He or she may be saying that he or she would like a mouth that looks as good and healthy.

Decide Patient Needs

Here, the dentist's professional skill, care, and expertise come into play. The dentist must decide the various treatment options based on his or her clinical and patient examinations. Many patients present routine, small-involvement needs that are easy to decide. The patients with complex treatment, psychological, and medical needs may require significant time from the dentist to decide the patient's needs.

Offer Solutions

In this step, a dentist uses his or her diagnostic and planning skills to decide the appropriate plan of treatment that addresses the patient's health or disease state and resolves the patient's treatment wants. Many adults learn best through methods other than oral communication. Audiovisual aids, such as videos, pamphlets, or flip charts, can help to show problem solutions for patients. The solution to a patient's needs is the technical

---

Box 18.2 Aids to Problem Solutions

- Printed material
- In-office videos
- Intraoral camera
- Physical models
- Web site

procedures that dentists do, but the solution to the patient's wants is the benefits of treatment.

Answer Objections

Many dentists are offended by patients who challenge them or question their treatment recommendations. Instead, they should view this as a positive step because the patient has not discounted what the dentist has said and recommended. Instead the patients are processing the information and trying to understand and internalize it. They must do this before they agree to treatment. They are interested but have significant questions that the dentist must help them to resolve. What if this crown has bad esthetics? What happens if the implant does not integrate? Are there alternatives that are less expensive? The objections often involve the four decision points: discomfort, trust, time, and money. The dentist should view each of these probing questions as an opportunity to educate the patient about the proposed treatment and to educate himself or herself about how the patient perceives the dentist. Some people want technical information about the procedures. They decide logically, trying to exclude emotions. Others want more assurance that the dentist can solve their problem. They decide on a "gut" or emotional level. By finding the type of objections, the dentist can often respond on an appropriate level that satisfies the patient's reluctance to go on with the suggested treatment.

Gain Commitment

The final step is to have the patient commit to act. Several techniques from the sales world work well in the dental situation. The dentist's technique may include a combination of these techniques, based on the individual circumstance.

- *Direct Close* The simplest way to do this is for the dentist to ask the patient if he or she is ready to go on with treatment. This is called a *direct close* in the business world. The salesperson asks the customer to purchase the good or service.
  "Mr. Jones, can I go ahead and schedule an appointment to start the reconstruction?"
- *Adjournment Close* This technique does not ask for commitment now. Instead, it gives the patient time to

think about it. This is especially useful when the dentist perceives that there are still unresolved objections that the patient needs to work through. This helps build trust and relationship in that the dentist is not using a "hard sell" sales technique.
  "Mr. Jones, I can see that this is an important decision for you. Do you need additional time to consider all of the implications? Should we discuss the details further at your next appointment?"
- *Concession Close* When the patient offers an objection, the dentist can make a condition of resolving the patient's objection that he or she makes the purchase. This is based on the idea of solving the patient's objections to satisfy their needs. Use an "If I … then will you … ?" statement rather than an "If you … then I will … " statement. This focuses on the dentist attempting to solve the patient's objection, rather than the objection itself.
  "Mr. Jones, if we can work out the financing for you, are you ready to go with the treatment?"
- *Testimonial Close* The dentist can use a satisfied patient to help convince this patient. Because a patient cannot prejudge services (until the dentist has delivered them), he or she may rely on others who have had similar services done. (Be sure that the testifying patient agrees or is anonymous.) In these cases, letters or before- and after-photos are valuable.
  "This patient had a similar case to yours. I think you will agree from the photos and her letter that the treatment was very successful."
- *Opportunity Cost Close* This technique stresses the cost of not going on with treatment. This shows the patient that the apparent cost is not as high as it appears when compared with future costs. Costs involve more than price (money). The costs may include future inconvenience, pain, additional cost, or disfigurement.
  "Mr. Jones, if we don't replace that tooth now, your teeth will drift, leading to gum problems, poor chewing, and a much more expensive solution in the future."

There is a big caveat in closing techniques. If a patient feels tricked or otherwise manipulated, they will not commit to treatment and may leave the practice. He or she may also tell friends and acquaintances, turning them against the dentist as well.

Controlling Costs in the Practice

chapter 19

A penny saved is a penny earned.
Ben Franklin

Objectives

At the completion of this chapter, the student will be able to:
1. Allocate typical costs in the dental office into fixed, step-fixed, or variable categories.
2. Describe the process of using standards in the dental office.
3. Describe the elements that contribute to dental office revenues.
4. Describe the elements of dental office costs.
5. Perform a basic break-even analysis
6. Perform a basic "What if ...?" analysis

Key Terms

basic profitability formula
break-even analysis
break-even point
cost allocation

fixed costs
practice cost analysis
practice revenue analysis
step-fixed costs

total costs
variable costs
"What if ... ?" analysis

Goal

This chapter examines the nature of dental office costs. It divides costs into type and defines the amount of control the practitioner has over each of those types of costs. The use of standards as an economic control mechanism is also discussed. Finally, representative data and measures for controlling costs in the dental office are discussed.

Business Basics for Dentists, First Edition. David O. Willis.
© 2013 John Wiley & Sons, Inc. Published 2013 by John Wiley & Sons, Inc.

Increasing income and controlling costs are the two methods to improve profitability in the dental office. Cost control is the easier to understand because a dollar saved saves through reducing costs adds directly to the bottom line.

Types of Costs

Dental practice costs fall into three basic categories: fixed, variable, or step-fixed. These differing costs can be displayed graphically, where it becomes more apparent how each type of cost behaves as production changes (Fig. 19.1).

Fixed costs do not change with production (Fig. 19.1). Whether a dentist produces $30 or $30,000 per month, fixed costs are constant. For example, rent, dental association dues, malpractice insurance, and many other costs remain constant, regardless the production. These may not be exactly the same from month to month but are generally consistent. Fixed costs consist of the following:

- *Office space and equipment* is the largest category of fixed costs. It consists of all costs associated with operating the physical space and equipment of the practice. These include rent, utility, tax, and repair charges associated with the occupancy of the building. Dentists should also include an estimate of the depreciation expense for office and equipment because this represents wear and tear on those assets, and any equipment replacement programs.
- *Other fixed costs* include bank charges, office insurances, advertising, and legal and professional expenses.

Step-fixed costs vary with production but only in discrete steps (Fig. 19.2). The existing staff will work harder as production increases. However, finally the load becomes too great, and dentists must hire an additional staff member to help the office run efficiently. Therefore, the cost jumps in a discrete step when the new person is

hired. Dentists hire staff members as entire people (or increments of people). These costs are considered "fixed" over their range so that when the dentist hires a new person, a new set of fixed costs is established. Unless a dentist hires an additional staff member or loses one of the present staff members, these costs will be relatively constant or fixed in the range of the analysis. For that reason, dentists often include staff costs with fixed costs.

Staff costs include direct wages, benefits, payroll taxes, retirement plan contributions, hiring and training expenses, and any other costs that are direct results of employing staff members for the office. Dentists can divide labor costs into clerical (front office), hygiene, and chair side assisting personnel and should categorize them individually for detailed analysis:

Clerical (front office) compensation
Chairside assisting compensation
Hygiene compensation

Variable costs change directly with the production level (Fig. 19.3). If a dentist produces $30,000 of dentistry 1 month, then his or her costs for dental supplies will be approximately 10 times more than a month in which he or she produces $3,000. If the dentist has no production, then theoretically he or she will have no variable costs. Variable costs change with production levels, not just collections. Dentists still must purchase supplies for procedures that he or she discounted or did not collect. In the dental office, variable costs consist of dental lab, dental supplies, and general office supplies. These costs often appear the month after they are purchased as a result of typical billing and inventory cycles. Nevertheless, conceptually, the costs are used in direct relation to the production. Each category should be tracked separately:

- *Dental lab* costs are associated with contract laboratory work. The costs of laboratory supplies in the

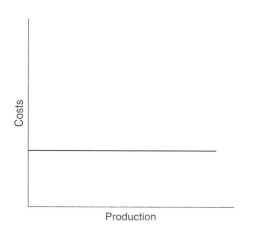

Figure 19.1 Fixed costs

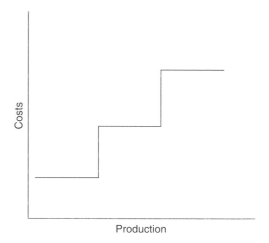

Figure 19.2 Step-fixed costs

office (stone, waxes, etc.) are considered dental supplies. If a dentist employs a laboratory technician in the office, he or she should include all costs associated with the laboratory operation (e.g., salary, benefits, supplies, and lab space rent) in this category.

*   *Dental supplies* are the materials dentists use when doing dentistry. They include expendable supplies (e.g., cotton rolls, anesthetic, alloy, and composite material) and small-instrument replacement.
*   *Office supplies* are the costs associated with materials for the front desk operation. This includes paper products, computer program fees, postage, magazine subscriptions, pencils, and other items used in processing patient visits.

Total cost is the sum of fixed, step-fixed, and variable costs (Fig. 19.4). (Step-fixed costs are considered fixed over their range.) Likewise, the diagram for total costs is the combination of these various types of expenses.

Owner's expenses are items that the dentist benefits from directly. The dentist could have taken them as profit from the practice but instead he or she elected (or were required) to pay for them, appearing to reduce the practice profit. Common examples include self-employment taxes, automobile expenses, continuing education programs, travel, meals, entertainment, and retirement plan contributions for the dentist.

Typical Dental Office Cost Allocation

Dentists can develop a list of common dental practice costs for use in financial analysis. One obvious place to begin is to examine the previous year's tax return. A Schedule C is a report of most dental office expenses. A complete checkbook register will also contain expenses grouped by category. The allocation of these costs into specific categories is somewhat arbitrary. Business office expenses, for example, vary slightly with an increase in patient visits through an increase in office supply usage and postage, although dentist may list them as fixed. Which specific category a dentist uses should result from the individual practice history.

Typical dental offices show the largest portion of costs in the staff (step-fixed) category, typically about 25 percent of collections (Table 19.1). Variable costs of production generally run about15 percent of production, with fixed costs accounting for the rest, at 25 percent of collections. (This results in the average overhead ratio of 65 percent of collections.) This explains why small increases in production and collection leads to a large increase in profit. Dentists have already paid fixed and step-fixed costs. The only cost of seeing a few additional patients is the variable cost of production (about 15 percent) leaving the rest (85 percent) as profit.

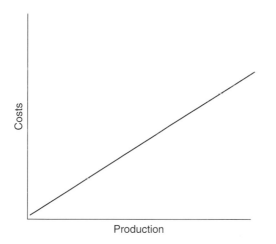

Figure 19.3 Variable costs

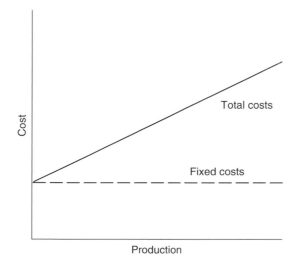

Figure 19.4 Total cost

Table 19.1 Business Office Expenses

Fixed Costs	Variable Costs	Step-Fixed Costs
Advertising	Supplies	Employee wages
Bank service charge	Dental laboratory	Employee benefits
Automobile expenses	Office supplies	
Dues and journals		
Insurance		
Equipment loans		
Legal and professional		
Rent or mortgage		
Repairs		
Travel or continuing education		
Utilities		

Break-Even Analysis

Proper allocation gives a more accurate understanding of practice costs than the simple traditional "percent overhead" figure. A valuable tool for putting this information to use is through the break-even analysis technique. This financial analysis technique relates the office's costs to the production and profit of a practice. Although, as its name implies, dentists can use it to detect the point of zero profit (the break-even point), it has a much wider use by providing insights into the cost behavior of the practice and the riskiness of many courses of action.

The basic equation used in the break-even technique is:

Collections – Variable Expenses – Fixed Expenses

= Net Income

The equation brings mathematical sense to an intuitive idea, namely, that all the money a dentist collects, minus all expenses (fixed and variable), leaves a profit or loss. If any of three of the numbers is known, the equation can be used to find the fourth number through substitution.

The break-even analysis may even be depicted graphically (Fig. 19.5):

Essentially, this is the cost structure diagram superimposed on a production diagram. The point of intersection between the revenue (collection) line and the total cost line is the break-even point. Any production above this point results in profit; any production below this point results in a loss. The production above the break-even point is "more profitable" because the fixed costs were paid and now only the lower variable costs are incurred. This also happens when a dentist takes an associate or in other ways offsets hours with another dentist. Only step-

fixed and variable costs remain. Any additional dentistry produced is on a better margin for the owner–dentist. The incremental cost of producing more is small in comparison to the initial cost ratio. This is also critical to understanding capitation or other reduced payment third-party plans. If there is slack chair time, then the only costs associated with the managed care production are the variable costs. However, if these patients replace traditional, fee-for-service patients, then the cost must also include the loss from the foregone production on those traditional patients.

As an example problem, assume that a dentist, Dr. Sample, wants to gain a better understanding of his office finances. He has asked his accountant to prepare an income statement for the previous year so that he can use the results for a more detailed analysis of the practice finances. From that statement, he allocated costs into the various categories and arrived at the following financial outcomes for the past year in his office:

Category	Amount	
Production	$460,000	
Collections	$446,200	97 percent of production
Fixed costs	**$107,088**	**24 percent of collections**
Step-fixed costs	$116,012	26 percent of collections
Total variable costs	$75,854	17 percent of collections
Total costs	$298,954	67 percent of collections
Total profit	**$147,246**	**33 percent of collections**

In the example, Dr. Sample produces $460,000 per year ($38,333 per month). He collects 97 percent of production. Using the formula and previously given cost data, his income for the year would be:

Collections – Variable Expenses – Fixed Expenses

= Net Income

$(0.97 \times \text{Production}) - (0.17 \text{ Production})$

$- (\text{Step-fixed Costs} + \text{Fixed Costs}) = \text{Net Income}$

$\$446,200 - \$75,854 - \$223,100 = \text{Net Income}$

$\$147,246 = \text{Net Income}$

Dr. Sample netted $147,246 by producing $460,000 of dentistry, collecting 97 percent of accounts, and paying all fixed and variable expenses. His actual production break-even point can be calculated, where net income is zero:

Collections – Variable Expenses – Fixed Expenses

= Net Income

$(0.97 \times \text{Production}) - (0.17 \text{ Production})$

$- (\text{Step-fixed Costs} + \text{Fixed Costs}) = 0$

$(0.80 \times \text{Production}) = \$223,100$

Production = $278,875

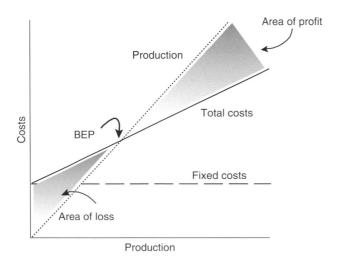

Figure 19.5 Break-even analysis

That is to say, if Dr. Sample were to produce $278,875 of dentistry this year ($23,240 per month), he would just pay all the bills but not make any profit, having a net income of zero ($0). If Dr. Sample wanted an income of $200,000 per year, the formula could be used to calculate the production required:

Collections – Variable Expenses – Fixed Expenses

$\quad$ = Net Income

$(0.97 \times \text{Production}) - (0.17 \text{ Production})$

$\quad - (\text{Step-fixed Costs} + \text{Fixed Costs}) = \$200,000$

$(0.80 \times \text{Production}) - \$223,100 = \$200,000$

$(0.80 \times \text{Production}) = \$423,100$

Production $= \$528,875$

Dr. Sample would need to produce $528,875 to gain the desired income. If he cannot do this given the present office configuration, then he would need to estimate new costs based on a different configuration, changing the formula values.

Categories of Cost Control

Cost control techniques can be grouped into general categories that are then applied to specific areas of the practice.

Know the Costs

Dentists need to have an accurate and detailed compilation of office costs. If a dentist has an accurate allocation in the office checkbook, this is an easy task. The dentist should look at the numbers on an annual and quarterly basis. More frequent than that, a dentist might develop false problems because of the normal ebb and flow of production, collections, and expenses over time.

Concentrate on Major Cost Items

Staff member costs typically are more than twice laboratory costs. Therefore, a 5-percent saving in staff leads to a larger return than 5 percent in the laboratory cost area. When a dentist has the major costs under control, he or she should work on the smaller-level costs. Remember, a dollar saved still increases profit, regardless the source of saving.

Also Look at Income

Profit comes from both cost and production. If dentists increase collections more than they increase costs, income increases. Dentists should negotiate reimbursement rates with insurers. Although the individual practitioner does not have as much leverage as a network of practices, he or she can often gain an increase. Most insurers will negotiate reimbursement rates. Dentists should eliminate less profitable (deeply discounted) insurance plans and should keep fees up to date through regular comparisons and increases.

Specific Cost-Control Techniques

These cost-savings techniques are described in detail in other sections of this book and they are briefly described by category here. No magic cost bullet suddenly makes the practice profitable. Instead, a dentist should keep an eye on small items that accumulate to large amounts. Some of these savings involve long-term costs, such as office rent. These may take years to see savings. Others are more immediate. Regardless, dentists should keep a constant eye on the costs of the business. Many do this through quarterly meetings with their accountant or practice financial advisors. A dentist should do an annual appraisal of general office costs, such as insurance.

Rent

Office rent is not controllable in the short term. In the long term, a dentist can negotiate different terms before signing a lease. Landlords like professional tenants. They are stable, profitable, and have a positive clientele. This gives the dentist some bargaining leverage when it is time to negotiate or renegotiate a lease. The dentist may gain a longer term on the lease at a steady price or may negotiate lower-rent escalators in future years. The dentist can probably push some expenses (e.g., snow removal) onto the owner. If the dentist is making significant leasehold improvements, he or she might negotiate the cost of those into the lease payment (the owner initially pays for them). This decreases the dentist's immediate out-of-pocket expense and time to claim depreciation expenses (though special tax rules apply here). The lease payment will be higher, as a result. If the landlord refuses to negotiate terms, the dentist should consider moving the office to a better location with better terms. If the dentist owns the space, he or she should look at leasing the space from a family partnership or other entity to recharacterize the rent as unearned income.

Upkeep

Dentists should know which upkeep costs the landlord pays and which the tenant pays. (These expenses often are exterior compared with interior expenses.) If, for example, the dental office shows water damage from a leaking gutter, the landlord (or owner or condominium association) may be responsible for repairing the problem and associated damages that have occurred in the dental office. The dentist should do upkeep and maintenance or hire a family member to do it. This not only keeps the payment within the family, it has a positive income tax effect and helps to teach children a work ethic and the value of a dollar. Upkeep items may include mowing the grass, small repair or painting jobs, cleaning the office, or decorating the office with seasonal decorations.

Equipment

Routine maintenance is always less expensive than replacing expensive equipment. The dentist should have an equipment-maintenance program for both large and small equipment in the office. This includes the furnace and air conditioner, compressor and evacuation system, and processor and computer equipment. Follow manufacturers' recommendations for handpieces, curing lights, and other small equipment. When a dentist has paid off the start-up loan, he or she should redirect some of that payment into an equipment replacement fund, so funds are available to replace or upgrade equipment. The dentist should consider tax savings by gifting equipment into a family partnership or other entity and lease back the equipment, keeping the income in the family, and making those expenses unearned income.

Total Staff Compensation Rate

A total compensation rate for staff members should be calculated annually. This is the total cost of employment (which is also the total compensation for the employee). It includes direct pay, any benefits, and all unwithheld expenses. The dentist needs to pay an appropriate total compensation. External comparisons (such as surveys) and internal comparisons (for employee equity) should be used. Paying an excessive rate does not guarantee a better employee. However, paying a substandard rate will almost guarantee a unsatisfied one. Start a cafeteria-type benefit plan. The employee gets to choose the benefits that are most important for him or her. The employee then pays for the benefit through salary reduction. The dentist should check with an accountant or financial advisor about health savings accounts (HSAs) or other health insurance savings plans. Dentists should also require employees to take time off when the office is closed for the dentist's vacations or for other reasons.

Employees should be paid on a wage (hourly) basis. Paying a salary only ensures that employees make a minimum amount. It does not limit costs for overtime. Many offices now give an annual bonus instead of a raise. The bonus is a one-time amount. The raise goes onto the employee's base pay and is carried forward forever, unless an employee's pay rate is cut.

Motivate Staff Members with Incentives Other than Pay

People work for many reasons. Only one of them is pay. The dentist should pay attention to the social aspect of the job environment and should promote skills development by employees. This skill development encourages performance through social and personal growth, rather than financial compensation.

Hire the Right People

Proper delegation of duties involves hiring lower-cost staff members, freeing higher-cost staff members to do more income generating work. Dentists should use part-time employees as needed and base their pay on either the time that they work or the functions that they do. Because employee turnover is so expensive, the dentist should take time to hire the correct employees. A dentist can use computer lists to generate potential employees or he or she can hire a spouse or other family member. The tax savings may be significant. The dentist should train and cross-train employees because if someone is sick, an expensive temporary employee may not need to be hired during that time.

Supplies

Dentists should keep an accurate inventory control system to end excess inventory costs or stock outs. They should make staff a part of the solution by encouraging the staff to shop wisely. Dentists should negotiate costs with suppliers. If a supplier has a special on a needed product, another supplier will often meet the discounted price, rather than lose the sale. Many offer convention specials, in which the supplier offers discounts for products bought on the convention vendor floor. The dentist should look into buying cooperatives. As corporate and chain practices increase, independent dentists are banding together to gain the economies of scale represented by the large networks.

Dental Lab

The greatest cost savings from the lab comes in doing the procedure correctly the first time. Remakes cost chair time and materials that can not be recovered. The dentist should use different labs for different procedures based on the quality and price of the specific procedures.

Promoting Staff Effectiveness

Part 1: Selecting and Hiring Employees

You're only as good as the people you hire.
Ray Kroc, Founder, McDonald's

Objectives

At the completion of this part, the student will be able to:
1. Describe the employment process for finding dental office employees.
2. Differentiate between a job description and a job specification.
3. Define the purposes of conducting a job interview.
4. Differentiate between legal and illegal job interview questions.

Key Terms

application
directive interview approach
employment interview
employment process
human resource
management

job description
job specification
job-related behaviors
nondirective interview
approach
observation of work

probationary period
references
resume
temporary placement services
working interview

Goal

The goal of this part is to prepare new graduates to select and hire staff members for the dental office.

Business Basics for Dentists, First Edition. David O. Willis.
© 2013 John Wiley & Sons, Inc. Published 2013 by John Wiley & Sons, Inc.

A properly trained and motivated staff is essential for survival in today's dental practice world. Although this at first appears to be a singular task, in fact, dentists must meet several steps or objectives along the way. These objectives include:

1. To hire the best applicants possible.
2. To compensate employees appropriately
3. To motivate employees to perform well.
4. To assess employee performance.

To accomplish these goals, dentists must organize and manage the staffing part of the practice. Staffing is a critical resource area (along with financial, technical, and physical areas). It should be called "Human Resource Management," to equate the importance with the other management areas of the practice.

Various types of dental staff members were described in the chapter on duty delegation. Each practitioner will need to decide the type and number of each category of employee. Because the dental staff is the single largest item of expense in most practices, the dentist should take care that the staff member will be fully used before making the hiring decision.

Attracting the Best Applicants

The obvious purpose of the employment process is to place the proper person in a given position so that the dental office can operate efficiently and effectively. This apparently simple process is founded on several background facts. A dentist must specify what the position entails, and he or she must also specify what characteristics and training is required of a person who would hold the position. The problem then becomes one of matching, finding the right person to fill the job.

The Job Description

The first step in the hiring process is to write a job description that explicitly lists the duties that the job holder is to do. The reason for doing this is to clarify the qualifications that are important for an applicant to possess. In addition, the dentist can discuss in more detail with each interviewee the tasks that he or she will do.

The dentist must first know what is entailed in performing effectively in the given position. What are the duties of the person who holds the job? Who will the person in this job interact with and what are the responsibilities associated with the job? The job description defines the duties of the job. The dentist should write this description so it is easy to understand, succinct, and yet detailed enough that a person who applies for or holds the position knows what is expected

of them. This description should consist of specific, observable job-related behaviors rather than attitudinal or general characteristics that are immaterial to performance on the job. A useful offshoot of developing a job description is that this essentially becomes the performance appraisal instrument. Because this consists of what a person should do on the job, assessing performance on these specific behaviors is easy. Perhaps the easiest way to write a job description is to have the person who presently holds the job write all the procedures that he or she does during a typical day or week on the job. This list of what a person does on the job should be the basis of the job description.

Recruiting and Advertising the Position

Recruiting involves the development of a pool of potential employees. Advertising is one obvious method to gather these people, either through newspapers or Internet bulletin boards. Another is through internal (staff) referral or through raiding or soliciting existing employees of other practitioners. Each approach has advantages and disadvantages.

Advertising is the most common form of identifying potential employees. Generally an advertisement is placed in the local newspaper (Sunday employment section) or on Internet lists. The ad should be specific for the job the dentist is filling, be positive in tone, and avoid misleading or discriminatory statements (Box 20.1). Several techniques can help an advertisement to stand out from the others. Simply making it larger, placing borders or white areas around it, or using bold or different type face can all draw a prospect's eye to the advertisement. Unless the dentist wants many calls or is looking for a fresh face, he or she should consider including the phrase *experienced* or the more restrictive *dental office experience required* included in the advertisement. The dentist may either want to have the applicant phone or send a resume to the office.

Box 20.1 What to Include in Recruitment Advertising

1. The location of the practice
2. The qualities that the dentist is looking for
3. The experience required
4. The skills required
5. The days and hours of the job
6. A statement about the practice that generates enthusiasm
7. Name of contact person, hours, and telephone number to call

Internet bulletin boards and lists are rapidly replacing newspaper advertising for many dentists seeking employees. They are inexpensive and common. Not everyone knows or uses these information sources. A dentist might miss many qualified potential employees, especially older workers, using Internet-only advertising.

Another common form of recruiting is by having existing employees of the practice identify friends or associates who may be searching for a change in employment. These people can then be contacted so that their interest can be determined. A dentist should not "raid" neighboring dentists of their staff people. If the potential employee is presently working for another dentist in the area, that person (employee) should initiate the contact and express an interest before the hiring dentist has any dealings with him or her. Although this may not eliminate ill will between the hiring dentist and the other dentist, it should reduce it. Some dentists offer a bonus or reward for the employee who identifies a new employee for the practice. If the present employees are happy and satisfied working for a dentist, they should be some of the best recruiters.

Other dentists may keep a list of acceptable candidates from previous job opportunities in the practice. Others may use a private placement service or a university-based work force service. The dentist should be aware that private placement services charge a substantial fee for finding an employee that a dentist can find just as easily.

Short-term and part-time employees can be found in similar ways. Temporary placement services will furnish employees on a daily basis. The dentist might use them as an opportunity to "try out" several people, looking for the person or the characteristics that he or she wants. These services are, again, expensive, but they do offer a solution to limited time needs for the practitioner.

Selecting the Best of the Applicants

When dentists have attracted a number of applicants, they need to select the best one for their office.

The Application

Unless a dentist wants the office staff to be unaware that he or she is hiring a new person, the potential applicants should phone the office. (The dentist should not use the primary patient lines in the advertisement and should have the applicants call a private number, if possible.) This allows the present receptionist to assess telephone communication skills. It also allows the receptionist to screen out unacceptable candidates by briefly describing the job and asking qualifying questions, such as salary requirements and experience. If the job has some undesirable component (e.g., evening hours 2 nights a week), the dentist should tell prospective applicants at this point rather than wasting everyone's time with an interview. If the prospect passes the basic screen, the dentist should have them come to the office and pick up an application, complete it, and return it by mail to the receptionist or have them send a resume to the office instead of an application.

Some dentists prefer to use experienced employees only. They simply do not want to take the time to train a person who is new to the job. Others believe that dentists should find a person who has the personal characteristics wanted; the dentist can then train the person to do the components of many dental office jobs. It is an individual choice. The dentist will obviously pay more for an experienced staff member and that person can help the dentist learn additional ways of conducting the practice. However, that person may have learned undesirable habits previously and may be difficult to control, believing that he or she knows more than the dentist about the way the office should run.

As a rule, new practitioners should hire an experienced receptionist. An experienced person can help establish the business systems that every office requires. Otherwise, a new practitioner and a new receptionist will be searching for answers that may be common knowledge for a more experienced person. Often, after several years, the established receptionist and the now more-confident dental practitioner will have control problems in the office (i.e., who is really the boss?). By then, the office should be running smoothly enough and the dentist should be knowledgeable enough to hire another receptionist that fits the office personality.

The application form should ask information about the individual's qualifications for and ability to do the job that the dentist has previously described. The dentist can gather information about an applicant's credentials, background, and qualifications more efficiently through a written format than through interviews. He or she can also determine a basic level of written and expressive abilities by having an "essay" section to the application form. Applications are better than resumes in that a dentist can ask specific questions that may be important to him or her. The dentist should also have the person fill the application out by hand to assess handwriting skills and neatness.

Many dentists prefer to have prospective employees send a resume, instead of filling out an application form. If a dentist requests resumes, he or she should review them carefully. The person who wrote the resume will obviously try to place himself or herself in the best possible light. The dentist should look for gaps in employment history or frequent jumps from one employer to another. The dentist should examine the form and neatness of the resume. People often place references on resumes. They are seldom useful because people are obviously only going to give as references people who support them. A dentist may get more useful and honest appraisals from former employers, although this is even doubtful in today's litigious society. Resumes may not give the dentist the specific information he or she needs about a particular candidate (e.g., can the person use a computer?) Nevertheless, the resumes are a good method for screening many potential applicants. Often business office applicants will have resumes prepared. Assistants or hygienists will usually not have a resume prepared and might not apply if that is required. The dentist may be missing a group of qualified candidates for these types of positions if a resume is required from them.

The Employment Interview

One means of gathering additional information is the employment interview, which is the final step in the employee selection process. The purpose of the interview is twofold: to aid the dentist in gathering information to select the best qualified applicant and to provide information so that the applicant can decide whether he or she wants to work for the practice. The dentist, therefore, may use the interview to "sell" the prospective employee on the practice.

As mentioned previously, the dentist should know as much as possible about every applicant. Before the interview occurs, the applicant should fill out an application form, which the dentist reviews before proceeding with the interview. Dentists do not need to restate any information that they can obtain from the application form during the interview. However, if there are any questions about the information on the application form, the dentist should discuss them during the interview. If, for example, the application shows a gap in the recent work history, the dentist should ask the interviewee to explain this unaccounted time.

Purpose of the Interview

The employment interview should be a required step in the recruiting and hiring process. The interview serves several useful purposes. These include:

- *Verify information on the application or resume* Most people will not actively lie on an application or resume. (Although one management study showed "inaccuracies" in nearly two-thirds of all applications examined.) Nevertheless, everyone wants to place their best foot forward. A person may, for example, not include a specific piece of employment history as a result of a probable poor reference from the employer. Other people may embellish their duties,

abilities, and responsibilities. The interview gives the dentist the opportunity to ask more in-depth questions of the applicant and to find missing information from the written application.

- *Find additional information that is not on an application or resume* Dentists can assess many skills and attributes from a resume. For example, does the person have the required years of experience, training, or background required of the job? Dentists cannot glean other attributes simply from the employment application. How well does the applicant communicate? Is he or she able to think quickly on his or her feet? How does he or she react when put in a difficult situation? Dentists can often deduce these and other traits and abilities during the employment interview when they are not evident from the application.

- *Let the applicant assess the dentist and the office* A prospective employee obviously wants to know about the office for which they will be working. The interview gives that person the opportunity to meet the dentist, the staff, and to see the physical and operational components of the dental practice.

- *Time to actively recruit the applicant* The marketplace for skilled dental auxiliaries is a competitive marketplace. An excellent staff member may have several possibilities for employment. Therefore, the dentist may have to convince the prospective employee that his or her office is the one for which the applicant wants to work.

- *Assess dental personnel and compensation policies* It is difficult to learn what a fair wage and benefit package is compared with what other dentists and other forms of comparable employment are paying. During the interview process, dentists find if they are "in the ballpark" regarding their compensation package. Many employees are looking for a particular situation (hours, benefits, etc.) that are not obviously apparent until asked. A dentist might satisfy that person through a minor adjustment to personnel policies.

Findings from the Interview

The dentist should try to answer three questions about each applicant.

- *Can the applicant do the job?* By reviewing the training and work experience of an applicant, the dentist should answer this question with a high degree of certainty. This question relates to information that should be readily available. However, the dentist should scrutinize these qualities closely to make an objective evaluation.
- *Will the applicant do the job?* This question is probably more difficult to answer than the first question. Even if the applicant has the skills to do the

job, a lack of motivation may impede job success. From the information obtained before selecting an applicant, an objective evaluation may not be possible. For these reasons, dentists should ask previous employers and educational personnel from whom the applicant received instruction how willing he or she is to do what is expected.

- *How does the applicant get along with people?* The dentist wants to know how the applicant will respond to him or her as the employer, to other personnel in the office, and to patients. In an organization such as a dental practice, there are many interpersonal relationships. An employee should relate effectively with other people. In the interview, the applicant should talk freely and easily. If the applicant has difficulty carrying on a conversation or shows a dislike for working closely with other people, the dentist should suspect that the applicant might have difficulty working in a dental office.

The Structure of the Interview

After reviewing the application form, the dentist is ready to talk with the applicant. An introduction is an easy way to begin an interview because it immediately lets the interviewee know that the dentist is the person for whom he or she will be working. In addition, it avoids that awkward situation in which both the dentist and the applicant are at a loss in beginning a conversation.

At this point, the interview may continue in one of two ways. The dentist may use the nondirective style or he or she may find that a more structured approach is appropriate (Box 20.2). In a nondirective interview, dentists do not try to direct the applicant's conversation. The nondirective approach can be helpful when the

interview is not yielding enough information. Dentists conduct this kind of interview in a conversational manner with the chief difference being that the interviewer listens and occasionally comments in ways that encourage the applicant to talk freely about any subject of interest. For example, the candidate may wish to talk about his or her scholastic background, but the interviewer may be more concerned with work experience. At this point, some direction may be necessary to elicit the kind of information in which the dentist is interested. Experience has shown that if dentists let applicants talk at length about matters that seem important to them, it is likely that most of the topics in which an interviewee is interested will be discussed.

The main advantage of these nondirective interviews is that it puts the applicant at ease and creates an atmosphere in which the applicant feels that the interviewer is accepting and understanding. They are also excellent means to assess the employee's organizational, communication and interpersonal abilities.

The primary disadvantage is that the interview may result in little exchange of information occurring between the interviewer and the applicant. If the dentist does not elicit any information that helps to make a choice among applicants, the dentist has wasted the interview time. Veteran interviewers can use this technique productively, but for the novice, a more direct approach is likely to be more productive.

In structured interviews, the interviewer assumes a more active role than in an indirect interview. The topics discussed are usually those of interest to the interviewer and rather than waiting for particular points to emerge during the interview, the interviewer usually imparts information or asks questions directly related to those points. Applicants for openings in a dental practice are usually interested in the following:

Duties to be performed
Types of personnel employed
Working hours
Scheduling of vacations
Number of holidays
Sick leave policy
Professional development
Insurance programs
Dental care at reduced cost
Salary level

Covering these points directly is easier for the dentist and less time consuming than using the indirect approach and hoping that points that he or she wants to discuss will arise. Therefore, in an interview the dentist should control the discussion and mention those things that he or she feels are important rather than waiting for the interviewee to ask questions about them.

Box 20.2 Sample Interview Structure

Introduction of participants
Description of practice
Job description
   Primary duties
   Secondary duties
   Wage (salary base)
   Benefits available
Office policies and procedures
Investigation of applicant
Discussion of qualifications and resume
Self-description
Asking for further questions
Plan of future action

Interview Questions

As a rule, whether the dentist uses a directive or nondirective approach, he or she should try to use open-ended questions whenever possible. Open-ended questions typically start with how, why, what, or tell me about. . . . Responses to these questions allow the dentist to assess the interviewee's communication skills and allows them to explain their answers in much more detail than a closed-end question. For example, the close ended question "Did you like your last job?" simply asks a "Yes" or "No" response from the interviewee. However, the more open ended "Tell me what you particularly liked about your last job" causes the respondent to give a discourse, rather than a simple one-word answer. The dentist will then be in a much better position to assess the person's communication skills. Box 20.3 gives many different questions that can be asked during an interview. It is not intended as the ultimate list of all possible interview questions, it is a list of suggestions on the types of questions that a dentist might ask to gain the most effect from and employment interview.

The dentist should listen to the answer of the question asked. Many people are so concerned with preparing to ask the next question that they fail to listen to what the interviewee is saying in answer to the previous question. Listen attentively. If something sounds strange or wrong, ask a follow-up question. If the person is struggling with an answer, allow them to struggle for a moment. In this way, the prospective employer can tell how a person may react under pressure.

Legal and Illegal Questions

People may legally ask any question of an applicant that pertains to the work or his or her ability to do the work. It is illegal to ask any questions that are discriminatory in nature, or that do not apply to the job. It is illegal, for example, to ask someone if they have any children. That has nothing to do with their ability to do the job. However, an applicant who has children in day care may not be able to work the extended hours required when an emergency patient calls. That affects job performance. Dentists must be sure to ask the question that is work related. The question, "Mary, do you have any children?" is illegal. Instead, dentists can ask, "Mary, due to the nature of dental services, we often have to work late, often until 7:00 pm. Is that a problem for you?" If Mary has day-care issues, that is a problem. She may have a spouse or other family member who can willingly pick the children up at day care before closing. Box 20.4 gives several examples of illegal questions.

Common Interview Pitfalls

Several practices and habits may lead to an interview being a frustrating experience for both the dentist and

---

Box 20.3 Sample Interview Questions

Experience
1. What did you particularly like about your last job?
2. What did you particularly not like about your last job?
3. Who did you get along with the least at your former job? What did you do about the problem?
4. Describe your previous employer's management style? How would you like to see it changed?

Training
1. What educational experiences would you like to do over again? Why?
2. Describe you present job duties and responsibilities.
3. How has your education, training, and experience prepared you for this job?

Skills
1. Why should you be hired for this position?
2. What skills and abilities do you bring to this position that other people do not?
3. What is the best skill that you bring to this job? Give an example.
4. If you take this job, in what areas do you feel that you would need additional training?
5. What should the other staff members know about you to work effectively with you?

Interests
1. What do you want to be doing 10 years from now?
2. Why did you select a career in _____?

Job Attitudes
1. Describe the perfect boss.
2. Describe the perfect employee.
3. Why did you leave your previous employer?
4. What are you looking for in a job that you are not finding now?
5. What is your greatest disappointment regarding your career to this point?

---

the applicant. To reduce these frustrations and make the interview more productive, consider the following suggestions:

- *The dentist should not allow interruptions during the interview* Staff members should hold calls and not interrupt the dentist's time with the applicant. This is both efficient and courteous.
- *The dentist should beware of dangerous first impressions* People often make an intuitive judgment of a person in the first minute after they have met. A familiar style of dress, smile, or tone of

Box 20.4 Acceptable and Unacceptable Interview Subjects

Name
- Acceptable questions: Whether applicant has ever worked under another name (if needed to verify information)
- Unacceptable questions: Maiden name of a married woman

Residence and Birthplace
- Acceptable questions: If applicant can furnish proof of citizenship
- Unacceptable questions: Citizenship, birthplace of applicant or applicant's parent; whether applicant owns home, rents, boards, or lives with parents

Religion
- Acceptable questions: Normal working hours and days required of the job to avoid possible conflict
- Unacceptable questions: Applicant's religious affiliation; church, parish, or religious holidays that are observed by the applicant

National Origin
- Acceptable questions: None
- Unacceptable questions: Applicant's lineage, ancestry, national origin, or parentage; nationality of applicant's parents or spouse

References
- Acceptable questions: Names of character or professional references for applicant
- Unacceptable questions: Name of applicant's pastor or religious leader

Sex or Marital Status
- Acceptable questions: None
- Unacceptable questions: Sex, marital status, or any item that could be used to determine them; if applicant is pregnant or planning to become pregnant; number of dependents or children; spouse's occupation

Arrest and Convictions
- Acceptable questions: Convictions that are relevant to the job
- Unacceptable questions: Number or types of arrests

Disabilities
- Acceptable questions: Any disabilities that would prevent the applicant from performing on the job
- Unacceptable questions: General inquiries as to whether applicant has any mental or physical disabilities

voice can lull an interviewer into a false first impression that cannot be overcome through the rest of the interview.

- *The dentist should not be too formal or too authoritative* The failure to exchange a few pleasantries and develop rapport makes it difficult for the applicant to relax and talk freely.
- *The dentist should plan the questions* The dentist should plan what he or she intends to ask of each applicant before the interview. Lack of planning on the part of the dentist may result in not obtaining information that could aid the dentist in selecting the best qualified applicant. The dentist should get as much information as possible before the interview, so that he or she can use the interview itself to build on this information.
- *The dentist should not talk too much* One purpose of an interview should be to find out if the applicant can express himself or herself verbally. If the dentist does most of the talking, it is unlikely that he or she could assess the verbal skills of the applicant.
- *The dentist should not mislead the applicant about the duties involved* The dentist may inadvertently do this if a clear job description is not available. He or she should be prepared to discuss duties and responsibilities in some detail. If a job turns out to be different from what the applicant expected, a new employee may quit within a short time.
- *The dentist should not make the interview too short* This makes it difficult to obtain anything but the most superficial information about the applicant. Lack of information frequently leads to errors in selecting the best qualified applicant.
- *The dentist should not allow the discussion to wander.* Discussions about mutual acquaintances or common interests may be entertaining, but they probably do not aid in judging the applicant's qualifications.
- *The dentist should not be too influenced by the applicant's physical appearance, dress, or grooming* Appearance only peripherally relates to the tasks normally expected of a dental auxiliary.
- *The dentist should avoid making assumptions* Just because a previous employee with a particular background did good work, the dentist should not assume that another person with a similar background would also be a satisfactory employee. Each person should be looked at individually.
- *The dentist should avoid biases* Age, education, and background are important only as related to job performance, so the dentist should avoid prejudging applicants on these qualities.
- *The dentist should use intuition carefully* The dentist should base a decision about a job applicant purely on intuition. Careful analysis and objective decisions should enter the selection process. The dentist should use intuition to complement these decision points.

Working Interviews

Many dentists have an employee work for a day in the office. This allows them to assess knowledge, skills, and abilities and to observe their interpersonal relations with patients and the other employees. It also allows the potential employee to assess the dentist's office as a place to work. The dentist must pay applicants for these "working interviews." If the employee is currently employed, it may be difficult to arrange a suitable time for such an interview. The dentist must also be sure that the employee understands that this is not regular employment but is only for the purpose of assessing skills and compatibility for the prospect of employment. Given these caveats, working interviews can be a valuable final step in the selection process.

The Hiring Decision

The decision of which of the final applicants to hire should be based on all the information that dentists can gather. It includes the application form, the interview process, reference checks, work history, and staff information. Personality and skill tests are legal (if they test attributes that are essential to the job), but their cost and low reliability make them impractical for the typical dental office. References should be checked, if only as a formality. Not many people will offer dissatisfied former employers as references. Few businesses are giving honest references on former workers (for fear of slander suits), but it is worth the small effort required for the dentist to pick up the phone and ask. A dentist may get lucky and find an honest evaluation. The dentist should call any previous dental employers; they will generally still give valid appraisals.

Once the dentist decides who to hire, he or she should move quickly! Really good employees seldom remain available for long. The new employee should be contacted (preferably by telephone) and offered the job. The dentist should be prepared to negotiate. The top applicant may have several other possible employment opportunities. The dentist should send a follow-up letter that details the expectations of staff in the office, the duties of the person holding this job, the pay rate, and any benefits that the person will receive.

Once the person accepts the job, the other final applicants should be contacted immediately and informed of the decision so that they can continue with their job searches. If more than one applicant had been acceptable, the dentist should ask that person if he or she can keep their name as an applicant if another opening becomes available. This may shorten the recruiting process in the future if the dentist needs to fill another position.

Probationary Period

Many offices hire employees into a "probationary" status that typically lasts 30, 60, or 90 days. Many dentists believe that they can try out an employee, then terminate him or her if the employee can not do the job duties or does not fit in with the other personalities of the office, without fear of legal repercussions. The dentist also does not pay employee-related benefits for the probationary period. If the employee passes the probationary period, they often are rewarded with a raise and qualifying for the employee-related benefit package.

Many large organizations have gotten away from probationary periods. They believe that their time is better spent in being sure that they select the right employee and train them appropriately. Most states support at-will employment, which means that dentists employ persons at their own will. Dentists can also fire these persons at their own will. Paradoxically, a probationary appointment may imply that once an employee passes the probationary period, he or she can only be fired for cause, essentially nullifying the at-will employment idea.

If a dentist wants to use a probationary period, he or she should probably call it a *waiting period*, which doesn't imply long-term employment and supports at-will employment. The office benefit policy can state when employees become eligible for various benefits, eliminating this justification for the period. A good hiring process will do more to insure excellent employees.

Integrating the New Employee into the Office

The employment process does not stop with job acceptance. The dentist must orient the new employee to the office procedures and possibly train or send him or her for education or certification. Taking time for orientation helps to encourage the employee's loyalty to the office, promote positive interpersonal relationships among staff members, and acquaint new personnel with all facets of the job. The following are tasks for new employee orientation activities:

- *The dentist should start a personnel file* This should include the person's resume or application, W-4 and K-4 (state) withholding forms, Social Security number, and any other necessary tax-related information or work permits.
- *The dentist should have the new employee fill out any benefit or insurance forms, if applicable* Give the employee pamphlets and policies that describe those benefits (again, if applicable).
- *If applicable, the dentist should verify and display the license or certification.*

- *The dentist should require the employee to read the Policy and Procedures Manual for the office* The dentist should review each section of that manual with the new employee and should do the same for the personnel manual. The dentist should have the employee sign that they have read and understand the manual.
- *The dentist should explain opening, closing, and emergency procedures* The dentist should have the employee sign for office keys, if applicable.
- *The dentist should give a detailed tour of the office so that the new employee can see where instruments and materials are* The dentist should show the new

employee where to store personal effects during working hours.
- *The dentist should introduce the new employee to all existing employees* The dentist should assign one employee who functions in a similar capacity to be the "information contact" so that the new employee knows who to ask office procedural questions.
- *The dentist should arrange for OSHA and Health Insurance Portability and Accountability Act (HIPAA) compliance* The new hire must have Hepatitis B vaccination within 10 days and must have the training required by OSHA and HIPAA when feasible.

Part 2: Compensating Employees

It's not the employer who pays the wages—he only handles the money. It is the product that pays the wages.
Henry Ford

Objectives

At the completion of this part, the student will be able to:
1. Describe basic principles involved in establishing a wage and benefit package for the dental office.
2. Define when an employee may be paid a salary and when he or she is an "exempt" employee.
3. Describe the benefits that employers are required to provide to employees.
4. Describe a flexible benefit plan for the dental office.
5. Describe an Annual Employee Total Compensation report.
6. Describe how to process staff pay checks.

Key Terms

benefit	pay equity
flexible benefit plans	required benefits
jury duty	salaried employees
maternity leave	Section 125 plans
military leave	total compensation
nonexempt employees	unpaid leave
optional benefits	wage
overtime	

Goal

The goal of this part is to prepare new graduates to develop a compensation system for the dental office

Dental practitioners compete with each other when recruiting staff for the office. The truly excellent dental office personnel will generally have several offices to choose from when looking for a new employment opportunity. Why would one choose one office over another? One reason may be the pay and benefit package of the dentists. A new practitioner probably cannot pay the top-dollar wage and benefit package that an established colleague or other business venture can. The dilemma that a starting practitioner will face is that he or she does not have the immediate cash flow to pay for the best employees, yet they need the best employees to become profitable.

How to set Staff Compensation Levels

Usually, dentists will pay the "going rate" for comparable employees in their area. The going rate is what most employers pay for similar positions with similar job requirements. This is in turn determined by technical skills or knowledge required, interpersonal abilities, and availability to work certain times. There also may be legal or licensing requirements (such as hygiene license or assisting certification) that limit the number of potential employees, driving up their cost to the dentist. In the end, supply and demand of the labor pool determines what dentists pay employees. If hygienists in the area typically earn $45 per hour, then a dentist will pay about $45 per hour for a hygienist. (There is a range around that average figure.) Various groups, including the popular dental press and organized dental groups, do periodic staff salary surveys. These are a good place for a dentist to start when looking for comparable wage levels.

When thinking of "pay," dentists should think of the total compensation package, which is composed of the hourly wage, legally required benefits, and any optional benefits offered. Wages and benefits are, to a certain extent, interchangeable. A wage of $20.00 per hour with no benefits may be comparable to a wage of $17.00 per hour with a health insurance plan. Every employee is different. He or she will value the balance between pay and benefits differently, according to his or her own needs. Benefits hold tax advantages for employees over straight pay. Many dental office employees would prefer part of their total pay to be in the form benefits. However, many others, especially low-paid employees, do not appreciate this and would rather have cash in hand. Benefits, like salary, help in recruiting, hiring and retaining employees. However, some employees poorly understand benefits. Often they do not understand their true value, and view benefits as employee "rights" rather than forms of additional compensation. Any paid time off (holidays, vacation) is additional compensation and comes from office profit. Unpaid time off decreases office production. To bring these confusing ideas together, many dentists compute the total compensation for employees each year at wage adjustment time. An example computation sheet is given in Table 20.1. Adding a staff member is a large investment, but if he or she increases office collections more than they cost, the addition is a good investment.

Staff Pay

Equity means fairness of the reward system. There are many reasons for promoting equity besides the altruistic desire to treat employees fairly. As a business, dentists compete with other businesses for the pool of labor in the community. Dentists compete with other dentists for the services of assistants, hygienists and receptionists. Dentists compete with the local bank and grocery store for the general labor pool. Although people work for many different reasons, one reason certainly is pay and benefits. Therefore, dentists must pay a competitive wage and benefit to hire and retain excellent employees.

Many pay issues are governed by the Fair Labor Standards Act (FLSA). This is a federal law that is carried out at the state level. So some state-to-state variation exists in the terms of the law. Dentists should check with the state's Bureau of Labor Standards (or similar state organization) for the exact interpretation in the state of practice.

Hourly Wage

Hourly employees earn an hourly wage. Their total pay is based on the number of hours that they work multiplied times their hourly wage. Most dental office employees earn an hourly wage for their work.

To figure out total pay accurately, dentists must have accurate information describing how many hours each employee worked for each day of the week. Either written pay records (pay sheets) or a time clock accomplishes this legally. If a dentist uses a written record, the person should record "time in" and "time out" for each session (morning and afternoon). Simply recording 8 hours is not adequate documentation. Also, the dentist should require each person to sign the time sheet or time card. This says that he or she agrees it is an accurate description of the time that they worked. Most office management computer systems have built in time clocks to help in recording hours worked. This also makes it easier to process payroll.

Salary

Salaried employees earn a fixed amount (salary) regardless how much time that they work (given some limitations). Some dentists prefer paying a salary for several reasons. The accounting is easier to calculate. Each pay period, the owner calculates how much Social Security tax, federal, state, and local (if any) income taxes, and voluntary employee contributions to withhold from each employee's gross pay. Salaried employees make the same gross pay and therefore have the same amount withheld each pay period, making this function easier. Some dentists erroneously believe that any salaried employee can work an unlimited time. (In fact, only "exempt" employees can work overtime without additional pay.) On the down side, a salaried employee gets paid for a full week's work, even if they work fewer hours.

Commission

Dentists may pay staff a percentage of the work that they produce. This pay scheme is valuable when the employee controls their own amount of production and when money motivates the employee to work harder. That is not always the case. A hygienist may be able to control patient volume, but a chairside assistant has much less control over how many patients he or she sees in a day. A commission is a much less effective way to compensate the assistant. A common problem is to decide which procedures should be included in the hygienist's base for commission. The periodic exam, for example, can only be done (in most states)

Table 20.1 Example Annual Employee Compensation

Employee Name: _____

Direct Compensation		Assumptions
Gross Pay	$41,600	Employee's wage rate=$20.00 per hour
Overtime	$900	Employee works 40 hours per week
Bonuses	$200	Employee worked 30 hours overtime (30 × 30=$900)
FICA (7.65%)	$3,182	Employee receives 2 weeks of paid vacation
Unemployment Insurance	$400	Employee receives six paid holidays
Retirement Plan Contribution	$2,080	Employee receive 5 sick days and 2 continuing education days
		Dentist makes 5% contribution to retirement plan
Employee Fringe Benefits		Dentist provides single health coverage ($400/month)
Medical Insurance	$4,800	Dentist provides a continuing education trip every year (value=$500)
Dental Care	$150	Dentist gave employees a $200 holiday bonus
Group Life Insurance		Dentist paid professional dues of $200
Dependent Care Allowance		Dentist provides routine dental care value=$150
Gifts and Awards		
Career Benefits		
Continuing Education Payments	$500	
Tuition and Travel Reimbursement		
Lodging and Meals		
Professional Dues/Subscriptions	$200	
Total Compensation	$54,012	
Total Hours Paid (52 × 40)	$2080	
Total Hours Not Worked	$154	
Total Hours Actually Worked	$1,926	
Nominal Compensation/Hour	$20.00	
Actual Compensation/Hour	$28.04	

by the dentist, so should not be included. Radiographs, although taken by the hygienist (on the dentist's equipment) must be read and interpreted by the dentist. Eliminating these procedures for compensation decreases significantly the hygienist's compensation and can lead to dissatisfaction.

The typical range dentists pay their hygienists is 30 to 35 percent of their production. The dentist is still responsible for ensuring the quality of work in the office. Associates are often paid based on a percentage of production as well. The specific percent varies tremendously across the country as supply and demand dictate.

Exempt Employees

Exempt employees are exempt from the wage and hour (overtime) laws. This means dentists must pay non-exempt employees overtime (at a rate equal to 1 1/2 times their wage) for any time they work more than 40 per week. Dentists may pay an employee a salary with no overtime (i.e., they are *exempt* employees) if they meet all three of these criteria:

a. They regularly supervise two or more 40-hour employees.
b. Their salary is at least $455 per week.

c. They spend less than 20 percent of their time doing the same duties as the people they supervise.

Professional employees are exempt as well. An associate dentist (and in some states, a dental hygienist) is considered a professional employee and, therefore, exempt from the overtime laws.

Given these restrictions, the only people who truly qualify as exempt salaried employees in a dental office are a dentist associate, a true office manager, and perhaps a dental hygienist. Dentists may pay dental auxiliaries on a salary basis. However, auxiliaries are still nonexempt employees. Because dentists must pay them overtime, it does not make much sense to put them on a salary. (The dentist loses if they work more or fewer than 40 hours per week.) Wage and hour laws vary from state to state. They are also subject to change by regulators. Therefore, the dentist should check with his or her state's labor cabinet before setting up a pay system.

Overtime Pay

The FLSA requires that dentists pay overtime to any employee who works more than 40 hours in a week. (Four states base their overtime on 8 hours per day.) Overtime pay is a minimum of "time and a half," or 1.5 times each employee's regular hourly wage for those hours worked more than 40 per week. Each workweek stands alone regarding overtime. That is to say, the employer cannot accumulate multiple pay periods (1 week the employee worked 42 hours, the next week, 38 hours) and not pay overtime. Dentists also may not legally substitute compensatory time (i.e., letting people take equivalent time off) for overtime pay, even if the employee agrees.

Determining the "base hourly wage rate" can be a bit tricky. What is (or is not) included in the regular wage is important because it determines overtime pay (Box 20.5). The regular pay includes all money received for employment, except reimbursed expenses, gifts, discretionary bonuses, and paid time off. A bonus is "discretionary" if it is not given it in exchange for action by the employee. So dentists should include a production

---

Box 20.5 Determining Overtime Pay

Mary, a dental assistant, is paid $10 per hour. This week she works 45 hours. To determine her gross pay for tax determination:

Mary is paid "time and a half" for any hours more than 40 per week. In this case, she is paid $400 base pay (40 hours × $10/hour) plus $75 overtime pay (5 hours × $15/hour).

---

bonus in the regular rate but not a Christmas bonus (unless it is based on production for the year). If a dentist has questions concerning overtime pay, he or she should check with an accountant about what be should included and excluded.

Paid Time Off

The FLSA does not require that employers pay for any time off for employees. This includes holidays, paid or unpaid vacation days, sick, or personal days. Most employers offer some of these as time off so that they will be competitive with other similar businesses when hiring employees.

Dentists need to decide their policy regarding staff working when they take time off from the office. When a dentist is not there, the office generates no income, and most employees have little to do. If a dentist is gone for a day (e.g., to a continuing professional education course), he or she can usually find enough work for the staff to do. This includes deep cleaning, checking inventories, maintaining equipment, updating periodic maintenance and other patient lists, contacting insurance carriers, making collection calls, and many other tasks that the office is behind on. If the dentist is gone for a week, the issue is more of a problem. Some dentists require staff members to take any vacation days when the office is closed. In small offices, it is a problem to let an employee take time off when he or she chooses because of the negative effect that has on daily operations. The employee is not there when the dentist needs him or her and there when the dentist does not need him or her. (One person may represent a fourth of the workforce.) Some have certain employees (e.g., the front office staff) work but not others (the clinical staff). Others who pay their employees a salary give employees the time off with pay.

Benefits

An employee benefit is something of value, other than cash money, that an employer provides for their employees. Benefits are valuable for employees because they are generally tax free. They are also generally a tax deduction for the employer. Law requires employers to provide some benefits. Others are optional.

Cost of Benefits to the Practice

Employers may pay for benefits to their employees beyond their hourly wage. Here, the cost of the benefit is tax deductible to the employer, and the benefit accrues to the employee without them having to pay income taxes on the value of that benefit. The tax deductibility helps to reduce the cost to the employer of providing the benefit, but it does not eliminate the cost. The employer still must pay for the benefit.

The benefits that dentists provide will depend, largely, by what is customary in the economy of the local community. The dentist will be competing with other dentists and other forms of employment in the area for excellent staff members. Early in a dentist's practice career, the practice is not as profitable as later, when the patient pool is larger, the dentist's skills have increased, and he or she has paid off the start-up loans. A dentist may have a difficult time, therefore, developing a compensation package that competes with other established dentists in the area. Nevertheless, that is exactly what the dentist needs to do to compete effectively. In these cases, the dentist should try to make the workplace environment an advantage. The dentist should sell the office as an excellent place to work. He or she probably cannot attract everyone as an employee, but neither do the established practices.

The Value of Pay and Benefits to Employees

Staff members want both pay and benefits, in varying amounts. Employee benefits can be powerful employment motivators. Many staff (or potential staff) members understand the value of employee benefits. Some (especially those with strong union family ties) believe that it is the dentist's obligation as the owner (management) to provide a complete benefit package for employees. Some, especially low-paid employees, often struggle to make ends meet and would rather have as much compensation as cash as possible. Those who make a higher wage (such as hygienists) may want more compensation in tax-advantaged benefits because their basic income needs are satisfied. Some may have family benefit plans through their spouse's employer. As a dentist develops their compensation package for employees, he or she will need to balance these competing desires. The dentist cannot satisfy all employee and potential employees without overpaying. One solution is a flexible benefit plan, which will be described later. The workplace environment and employee motivation techniques (in the next chapter) also affect employee job satisfaction.

Required Benefits

Some benefits are required by federal or state laws.

Required Insurances

The law requires the employer to carry (and pay for) certain insurances on his or her employees. The three required insurance benefits are:

1. **Workers' compensation** provides an income to workers who are temporarily unable to work as a result of an injury on the job. This is an insurance that the owner must purchase and carry on his or her employees.
2. **Unemployment insurance** provides income to employees who lose their job through no fault of their own (e.g., layoffs, plant closings). This is a federally mandated program administered through the state through unemployment taxes.
3. **Social Security** provides income to retirees and disabled people. It is a federal program jointly funded by the workers, employers, and self-employed people. Social Security provides income when a family's earnings are reduced or stopped because of disability, death (survivor protection), or retirement. The government requires an employer to participate in the Social Security system through matching contributions on employees' wages.

Time off from Work

Federal, state, and local laws require an employer to offer several types of unpaid leave.

1. *Jury duty* is function of good citizenship. The employer must allow people time off if the courts have called them for this duty. The employer must hold a comparable job open for someone who does jury duty, but the employer does not generally have to pay the employee for the time on jury duty. (Some states [AL, CO, CT, LA, MA, PA, NE, TN, and DC] presently require employers to pay employees for time served on juries.) The employer may also require employees to return to work if their jury duty ends before normal work hours.
2. *Military duty* is also a function of good citizenship. The employer must allow people the time if they are in the military reserves to fulfill their obligations. The employer may fill the position, either permanently or temporarily, but he or she must have a comparable position available for the employee when they return from active duty to work.
3. The employer must allow *maternity leave* of 6 weeks for women who will give birth to a child. If their doctor says they must have more time, the employer must grant it. Further, the employer must hold a comparable job for a woman to return to, although it can temporarily be filled in her absence.

Table 20.2 "Unwithheld" Expenses

Type	Percentage
FICA (including Medicare)	7.65%
SUTA (state unemployment)	2.80%
FUTA (federal unemployment)	0.80%
Workers' compensation	0.50%
Total unwithheld expenses	**11.75%**

Contracts and Benefits

Laws or contracts may require certain other benefits. They include:

1. Depending on the particular *retirement plan*, tax laws may require the employer to include employees in the plan. These plans may require the employer to provide all of the funds for an employee's retirement account or match the amount the employee elects to save for retirement.
2. Certain *group health plans* may require minimum group participation.
3. *Occupational Safety and Health Administration (OSHA)* has requirements that the employer must meet regarding worker safety. This includes a worker's protective gear and clothing, supplies, vaccinations, and medical tests related to his or her job.

Unwithheld Expenses

The cost of a worker's wage is only one part of the total compensation package. The required benefits are an additional cost to the employer. These are called *"unwithheld" expenses* because they are additional expenses to the employer but they are not withheld from the employee's pay (e.g., federal income taxes). For every dollar of payroll, these unwithheld expenses typically cost the owner approximately an additional 12 cents (Table 20.2).

Optional Benefits

The employer may provide many benefits to workers. Generally, these are business expenses to the employer and are, therefore, tax deductions for the employer. Besides the legally required benefits, any paid holidays, and vacation, sick, or personal days are also costs to the employer above the pure cost of employment (plus the lost production and income). When the price of retirement plan participation and even a modest benefit package is added, the total compensation package often runs 20 to 40 percent above the pure salary cost of an employee. Many employers give employees a detailed description of the entire cost of employment (see Table 20.1). The purpose is not to defend a wage.

Instead, it is to make employees aware of how much they are actually making because such a large portion of their compensation may be in unseen benefits.

The employer may pay for benefits for employees, besides their hourly wage. Here, the cost of the benefit is tax deductible to the employer, and the benefit accrues to the employee without them having to pay income taxes on the value of that benefit. The tax deductibility helps to reduce the cost to the employer of providing the benefit, but it does not eliminate the cost. The employer still must pay for the benefit. As an alternative, in a properly structured plan, the employer can withhold from the employee's gross pay the money needed to pay for a given benefit. The employee then, through a salary reduction, pays for the cost of the benefit. This decreases the staff member's direct pay, which also decreases the unwithheld amounts that the employer contributes. So every dollar that an employer converts from salary to benefit saves him or her an additional 13 to 24 percent. As a final alternative, the employer may choose to share the cost of the benefit with the employee through a combination salary reduction and additional compensation plan.

The employer must pay for certain other costs associated with employees (besides the required benefits listed previously). If the employer requires staff to attend a continuing education course, he or she must not only pay for the course, but also pay normal wage rates for the time that the employee attends. The employer must also reimburse meals, tuition, and travel expenses. If an employee voluntarily attends a course on nonwork time, the employer does not have to pay or reimburse, even if it is practice related.

There is a long list of benefits that an employer can offer to employees. These vary greatly across the country and within regions. Benefits should be set based on what is common in the practice area so that dentists can compete effectively for employees. A dentist will probably not provide all of the benefits detailed here—the cost would be too great—but it gives dentists and idea of commonly provided benefits in dental offices.

Paid Vacation Days

Many dental practices nationwide (about 90 percent) offer paid vacation days. Typically, employees may receive 1 week of paid vacation after a year of employment, 2 weeks after 5 years, and 3 weeks after 10 years of employment. Dentists often require that employees take these vacation days when the office is closed.

Paid Sick or Personal Days

Many dental offices (about half) offer additional sick or personal days for staff members. Others require staff to use vacation days (or generic time off) for sickness or personal reasons.

Health Insurance

About half the dental offices offer health insurance as an employee benefit. They often do this through some sharing arrangement, such as a salary reduction or contributing up to a certain amount to go toward the health insurance premium. This is an expensive benefit, but one that many employees require in the workplace.

Dental Care

Almost all offices offer dental care for their employees, either free of charge or at a reduced rate. Some require that employees pay any direct costs, such as laboratory bills. Some offer the benefit to immediate family members as well.

Retirement Plan Contribution

About half the offices provide a contribution to a retirement plan. There are many types of plans and the contribution amount various greatly.

Continuing Education

More than half of the practices pay for continuing education for their staff members. This improves the abilities of staff members and increases their sense of personal fulfillment on the job.

Bonus Plan

About a quarter of the dental practices offer some form of a bonus plan, where the staff can make additional income through meeting targeted goals. Some employees respond to the desire for additional income.

Flexible Benefit Plans

Each staff person is going to have their own set of needs, wants, and desires regarding a benefit plan. For example, the worker whose spouse works at a Fortune 500 company and receives a complete benefit package will have an entirely different set of benefit needs than the single parent. Many of these benefits, such as health insurance, are costly to provide to employees. Others, such as paid time off (vacation or sick days) result in payments to the staff member and lost production from not having that person in the office. Giving all benefits to all employees would therefore be prohibitively expensive, even for a well-established practitioner. One solution is to develop a flexible benefit or "cafeteria" plan. In these plans, an employee who does not need health insurance could decide to have dependent care expenses withheld for their children who are in day care. These plans consist of a group of benefit possibilities that employees may choose among, similar to choosing a meal at a food cafeteria. The employees probably cannot get all of the benefits, but they can get the ones that are most important to them. An employee may choose health insurance, another dependent care allowance and life insurance, whereas a third employee may choose to take no benefits and instead take the entire amount as taxable income. Tax laws are explicit on this topic but are subject to change. Dentists should consult with an accountant or tax planner regarding their current deductibility.

Benefits cost the employer less than paying an equivalent amount in wages. This is because the employer does not have to pay the unwithheld expenses. Benefits also hold a significant financial advantage for employees in that they do not have Social Security/Medicare taxes withheld and because they gain the full value of the benefit without having income taxes withheld. For example, assume an employee wants a health insurance package that costs $200 per month ($2,400 per year). His or her gross pay is $10 per hour ($20,000 per year) and the tax rate is 25 percent. Two options are available. The first option is to receive full pay, less taxes, and then buy health insurance with after tax dollars. The second option is to have the amount withheld from his or her paycheck as part of a tax-free, flexible benefit plan, and then receive the difference, less taxes as pay. Table 20.3 shows the practical effect for the

Table 20.3 Three Types of Benefit Plans and Total Cost of Employment

	No Benefit Plan	Flex Plan	Employer Paid Plan
Gross pay	$20,000	$17,600	$20,000
Pretax insurance	$0	$2,400	$2,400
Taxable income	$20,000	$17,600	$20,000
FICA taxes (@ 7.65%)	$1,530	$1,346	$1,530
Retirement plan contribution (@ 5%)	$1,000	$880	$1,000
Net, pretax cost of employment	**$22,530**	**$22,226**	**$24,930**

This table shows the effect of three types of benefit plans on employer's total cost of employment. It assumes that the employee needs health insurance (@ $2,400/year), has a gross pay of $20,000, and the dentist also has a retirement plan in which he or she contributes 5% of each employee's pay.

employee. The employee has an increase in net spendable income of $600 simply by having the insurance taken out as a pretax benefit instead of paying for it with posttax dollars. The employer saves approximately $282 through the second option because he or she pays the unwithheld expenses (11.75 percent) on the reduced taxable income. This sounds like the perfect "free lunch," with both sides winning. In fact, the government, through the tax deductibility of employee benefit plans, ends up subsidizing the difference in cost.

These 125 Plans (named for Section 125 of the Internal Revenue Code) allow the employee to choose between cash salary (taxable) and nontaxed benefits. Because the employee may take the compensation as cash, the employer can finance the entire cost of the benefit through employee salary reductions. These plans offer significant advantages (such as flexibility and cost control) but have the disadvantage that the employee may lose the money that they have allocated to the benefit plan if not used by the end of the plan year. (This is the "Use It or Lose It" rule.)

Flexible benefit plans are easy and inexpensive to operate. (The employer will want to get a benefit specialist to set up the plan.) The unwithheld expenses that he or she does not pay on benefits offset the administrative costs. For example, if three employees reduce their salaries by $200 per month, the employer does not pay the unwithheld expenses on $7,200 of employee salary per year. That translates into a total savings on employee taxes for the employer of approximately $850. The more that employees shelter, the more money is saved in employer taxes. However, the employer should not view these flexible benefit plans as a tax "gold mine." The administrative expenses will often about equal the tax savings. A flexible benefit plan allows the employer to compete effectively for employees by offering a benefit package that meets each employee's most important benefit needs at least cost to the employer. As a result, the employer should have better, more loyal employees.

Table 20.4 Three Types of Benefit Plans and Employee's Take-home Pay

	No Benefit Plan	Flex Plan	Employer Paid Plan
Gross pay	$20,000	$20,000	$20,000
Pretax insurance	$0	-$2,400	$2,400
Taxable income	$20,000	$17,600	$20,000
Taxes (@ 25%)	-$5,000	-$4,400	-$5,000
Posttax insurance	-$2,400	$0	$0
Net, spendable income (employee)	**$12,600**	**$13,200**	**$15,000**

This table shows the effect of three types of benefit plans on employee's take-home pay. It assumes that the employee needs health insurance (@ $2,400/year), has a gross pay of $20,000, and is in the 24% marginal tax bracket.

Processing Staff Pay Checks

Writing staff pay checks involves several steps beyond the typical office expense check. Some offices hire a payroll company to process staff pay checks. Many others use a computer program (such as Quick Payroll) to process checks. Still others use the forms and material sent by the IRS. Each works. The deciding factors are the number of checks to process and the comfort level of the doctor or bookkeeper in payroll issues. This discussion focuses on the theory of payrolls so that dentists will understand how to use any payroll system.

When dentists prepare a payroll check for an employee, the IRS requires that they estimate the income tax that the employee owes, withhold it from the employee's pay, and send it to the IRS. At the end of the year, the employee calculates his or her actual tax liability and compares it to the amount that the employer withheld along the way. If the employer withheld too much, the employee gets a refund of that amount. If the employer withheld too little, then the employee owes extra tax to make up the difference.

At the end of the month (or quarter depending on the agency), the employer sends each taxing agency a check for all the taxes that withheld from all employees for the payroll period. The dentist can use the general office checking account and does not have to have a separate or special account for holding this money. At the end of the month, the dentist sends the US Treasury all the taxes withheld from all employees for the month (federal income, Social Security, and Medicare taxes) and his or her matching amounts for Social Security and Medicare (Table 20.5). The employer can make one

Table 20.5 Processing Staff Pay Checks*
An employee, Susan, is paid $20.00 per hour and works 40 hours this week. She has $100 withheld weekly for medical insurance. Her paycheck for the period would be:

Gross pay[a]	$800.00
Health insurance	$100.00
Taxable income	**$700.00**
Federal income tax withheld[b]	**$52.00**
Social Security withheld[c]	$43.40
Medicare withheld[d]	$10.15
State income tax withheld[e]	$42.00
Local income tax withheld[f]	$10.50
Net pay	**$541.95**

*Assumptions: [a]Gross pay = $20.00 × 40; [b]from Tax Table (Circular E); [c]$700 × 6.2%; [d]$700 × 1.45%; [e]$700 × 6% (state income tax rate of 6%); and [f]$700 × 1.5% (city income tax of 1.5%)

The employer should write Susan's check for $541.95 and should keep the remainder ($158.05) in an account along with other employees' withholdings to pay to the various taxing agencies. The employer should add $53.55 (7.65% of $700) as the matching portion of FICA and also pays the health insurance premium for Susan.

online payment, which the IRS electronically deducts from the office checking account. State and local tax agencies have similar rules and procedures.

To know how much tax to withhold, the employer should have each employee complete a Form W-4 annually. (These forms can be downloaded from the IRS Web site or gotten from an accountant.) This form declares the marital status and number of exemptions claimed by the employee. The employer then looks up the gross pay in the appropriate table and deducts the given amount from the employee's gross pay for taxes. (Again, computer systems have the tables built into their software.) It does not affect FICA or Medicare taxes. It does not affect the tax owed by the employee, only the amount that the employer withholds along the way. The IRS sends a publication (Circular E) to all employers that describes these withholdings and gives tables that dictate how much the employer must withhold from each employee's check. (The employer does not have a choice. He or she must follow the tax withholding table amounts.). Many states, counties, and cities have similar income tax or occupational tax requirements of employers. They will also send the employer tax tables that describe how much to withhold from employees' paychecks for their various taxes. Payroll computer programs have these tables built into them to make the calculations easier. Because tax rates and rules change frequently, the employer should be sure to have an updated payroll package or the wrong amounts may be withheld.

Besides income tax, employers must also withhold Social Security and Medicare taxes and send these to the federal government. These payroll taxes are collectively called Federal Insurance Contributions Act (FICA) and this money funds these programs. Employers withhold a certain amount from employees' pay (earned income), then match it with additional company money, and send the entire amount to the government. Currently, employers withhold 6.2 percent for Social Security and 1.45 percent for Medicare from wages for a total withholding of 7.65 percent. The employers then match this amount (totaling 15.3 percent), and send this to the government. There is an upper limit on the Social Security portion (currently about $110,000 adjusted for inflation). So any earnings beyond this amount are only subject to the Medicare portion of the tax.

To begin processing the payroll, the employer needs to know the number of hours worked for the week and the hourly wage for each employee. The employer finds the hours worked for each employee from a time clock or other record. He or she then decides the hourly wage through annual performance appraisals and reviews. The gross wage is simply the hours worked times the per hour wage. If there is an employee benefit plan, tax-deductible amounts for benefits is subtracted first, which leads to a taxable income. In this way, taxes are not withheld from benefits. From this, subtract table amount for income tax withheld and calculated amount for FICA. This results in the employee's net pay. The employer then writes the check to the employee for net pay, leaving the withheld amounts in the checkbook.

If a dentist operates as a corporation, then he or she is an employee of the corporation. When the dentist pays himself or herself, amounts are withheld, just like any other employee. If a dentist operates as a proprietor, partnership, or disregarded entity, then he or she is an owner, not an employee. Instead of withholding taxes, the dentist estimates his or her tax liability and pays it quarterly to the government. Instead of FICA, the IRS imposes a similar tax on the earnings of self-employed individuals called SETA from the Self-Employment Tax Act. It is similar to FICA in the amount. It is calculated using a special form (Schedule SE).

The Cost of a Staff Member Leaving

Staff compensation is the single largest expense item for most dental practices. If a staff member leaves the practice, the practice incurs additional and hidden costs. These include lost production from not having the employee, additional pay for other employees to cover the lost time, cost of advertising the position, time away from production for interviews and selection, and lower production while the new staff person acclimates to the job. Many management experts have calculated that it often costs from 3 to 4 months' pay to replace a person who leaves. For a typical chairside dental assistant, that translates to $8,000 to $10,000. If the employer can make this a smooth transition, then he or she can keep these costs on the lower end. It obviously costs more if an employee walks out with a full schedule of patients, rather than giving several weeks' notice so that the employer can begin the replacement process. The employer must balance the cost of turnover with the cost of paying additional wages and benefits.

Part 3: Motivating Employees to Perform Well

There are no bad regiments. Only bad colonels.
Napoleon

Objectives

At the completion of this part, the student will be able to:
1. Differentiate between leadership and motivation.
2. Describe the three factors that affect a person's performance on the job.
3. Describe the major motivation perspectives and give examples of their application in the dental office.
   The work ethic
   Theory X and Theory Y
   Need theories
   Equity Theory
4. Define guidelines for a proper incentive plan.

Key Terms

ability	leadership
coercive power	legitimate power
content perspectives	motivation
environment	need theories
Equity Theory	reward power
inputs	Theory X
rewards	Theory Y
expert power	work ethic
incentive plans	

Goal

The goal of this part is to describe how to motive staff in the dental office.

Before deciding a particular wage and benefit package, it is important to understand why some people are motivated in the office and others are not. This is such an obviously important issue that management experts have been doing research in this area for many years. Most now believe that pay and benefits simply act as a baseline or threshold that employers must meet to develop a motivated worker. The motivation itself comes from the achievement, growth, and recognition gained from the job. Employers must have both factors covered to have the truly satisfied and motivated worker. According to this theory, a dissatisfied worker is guaranteed if they are not paid enough. However, simply paying an adequate, or even excessive, wage will not

Box 20.6 Three Factors of Job Performance

Ability
Environment
Motivation

produce a more motivated worker. It may lead to a worker who is less likely to leave because of the high pay. Still, it does not make the person a better or more motivated worker.

Researchers have developed many other theories to explain what motivates employees in the workplace. Motivation refers to all the forces that direct, energize, and maintain a person's effort on the job. Highly motivated employees work hard to achieve performance goals on the job. If they have adequate skills, resources, and freedom on the job, they will show a high job performance. To be effective motivators, the dentist must know what behaviors he or she wants and then stimulate and challenge employees to do those behaviors.

Three factors determine a person's performance on the job (Box 20.6). The first is ability, or physical and mental preparation to do the job. This includes all forms of training and experience. This is assessed through the application and interview process and by licensing and training credentials. The second factor is the environment. Without the proper setting, tools, and materials, a person cannot properly do a job. Employers control the work environment to help the work process. The third factor that determines job performance is motivation, or desire to do the job. Employers must motivate through daily interactions with the people involved.

Leadership

People often think of leadership as an innate ability that certain people possess and others lack. Research has shown, however, that leadership, rather than being a genetic or personal trait (like blue eyes or black hair) is instead a style or behavior that people display. Leadership is the process of creating a vision, having the power to translate that vision into reality, and then sustain it over time. Leaders inspire people to perform; managers see that the organization runs smoothly. In the dental office, the dentist will fulfill both of those roles.

Leadership means working with the employees of the office (dental team members) to have a common office goal and then getting the people to "buy into" the goal and work toward meeting the goal. It is the human factor that binds the work group together and makes it function at its peak. Leadership involves power but is

Box 20.7 Types of Leadership Power
Legitimate
Reward
Coercive
Expert
Personal

Box 20.8 Reasons People Work
Compensation
Pay
Benefits
Psychological reasons
Social reasons

not necessarily pure power. It is the employer's ability to influence the people that work for him or her (Box 20.7). As the owner of the practice, the owner has *legitimate* power over the people who are hired to work. The employer can legally fire or reprimand employees and set work conditions (such as hours of employment). He or she also has *reward* power in that the employer establishes pay scales and offers raises and issues recognition and praise for performance. Conversely, the employer may also punish noncompliance by using *coercive* power. Because a dentist has special skills, training, knowledge, and certification (licensing), he or she also has power as an *expert* that other employees do not have. *Personal* power comes from the influence that an employer may (or may not) have over others through the force of individual personality.

Leadership then involves getting the people in the office to perform as the employer wants them to perform, by influencing their behavior with the employer's behavior. The effectiveness of the employer's leadership depends on several factors. The employer's background, experience, personality, and style will obviously affect his or her effectiveness as a leader. An equally important factor is the background, experience, and personality of the followers in the office. If there is not an appropriate match, then the interaction is destined to fail. Finally, the leader who understands a subordinate's task is in a much better position to select an appropriate leadership style and strategy to fit the particular situation. To understand these interactions, the employer first has to understand himself or herself.

Why People Work

Many dentists believe that a person will work harder if they are paid more. Many also believe that pay is the only reason that people work. However, modern management proposes that people work for reasons other than just pay. (After all, many people put in many hours in volunteer work for organizations that pay nothing!) Although people must meet their financial needs, they also work because of the friendships they form on the job and the sense of personal accomplishment and value that they can gain from doing a job. It follows, then, that if people

work for these other reasons, they may be motivated to work harder or do better by arranging the job so that they can accomplish these needs.

Modern management experts believe that people work for three reasons; compensation (pay and benefits), psychological reasons (personal growth and fulfillment), and for social reasons (friendships and relationships in the workplace) (Box 20.8). As the dentist–manager of the practice, the dentist must control each of these motivation factors to develop and encourage excellent employees. That is a difficult task in itself. To make the problem even more difficult, different employees want different amounts and types of fulfillment in each of these areas. Obviously, motivating employees to work at their peak level can be a complex problem.

Compensation

People often use pay as a comparative indicator of success. Even people who do not need the money resulting from work use their earnings as a supplement to family income or to fund special needs or savings plans. So, people will not work unless the pay is adequate, but adequate pay alone is not a good job motivator. But pay is only a short-term motivator. If someone receives a raise, he or she will work harder for a while, but the new pay level soon becomes the norm and he or she returns to the previous work level. If an employee views the raise as recognition for work well done, then the recognition can become a longer-term motivator on the job.

Psychological Reasons

People want to believe that they have a purpose in life and that their lives have meaning. An important job or a job that contributes to others' well-being helps to bring meaning to what people do. Some people define themselves by the job they hold. They have strong psychological reasons for their work. Everyone continues to grow their entire lives, in knowledge, skill, and abilities and in spiritual and emotional ways. Many people look to their work environment to provide some of that growth, both professional and personal.

Obviously, the practice needs certain tasks to be done. The purpose of the practice, after all, is not to provide a country club atmosphere or a self-help venue for its employees. However, if dentists understand what excites people about their jobs, the employers can structure the job or work setting to encourage motivated people to work better. This leads to a more successful practice.

Social Reasons

People often form friendships and personal relationships with coworkers. The daily interaction with a group of people is itself a social function that many people enjoy in the workplace. Because people spend such a significant portion of their adult waking lives in the work setting, many look for and appreciate close personal relationships that develop. Staff members may meet socially outside the office, and their families may become close as they share personal and family triumphs and failures. This helps lead to a cohesive work group in the office.

The owner–manager–dentist is in a difficult situation regarding social interaction. He or she wants to promote a cohesive team atmosphere in the office, but he or she is still the boss. The employer is responsible for staff direction, evaluations, raises, and discipline. Therefore, he or she has a fine line to walk between being friendly (pleasant, warm, concerned, engaging) with the staff and being friends with the staff. (It is difficult to discipline or fire an employee, much less a friend!) The employer should keep a certain formal distance between the boss and the workers. This helps insulate him or her from staff members claiming that the employer shows favoritism toward a particular staff member and helps remove claims of harassment.

The Work Environment

Many dentists believe that job motivation is a trait that a person either possesses or does not possess and that the dentist can do little to influence motivation. The experience and history of US business do not bear out this belief. Most people want to do well on the job and are willing to work hard if they are reasonably sure that their hard work will result in a meaningful payoff (financial, social, or personal). This is the point that owner–dentists can affect the environment, by setting goals and reward systems that allow and encourage motivated people to succeed in their jobs. The employer can encourage those workers who value personal development to take continuing education courses and report to the group important items learned. He or she also can encourage work-related social activities for

those who value aspect of his or her job. For those motivated more by money, the employer can establish a pay system that rewards taking on additional duties or additional work.

So the way that a manager arranges job tasks and the work environment profoundly affects the motivation of employees. As the manager of a small business (i.e., the dental practice), the dentist is responsible for formulating policies and an environment that enhances the productivity of the practice. Employee work habits, turnover, tardiness, and performance affect productivity. By learning which factors lead to enhanced motivation of employees, employers can understand what causes workers' behaviors (good and bad), predict the effect of policy changes, and direct workers' behaviors to meet the business' needs better.

The basic paradigm of a motivation system is to define the objectives of the job as to the practice needs, identify a person's needs, and then set a system that encourages constructive behavior on the job by rewarding proper behaviors and punishing or extinguishing improper behaviors. This assumes that the dentist can identify clearly defined, challenging-yet-attainable goals, that there is an effective ongoing system for monitoring attainment of those goals, and that constructive methods of thoughts about performance are present.

Employee Motivation Concepts

Researchers have proposed that several theories help explain what motivates people on the job. If employers can learn what motivates people on the job, then they can structure the job to have more motivated employees. None of these theories explain all of the motivation (or lack of motivation) that are seen in the workplace. However, they are all helpful in explaining some motivation that is seen or in explaining certain cases of motivation, or demotivation.

The Work Ethic

Dentists are highly motivated, successful workers. The practice of dentistry is inherently interesting and rewarding work with high levels of responsibility, growth, and self-fulfillment for the dentist. Dental schools have screened dentists for success and work habits through the educational process. The work has a value by itself. In this sense, it is a terminal value, like honesty. People think that a strong work ethic is internalized among good people. However, people value the meaning of work differently. Some people do not believe that work is a terminal value (i.e., a desirable activity by itself), but instead, that it is an instrumental value

Box 20.9 The Work Ethic

Terminal value	<--------> Instrumental value
Career	<--------> Job
Internal motivation	<--------> External motivation

Table 20.6 Theory X, Theory Y

Theory X	Theory Y
Workers	
Dislike work	Work is a natural activity
Lazy, indolent, lack ambition	Self-directed, seek responsibility
Prefer external control	Prefer internal control
Managers	
Close supervision	General supervision
Directive	Supportive
Authoritarian	Participative
Boss centered	Employee centered
Task oriented	Relationship oriented

(i.e., produces desired consequences). Although these people may be hard workers while on the job, they see the job as a means to the end, rather than an end unto itself. These people view their work as simply a job. They work so that they can get paid; their motivation is external to them. Others view their employment as a career. They have long-term outlooks and long-term employment goals. Their work fits into a life script; their motivation is internal (Box 20.9).

These two conflicting views can be seen in the extreme examples of a "workaholic" who places an exaggerated importance on work, to the teenager who works only to buy clothes and gas for their car. Obviously, rewards needed to motivate will vary with the worker's perceived importance of work. This perceived importance or "work ethic" is not an entirely fixed internal response. It is some personal combination of moral obligation, productivity, pride in work, commitment to employers, and an achievement orientation that others can influence, to a degree, by the work environment. In other words, rewards may influence the extent to which workers perceive work to be important.

Theory X, Theory Y

Douglas McGregor developed a related idea concerning a manager's perceptions of human beings at work that he detailed in his 1960 work, *The Human Side of Enterprise*. He described two opposing views of how managers perceive that people approach work. One he called Theory X; the other, Theory Y. Theory X and Y are not distinct types, but a continuum, with each theory on one end. Theory X adherents believe that workers are lazy, indolent, dislike work, lack ambition, dislike responsibility, are easily duped, and prefer to be directed. Theory X managers, therefore, are more authoritarian, task-oriented, boss-centered, and use external controls. Theory Y adherents, on the other hand, believe that work is a natural activity for most people, that they are internally motivated, and willingly seek and accept responsibility. Theory Y managers are more democratic, participative, employee-oriented, and people and process oriented (Table 20.6).

McGregor believed that Theory X is a destructive, self-fulfilling prophesy. Theory X beliefs lead to policies and practices that tightly control employees. (In the previous system, they believe that workers see their work as a job.) This leads to withdrawal and resentment by the workers. The manager then observes these negative behaviors that reinforce their beliefs in the nature of people, leading to tighter controls.

Obviously, a dentist–manager's view of the nature of workers will profoundly affect the techniques used to motivate staff members and, in turn, the workers' response. A dentist who views workers through Theory X will have much tighter control and use more external rewards than the Theory Y-oriented dentist. This highly controlling, distrustful atmosphere may be appropriate in certain situations, but the dentist must be willing to realize the almost inevitable results: employee resentment, turnover, and dissatisfaction. The Theory Y dentist, on the other hand, must also be aware of the limitations of the system. Too often, ideas of efficiency, production, and results are considered secondary to the people's growth and enjoyment of work. Purely internal rewards may not be enough to get total results.

Need Theories

Need theories are based on the supposition that everyone has needs or internal stimuli that they want to satisfy. Jobs have various attributes that may or may not correlate with a person's needs. Because actions are based on some intrinsically (within the individual) determined need, it is assumed that everyone will react similarly. This perspective, then, assumes that attitudes, job characteristics, and behavior are related. People's behavior is an attempt to satisfy needs. Incentives reward people for satisfying those needs. Needs determine the motivational value of incentives. The job of the manager is to decide what those needs are and then to structure the work environment to allow people to satisfy those needs best.

Abraham Maslow developed the best-known idea of human motivation. Maslow believed that people have essentially five different levels of needs, or internal stimuli. These are physiological, safety, belongingness, esteem, and self-actualization. One well-known simplification of

Table 20.7 ERG Theory

Alderfer's Levels	Components
Growth (Personal)	Self-esteem; self-actualization; achievement
Relatedness (Social)	Social and interpersonal relations; esteem of others
Existence (Pay and benefits)	Physical safety and human existence

Box 20.10 Equity Theory

$$\frac{I_s}{O_s} = \frac{I_o}{O_o}$$

I_s Input of Self
I_o Input of Others
O_s Output of Self
O_o Output of Others

Maslow's Hierarchy was proposed by Clayton Alderfer. His modification collapsed the five levels of needs into three: existence, relatedness, and growth, and is known as ERG Theory (Table 20.7). He believed that all three levels influence work motivation but not equally. Existence needs are satisfied primarily by extrinsic rewards (e.g., pay, fringe benefits). Relatedness is satisfied through friendships and interaction with coworkers. Growth needs (the highest preference needs) are intrinsic motivators and are encouraged through the opportunity to learn and advance and through positive responses. People can respond to different levels simultaneously. For example, money (E), friendship (R), and learning new skills (G), may all be motivators for a person. Alderfer's theory forms the basis of the initial proposition of this part, that people work for compensation (existence), social reasons (relatedness), and personal reasons (growth).

The implications of ERG theory for dentists are important. Dentists cannot change employees' needs, but they can react to them by manipulating the incentives (means) to satisfy them. Dentists must tie existence needs to incentives to work. Formal and informal groups and formal titles and office organization will meet relatedness needs in the dental office. The dentist can influence all these. The dentist can meet growth needs by creating a proper climate that will encourage and enable employees to develop to their full potential.

Dentists may see the effects of unrecognized needs in the common dental office problem of staff members (often hygienists) having basic existence and relatedness needs being met and still being unfulfilled in the job role. Often, this situation is a result of the staff member wanting to fulfill those higher level needs represented by growth or actualization. If no one allows and encourages these people to expand their roles, continued unhappiness and eventual departure are the almost inevitable results.

Equity Theory

Equity Theory is based on group influences (Box 20.10). It asks whether people feel that they are being treated fairly compared with others, based on the value of their contribution. Each person has expected outcomes (rewards) from the work setting. These may be external (pay, promotion, benefits) or internal (recognition, social relationships, satisfaction). To get those outcomes, people realize that they must have certain inputs. These may take the form of time, expertise, effort, education, hours worked, certification, or loyalty. Equity theory assumes that people compare themselves with others and assess the fairness of the outcome considering the inputs required. This "other" may be a specific person or group of people, or it may be a composite of a given workforce. Based on this subjective and personal comparison, employees will decide that they are equitably rewarded, under-rewarded, or over-rewarded for the input required. If the employees feel that they are under-rewarded, they will likely put forth less effort (lower inputs), ask for a raise (increase inputs), rationalize the difference, get others to change their inputs or outcomes, or seek new employment. If employees feel that they are overcompensated, they may increase their effort to balance the outputs, or simply justify the higher reward.

Equity Theory has clear implications for the dentist for managing a dental practice. This theory is based on group and social norms, which are prevalent in small businesses. It involves a person's perception of values of inputs and outcomes. Those perceptions, although not necessarily the truth, are reality for that person, and they must be viewed as such. The accuracy of a person's information becomes important. People may view the group to which they compare themselves entirely differently from the dentist. This raises the problems of job values and comparable worth of different jobs in the office. Finally, for rewards to motivate, they must perceive them as fair and equitable, or the difference will simply exacerbate the problem.

Equity Theory probably has more implications for pay practices than any aspect related to practice management. Auxiliaries in a practice will compare earnings, and any discrepancy between what a person earns and what a person believes they should earn may result in problems. Consequently, the dentist should pay particular attention to designing a compensation system that is equitable and well understood by the employees. Dentists should tell the employee how the dentist relates performance to possible pay increases and what level of performance will result in a salary increase.

Employees compare their wages to other people in the dental office. Although it is easy to make a policy that, "All pay issues should be strictly confidential," it is quite another to keep that confidentiality. Eventually, everyone in the office will know what everyone else is making. They will then compare their pay to others to see if they are being treated, in their mind, fairly or equitably. If the employees do not understand how salaries are determined, feelings of resentment and hostility may arise because of a lack of knowledge about how the dentist decides salaries. The hygienist may make $5 an hour more than an expanded duty dental assistant (EDDA), but an employee may see that as reasonable given the additional training and certification required of the hygienist. However, if another assistant makes 50 cents an hour more but has no additional skills, training or work habits, the same employee will see that as inequitable and cause employee job dissatisfaction. This comparison of other employees in the office is called *internal equity*.

Employees make the same types of comparisons with alternate forms of employment in the same geographic area. This comparison is called *external equity*. A staff member may know other dental assistants who are working for other local dentists and make different wage and benefit rates. Or a person with the general training and skill level of a dental assistant may work at a local bank or grocery store for $3 more an hour and a complete benefit package. Both external comparisons lead to equity considerations that are outside the control of the practitioner.

Employees may feel either or both types of equity problems simultaneously. Both internal and external types are important to employees and therefore are important in wage rate determinations. The prevailing economic conditions, general wage and benefit rates, and the local unemployment rates all affect the amount that dentists need to pay to attract productive employees.

Incentive Plans: Using Money to Motivate

Many dentists believe that money motivates all employees. All they need to do is to establish a bonus or incentive plan and all of the employees will work harder to make more money. Often a bonus plan can help the office to increase productivity. Unfortunately, this idea is not a panacea for poor management. Dentists must carefully structure incentive plans or else the plans may backfire and cause more problems than what was started with.

Guidelines for Incentive Plans

Each Incentive Plan Must Have a Specific Goal

Most employers have the simple goal of "increasing production." However, they must accurately identify the real problem. The problem may be a lack of new patients or a poor collection policy. If an ineffective recall system, poor scheduling, or poorly performing employees are the cause of low production, the dentist should address the problem first. By establishing goals and rewards that address the specific problem, an incentive plan can help to achieve the ultimate goal of increased production.

Each Plan Must Have Appropriate Rewards

The dentist must be sure that his or her incentive plan has a proper reward system for the employees. Not all employees are motivated by money. (In fact, many employees are internally motivated.) Certainly, the prospect of making more money motivates some employees to work harder. Others may not feel that the rewards are worth the extra work, time, and effort required. They may be motivated by the possibility of extra time off, office trips, or additional continuing education courses. When offices have employees who are motivated by different incentives, establishing an effective bonus plan can be difficult.

Staff Members Must Have Control over Critical Factors Needed to Meet the Goal

If the dentist is slowing down production (because he or she enjoys talking with patients), staff has no real control of the problem (dentist's style). They can, therefore, do nothing to increase production (schedule effectively). Staff performance must be the critical factor that is causing the lack of goal attainment.

The Dentist Must Be Ready to Manage Collateral Problems

Every action in the dental office has collateral, or unintended, side effects. The employee focus becomes attainment of the goal, not necessarily the work itself. If the dentist wants to see additional patients and the schedule is full, he or she should be ready to work longer hours or through lunch.

Incentive Plans Lose Their Effectiveness over Time

The lack of money can be a demotivator, but money will only be a short-term incentive. Soon employees grow to expect the bonus as pay. A guaranteed bonus decreases the motivation to work hard to achieve the bonus. However, constantly increasing the goal leads to staff frustration as dentists expect them to achieve ever higher levels of production.

Developing Incentive Plans

Given these problems with incentive plans, dentists need to follow certain steps if they want to develop an effective plan.

Make Sure Management Systems Are Well Constructed

The dentist should make sure to do everything that he or she, as the practice owner and manager, can do to increase production. The dentist should have an excellent scheduling system; have employee job descriptions, performance appraisals, and compensation policies in line; and make sure credit and collection policies are effective.

Be Sure Incentive System Is Easy to Administer and Understand

The dentist can probably pick out one or two numbers (from the end-of-month computer report) and decide if he or she has met goals. The dentist also needs an easy method of dividing the bonus. Is it equal shares, based on pay, or based on hours worked?

Identify Goals to Achieve

Most offices simply say they "want to increase production." Is that really the goal, or is the real goal to increase staff productivity to increase doctor take-home pay the actual goal? Some goals are best for individuals, others for groups. If the goal is to increase recall effectiveness and the hygienist runs the recall system, the dentist does not need to involve others in the incentive system. Conversely, a goal of increasing new patient visits will probably need to involve everyone in the office.

Identify What Motivates Employees

The challenge may motivate some employees. Additional vacation days, additional money, or an office vacation may motivate others. The dentist should talk with the employees and come to a consensus on what will get the employees to buy into the incentive plan. The dentist should set a reward system that is achievable but is also difficult to attain.

Follow-up

Employees need to know how well they are doing in meeting the goals. When the dentist and staff meets the goals, all should celebrate and be congratulated. If the goals are not met, the dentist should sit with everyone and develop a plan to meet them the next period. The dentist should be careful that incentives do not become entitlements.

Part 4: Assessing Employee Performance

Start with good people, lay out the rules, communicate with your employees, motivate them and reward them. If you do all those things effectively, you can't miss.
Lee Iacocca

Key Terms

constructive discharge	unjust dismissal (wrong
implied contract	termination)
performance appraisal	whistle-blower
review (PAR)	
progressive discipline	

Objectives

At the completion of this part, the student will be able to:
1. Describe how to develop a performance appraisal review.
2. Describe the process for terminating employees.
3. Describe the areas a former employee might successfully sue for wrongful termination.
4. Describe the use of performance appraisals in the dental office.
5. Describe the progressive discipline system.
6. Describe how an employee might try to "get even" for being fired.

Goal

The goal of this part is to prepare new graduates to hire, compensate, and motivate staff for the dental office.

Most employees want to do well on the job. Both intrinsic and extrinsic rewards are valid goals toward which workers strive. They need and want fair and accurate appraisals based on standards of performance that explain what the dentist expects of them. Dentists should not compare employees with each other but rather should evaluate them based on how well they perform on the job. Appraisals should identify individual outputs or goals. They must also be honest to be effective. If employees perceive the appraisals as dishonest, (e.g., performance was not adequate but was rated as adequate), then the employees will be ineffective. Appraisals should evaluate levels of skill, knowledge, responsibilities, and special certification but not the worth of the job itself. Employees should not view appraisals as punitive but as suggesting ways to improve. A formal system of response must be incorporated so that the employee can relate personal performance to the review.

Given these requirements for fair and accurate performance appraisals, it is little wonder that both managing dentists and workers view them suspiciously. Everyone appraises each of their associates continually and informally. (Coffee room gossip frequently concerns people who are not present.) Dentists also continually assess (informally) the appearance, behavior, and motivation of workers. Yet when dentists begin a formal system of review, there is often initial resistance both from staff and from the owner–dentist. Employees fear job appraisals for reasons of job security and reprisals. Dentists are fearful because of the time needed, the responsibility for objectivity, and the loss of personal power to a "system." Once a proper system is in place and working, however, both employees and dentists generally find their fears to be unfounded.

Performance Appraisal and Reviews

Performance appraisal and reviews (PARs) have two general purposes. First, they justify personnel actions. By objectively appraising work done, the manager has a strong basis for personnel actions. These include promotion, rewards for past performance, probationary reviews, and warnings for unacceptable behavior. Second, PARs help counsel employees. Managers can better use staff by improving performance, assigning work more efficiently, meeting employees' needs for growth, recognizing potentials, and identifying training needs.

The result of the performance appraisals should not be a surprise to an employee. Dentists should give immediate, constructive feedback every day of practice. If an employee does a particularly good job at a task, the dentist should praise them on the spot. The dentist should let the employee know (sincerely) why this was such good performance and how much that means to the success of the practice. The employee likely will repeat this behavior or action. Conversely, if someone does a poor job, the dentist should tell him or her on the spot (in private) why the behavior or performance was unacceptable and what he or she can do to improve their performance. Most employees will try to improve.

PARs have several spin-off uses as well. They help in the selection/hiring process. Selection of the best person for any job is a difficult task. To find the best person, employers first identify job-related behaviors and qualifications so that they can find someone who meets those criteria. This is the basis of PAR systems. Instead of an informal, intuitive idea of traits needed, dentists generate a list of specific characteristics from the review process. They can use properly conducted PARs as contracts. Dentists can, by using PARs for feedback, goal setting, rewards, punishments, motivate employees to accept change. Dentists are on much more solid legal ground when they take personnel actions if a PAR system is in use. They can objectively show reasons for promotion, raises, and dismissals. The use of PAR systems can improve employee involvement in the practice. Employees who do tasks often define acceptable behaviors better than the managers who oversee them. By defining goals and objectives and gaining the active participation of employees in the process, dentists improve the performance of the whole organization.

Constructing the Performance Appraisal and Review

Dentists must properly construct performance appraisals to be effective. Done poorly or under unsatisfactory conditions, the PARs may be detrimental to employee motivation and performance. Dentists should the following guidelines for effective performance reviews:

- Before conducting the review, the dentist should determine the purpose (coaching, salary appraisal, criticism) and ensure that objectives do not conflict with each other.
- The dentist should be sure that the staff members know what is expected of them in their jobs. Many dentists use the employee's job description as the basis of the performance appraisal. This document describes what tasks the employee does on the job. It is outcome related, not attitudinal. That is to say, it looks at job behaviors (what people do on the job), not attitudes (whether or not they like their job).
- A PAR should reflect all of the duties involved in the job, but only those duties. Components should be weighted to represent their importance.
- The dentist should set standards of acceptable behaviors and should present employees the "who, how, what, and when" of performance. Both acceptable and unacceptable behaviors should be specified.
- The dentist should give an immediate, constructive response so that employees know the results of the appraisal. Writing down a verbal appraisal gives direction to the employee and is a strong base in future disagreements.

- The dentist should develop tangible and identifiable rewards, punishments, or assistance for outcomes or specific behaviors.
- The PAR should be an ongoing, long-term system for performance improvement rather than a one-time punitive system. Follow up with "mini-reviews" of problems identified during the formal review. If the PARs are used simply to dismiss employees, employees will perceive it as such and they will lose all effectiveness.
- The dentist should seek the employee's input during the review about his or her performance and problems on the job. The dentist should ask for ways that could make the job easier (and therefore the office more efficient). Many dental staff members doubt that their dentists truly listen to their job problems, so it is important that dentists listen.
- The PAR should not replace continual immediate reactions in the workplace. If a staff member does a task particularly well or poorly, that should be notice and commented on at the time. The dentist can then reinforce it at PAR time. The dentist should keep a written log throughout the year of staff members' performance to help at review time.

The dentist should consider several other issues before starting a PAR system. He or she should have well-defined, written philosophies and goals. Unless the dentist clearly defines the target or performance, employees can not aim for it. Institution of such a system may require changes in the dentist's philosophy, policies, or procedures. Additionally, the dentist needs to remember that a PAR system is an ongoing review process, not a one-time effort, and should be willing to reward through salary increases and other methods of compensation those people who perform well. Finally, the dentist need to be willing to spend the time and energy needed to develop and carry out such a system.

Disciplining Employees

Most employment experts suggest that the proper way to discipline employees involves a system called "Progressive Discipline." In this system, the dentist provides and records feedback that is given to an employee about his or her performance, suggesting ways to improve faulty performance. If the employee does not improve performance, then each round of discipline becomes progressively more severe until the dentist fires the employee.

Progressive discipline encourages employees to improve performance. It also documents their poor performance. In the progressive discipline scenario, the dentist gives an employee who is not performing to expectations a verbal reprimand, with methods to improve their performance. The dentist notes that

reprimand in the employee's personnel file. If the employee continues to perform poorly, the dentist gives a written notice (again with a copy in the personnel file) and methods to improve. If the employee shows no improvement, the dentist suspends him or her for several days with warning of possible termination. Continued poor performance leads to firing. By using this method, employees cannot reasonably claim that they did not know that their performance was below standard or that their job was in jeopardy. It is also fair in that it encourages the employee to improve performance; it does not simply threaten them.

Progressive discipline requires that the dentist keeps written documentation of all warnings to employees about their performance. Fortunately, this is not as big a problem as it initially sounds. As the discipline becomes more severe, the documentation should be more thorough. (Initial counseling may warrant a two-line note, jotted down in the employee's personnel file.) Written documentation should include the following.

1. The reason for the problem
2. Corrective action to improve performance
3. Employee comments
4. Employee's signature and date
5. Employer's signature and date

This system provides documentation of employee performance problems in the case that the employee files charges for a breach of employer responsibility. It also helps keep discipline consistent from employee to employee. Through the act of counseling, many employees will improve their performance so that they do not need additional disciplinary steps. Finally, the dentist may find areas of policies and procedures that need to be revised to make the office work environment more effective.

It is important that dentists take action in all situations of poor job performance. Failure to take action tells employees that the dentist has no standards for work in the office. If a dentist does not take notice of an employee's sloppy work practices, then the others see that it does not matter if they are sloppy too. The end is lower standards and bad service to patients. Taking no action is a decision that may also prevent a dentist from taking action in the future in a similar situation. If the dentist suddenly treats one employee differently than other for a similar act of poor performance, then he or she is opened up to charges of unfairness in the workplace.

Guidelines of Progressive Discipline

Several things to remember if the dentist decides to use a progressive discipline system in the office:

The goal of the system is to catch poor or marginal performance early, and then help employees to improve their performance in areas where problems have been problems. Early coaching becomes important. The dentist may require an employee to take a continuing education course or do other study, practice, or demonstration to improve his or her skills. Punishment is appropriate for employees who do not improve performance.

The dentist may repeat a step if he or she believes that it will help to improve performance. For example, the dentist may decide that a significant amount of time has passed since the last warning and that another warning is in order. If repeating the warning and remediation works, then the dentist has solved the problem without escalating to a higher level. The employee should understand, however, that repeating a step may lead to higher forms of discipline.

The dentist may skip steps for serious offenses or breaches of office policy. He or she will generally use all of the steps for more routine problems, such as attendance or general work performance problems. The dentist's judgment of the severity of the offense and remediation (if any) will help to define the steps to use.

Several behaviors are often excluded from a progressive discipline system. Employees are generally immediately fired for any of the following offenses:

- Reporting to work intoxicated or impaired on alcohol or illegal drugs
- Stealing from the practice or another employee
- Lying on an employment application or other practice documents
- Violating confidentiality of practice or patient information
- Causing a fight in the work place
- Bringing a weapon to work
- Intentionally harassing someone (including sexual harassment)
- Insubordination
- Extended unexcused absences

The dentist should talk with the employee about the problem and explain what acceptable behavior is and what the consequence of failure to act properly is.

Counseling should be done in a friendly yet firm way. Tell the employee the problem and try to identify a solution for the problem jointly. The dentist should be sure that the employee has a way that he or she can solve the performance problem. Often documentation of counseling is brief, but the dentist should save it in the employee's personnel file in case the performance problem continues or escalates.

If an employee is suspended from work, the dentist should tell the employee the length of the suspension and that it is a suspension without pay. Usually one to several days is enough to set the stage and impress the employee with the seriousness of the problem. (Some states require that dentists suspend professional people [associate dentists or some hygienists] in week-long time blocks. Dentists should check with an attorney familiar with the state's employment law.)

For serious problems (anything more than a verbal warning), the dentist should require the employee to sign the form, acknowledging that the problem has been discussed, and the corrective steps required. This does not mean that the employee agrees (they do not have to agree with the dentist's assessment), but that the dentist has discussed the problem with him or her. If the employee disagrees or wants to offer an explanation for his or her actions (there ore often two sides to a story), have then the dentist should write those on the back of the disciplinary record form. If an employee refuses to sign the form, the dentist should record (on the form) that the employee refused to sign.

Some management experts suggest that the dentist not include the progressive discipline plan in the employee manual. If a dentist does, he or she should contact an employment lawyer first to check on the language and wording in the policy. The policy probably will not be used often, so if the rules are not followed exactly each time an incident occurs, the dentist might be in trouble. Employers should treat employees equally. If the dentist does not warn one employee about a particular performance problem but warns another, the progressive discipline process may not protect the dentist.

Terminating Employees

Terminating (firing) an employee is perhaps the least enjoyable job a business owner can have. The dentist should view firing an employee as the last option for personnel issues. If the recruitment and selection process has worked properly, if the dentist has given specific direction and performance response to employees, and if the compensation system is fair and equitable, firing should seldom be an issue. However, this is not always the case.

The practice may be better off by not having a particular employee around. If a staff member is not performing adequately, if the dentist has given him or her notice and methods of improvement, and if the employee continues to perform inadequately, then firing may be in order. If an employee is found in gross violation of established laws, rules, or policies (e.g., stealing, alcohol impairment on the job, continual insubordination), firing is necessary. Finally, if a personality conflict has developed that severely impairs the effectiveness of the office team, dismissal may be in order.

Guidelines for Terminating Employees

If all attempts to salvage an employee through a progressive discipline process have failed and the dentist decides it is time to fire that employee, these guidelines should be followed.

- The dentist should decide beforehand will be said and should have all information concerning the problem ready.
- The dentist should carefully select the day of dismissal. Most management experts suggest not to fire someone on Friday or the day before a holiday. This gives the person the weekend to stew and possibly plot revenge; the dismissed employee should be able to look for another job quickly.
- All paperwork should be in order. The dentist should be sure that time records are accurate (and not forged) and see if the person is due any vacation days or other benefit. If so, the employee should be compensated for them. The dentist should not provoke the employee or give him or her any reason to involve the wage and hour cabinet.
- The dentist should be firm and businesslike, but sympathetic. He or she should not berate the employee for work that was not done properly and should not argue with the employee over the validity of the information. The decision is final.
- The meeting should be no more than 15 minutes. It should be kept private and brief. The person's final pay check, including compensation, any benefits owed, or severance pay should be ready to be given to the employee.
- The employer should inform the employee what will be said regarding future references from other potential employers.
- The employer should encourage the employee to seek employment counseling or job placement services and can provide the names of several agencies to give the person.
- The employer should take care of housekeeping duties, such as office keys, instruments, personal effects, or other materials that either person must return.
- The employer should manage the effect of the firing on the other employees. If the other employees are not aware of all of the problems, they may be wondering if they are next to be fired. If they are aware of the problems, this will be less an issue. The dentist should not discuss shortcomings of the released employee with the other employees; this invites defamation and slander actions.

Legal Issues in Dismissal of Employees

Three primary issues are involved in firing employees. They are unemployment compensation problems, wage and hour laws, and legal suits related to unjust dismissal. Of these, the unemployment issue is by far the more common. The unjust dismissal case, although far less common, is far more serious. Wage and hour law problems are in the middle on both counts.

Unemployment Insurance

Unemployment insurance premiums are dependent on an employer's employment history, just as automobile insurance depends on a driving record. When a former employee collects unemployment compensation, it is credited against the employer's "account." Premiums may vary as a result. Unemployment compensation is available to people who lose their jobs through no fault of their own. People cannot collect unemployment if they quit a job, if someone fired them for unwillingness to work on the job, or other due cause. If the person tries to collect unemployment or contests the firing (saying that they were not fired for cause), the unemployment department may call the employer into a hearing on the matter. This is where excellent records help. If the employer has documented the problem through performance appraisals, written warnings, and suggested improvements, he or she will have no problem. Without these records, the employer may see his or her unemployment insurance rates increase.

Wage and Hour Laws

The federal government sets employment rules through the FLSA. Each state has a "Wage and Hour Cabinet" or commission (they go by slightly different names) that enforces the national wage and hour laws in their state. Generally, they only become involved with an office if someone files a grievance against that employer. (They occasionally make routine "field audits.") If an employee (or usually, a former employee) files a grievance concerning employment practices, they may require an employer produce evidence to refute the claim. This is one of those cases in which the employer is, in reality, considered guilty unless he or she can prove his or her innocence. Excellent employee records are important. The cabinet may use all call time sheets, pay records, office policies, and vacation schedules into the review. If the employer has kept excellent records and has followed the laws about fair employment in the state, he or she should have no problems. If the employer cannot refute the claim, he or she may have to pay back overtime, vacation, or benefits plus penalties.

Unjust Dismissal (Wrongful Termination) Suits

According to the doctrine of employment-at-will, if an employee does not have a specified term of employment (such as in a contract), then that employee works "at will." Either side can end the employment relationship anytime for any reason (at the will of either party). The corollary of this doctrine is the *fire at will doctrine*, which says that an employer can fire an employee (noncontracted) any time for any reason. Although these general principles are still in force, the courts have eroded them over time, as legislatures have limited the right of employers to fire employees. Four areas have been singled out that may result in a wrongful termination lawsuit (Box 20.11).

1. *Antidiscrimination* An employer may not fire an employee for a "wrong" reason. Several different laws contribute to this list, but it generally it includes race, color, national origin, gender, age, disability, pregnancy, and religion. Although written statutes protect many of these groups only for large employers (15 or more employees), often courts hold the small employer to the standards of the larger employers. Many state and local laws apply these standards to all employers in their jurisdiction. So the essence is, do not discriminate in hiring or firing practices.
2. *Oral contract* Oral contracts are just as binding as written contracts. The problem with oral contracts is that when it is time to interpret them, each side has a different memory of what was said. However, if the court finds that an employer made an oral promise of job security to an employee, the court will probably find that it is a legally binding contract.
3. *Contrary to public policy* An employer may not fire an employee if he or she is being fired for actions that are in the public's interest. This includes items such as jury duty or military duty. It also covers employees who raise questions about work procedures that are illegal or especially dangerous. This is the basis for the whistle-blower court decisions. In these, employees who have been fired for telling of their company's illegal or immoral actions have won wrongful termination suits.
4. *Implied contract* Often, the employees' handbook, office manuals, employment applications, or performance appraisals contain language that implies job security. These "implied contracts" are not direct agreements, but sometimes the courts interpret them as a form of promise, or contract. Such documents should include language that advises that an employer is an at-will employer and that none of the documents are or imply a contract.

Box 20.11 Examples of Wrongful Termination

Antidiscrimination
An assistant is pregnant. The dentist terminates her because she does not plan to return after having the baby; the dentist wants to go ahead and get a "steady" employee. Her wrongful termination suit will probably win.

Oral Contract
A dentist has told an assistant that as long as performance is good, employment is guaranteed. As a result of the closing of a local plant, the practice is in steep decline and the dentist terminates the assistant. Even though the economic problems of the practice were not foreseen, the oral contract is binding as long as the assistant's performance is good.

Public Policy
The dentist has instructed an assistant to scale "small chunks" of calculus when necessary, even though this is contrary to the state's dental practice act. The hygienist threatens to inform the state board of dentistry if the practice continues. The dentist fires the hygienist, citing a bad attitude and not being part of the team. The wrongful termination suit will probably be upheld because the hygienist was acting in the public's interest and according to law.

Implied Contract
The office manual states that employees will be retained if their performance appraisals are good. If the dentist terminates an employee who has good performance appraisals, he or she may be subject to wrongful termination suits based on this principle.

Constructive Discharge

Many employers try to get around these problems by forcing or enticing the employee to quit. The employer may do this by offering a good letter of recommendation or a severance bonus if the employee resigns. The employer might assign the employee excessive overtime or work or give a pay cut with the intention that the employee will become dissatisfied and quit. Often employers take this approach when they fear a wrongful termination suit or other problem resulting from the firing. The courts generally rule that this is a constructive discharge, or in fact, firing. They often uphold a constructive discharge claim when evidence shows that the circumstances the employee was under were "unreasonable" and the employer was trying to make the employee quit. Damage awards in these cases are similar to wrongful termination awards.

Retribution by a (Former) Employee

A former employee may try to "get even" with an employer for being fired. Some are legal, others not. Besides the previously mentioned FLSA, a former employee may file a complaint with OSHA claiming an unsafe workplace. The former employee may call the state's board of dentistry and lodge a complaint against a practice. If the employee knows that an employer has cheated on taxes (e.g., not reporting cash income from patients), the employee can turn the employer into the IRS and receive a bounty of 25 percent of all back taxes, penalties, and interest collected. This is in addition to the aggravation that the former employee knows he or she has caused. In these cases, prevention through best business practices and records are the best defense.

Former employees have also been guilty of mischief, from trivial to major. The employer should be sure to collect office keys at the time of firing to avoid internal mischief or theft. If an employer has any question of a fired employee's (or spouse's) intent, the locks on the doors should be changed immediately. If there is a security system in place, the access codes should be changed. The employer should also have a current back-up of the computer system data to avoid mischief or data catastrophes and have the back-up off site. The employer should further be prepared for possible slanderous or libelous statements from the disgruntled employee.

Maintaining Daily Operations

chapter 21

Part 1: Office Operations

Efficiency is doing things right; effectiveness is doing the right things.
Peter Drucker

Objectives

At the completion of this part, the student will be able to:
1. Compare efficiency and effectiveness.
2. Describe what factors affect capacity.
3. Describe how to affect capacity used.

Key Terms

capacity	effectiveness
capacity utilized	efficiency

Goal

The goal of this part is to describe several techniques that improve the efficiency of office operations.

Business Basics for Dentists, First Edition. David O. Willis.
© 2013 John Wiley & Sons, Inc. Published 2013 by John Wiley & Sons, Inc.

Efficiency and Effectiveness

In operating a productive practice, dentists need to be both efficient and effective.

Efficiency

Efficiency looks at how cheaply something is done. The focus is costs. The intention is to save money, time, or effort regardless quality. To become more efficient, people simply must lower costs. Efficiency measures productivity at the individual process level, regardless the collateral effects of the decision (Table 21.1). It often requires conforming to norms. In this way, the process is no worse than others in the industry. It examines internal, technical issues. The result is to improve profitability by working harder and quicker.

In dentistry, efficiency comes from doing procedures correctly the first time, without remakes. Not only does the dentist have the cost of additional materials, staff, and lab charges, but he or she has also lost the additional production he or she could have during the time spent with the remake. Clinical decision making is the prime factor that increases clinical speed.

Effectiveness

Effectiveness looks at how well something is done. Here, the focus is the benefit or outcome of the process. The intention is to improve quality at a higher level than the individual process, thereby raising performance levels. It measures how well the job gets done, or the correctness of a product or service. Effectiveness then is a quality measure, not a cost measure. It examines external, strategic results. The outcome of effectiveness is improving profitability by working smarter.

As an example of the difference in a dental practice, dentists can be more efficient (lowering costs) if they use a foreign lab. However, dentists may be less effective in crown and bridge work because of more remakes and lower patient satisfaction that result. So here, effectiveness trumps efficiency. Using the foreign lab costs less, but dentists are not doing their job as well. So simply doing something less expensively does not necessarily lead to more profit. In all of office decisions, dentists must be sure that they are both efficient and effective.

Table 21.1 Efficiency versus Effectiveness

Efficiency	Effectiveness
How cheaply you do something	How well you do something
Costs	Quality
Process	Outcomes
Working harder, quicker	Working smarter

Capacity

Capacity is the ability of the office to see patients. It is the maximum number of patient visits (or appointments) that the office has available for a given period. The way dentists plan and organize the office ultimately decides the ability to see patients. This configuration can (and should) change over time. As the practice matures, the number and type of patient visits change. Although capacity defines a dentist's ability to see patients, marketing brings those patients in and fill available chair time. Both sides (driving demand and then seeing those patients generated) need to be satisfied for success. The dentist's practice philosophy guides the changes made in the operational and marketing systems to achieve goals.

What Determines Capacity

Capacity is affected by all of the management decisions dentists make in the office.

Number of Operatories

The number of operatories has an obvious and important effect on the dentist's ability to see patients. However, the dentist must be sure that proper staffing levels support the operatories. Seven operatories will not let a dentist see more patients than one operatory, without staff support. The additional six operatories become nothing but expensive waiting rooms. Generally, dentists assign one chairside assistant to one operatory. The assistants are responsible for chairside assisting during patient procedures, set up, break down, and disinfection of the operatory between patients.

Operator Speed

The dentist's speed when doing patient procedures determines the length of appointments and therefore the number of available appointment slots. Operator speed is not really dependent on "hand skills" and physical speed. Speed in completing patient procedures depends on the dentist doing the procedure correctly without remakes. This means that the dentist and staff are knowledgeable about each step of every procedure and that they take their time to do procedures correctly, as opposed to just doing them quickly. Operator speed then increases automatically with experience. As staff members become more accustomed to the dentist and better trained in specific procedures, the dentist can move more quickly through procedures without internal "wait time" for mixing materials, repositioning patients, or other small inefficiencies. That training does not just "happen." It is the dentist's responsibility to ensure that staff training is an ongoing office function.

Office Hours

The more hours that a dentist is open, the more appointments are available. There are some limitations. Most people want time away from the office for personal and family enjoyment. So although working 80 hours a week opens many appointment slots, most dentists are not willing to make the sacrifices involved in the trade off. (The typical practicing dentist works 35 hours per week, according to the American Dental Association [ADA].)

Many patients want to come to the dentist during nontraditional hours (evenings and weekends). If a dentist keeps "bankers' hours" (9 to 5 Monday through Friday) then he or she may lose some patients to other dentists who are open during those "off" hours. Although the marketing and operational considerations encourage use of off hours, staff considerations do not. If staff works more than 40 hours per week (in most states), then they must receive overtime pay. Staff members generally do not want to work evenings or Saturdays for the same reasons dentists do not. (They would rather spend time in personal or family pursuits. They may have children in day care or after-school programs.) So although there are reasons to work extended hours, the dentist must consider trade-offs.

Early in a dentist's practice life cycle, he or she needs to generate patients for the practice. To do this, the dentist may keep more off-peak hours (evenings and weekends). If the available appointments cannot be filled, he or she may close the office for some traditional business hours to decrease costs. As the practice becomes more mature, the number of patients waiting for treatment increases. The dentist can then cut back on off-peak hours, forcing patients into the more traditional appointment slots. If the patients cannot make these appointments, they may go elsewhere for treatment, but the dentist will generally have other patients waiting to fill the appointment slot.

Number and Types of Staff Members

Operational decisions do not affect facility costs greatly, unless the dentist decides to expand the office to increase capacity. The dentist pays rent regardless the number of hours worked. Utility costs may be higher with additional or evening hours, but the lights are on for all working hours regardless. The biggest cost item is staff cost. If a dentist has existing staff members work additional hours, he or she may have overtime costs. The dentist may have to offer differential pay to induce someone to work nontraditional hours. He or she may also have extra costs as the result of hiring additional part-time staff members.

Many dentists hire part-time staff. They may hire them to work during a busy time of the day (e.g., evenings) or to do a particular function in the office (e.g., collecting accounts). With either type, dentists only hire people for the times that they are needed most, improving office efficiency.

Chairside Assistants

As a rule, a dentist needs one chairside assistant for each operatory. (If a dentist has seven operatories and one assistant, he or she cannot see many more patients than with one operatory and one assistant.) Fewer assistants lead to the extra chair being unused, more and the additional staff are not as needed.

Expanded Functions

If the practice state allows expanded functions by trained (or certified) dental assistants, then additional operatories can significantly increase capacity. These staff members can be completing intraoral procedures while the dentist sees additional patients.

Receptionists

Receptionists are necessary for smooth and efficient operation. A lack of receptionists will decrease recall patient visits (because the receptionist is too harried to manage the recall system effectively). This also leads to a decrease in overall patient visits (as a result of inadequate scheduling procedures.) As a rule, one receptionist can handle up to 1,000 patients per quarter (18 to 20 per day) with no decrease in effectiveness. As the number of patients increases above this number, office capacity decreases unless additional receptionist help is hired.

Hygienists

Hygienists increase capacity by freeing the dentist to see other patients (if there are adequate chairs available). If the office does not have enough operatories available, then the hygienist merely trades chair time with the dentist. The total capacity remains the same. They contribute to increased production and profit in the office. Hygienists also generate demand for the practice by seeing additional diagnostic (recall) patients that have other work to be done.

Owner Wants, Needs, and Desires

The owners' wants, needs, and desires heavily influence office capacity. Some dentists do not want a large, "run and gun" practice. They prefer a more intimate, personal style of practice. Neither extreme is right nor wrong, merely personal preference. Regardless of the practitioner's desires, an efficiently run practice that fully uses available capacity will be more profitably than a less efficiently run one.

Office Systems

The way that office systems are structured also affects capacity. If a dentist organizes patient scheduling around 10-minute blocks, then he or she can see more patients than if 15-minute blocks are used (assuming adequate patient demand and operator ability). If the instrument management system is not able to provide enough sterile instruments sets, there will be a capacity limitation.

Capacity Utilization

Capacity utilization measures the actual use of potential appointment time. It is calculated by dividing capacity (potential patient visits) by the number of actual patient visits for a period. The result is the percentage of available appointments (chair time) that were actually filled. Ninety percent use and above is very good; 80 to 90 percent is OK; and below 80 percent shows that the office resources are not well used. Early in the practice cycle, capacity utilization may be lower as available appointment time goes unused. As capacity utilized increases above 90 percent, it signals the need to expand capacity or to become more efficient to increase profit.

Capacity utilization is the primary measure of office efficiency. It does not depend on the number of operatories (chairs) or staff. (Both an eight-operatory office and a one-operatory office should have their capacity well used.) Because a significant part of dental office costs are fixed, it becomes important to use those fixed costs efficiently. Both large or small offices can be efficiently operated. This measure suggests if this is happening.

Increasing Patient Visits

Patient visits then are the driving force of a profitable dental practice. The key to maintaining efficiency (high capacity utilized) is to increase capacity as dictated by patient load. There is a need to anticipate growth in patient visits. (Dentists do not want to turn people away because they do not have the capacity to see the patients, especially early in the practice life when they are trying to build patient pool.) So the dentist increases capacity in anticipation of additional patient visits.

A practice's service mix describes the types of dental procedures that the office does. Patient visits are divided into three types: diagnostic, basic services, and complex (major) services. Diagnostic visits involve new patients and routine recare (recall) procedures. They are where the dentist identifies additional work that a patient needs. Basic care includes restorations, endodontics, and surgical procedures. These visits prepare the way for the complex visits, which generally involve laboratory work and multiple-visit procedures. Each type of visit is necessary for a profitable practice. Expanding the service mix (by taking continuing education to increase or improve the types of procedures done) increases the number of patient visits within the office.

Marketing efforts, both internal and external, are a common way to generate additional patients. These include making more nontraditional hours available, changing credit and collection policies, and increasing insurance plan participation. Aggressive dentists may buy another practice or merge practices to increase patient pool.

Daily Scheduling

Hours

Dentists typically work about 40 hours a week, 32 of them in direct patient contact. Most offices do not work more than a 9-hour day; they find longer days too exhausting, although a few offices work fewer, longer days. For example, some work three 12-hour days. Most state employment laws require that a lunch break (unpaid) is provided after 4 hours of work. This varies from 30 minutes to an hour.

Many offices schedule early or late hours to accommodate patients. If a dentist does this, he or she should be sure not to work late one day and open early the next. This simply does not give people enough time from work. Evening hours are lucrative. Many patients who work (and have dental benefits) enjoy the evening-hour appointments. Saturday hours can be lucrative. Often, patients schedule these visits with good intentions, but when the time comes, they find that they would rather have the time off. They then cancel or do not show for a visit, leaving the dentist and the staff in the office on a beautiful Saturday.

Daily Huddle

The daily huddle is a short meeting at the beginning of each day. During the meeting, the staff discusses the schedule for the day, looking for potential conflicts or problems. For example, if the office has one nitrous oxide oxygen analgesia unit and two patients require the service, then one of them needs to be rescheduled. This is also the time to discuss if periodic maintenance patients require radiographs, to ensure that all patients have been contacted for appointment reminder, and checking to be sure that the laboratory has returned cases for scheduled patients. Each of these checks avoids a scheduling problem and improves patient flow and treatment.

Ways To Become More Efficient

Dentist can become more efficient without changing the capacity of the office. A dentist can streamline processes, using new or improved procedures to replace old ones. New materials may set more quickly or allow fewer steps in a process, decreasing time required for placement. Using a new technology (such as digital radiography) allows for less time in treatment. Over the long haul, dentists can save more in time (and additional procedures) than the technology costs to install. Adding a staff member is a large investment, but if he or she increases office collections more than he or she costs, the addition is a good investment.

If the capacity of the office is not fully used, then the primary focus should be on increasing the percent of capacity that is used. A dentist can do this either by increasing patient visits or decreasing capacity (and the associated costs). Increasing visits involves all of the internal and external marketing efforts that are described elsewhere in this book. Dentists should also check scheduling to be certain that they are using the time available best to advantage. Dentists can decrease capacity by decreasing hours, making the time that they and the staff are in the office more productive. (Dentists do not want to decrease hours to the point that it becomes difficult for patients to schedule appointments.) Dentists can also decrease capacity by decreasing the number of staff members or the hours that they work.

If the office capacity is fully used, then there are different solutions to the efficiency question. If there are adequate patients and a dentist has not reached maximum capacity, then he or she can increase capacity through moving to a new office space, adding operatories, adding staff to maximize the use of the space, or increasing hours that patients are seen. If, on the other hand, a dentist's capacity is as large as he or she wants it to be, then he or she should increase efficiency and profitability. A dentist can do this by some combination of an increase in fees, a stricter credit and collection policy, and changing insurance plan participation (eliminating lower-paying plans).

Part 2: Office Accounting Systems

Don't go around saying the world owes you a living; the world owes you nothing; it was here first.
Mark Twain

Objectives

At the completion of this part, the student will be able to:
1. Describe the elements of common dental office accounting systems.
2. Describe the purposes of the income accounting system.
3. Properly enter charges, payments, and adjustments.
4. Accurately compute current balance and accounts receivable.
5. Accurately "proof" the day sheet posting, accounts receivable, and month-to-date figures.
6. Accurately enter and compute typical transactions including:
   Charge and payment
   Patient payment
   Insurance payment
   Medicaid payment and adjustment
   Professional discount
   Returned check
7. Posting to the wrong account correction
8. Properly write checks and record them in the check register.
9. Describe how to prevent embezzlement in the dental office.

Key Terms

account guarantor	credit card
account ledger	checkbook register
account payable	payroll stub checks
account receivable	embezzlement
annual report	end-of-day (EOD) procedures
assignment of benefits	end-of-month (EOM)
audit trail	procedures
back-ordered supplies	end-of-year (EOY) procedures
bank deposit	first in, first out (FIFO)
bank deposit verification	holdback (discount)
bookkeeping	monthly ledger
bulk payment	negative account balance
business analysis summary	office credit card
cash control	packing slip
cash flow	peg board
cash transactions	petty cash
charges	positive account balance
production	posting
adjustments	previous balance
production or charge	reconciling the bank
(credit or debit)	statement
payment or collection	routing slip
(credit or debit)	shipping invoice
credit card transactions	specific allocation
credit memo	statement
current balance	walkout statements
day sheet	third-party carriers
disbursements	transaction history
binder checkbooks	

Every business must have a system for recording all the business transactions that occur each day. A dental office is no exception. It is a business. The compilations of those financial transactions are the "books" of the practice. Most dentists delegate part of the bookkeeping

Goal

The goal of this part is to establish office accounting systems for tracking income and disbursements.

function to staff members, professional bookkeepers, or accountants. However, understanding office bookkeeping is important for several reasons. When a dentist is starting practice, he or she needs to establish a bookkeeping system that provides accurate information that it can be used to improve the practice. Having other people do these functions can be expensive; until a practice has grown, a dentist may decide to keep his or her own books to decrease expenses. Finally, a dentist needs to understand bookkeeping systems so that he or she can review them regularly to assure their accuracy. Embezzlement is a sad but all-too-frequent occurrence in offices where the dentist trusted staff members and did not adequately oversee the bookkeeping function.

A dentist needs to keep books of practice income or charges to patients for services that are done. Some patients will pay on the day services are rendered; other payments will arrive in the mail. Besides these routine transactions, dentists will need to record other transactions from time to time (e.g., no fee, a reduced fee, write-offs). Transaction records will give a dentist information about each patient's status and overall information about the financial condition of the practice. The dentist also needs a series of "books" that account for expenditures or the money that goes out of the office. This system should keep a running tally of how much money is available, who the dentist owes money to, and the categories of spending for management information and tax reporting purposes. Finally, the dentist will need to combine the income and expense information into a series of books for tax-reporting and management analysis. The dentist will work with an accountant, tax expert, or management consultant to use this information to improve practice performance and to reduce tax burden.

Fortunately, computerized systems have become the norm for dental office patient accounting. These systems replace the physical books of paper systems with computerized databases. The functions in these two types of systems are similar. The dentist still needs to know the terminology and understand how to record items so that he or she can use the system effectively. If the dentist simply turns over the entire accounting function to a staff member without adequate oversight on his or her part, the dentist is inviting the problems of errors and embezzlement. Each of the major computer systems has a report function built into their software. The systems can print out more reports than a dentist can likely use. The problem is deciding which of these reports is useful. The chapter on financial analysis and control describes the data that needed. The computer program can then deliver the data for a dentist's use. The price and power of these systems make them cost effective for even the individual practitioner. The dentist should use an established computer system rather than trying to

---

Box 21.1 Dental Practice Accounting Needs

Determining Income
  Cash and checks
  Insurance payments
  Credit card payments
Who Owes Money
  Patient accounts and receivables
  Third-party accounts and receivable
Recording Expenses
  Expenses by categories
  Tax purposes
  Management purposes
  Checkbook balance

---

develop his or her own. Unless computer programming is a hobby and the dentist wants to spend his or her recreational hours writing computer programs, time can be better spent working in and developing the office.

Dental offices have three primary office accounting functions (Box 21.1). The first is to record and account for money that is collected from patients, insurance companies, or others for the services provided. Secondly, the dentist must also track those who do not pay at the time of service, instead owing for all or part of the fee for the service. The dentist accomplishes both through the office management system (e.g., Eaglesoft, Dentrix, Softdent). The final function is to record the payments that are made to others for material and services that are used in the office (e.g., lab services, supplies, payroll). The dentist generally accomplishes this through a readily available commercial program, such as Quick Books. (Some management programs have primitive checkbooks built into them, but the common commercial programs are so powerful and easy to use that most practitioners use them.)

The system described is for patient financial records, not treatment records. These are two separate issues and a dentist will have two separate systems for them. A computer program may cross-link patient charts (for treatment histories) and accounts (for financial histories), but they serve two different functions.

Most service industry businesses (such as dental practices) elect to use "cash basis" accounting. (The other method "accrual basis" is used more in larger and manufacturing businesses.) When using cash-based accounting, income is recognized when it is received (i.e., when the check crosses the receptionist's desk) and an expense is recorded when it is paid (i.e., when the check is written). A dentist will use the cash basis for both income and expenses. (This does not mean that a dentist only accepts cash payment, but that all transactions are considered like a cash transaction, whether it is cash, check, credit card, or other form of payment.)

Accounting for Income

Businesses that have many cash transactions use a simple cash register to record their daily transactions. Dental offices do not have the number of cash transactions that a fast-food outlet or retail store has, so the dental office will have a different method of recording or registering payments.

Purposes of Income Accounting Systems

Generally, any income accounting system used in the dental office serves five main purposes.

Office Communications

It is a method of communication between the front office and the production areas of the office. The receptionist needs to inform the production area assistants who will be coming and what procedures for which to prepare. After the visit, the doctor, assistants, or hygienist inform the front office personnel what procedures they did and what the plan is for the next anticipated visit (if any). Many dentists do this in person by walking the patient to the front desk and communicating verbally with the receptionist and patient. Others prefer a more efficient written method. If a dentist saves 1 minute per patient and sees 20 patients a day, he or she can either see an addition patient in the time saved (making additional income) or leave the office 20 minutes earlier. Either way, the dentist wins.

At the beginning of the day, the receptionist should provide copies of the day's schedule in the operatory area (or each operatory) and in the sterilization area. The receptionist then prints a "routing slip" for each patient and places them in the sterilization area. This routing slip specifies the procedure to be done and often other information such as balance due and medical history alerts. Through this communication, the assistants can prepare appropriate instruments and trays for the given procedure for each patient. Routing slips are generally then placed with the tray and taken into the operatory. At the completion of the visit, the office staff or doctor notes on the routing slip what procedures they did and variation from the usual fee (if any). (Offices with networked computer systems often provide this information directly in the sterilization area and operatories, saving time, paper, and possible error.)

Documentation for Patients

An income accounting system provides a receipt to patients, showing the procedures billed today, evidence of any payment received, and their new balance. When dentists enter a procedure onto a patient's account, accountants say that they have "posted" it to the account. The receptionist completes the receipt after posting the procedures and asking for (and hopefully gaining) payment from the patient for the new current balance (previous balance+charges – adjustments). The receptionist then prints a "walk out statement" for the patient that records this information as he or she walks out of the office.

Insurance Billing

An income accounting system provides information for third-party carriers (insurance companies) for billing and payment purposes. The more quickly accurate information is sent to them, the more quickly the dentist or the patient will receive reimbursement. The dental office may transmit this information to the insurer either through a mailed paper form or electronically through the Internet.

Transaction History

An accounting information system gives a listing of the transaction history (charges, adjustments, and payments) for each patient within the account. The account is the billing unit. The dentist sends one bill to the account guarantor of each account because they are responsible or have guaranteed to pay the account. Each account may contain one or many patients. For example, the father may be the guarantor for an account that contains the spouse and their five children. Or in a divorce situation, the father may be the guarantor for an account in which the child is the only patient on that account. The mother may have custody of the child, but the father is responsible for paying for health care for the child. If the mother is also a patient of the practice, she may be her own account guarantor and the only patient on that account. In a case such as this, the dentist sends the child's bill to father but sends the mother's bill to her.

The account or account ledger is the history of all the financial transactions for the account. The current balance is the amount that the guarantor presently owes the dentist for all transactions on the account. A positive account balance says that the guarantor owes the dentist. An account may show a negative account balance if there has been an overpayment. Generally this occurs when third-party payers overpay, or a dentist changes treatment planned procedures, which have already been initiated. (For example, the endodontic procedure that a dentist initiates changes to a less-expensive extraction, although the patient had already paid for the endodontic procedure.) In these cases, the dentist may write either the patient a check for the overpayment, or if the patient desires, the dentist can retain the patient portion of the negative balance to credit it toward future work. Insurance companies will always want the check for a negative balance.

Daily Transaction Journal

Finally, the accounting information system provides a day sheet or a record of each day's transactions for the practice (and each practitioner, if a multipractitioner office) that summarizes the charges made, payments received, and any adjustments made. The computer program accumulates the day's transactions to form a monthly ledger. The program then accumulates monthly ledgers into an annual report. Some dentists rely on their computer backup procedure to ensure that their records are complete. Others print out a copy of the day sheet and keep it in a binder as an additional data backup procedure.

Components of Accounting Systems

Computerized accounting systems are composed of a series of related databases. Databases are computer programs, which save large amounts of information concerning a specific item, and then allow the program to relate that information to other, similar cases. The common databases used by these systems include account information, patient information, third-party database, procedure database, practice history database, and specific databases.

Account information defines each account and the guarantor for each account. The account information relates each patient associated with the account, but the program stores the information about each patient in a different location. Generally the program stores transaction histories with each account.

Patient information defines the patient elements (e.g., name, address, age, etc.) and ties them to an account.

Third-party database establishes the third-party carriers, their addresses, and, generally what each plan pays for each procedure.

The *procedure database* defines the procedures that dentist do, usually by specifying ADA code procedure numbers. This file also includes the normal fee for each procedure and the fee allowed by each insurance plan.

A *practice history database* holds daily and monthly activity reports (day sheets and monthly summaries).

Programs include *specific databases* that store information for the individual program. Examples include dunning messages (little notes that appear on patients' bills), schedule databases, prescription databases, medical history messages, and many other types of information.

These computer programs use each database as needed, pick up the information that they require from that database and then move to the next database, adding required information. For example, if a dentist does a two-surface alloy on a patient who has insurance, the program first identifies the patient from the patient database. It then relates that patient to the account, checking to see the balance of the account. It finds the insurance information from the third-party database, which tells the main program how much the dentist expects the third-party carrier to pay for this specific procedure. It checks the procedure code file to decide how much the dentist normally charges for this procedure. The main program then calculates the amount that the patient should pay, enters any payments made, and saves that information in the updated transaction file for the patient and on the day sheet for the practice.

Accounting Terminology

A charge is the dollar amount that a dentist requires to do the service. It is the same as his or her production figure. Payments may come from the account guarantor or patient as cash, check, or charge card or may come in the mail from third-party payers, such as insurance companies or employers. Adjustments are the amounts for which a dentist decides not to bill. This may be as a result of the patient being a friend or family member or may be required by a managed care insurance plan. A production (or charge) adjustment is a change in the amount of a patient's account as a result of changes in procedures done. A payment (or collection) adjustment is a change in how much money the dentist expects to collect from the patient. Either production or collection adjustments can be credits to the account (decreases the balance due) or debits from the account (increases the balance due.) In the previous example, the dentist had initiated and charged an endodontic procedure but then changed this to an extraction. The dentist has a charge credit (negating part of the endodontic procedure) and a new charge for the extraction. If a dentist does a procedure on a family member or a managed care patient, "writing off" 50 percent of the amount due, the dentist enters a payment credit because the production remains unchanged. When the computer calculates the new "current balance," it uses the formula: Previous Balance + Charges – Payment – Adjustment = Current Balance (Box 21.2).

A credit is an accounting entry that decreases the account balance. A debit is an entry that increases the account balance. Adjustments may either be related to production (or charge) or else to payment (or collection) adjustments (Table 21.2). Either type may be a credit or debit to the account. The dentist wants to keep the types separate so that he or she can keep an accurate tally of office production and collections. The dentist also wants to have a separate payment adjustment for each type (e.g., Delta Dental, Aetna) so that he or she can track the

Box 21.2 Income Accounting Formula

Previous Balance
+ Charges
− Payments
− Adjustments
Current Balance

New Previous Balance = Old Current Balance

Table 21.2 Types of Adjustments

	Credit (Decreases Balance)	Debit (Increases Balance)
Production (Charge)	Entry error Redo a procedure	Entry error
Payment (Collection)	Cash courtesy Bad debt write-off Patient refund Insurance refund	Insurance did not pay full amount

discounts for each plan. This way the dentist can calculate the overall reimbursement rate for the different plans. The chapter on dental insurance discusses how to do this.

Income Accounting System Procedures

Patient Encounter Procedures

Specific patient encounter procedures vary by office and the amount and use of technology in the office. The essentials remain constant.

At the beginning of the day, the people working in the sterilization area and each operatory need to know who is coming in and what procedure is planned at the visit so that trays, equipment, and operatories can be set up appropriately. There are three common methods. If the office uses a paper schedule system, the receptionist makes a photocopy of the day's schedule and posts it in the sterilization area and each operatory. (No one should display them for patient privacy [HIPPA] security.) If the office uses computerized scheduling with computers in each area, then the staff can pull up the day's schedule on the computer system or print out a copy of the day's schedule. Finally, many offices print out a routing slip for each patient planned for the day. Sterilization areas use the routing slip to set up trays. They then place the slip with the tray that goes to the operatory.

Patient Walkout Procedures

Once the dentist does the dental procedure, he or she needs to tell the front office what he or she did for charge purposes and what is planned at the next for scheduling purposes. If each operatory has a computer station, many offices have the staff directly enter the procedure on the patient's ledger. By the time the patient arrives at the front desk to leave, the receptionist then has the patient's bill ready, waiting for payment. If an office uses a routing slip, then staff enters the procedures for the day and plans for the next appointment on the slip. The patient then walks the routing slip to the front desk, where the receptionist enters information on the patient's ledger and asks for payment, and schedules the next appointment. When the patient returns to the reception desk, the receptionist enters the day's procedures, determining the total amount owed and an estimate of insurance coverage (if any). The receptionist should then ask the patient for payment, entering any payments into the system and then he or she should print a walk out statement, which details the day's procedures, charges and payments, and an account summary. Finally, if the office uses mailed insurance forms, the receptionist should then printout an insurance form of the day's procedures to put in the mail.

End-of-Day (EOD) Procedures

Day sheets should be closed and "proofed" each day. Proofing means that the dentist verifies or proves the correctness of the entries and the mathematics. Proofing is important to ensure the accuracy of the accounting and to guard against the possibility of staff embezzlement. Day-end proofing includes proof of posting, accounts receivable proof and control, cash control, and bank deposit verification. Proof of posting verifies that staff members have entered the day's transactions correctly, that they have accounted for adjustments properly, and that they have credited payments correctly. Accounts receivable proofing verifies the accuracy of the total accounts receivable and keeps a running tally of the amount. Cash control checks that staff has accounted for all cash transactions. This cash may be as patient cash payments or in "petty cash." The bank deposit verification assures that the staff have included all payments in the bank deposit for the day. EOD checking takes just a couple of minutes each day, but it is simply expected business practice on the part of the dentist.

The dentist should be sure to close the day sheet at the end of the day's operation and not later. If staff members have made entry errors, they need to address them quickly so that their effect will not multiply throughout subsequent days. Computer systems will not make mathematical errors, but data entry errors are still a problem. (The receptionist may have entered a collection credit instead of a collection debit.) The receptionist or office manager will generally make all entries. The dentist should verify all entries and the proofing procedures each day. Again, this is not paranoia, simply sound business practice.

By the end of the day, several procedures must be completed.

1. *The receptionist should have completed a bank deposit ticket* Generally, the banks prefer their own preprinted deposit tickets rather than the ones printed by the computer system. The front office should stamp all checks as they receive them with the dentist's stamp (available from the bank) that states "For Deposit Only, to the Account of Dr. XXXX, Account # 111-222-333-4."
2. *The deposit ticket total matches*, exactly, *the day sheet "receipts" total* The purpose is to verify that they report all money taken in for the day.
3. *Check the office schedule against the day sheet* Verify that all patients seen in the office for the day have a corresponding entry on the day sheet. This forces a numbered receipt for each patient visit. The dentist should check that all procedures that were done (and charged for) were charged the "usual and customary" amount, unless the dentist has specifically authorized an adjustment.

   If a patient pays in cash, the transaction should appear in the payment section of the day sheet. Even if a patient has a "no charge" visit, the receptionist should give him or her a walk out statement to:
   Verify their previous balance, if any.
   Ask for payment.
   Ensure all patient cash transaction have been recorded.
4. *Verify the "proof of posting"* The dentist should check that the numbers add up as they should. If the staff knows that the dentist regularly look at the numbers, they will be much less likely to take liberties with the money.
5. *Take the day's deposit to the bank* The dentist should take the day's receipts to the bank each day. (This may not be possible if he or she works late hours.) The dentist wants the money in his or her account quickly. The dentist also wants all checks, and especially significant cash, out of the office quickly. In that way, if the dentist is the victim of a break-in or robbery, he or she will lose less.
6. *Occasionally verify the mail* The dentist should occasionally (unannounced) open the mail and post checks to patient ledgers himself or herself. This verifies the accuracy of posting and decreases the likelihood that a front office worker might try to embezzle personal or insurance payment checks from the dentist.
7. *Close the day* Once the dentist has verified that all the day's numbers are correct, he or she needs to close the day in the computer system. The computer system will have routines for doing this. Essentially, closing the day accomplishes the following procedures:

Totals all numbers entered into the system for the day. These include production, collections, adjustments, and other accounting numbers.
Resets the accounting numbers to zero for the new, upcoming day.
Prints out a paper copy of the day sheet for the office financial records.

8. *Back up the computer* The dentist should back up the computer (data) on a daily basis after all other functions have been completed.

End-of-Month (EOM) Procedures

The office needs to do a couple of additional procedures at the end of each month. Again, management computer systems have built in procedures that do these functions.

1. Close the day. The dentist should be sure that he or she has closed the current day to include any transactions from the current day on the monthly totals.
2. Add up the month's totals for all running tally numbers (production, collections, etc.) and store them.
3. Reset those numbers to zero for the upcoming, new month.
4. Print out a paper copy of monthly totals.
5. Age accounts. Most offices age their accounts when they run the end-of-month procedure.

End-of-Year (EOY) Procedures

EOY procedures are similar to end of month, except that they account for the entire year. The system will guide the user through the procedure.

1. Close the month. The dentist should have closed the current month to include transactions from the current month on the yearly totals.
2. Add up the year's totals for all running tally numbers (production, collections, etc.) and store them.
3. Reset those numbers to zero for the upcoming, new year.
4. Print out a paper copy of annual totals.
5. Back up the computer's data. Most offices run an additional (safety) back up for the entire year and store it with the tax records.

Types of Patient Payments

Patients should be encouraged to make payment when the procedure is completed. This may be in the form of cash, check, or credit card. The receptionist informs the patients of the total amount owed. He or she then receives the payment and enters the payment into the computer system and prints a walkout statement. After the receptionist gives this to the patient for verification, he or she stamps the back of the check with a bank deposit stamp and places it and any cash in a secure area of the desk.

Cash

The dentist should deposit all money taken into the office in the office bank account. If he or she takes any cash from patient payments for personal use, the dentist should be sure to use the accounting system totals for income tax determination, rather than the checkbook or bank statement. Dentists face a real temptation to pocket cash money without entering it into the accounting system. People may know others who do it and get away with it. However, the risks are not worth the little extra income (income tax savings).

Note: It is not a good idea to take cash money for personal use without reporting it to the IRS as taxable income. The IRS takes a dim view of people who intentionally do not report income. If a dentist does this, several negative things may happen:

1. If the dentist does not include cash payments as income, he or she will be guilty of income tax evasion or tax fraud, not just a "mistake," if the IRS catches him or her. Conviction is a felony and carries jail terms (not just monetary penalties).
2. Employees will see that it is OK to take cash (i.e., steal). They may similarly be tempted. Because a dentist may simply "rake the cash drawer," he or she may have no idea how much cash is there or even how much is supposed to be there. So the dentist may have no idea how much cash may be missing.
3. A disgruntled or fired employee may "get back" at the dentist. If the former employee reports the dentist to the IRS for tax evasion, the former employee gets a "reward" or bounty of 25 percent of any back taxes and penalties that the dentist owes. An employee that knows this about a dentist can be difficult to fire or control in the office.

Patient Payment by Personal Check

Many patients pay with personal checks. They should make out the check to the dentist's name or the name of the office or practice (if it is different). The front office should staff stamp each check (on the back in the "endorsements" section) when it is received. This stamp has "For deposit only" with the bank and account number. (Banks will generally send businesses these stamps, although there may be a small fee.) That way, if someone steals a check, he or she can not cash it; it can only deposited into the dentist's account.

Patient Payments by Credit Card

Many offices allow and encourage patients to make payment by credit card. From an accounting perspective,

these payments are no different from any other. These should be included a payment on the day sheet and patient accounts.

The dentist will set up a merchant account with a bank to oversee credit card transactions. (Banks offer different rates, fees, and options, so the dentist should shop around.) The overseeing bank may hold these payments in a separate account or may deposit them directly in to office checking account. When the dentist transfers this money to the checking account, the dentist does not have to report it. He or she has already counted it as income when it was entered into the accounting system. Other banks will directly deposit the credit card transaction amount into the checking account the day it occurs. The bank will then summarize the transactions in an EOM statement.

Credit cards charge a fee for each transaction and often a monthly service fee. (See the chapter on credit and collection procedures for a detailed discussion.) The banks call this a "holdback" or "discount." The dentist does not need to enter each transaction fee into the checkbook but rather the entire monthly discount amount. It should be entered as a bank expense in the checkbook.

Accounting for Traditional Insurance Payments

If a patient has dental insurance that covers all or part of the fee, then the accounting becomes a bit more complex than a simple cash transaction. The big question is whether or not the dentist accepts "assignment of benefits." This means that the insurer will send (assign) the benefit (payment) directly to the practice instead of the patient. The chapter on credit and collection policies discusses this in more detail.

If the dentist does not accept assignment of benefits, the accounting is easy. The dentist should charge the patient (actually the account) the full fee and collect as fee for service. The dentist then prints a completed insurance form for the patient to submit, and the patient is responsible for getting reimbursed from the insurer.

If the dentist does accept assignment of benefits, then he or she collects from the patient only the portion that the insurer does not pay. There are two options here. First, the dentist can submit the insurance form to the insurer. The reimbursement will be sent to the dentist. The dentist waits until the insurance "clears" and then charges the patient the difference. The second option is to estimate (through the computer system) what the insurer will pay and charge the patient their expected amount immediately (at time of service). When the insurance company sends payment for its portion, the dentist reconciles his or her estimate with the actual payment. If there is a difference, the dentist either charges or reimburses the difference, depending on whether the total payments are too large or too small. The claim should be closed in the computer system so that it will not continue to track the claim as open (unpaid). The second option speeds cash flow through the practice, but it may require some adjustments after the insurance clears. The dentist also needs to be sure to keep accurate and up-to-date information on all the plans in the computer.

With any of these systems, the dentist should get a pretreatment estimate of benefits from the insurer, especially for large cases or insurance plans with which the dentist is not familiar. The insurer will send an explanation of benefits (EOB) to dentist and the patient. This estimates the patient's coverage (what the insurer will pay for the procedures) that the dentist has submitted for this patient. It is not a payment or even a contract for payment. It is a good faith estimate of what the insurance company will pay. It can (and occasionally does) change from the time the dentist receives the estimate and submits the claim for reimbursement. This does not allow or disallow treatment. That is between the dentist and the patient. The insurance simply pays (or not) for certain procedures, according to the contract with the patient or employer. The pretreatment estimate defines this payment so that no one is surprised.

Insurers will often send one check for payment for services done for several patients. These "bulk payments" will have a form (explanation of payments) with them that details the patient payments included, what procedures the payments cover, and the amount of each payment. When the dentist receives these bulk payments, he or she should be sure to allocate them to the proper procedures on the correct patients.

Accountings for Managed Care Payments

If a dentist participates in a managed care program, he or she will have signed a contract agreeing to the terms of the program, one of which is a reduced fee for procedures. Two options exist for these payments, depending on the specific program(s) with which the dentist participates. In one, the dentist charges and collects from the patient a contractually agreed price for each service. In this case, the dentist enters the full fee value as the charge and then adds a collection adjustment of the difference between the full fee value and the contractually agreed fee. This is listed as a "managed care adjustment" or discount. In the second method, the dentist submits the full fee value to the managed care insurer like a traditional insurance plan. The managed care insurer then sends payment along with an explanation of payment that details how much it reimburses and how much (if anything) the dentist may charge the patient. The difference between the full fee and the total payments (from the insurer and patient, if any) is the managed care adjustment. The chapter on third-party plans describes the financial impact of managed care participation on the dental practice.

Tracking Who Owes Money (Accounts Receivable)

Immediate payments are easy to account for on the day sheet. A bigger problem comes when patients do not pay immediately or have a third-party that pays all or part of the bill. The dentist needs to track the amounts that patients and insurers owe so that the dentist can be sure that he or she is paid properly. (See the chapter on credit and collection policies for a discussion of how to set financial policies for the office.)

All management computer systems have a method for tracking accounts receivable. These are generally called *account aging reports*. These reports categorize accounts by the time since the patient made the last payment. The generally accepted categories are 30, 60, 90, and 120 days. So an account that falls into the 60-day category has not had a payment made in at least 60 days and possibly as many as 89 days.

Simply printing the report does not solve any problem. The dentist has to use the information on the report. This means calling patients, writing letters, or denying future appointments until the patient brings the balance up to date. The older the account, the more difficult it is to collect. So the real value of these reports is to prevent problems by identifying slow payers early so that they can be encouraged to pay what they owe.

For patients who have insurance, there are two theories for determining aging of accounts. (Most dental office software will let a dentist choose which method to use.) The dentist can "start the clock" for payments when the procedure is billed or start it when the insurance has cleared and th dentist is certain what the patient's portion of the bill is. If a dentist uses the first method, he or she needs to have good information about the patient's insurance plan so that the patient's portion can be accurately estimated. This becomes less of a problem with plans that are common in the dental office; more of a problem with seldom-used plans.

The dentist also needs to keep track of insurance forms and pretreatment estimates that he or she has submitted to insurance companies. If the dentist does not get a response from the insurance within 30 days (some offices use 2 weeks) then the dentist (or staff) should follow up with a telephone call to find out what the problem is. Insurance companies are not usually in a hurry to pay out money, so claims and pretreatment estimates may sit on someone's desk if they have a question. The dentist's computer program will track "open" (unpaid) claims and pretreatment estimates that insurers have not returned; he or she should use this feature regularly.

Multipractitioner Offices

Accounting for income becomes more complex in multipractitioner offices. The problem becomes allocating charges and payments to particular providers, rather than the office as a whole. (If the providers are all on salary or other fixed compensation, then there is no need for allocation; simply tally the office totals no matter who provided the service.) There are two common methods of allocating payment to providers, first in, first out (FIFO) and specific. FIFO is an accounting term that means that the payments go to the first procedure completed on the transaction history. Specific allocation states that the dentist will credit the payment to the nearest specific procedure.

For example, Dr. Alpha sees Mrs. Jones and does $300 worth of dental procedures. The next visit, Dr. Baker does a $400 procedure, which requires a $200 down payment. Mrs. Jones pays $300. Who gets credit for the $300 payment? The FIFO procedure says that Dr. Alpha gets credited. Because those procedures were the "first in" the account, they should be the "first out" as well. (This says that the well is filled from the bottom up.) The specific method says to credit Dr. Baker because the requirement for the down payment takes precedence over the age of the receivable. Either way works; the dentist needs to be sure to list in advance which method the office will use. (The FIFO method is more common.)

Recording Expenses: Payments to Others

The dentist also will need a system to record and categorize expenditures for the office. He or she needs this information for two purposes: to know how much cash is in the account and to record expenses for tax and management purposes. Most dentists have two methods for paying office expenses: a credit card and checkbook.

Checkbook Systems

The office checkbook is the system for managing cash in the practice. The dentist should have two checking accounts: one for the office that contains only office expenditures and another personal account that has only personal expenditures. This way, the accounting becomes much easier because the dentist does not need to decide, after the fact, if an item is an office expense or not. All checks written from the office account are business expenses. Be sure that the categories that are established for the checkbook register are the same ones used for tax reports and management information. That way, the entries will not have to be recategorized when the reports are run. (Table 21.3 gives an example of the categories.)

Dentists deposit all income (cash payments, personal checks received from patients, insurance checks, and credit card payments) into the office checking account. (The total amount of daily deposit should be the same as the daily receipts on the computer system.) Dentists then make all office payments from the checkbook and pay the office credit card with a check from the office checking account. If the dentist borrows money, it adds to the checkbook balance, but it is not considered income.

The check register is the mechanism for recording and allocating office costs. Registers may be paper products (they are available from any office supply house) or they may be part of a computerized check system. Check registers identify checks issued for the month and allow the dentist to categorize each expenditure for tax reporting and business management purposes. The purpose of the register is not to keep a running tally or balance of the checking account. The dentist should do that in the checkbook on the check stubs. Instead, the register allocates or categorizes expenses into categories. Summarize the categories for the month and "post" them to an annual report.

The annual report is a summary of all office expenses for the year, broken down by category. These categories are the same as on the checkbook register. The annual report is what the dentist takes to the accountant for processing of taxes. If a dentist has done a good job in these bookkeeping chores, he or she will save hundreds or thousands of dollars in tax preparation fees.

Types of Checkbooks

Binder Checkbooks
Some dentists have checkbooks that fit into three-ring binders, which the bank has provided. The least expensive method is to get the checkbook from the bank and then purchase a good register from an office supply company. Bank checks come in two styles. If a dentist processes his or her own payroll, he or she should get the type called "payroll stub checks" that have an extra section for recording tax withholdings on employees' checks. The dentist will keep meticulous records of employee withholdings on a separate payroll record. Nevertheless, it is important that employees see the total amount of their pay (gross), and all the money that various taxing agencies require that employers withhold and pay for them. Although this will not necessarily make employees happier about their pay level, the lack of this information can cause confusion and dissatisfaction.

Table 21.3 Listing of Accounts for Office Checkbook

Category	Line # Schd. C	Deductible ?	Category	Line # Schd. C	Deductible?
DENTAL SUPPLIES			OFFICE SPACE AND EQUIPMENT		
Dental Supplies	27	Yes	Equipment Lease	20a	Yes
LABORATORY CHARGES			Loan Payment[1]	16a	Yes/No
Dental Lab Charges	27	Yes	Office Rent	20b	Yes
OFFICE EXPENSES			Repairs	21	Yes
Office Expenses	18	Yes	Utilities	25	Yes
Office Supplies	22	Yes	STAFF COSTS		
Postage and Shipping	27	Yes	Associate Expense	11	Yes
Office Cleaning	18	Yes	Employee Benefits	14	Yes
MARKETING			Pension / Profit Sharing	19	Yes
Advertising	8	Yes	Temporary Services	27	Yes
Professional Relations	8	Yes	Uniforms	27	Yes
LEGAL AND PROFESSIONAL			Wages (Net)	26	Yes
Accounting	17	Yes	Withholdings Paid	26	Yes
Legal Services	17	Yes	TAXES		
Management Consultant	17	Yes	FICA (Payroll) Taxes Paid	23	Yes
INSURANCE			Licenses	23	Yes
Office (Business) Insurance	15	Yes	Property Taxes	23	Yes
RETURNS AND ALLOWANCES			Unemployment Taxes Paid	23	Yes
Returns	2	Yes	OWNER'S EXPENSES		
MISCELLANEOUS			Automobile Expenses	10	Yes
Miscellaneous	27	Yes	Continuing Education	27	Yes
Bank Charges	27	Yes	Draw		No
Other Interest Expense	16b	Yes	Dues and Publications	27	Yes
			Meals and Entertainment	24b	Yes
			Personal Insurance		No
			Personal Taxes Paid		No
			Travel	24a	Yes

Notes:

This only lists expense categories. Income categories (patient payments, loan proceeds, interest expense etc.) are not included here.

[1] "Loan Payment" is part interest expense and part principal payment. The interest portion is deductible. The principal portion is not deductible. Depreciation is a noncash expense and not included in the checkbook.

Computer Checking Systems

Many dental office management programs have check writing and register elements included. Most dentists use commercially available accounting systems such as Quicken/QuickBooks. These systems can print the physical check itself, keep an accurate register, determine staff pay and withholdings, produce financial statements, and transfer funds electronically. They are the most effective method available today for tracking expenses in the office. They all operate using the same principles and nomenclature as traditional checkbook systems.

Electronic Checks (E-Banking)

Many banks allow and encourage patrons to use electronic bank services. These systems are especially useful for accounts from which someone regularly write checks (like many dental offices). In these systems, a payee (who to send payment to) is set and a payment amount is added online. Statements are available at the end of each month. Specific systems differ greatly. Banks have different options and requirements, and a dentist should explore all options.

Procedures for Writing and Entering Checks

Regardless the type of system used, there are standard procedures for writing checks and keeping an accurate checking account.

1. *Verify the accuracy of the order* If a dentist receives a box of supplies or other articles, he or she should thoroughly examine all of the items and compare them to the enclosed "shipping invoice" or "packing slip.". If items are incorrect or missing, the dentist should call the supplier immediately to see that they ship the correct items. Further, the dentist should keep a list of items that are "back ordered" (the supplier was out of stock, but will send them when they are in stock) so that he or she does not order them again or pay for them twice.

2. *File (Save) the invoice* An invoice is the charge for payment from the supplier. It lists the material or services provided and the charges for each. Invoices are proof of the expense. Most practitioners keep invoices in an "accordion file" (available at all office supply

stores). Some arrange them by category of expense (e.g., dental supplies), whereas others keep them by month, relying on the check register for accuracy of category totals. The monthly file is probably easier, if a dentist keeps an accurate check register for allocation of expenses.

3. *Wait for the statement* Some suppliers send an invoice with each order (especially ones that are used infrequently). Their invoice states "pay from this invoice" or something similar. These suppliers generally do not send a statement. Others (especially those with whom the dentist has several orders through the month) will send an end-of-the-month statement and mail an invoice for each order. The dentist has to learn which supplier operates in which manner. A statement of the account summarizes all of a dentist's invoices and payments for the month and presents a new monthly total due. The dentist should verify that all the invoices entered on the statement are correct and that they have entered any credit memos. (A credit memo is like an invoice but gives a credit on an account for returned items or overbilled amounts.)

4. *Write the check* Complete the entire check. Enter the corresponding invoice number or account number on the check. If there is ever a question of whether an invoice was paid, the dentist can look at the canceled check to verify invoice number. If this is a pay check for an employee, the dentist should note the dates the paycheck reflects.

5. *Enter information into the register* If a dentist is using a paper system, he or she must reenter the information from the check on the register. Computer systems prompt the dentist do this. The payee is the person, or organization to which the check is being written. It may be a staff member, supplier, or self, as the dentist's own draw. Checks are numbered consecutively. If the dentist makes a mistake on a check, then he or she should write *void* in the register for the payee and should also write *void* clearly across the check and then destroy the check. The dentist should then go to the next check.

The dentist should enter the check's amount in the appropriate category of the register. (Enter all dental supplies, for example, under the "dental supplies" category.) The categories should be the same as the categories on the current Schedule C tax return.

The dentist should list his or her personal draw in a separate category. When money is transferred from the office account to a personal account, the dentist is taking a draw on the assets of the practice. It should be categorized as a "draw" in the check register. This is not a tax-deductible expense item. (If the dentist practices as a corporation, he or she is an employee. In this case, the dentist's salary is deductible to the corporation like any other employee.) If the dentist writes personal or nonprofessional checks from this account (such as life insurance payments), he or she should post them as a draw as well. This is so that nondeductible expenses are not deducted on tax returns.

If the expense does not fall into a predetermined category, it should be placed in the "sundry" or "miscellaneous" column or category. Again, only professionally related expenses should be entered in the body of this register.

Accounting for Credit Card Purchases

Dentists should have a credit card (MasterCard, VISA, etc.) that they use only for office purchases. (They should obtain a separate credit card for personal purchases.) Generally, the higher the interest rate, the lower the annual fees; the reverse is also true. If a dentist routinely pays off his or her credit card balance the month it is due, he or she should get a card with lower annual fees. If the dentist does not routinely pay off the balance, then he or she should pay the higher annual fee in return for lower monthly interest rates. The dentist should consider getting a card that pays for frequent flyer miles, if he or she pays off the credit card regularly. If the dentist makes many office purchases (e.g., office supplies, lab and dental supplies) with this type card, he or she may have several free trips each year. If the dentist uses the frequent flyer miles for business-related trips (e.g., continuing education), the trips are not considered taxable income by the IRS. Personal use may result in assumed income by the IRS.

The dentist may make business-related purchases with an office credit card. He or she wants to be sure to include the cost of these business expenses as deductions for tax purposes. The dentist should write one check from the office checkbook to the issuing bank for monthly credit card purchases. He or she will then need to allocate the purchases to correct categories. For example, the dentist may have purchased professional supplies, advertising materials, and paid for continuing education courses with the credit card. The dentist should write one check to the bank to pay for the credit card purchases but should categorize those separate purchases for tax and management information. If the dentist is using a computerized accounting system, he or she will generally run separate accounts. The dentist should use all of the accounts when determining and printing monthly and year-end reports. If a paper system is used, he or she will need to run a separate sheet for credit card purchases, adding them to the register allocations for tax reporting purposes.

Reconciling the Bank Statement

The dentist will receive a bank statement each month that details the initial balance, all checks written and deposits made for the month, and an ending balance. The dentist should check the accuracy of the statement.

(Banks do make mistakes!) This is called *reconciling* the statement to the checkbook. The procedure follows.

1. The dentist should verify that all transactions (checks and deposits) have "cleared' or have been processed by the bank. He or she should be sure that the bank recorded the amount of the transaction correctly. The dentist may have written some checks that the payee has not yet cashed, or he or she may have written checks since the bank issued the statement.
2. The dentist should subtract the amount of the checks that have not cleared from the ending balance and add the amount of any deposits that are not recorded.
3. Then any bank charges should be subtracted and any returned checks added.
4. This should equal the current checkbook balance. If not, the dentist needs to check item by item to detect the sources of the error.

Petty Cash and Cash Control

Many business checking accounts are not interest-bearing accounts. That is to say, the bank does not pay the holder interest on money in checking accounts. (The dentist should see if the bank has a "sweep" or other type account that does pay interest on checking account balances.) The dentist needs to manage the money in his or her bank accounts to maximize the interest earned from these assets. He or she should be sure to keep an accurate balance of the amount in the checking account so that he or she does not fall below the minimum balance, which generally initiates fees. However, the dentist does not want to keep too much money in an account that does not pay interest. If the account does not pay interest, he or she should have a separate account (often a money market type account) that does. Any extra cash should be swept (transferred) into the interest-bearing account, earning interest. The dentist should make frequent deposits, daily if possible, to earn interest on that amount as well. He or she should also delay payments to others (checks) so that money is kept as long as possible. (The dentist should not be late with a payment, initiating interest or penalty charges, but there is no reason for the payment to be there early either.)

Most offices have a petty cash drawer or box. Petty cash is used for small purchase items, such as postage due or delivery charges. The dentist should track the petty cash and make one person responsible for the petty cash account. The dentist should make the responsible party understand that this is not "free" money, but that he or she is responsible for it. The dentist should have a simple book that lists all petty cash expenditures. That way, he or she can keep an accurate listing of how much petty cash has been used and who has used it.

Protecting Against Embezzlement

It is a sad fact that many dentists fall prey to embezzlers. *Embezzlement* sounds like an innocuous, white-collar crime, but it is really another word for "stealing." Some statistics show that as many as one in three dentists may be victims. Embezzlement may be as innocuous as taking a book of postage stamps (worth $30) or may involve purposeful and systematic theft of thousands of dollars from the practice. The best defense against embezzlers is to be constantly aware, to know their patterns, and to be involved enough in the day-to-day office finances to discourage any would-be embezzlers.

Research has shown that typically the employer thought of an embezzler as a "model" employee. Embezzlers work long hours (to cover their tracks) and to relieve the dentist of all need to be involved in the finances (to keep them ignorant of the problem). Embezzlers maintain a high degree of control of the systems, seldom taking vacation or allowing anyone else to help with "their" functions in the office. They generally present apparently thorough and complete reports, but they seldom show any account cards, bank statements, or other details of the accounting systems. All of this is allegedly to free the dentist from having to "worry" over accounting problems. In fact, it is to keep the dentist from discovering problems with the "books" of the practice.

Intelligent, enterprising, and unscrupulous people can devise many ways to steal from a dentist. Cash transactions are difficult to trace, especially if the office does not issue a numbered receipt for every transaction. Staff can alter or destroy cash receipts, pocketing the money. Staff members have made checks out to their own debtors, having the practice unknowingly pay off a personal debt. Other staff members have made fraudulent adjustments to a patient's account when they pay with cash, pocketing the adjustment. Some give favors to patients in return for kickbacks. False patient accounts are a likely source of embezzlement. For example, one employee even set up a new joint bank account with the employee and dentist's names on the account. The employee then deposited patient checks in the new account and withdrew money from the account. All of this was unknown to the dentist.

To avoid embezzlement, dentists must actively protect themselves through preventive measure. The dentist should always assume that he or she might be a victim of staff embezzlement. He or she does not need to be paranoid, but being involved with the accounting is a responsibility of being a business owner. The dentist can take several steps to decrease the likelihood that someone will embezzle from him or her. First, the dentist should lead by active example. He or she should act legally and ethically, that he or she does not take cash from the office without a proper accounting, and that the dentist expects others to behave similarly. The dentist should recruit and hire trustworthy and ethical people to manage the office finance systems. He or she should thoroughly check the references and background of the people that are hired. The dentist should set up the office job duties so that two or more people share some financial duties of the practice. He or she may have different people making collection calls, processing the mail-in and insurance checks, or preparing bank deposit slips. This form of check and balance discourages a would-be embezzler because others are looking at the details of the accounting system. Finally, the dentist should insist that employees take vacations and maintain regular working hours. Although an employee who never takes vacation and is willing to stay late (while the dentist is not there) sounds like a dream worker, they are, in fact, a problem waiting to happen. The dentist should be sure that each patient encounter has a corresponding transaction slip (or walk-out statement). At the end of each day, the dentist should check the day sheet to verify all patient transactions, especially adjustments. He or she should check the deposit slip against the day sheet to be sure that all money collected is going to the bank.

Periodically (and unpredictably), the dentist should audit the financial records of the practice and should be sure that everyone in the office sees him or her doing the audit. The dentist should ask for detailed records (appointment books, ledger cards, bank deposit slip etc.). Although he or she may not find a problem, the fact that the dentist is looking will discourage many people from even trying to steal. All computer systems have some form of an audit trail. An audit trail lists all computer transactions, even if someone has deleted or overwritten them. There is a history of those changes that no one can erase. If a dentist suspects embezzlement, the first place to look is the audit trail to see if anyone has altered or deleted transactions.

The dentist can do several things about accounts payable and disbursements to discourage embezzlement. The doctor (or spouse) should sign all checks drawn on the practice and should not grant signatory authority to a staff member. (The dentist can have the staff member write or print out the check. However, the dentist must verify and sign it.) A rubber stamp authorizing signature is an invitation to someone to act fraudulently. The dentist should maintain a copy of every invoice and mark the check number on the invoice.

Box 21.3 How to Prevent Embezzlement

- Be active in leadership and involvement
- Hire the right people
- Be involved with the accounting systems
- Review financial records regularly
- Sign all checks
- Periodically audit the system

Example Patient Accounting Transactions

The following are accounting transactions for the cases given. These are the most common transactions in the office. They show the difference between production and collection transactions and credit and debit transactions (Table 21.4).

Table 21.4 Example Patient Accounting Transactions

	Date	Family Member	Professional Service	Charge	Payment	Charge Adj	Payment Adj	Balance
A	9/12	Mary	Restoration	$150	$150			$0
B	9/13	Chris	Crown	$1000	$200			$800
	9/22		Ins Check # 223344		$500			$300
C	9/13	Larry	Prophy	$80	$60		$20	$0
D	9/14	Betty	Restoration	$150	$100		$30	$20
E	9/15	Joe	Ex, Rad, Pro	$135			$135	$0
			Rest	$150	$65		$85	$0
F	9/20	Sam	Surgery	$300	$300			$0
	9/21	Sam	Posted in Error			<$300>	$300	$0
	9/21	Samantha	Surgery	$300	$300			$0
G	9/6	Louise	Rec, Pro	$95	$19			$76
	9/20		Ins Check # 45678		$79			<$3>
H	3/6	Tom	Restoration	$185	$50			$135
	8/10	Tom	Bad Debt				$135	$0
I	7/12	Sarah	Rec, Pro	$95	$95			$0
	7/19	Sarah	Bad Check				<$95>	$95
	7/19	Sarah	Bad Check Charge			$20		$115
	7/26	Sarah			$95			$20
J	7/19	Bob	RCT	$600	$600			$0
	7/25	Bob	RCT			<$600>		<$600>
	7/25	Bob	Debride, Ext	$175			$425	$0

A Mary has a restoration and pays for it at the time of the visit. Her new balance is zero (0).

B Chris has a crown on #3 ($1000 total charge). Chris pays $200, leaving a balance of $800. Chris's indemnity insurance company pays $500. Chris new balance is $300.

C Larry receives a dental prophylaxis. A professional courtesy discount of $20 (a payment credit) is given. He pays the rest and has a zero (0) balance.

D Betty has a restoration done. The regular fee is $150. Her insurance plan allowable charge is $120. The required $30 is adjusted. Betty pays $100. Her balance is $20.

E Joe has a capitation plan for his third-party plan. The contract specifies that dentists provide exams, radiographs, and prophylaxis (a $135 value) at no charge. The dentist then must only charge him $65 for a restoration (full fee $150). The rest is adjusted off his account (a payment/collection credit).

F The dentist incorrectly entered periodontal surgery and payment on Sam Smith's ledger. It should have been entered on Samantha Smith's account (a different account). It is entered as a "negative charge" (production debit) and a payment (payment credit) and reentered, correctly, on Samantha's account.

G Louise had an exam and prophylaxis. The total charge was $95. The dentist expected the insurance to pay $76. She paid her portion, $19. The insurance check came 2 weeks later for $79. Louise now has a negative balance due of $3. The dentist could write her a check for $3, but she would rather just leave it on her account and use it against her next visit. This would be a payment credit if the dentist wrote the check.

H Tom had a restoration on #30, total charge $185. He paid $50 that day. Five months later, the dentist sent Tom's account to the collection agency. The dentist "wrote off" his bad debt (a collection or payment credit of $135).

I Sarah had an exam and prophylaxis, total charge $95 (production debit). She paid with a check which "bounced" (payment debit). The bank returned it a week later marked *insufficient funds*. The office policy is that there is a $20 charge for all "bounced" checks (payment debit). The dentist called Sarah; she assured us the problem was taken care of and to redeposit the check (payment credit). This time, the check was good. She owes the dentist $20 for the bad check.

J The dentist started a root canal on Bob. He paid in full at the initial appointment. When he returned for completion, the dentist found a crack running through the tooth, making it unrestorable. The dentist extracted the tooth and rebated the cost of the endodontic therapy, charged him $100 for the debridement (previous appointment) and $75 for the extraction. The dentist wrote him a check for the difference ($425).

Part 3: Instrument Management Procedures

One only needs two tools in life: WD-40 to make things go, and duct tape to make them stop.
G. Weilacher

<table>
<tr><td colspan="2">**Key Terms**</td></tr>
<tr><td>cleaning instruments</td><td>instrument sets</td></tr>
<tr><td>clinical surfaces</td><td>noncritical instruments</td></tr>
<tr><td>critical instruments</td><td>semi-critical instruments</td></tr>
<tr><td>dental health care personnel</td><td>sterilizer monitoring</td></tr>
<tr><td>(DHCP)</td><td>supply tubs</td></tr>
<tr><td>housekeeping surfaces</td><td></td></tr>
</table>

Objectives

At the completion of this part, the student will be able to:
1. Describe the goals of an instrument management plan for the dental office.
2. Differentiate between the classifications of risk potential for dental instruments.
3. Describe the types of surface disinfectants.
4. Describe the proper sterilization procedure for the dental office.
5. Describe office design considerations for instrument sterilization procedures.
6. Describe procedures to properly sterilize instruments in the office.
7. Describe a sterilizer monitoring program for the office.

Goal

The goal of this part is to discuss an instrument management system for the office so the new dentist can effectively manage this office function.

The instrument management plan for the office should accomplish several goals, as outlined in Box 21.4. The first goal is to prevent spread of disease between patients and staff members. How dentists handle clean and dirty instruments has an obvious relationship to these goals. A properly designed instrument management plan also keeps instruments in good repair. Dentists buy only the instruments that they need so that they keep costs as low as possible.

Center for Disease Control and Prevention Background

The Centers for Disease Control and Prevention (CDC) dictates instrument management procedures through their "Guidelines for Infection Control in Dental Health-Care Setting– 2003." The Occupational Safety and Health Administration (OSHA) has adopted these CDC guidelines in their recommendations for worker safety in the office. This section does not try to describe that report in detail but discusses how it is applied effectively in the dental office. The entire report can be found at the following Web site, http://www.cdc.gov/mmwr/preview/mmwrhtml/rr5217a1.htm (Table 21.5).

Dentists must closely link any instrument management plan to the OSHA plan for office. Because of the potential for sticks by dirty sharp instruments, dentists must have a plan in place that protects staff from injuries and follows up in case of an injury. The section on OSHA compliance discusses these issues.

Many new dentists assume that staff members, especially those who have been "in the business" for many years know how to manage instruments. That simply may not be the case. They may not have been trained, been trained improperly, or they may have been trained before many present guidelines were promulgated. Regardless, it is the dentist's responsibility as owner and manager of the practice to ensure that all staff members know and follow proper instrument cleaning and sterilization procedures.

Box 21.4 Goals of Instrument Management Plan

1. Prevent cross-contamination
2. Assure worker safety
3. Provide enough instruments for operation
4. Maintain instruments properly
5. Allow change in instrumentation
6. Keep costs low
7. Be compliant with regulations

Types of Patient Care Items

The CDC has classified instruments according to their potential for spreading infection in the dental office. Depending on the classification of the instrument (Table 21.6), they require different types of sterilization or disinfection. If a semi-critical item tolerates the sterilization procedure, it should be sterilized. If not, a high level of disinfection is acceptable.

Table 21.5 Classification of Risk Potential for Spreading Infection

Category	Item Definition	Examples	Transmission Risk	Method of Processing
Critical	Penetrates soft tissue Cuts hard or soft tissue	Burs, surgical instruments	High	Sterilization
Semi-Critical	Touches mucous membrane or non-intact skin	Bite blocks, X-ray blocks	High Moderate	Sterilization High disinfection
Noncritical	Contacts intact skin	Facebow	Low	Clean and disinfect

Table 21.6 Surface Disinfectants

Category	Definition	Examples	Uses
High-level disinfectants	Destroys all microorganisms except bacterial endospores	Glutaraldehydes, hydrogen peroxide, hypochlorites	Heat-sensitive items, immersion only (do *not* use on environmental surfaces)
Intermediate-level disinfectants	Destroys bacteria, most fungi and viruses; tuberculocidal	EPA-registered hospital disinfectants with claim of tuberculocidal activity, iodophors	Clinical contact surfaces; noncritical surfaces with visible blood or debris
Low-level disinfectants	Destroys bacteria, some fungi and viruses; *not* tuberculocidal	Quaternary ammonium compounds; EPA-registered hospital disinfectants *without* claim of tuberculocidal activity	Housekeeping surfaces

EPA, Environmental Protection Agency

Patient care devices that do not require sterilization are subject to one of three levels of disinfection: high, medium, or low. Environmental surfaces (floors, cabinets, etc.) require one of two levels of disinfection: medium or low. Table 21.6 describes these levels of disinfection.

Dental Office Requirements

Instrument Sets

Modern dental operatories contain small storage areas. Dentists house instruments in the sterilization area and take them to the appropriate operatory as needed for each patient. This allows smaller operatories with less cabinetry. It also requires fewer instrument kits because dentists do not need to store multiple copies of each kit in each operatory. As the number of procedures increases or change over time, instrument kits can be added or changed in response.

There are two major methods of distributing instrument sets to the operatories, trays, and cassettes. The staff must package instruments from trays for sterilization and then reset fresh trays with sterile instruments. This involves additional staff time and increases the possibility of injury each time they handle instruments. Cassettes have the advantage that human hands do not touch the instruments. The entire cassette is placed in the cleaner and then the autoclave. Cassettes carry a higher initial cost than trays. Dentists also need a larger (more expensive) autoclave to accept cassettes (particularly large cassettes) over bagged instruments.

Cassettes can be color coded or have colored tape or other markers applied to show the types of instruments contained (e.g., operative).

Plastic tubs (color coded) contain all the special materials needed for a given type of procedure. These materials and equipment are *noncritical* instruments that do not need sterilization after use. Those that need sterilization are placed into a separate tray or cassette for processing. For example, an endodontic tub contains sealers, points, and other supplies used in endodontic procedures.

Number of Instrument Sets and Types Needed

Several factors dictate the number and type of instrument setups that dentists need. A dentist does not want to run out of instrument set ups or have too many set ups because they are expensive. First, the dentist determines the office instrument processing cycle. Many offices process once per day. Others process twice daily (at lunch time and again at the end of the day). Larger offices that have a dedicated sterilization clerk process

instruments continually. Next, the dentist estimates the maximum number of patient visits per processing cycle. If the hygienist sees a patient for an hour and instruments are processed every 4 hours, the need is a minimum of four hygiene setups. If the dentist might do two endodontic procedures in a cycle, then he or she needs a minimum of two endodontic setups. Once the dentist decides the minimum number of instrument sets that are needed, he or she should add 50 percent. (For example, if the dentist decides that he or she needs six operative sets, he or she should get nine.) This covers a particularly busy day, processing backlogs, or the possibility of a set being dropped or otherwise deemed unusable.

Instruments within the Sets

The dentist needs to decide the specific instruments that he or she wants within each set of instruments. He or she should use the minimum number that gives excellent results. Dental suppliers have sets of instrument markers (small plastic rings that fit securely on dental instruments). The dentist should get a different color for each type of set-up (e.g., blue for operative, green for prophy). Within those set-ups, the dentist places the instruments in the order in which they are generally used. Place the color-coded bands on the instruments in a descending order (as seen in the accompanying picture). By this method, staff can easily put the instruments in the proper order and decide if any instruments are missing during processing (Fig. 21.1).

Staff Considerations

As previously mentioned, OSHA requirements dictate instrument processing procedures. Dentists must train and monitor dental health care personnel (DHCP) for

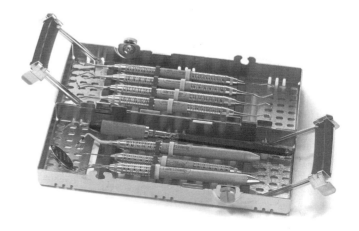

Figure 21.1 Example instrument set
Courtesy of Hu-Friedy Mfg. Co., LLC, Chicago Ill.

properly performing procedures. They must wear personal protective equipment (PPE) and thick protective gloves (not patient care gloves) when they process instruments.

Larger offices often have staff members whose only job is to process instruments. In these offices, instrument processing will be a continuous procedure. Many smaller offices do not need to process instruments constantly. Instead, they process instruments at several points in the daily routine, often at lunch or the end of the day. Some offices make each staff member responsible for cleaning and packaging his or her own instruments. Others make one staff member responsible for the entire processing.

Office Design Considerations

The design of an office should provide for easy transportation of instruments to and from the sterilization area. Therefore, it should be centrally placed near the operatory patient areas. Ideally, it should have a separate traffic pattern from patients so that patients cannot contact dirty instruments or wander into the sterilization area.

The size of the sterilization area will obviously vary with the available floor space, number of operatories, and normal patient flow. It should have large counter space (at least ten linear feet) and be divided into "dirty" and "sterile" sides. Dirty instruments stay only on their side, and sterile instruments on theirs. (Some offices use signs or tape on the counters to designate clean and dirty areas in the sterilization room.) Storage for dirty instruments (trays or cassettes) should never mingle with storage of clean trays or cassettes. Storage cabinets should ideally have clear plastic doors and be easily taken apart and cleaned. A large, deep sink with spray attachment must be found on the dirty side of the counter.

For optimal work flow and aseptic technique, the instrument processing area should allow instruments to flow in a single loop. Staff brings contaminated instruments into the area, cleans, packages, sterilizes, and stores them in a continuous process, similar to an assembly line. The more automated the process becomes, the less chance for operator error in processing.

The sterilization area should be a separate area, not shared or mingled with other functions. Some offices that are cramped for space combine the dental lab or general storage areas with the sterilization area. This obviously invites cross-contamination. Although space limitations may dictate some compromises, the dentist should try to keep a dedicated area for instrument processing. OSHA guidelines require an approved eyewash station in the instrument processing area. It should also have compressed air and vacuum lines for cleaning and lubricating handpieces before sterilization.

Sterilization and Disinfection Procedures

Operatory Breakdown

The DHCP should place all sharps into an approved and labeled sharps container. All soaked or saturated material and all tissue (teeth or surgically removed tissue) should be placed into appropriate biohazard bags. They may put all other waste into the waste system. Instruments should be placed in covered containers before transferring them to the processing area. DHCP should disinfect smooth surfaces and remove and discard barriers. The dentist should be sure to schedule enough time (10 minutes) at the end of each appointment for operatory break down and set up.

In the dental operatory, surfaces that do not touch the patient can still become contaminated with saliva, blood, or other infectious residue. Their likelihood of having any infectious residue dictates their cleaning method. CDC classifies them as either clinical or housekeeping surfaces (Box 21.5).

Housekeeping surfaces, such as floors, walls, and sinks, have limited risk of disease transmission. Dentists decontaminate them with less-rigorous methods than patient care or clinical surfaces. Most of these surfaces need to be cleaned only with a detergent and water or hospital disinfectant approved by the Environmental Protection Agency (EPA). Thorough cleaning once a day is more important for these surfaces than disinfection.

Clinical surfaces are touched during procedures with contaminated gloved hands or are spattered or sprayed during procedures. Examples include light switches and handles, drawer pulls, pens, and curing light triggers. Barriers are the most effective method of preventing contamination on these surfaces, especially those that are difficult to clean (such as knobs on operating equipment). If barriers are not used, the surface requires thorough cleaning followed by an EPA-registered hospital disinfectant.

Box 21.5 Operatory Surface Asepsis

Type
   Clinical contact
   Between patients
   Housekeeping
   End of day
Methods
   Barriers
   Preclean and disinfect

Receiving and Cleaning

The receiving area is where instruments are stored before they are processed. Staff discards any disposables not previously removed from the trays in the operatory. Cabinets above the counter, with shelves for cassettes, trays, or instruments provide a safe storage until staff can complete the cleaning procedure (Fig. 21.2). If instruments cannot be processed immediately, they should remain wet so that material does not dry onto them. Many practices use puncture-resistant plastic holding tubs for this purpose. The solutions used include enzymic cleaners or detergents. Individual instruments should be placed into wire mesh baskets to reduce the chance of an accident.

Cleaning should remove the obvious material (e.g., blood, cements, material) that the staff members did not remove previously. Cleaning does not sterilize the instruments; it only prepares them for sterilization. In most practices the cleaning area includes a large, deep stainless steel sink with a spray attachment.

There are three methods of cleaning, hand scrubbing, ultrasonic, and dishwasher-style cleaning systems. Hand scrubbing has fallen out of favor because of the obvious problem of potential worker injury. Ultrasonic cleaners are often plumbed directly into the existing sink drains. Many are recessed into the counter top to improve the ergonomic transfer of cassettes at elbow height. The dentist should be sure than the ultrasonic cleaner is large enough to hold the largest cassette. Instrument washers are devices approved by the Food and Drug Administration (FDA) for cleaning instruments and cassettes. They operate similarly to a home dishwasher.

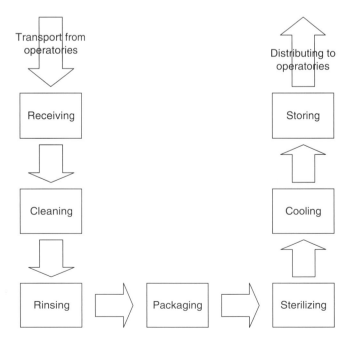

Figure 21.2 Instrument processing cycle

When DHCP are ready to process instruments, they remove them from the holding solution. They gather instruments from trays (in tray systems) and bind them with a rubber band. They then place them in the ultrasonic cleaner or washer-disinfector. They remove cassettes (in cassette systems) from the holding solution and place them into the cleaner. DHCP then run the ultrasonic or washer-disinfector according to manufacturers' instructions. After the cycle is complete, the DHCP removes cassettes or bundles of instruments and places them in the sink to rinse them thoroughly to remove chemical or detergent residues. They then place them on a rack or towels in the next area to dry.

Packaging

When the instruments have dried, DHCP inspect and clean any instruments that have any remaining material stuck to them with a brush. At this time, they replace any broken or damaged instruments. They also sharpen cutting instruments that have dulled. They then place the instruments in their proper place in the cassette, close the cassette and place it in an appropriate sterilizer bag (along with a sterilizer monitor strip), seal and label the bag. After this, no one reopens the cassette until it is next used in the operatory. In tray systems, the staff member removes the rubber band holding the instruments and verifies their cleanliness, replacing or sharpening as required. They then package the instruments in an appropriate sterilizer bag (along with a sterilizer monitor strip) and seal the bag. All instruments and kits that they have sterilized should be placed in a bag before sterilization. DHCP should always wear heavy-duty puncture resistant gloves whenever they are working with instruments.

Sterilization

Bags or bagged cassettes are then sterilized according to the sterilizer manufacturer's directions. The DHCP should take special care to load the sterilizer according to the manufacturer's directions. It is important that the sterilizing agent (steam or vapor) circulate properly within the sterilizer to insure proper function. At the end of the cycle, the instruments should cool in the sterilizer to avoid burns. If this is not possible (because of time constraints), the dentist should have the staff member use tongs to remove instrument packages and let them cool on the countertop. A *hot* sign should be kept so that hot instruments are properly marked.

Handpiece Sterilization

Dental handpieces are critical instruments that require sterilization. They are also expensive instruments that must be properly cared for and maintained. Fortunately, modern handpieces will last many sterilization cycles, if they are properly cared for during the process. Handpiece sterilization involves several steps.

1. Instruments must be purged. All water must be blown out of the handpiece.
2. They must be lubricated. Lubricant must be sprayed through the handpiece into the turbine area to lubricate and protect before sterilization. (Manufacturer's directions should be followed closely.)
3. They must be bagged and indicator strips added.
4. They must be sterilized.
5. They must be stored properly (usually in an upright position).

Despite best efforts, the dentist will need to have handpieces repaired periodically because of wear and tear from the sterilization process. This is a cost of doing business.

Sterilizer Monitoring

Most states require that dentists monitor the effectiveness of their sterilization procedures. Each state's laws vary regarding frequency and type of testing but generally follow the CDC guidelines, which include:

1. Use mechanical monitoring every load. Staff should check the timer and indicators on the autoclave to be sure that it has operated according to specifications. Many modern sterilizers have printouts for each load as a record of effectiveness.
2. Place a chemical indicator inside every package. Most offices use a color-change test strip with each load (or in each bag) to assure that the proper amount of heat has penetrated the load.
3. Monitor each sterilizer with a spore test once per week. Subjecting live organisms and spores to the sterilization cycle accomplishes the actual monitoring. Dentists then send these to an appropriate lab to be cultured. If nothing grows, the procedure was effective. Several businesses contract with health care facilities for this monitoring function.

Storage

Staff members then stores sterile instrument packages in the clean side of the sterilization area in a way that ensures their sterility is maintained during storage. If trays are used, instruments are generally set on trays and the set trays stored, rather than setting trays at the time they are needed. (Schedules have a way of falling apart and days become hectic.)

Distribution

Staff uses the daily schedule as a guide to setting trays and tubs for patient procedures. After they dismiss a patient and disinfect the operatory, they then carry the appropriate tray (and tub) for the upcoming patient to the operatory. They wait to open sterilization packs in the operatory in front of the patient. Not only does this reduce contamination of the instruments, opening them in the presence of patients reassures them that the instruments are sterile.

Other Office Instrument Issues

Dental Waterlines

Biofilms often form from oral fluids being sucked back into dental instruments (e.g., handpieces, ultrasonic scalers, three-way syringes). There are presently no federal regulations, per se concerning dental office waterline management. There is presently no epidemiologic evidence that shows waterlines in dental offices pose a safety risk to patients or DHCP. However, the CDC considers exposing patients or staff to water of uncertain microbiological quality to be a concern. They recommend that water used as a coolant/irrigant in nonsurgical procedures meet the standards for drinking water as established by the CDC and American Public Health Association. Manufacturers have engineered many modern dental units to prevent contamination. The DHCP should be sure to follow the manufacturer's recommendations. CDC further recommends that all instruments connected to the public water lines should be run for 20 to 30 seconds at the end of a procedure to physically flush any patient-generated material that might have entered the instrument or waterlines.

Mercury Effluent

When a dentist removes an amalgam restoration, the pieces of the old filling, dust, and slurry from the procedure are all collected through the high-speed evaluation system. This usually then empties into the local sewer system and, after treatment, into public water supplies. Heavy metals, such as mercury, are well-known health hazards, even in small amounts. Consequently, many people are concerned that dental offices are adding a significant amount of mercury to the public water treatment system. Some offices have added a mercury trap that captures the mercury and other metals before they enter the public sewage system. This may be a requirement for all dental offices in the future.

Part 4: Office Supply and Lab Management

Inventories can be managed, but people must be led.
Ross Perot

Most dental offices have an "inventory" of materials and medicaments that they use when treating patients. These are really supplies because inventory is a product that will be sold to customers. These are accounted for differently for tax determination, but for these purposes, they can be thought of similarly.

A well-designed and implemented inventory system satisfies several purposes. It ensures that the dentist has supplies when he or she needs them. If the dentist "stocks out' and does not have impression material for a large case, the dentist will lose the income and possibly the goodwill of the patient. Dentists need to be sure that supplies are current and have not expired. Many materials have expiration dates associated with them. The material may not perform as expected if it is too old. This system should help to control supply costs and let the dentist change materials without undue cost or time.

Dentists have several types of supplies that are routinely used in the office. The ones often most thought of are dental materials. These include all of the cements, restorative materials, medicaments, and operating supplies used in patient care. Dentists also need general office supplies, such as paper hand towels, toilette tissues, cleaning supplies, and hand soap. Finally, dentists need business office supplies, such as stationery, copy paper, pens, paper clips, and toner cartridges. Each of these categories of supply may be purchased from a different vendor. A large wholesale store may provide the best price on paper products, whereas an office supply store may have the best selection and price for the office supplies.

Inventory Systems

In the ideal inventory system, supplies are ordered with just enough lead time to fill and ship the order (Fig. 21.3). The dentist runs out of supply just as he or she receives the order to replenish the supply and put it on the shelf. This keeps supplies fresh and cuts storage costs to a minimum. In the real world, dentists can not live nearly this close to the line. They do not know precisely how much material is needed and when it is needed. Suppliers may run out of a product to send and back order the supply. They may delay shipping, or find that some of the current supply does not perform adequately. So although this inventory system is the ideal, dentists know that they will carry some excess supply, as shown in the diagram of a realistic inventory system (Fig. 21.4). We want to reduce excess inventory and storage costs, to a reasonable extent.

Dentists can buy supplies in bulk, that is, to say in a large quantity that lasts a long time. The advantages are the lower cost per unit that vendors offer for quantity purchase and freedom from worrying about running out of supply for an extended time. However, especially bulky items may lead to increased space and cost of storage. Materials that have a shelf life may expire and be wasted. So there is an obvious balancing act here.

Any chemicals or materials come with a Material Safety Data Sheet (MSDS). Generally they package them with the product, although sometimes, the dentist needs to go online to get the sheet. OSHA requires that the dentist keeps these in case a patient or staff member has an accident with the material. These sheets have required emergency procedures and antidotes for the chemicals in the product. Emergency department personnel can then provide appropriate care based on the contents of the MSDSs.

Some materials (e.g., composite restorative material) require refrigerated storage to achieve optimum shelf life and performance. In these cases, OSHA requires that dentists have a refrigerator that is separate from any that staff uses to store food products (e.g., lunches.) In this way, dentists avoid any potential cross-contamination.

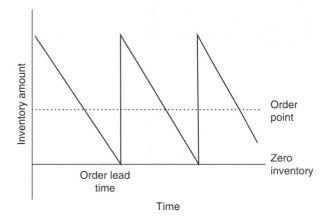

Figure 21.3 Ideal inventory system

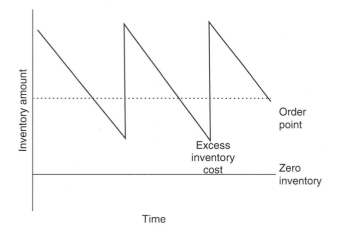

Figure 21.4 Realistic inventory system

Dentists generally want to rotate their stock of supplies. This means that the newest material is placed at the "back of the line" of supply. This ensures that the dentists use the older supplies first, which helps prevent supplies from passing their expiration date.

Ordering Supplies

A couple of common ordering systems exist. In the first (informal) system, a designated staff member checks the inventory weekly, noting any supplies that are running low. They then list needed product for order. The informality of this system leads to some obvious caveats. A different person generally looks at clinical and business office supplies. Each person needs to know how much of a material is typically used, so he or she can decide an accurate order point. This may take some experience and growing pains as the person acclimates to the job. The dentist might set rules such as "Order impression material when the second to last box of material is opened" to give guidance to an employee who is learning to manage the inventory system.

A more formal system requires a card for each inventory item. Staff members place a small colored dot sticker on the box of supplies at the reorder point. They rotate stock and when they pull the box with the sticker from inventory, they pull the card and place it in a "to order" box.

Once the office decides to order, the dentist must decide from whom to order. Dental suppliers want to be a dentist's "full service" supplier, providing dental materials, equipment, office supplies, equipment repair, computers, software, and management advice. In short, the suppliers want to provide all of a dentist's support services. When supply houses find that a dentist has entered practice, they will generally send a sales representative (or rep or detail man) to the dental office in hopes of gaining business. These representatives take orders for supplies, bring samples of new materials, return incorrect orders, and make a dentist aware of special offers. It is advantageous to have one (or two) suppliers that the dentist's primary suppliers. If a dentist suddenly finds that he or she has run out of a supply, or a piece of critical equipment stops working, a supplier will more likely work extra to see that the dentist is satisfied if the dentist has a primary account with them. The dentist can order materials from mail order or online suppliers. The price will probably be less because the supplier does not have the expense of representatives driving to the office regularly to take orders. The dentist may have a problem if a piece of equipment breaks or if the supplier back orders a supply or for another reason the dentist needs immediate service of a supplier.

Dentists can buy common paper and office supplies from warehouse clubs for less than the dental supplier. However, there is a convenience factor for the "one-stop shopping" that the supply houses offer. If the dentist accumulates several small orders into one larger order, he or she often saves through lower shipping costs. The dentist also can negotiate with vendors. If he or she finds something that the dentist wants from a competing vendor, he or she should show the special price to the supplier and ask them to meet the price. Often the supplier will. Dentists should watch for specials from vendors. They will often offer free material or additional products if the dentist purchases during a convention or dental meeting from the convention floor.

Receiving Supplies

When the order arrives from the supply house, the dentist should verify that they shipped all material as ordered. Each shipment should contain a packing slip that details all items shipped in the package. Often they include an invoice as well, though sometimes they send the invoice separately. An invoice, or bill, is a document that the seller provides that details the products, quantities, prices, and payment terms for the goods.

If something is missing or shipped incorrectly (wrong item or size or damaged goods), the dentist should call his or her sales rep and inform the rep of the problem. The dentist does not want to pay for items he or she did not order, and he or she does want the items that were ordered. Different supply houses have different procedures for returning incorrect or damaged merchandise. Many dentists will have the representative pick up the supply on their next visit. The representative will issue a credit memo for the material that was incorrect. The dentist should track these to be sure they are on his or her monthly statement. If the vendor is out of an item, he or she will say that it is back ordered, which means that it will be sent when it is received from the manufacturer.

Paying for Supplies

The large supply houses send the dentist a monthly statement that has each invoice noted and a total of all charges for the month. The dentist should pay for the supplies when this monthly statement is received, not from each separate invoice. This statement has all of the invoices from the month collected. In this way, the dentist only pays once, even if he or she has made and received several orders during the time. Often the dentist can pay supply invoices by credit card. (The practice depends on the vendor.) This practice allows the dentist to pay for the supplies later and increases the rebate tally on the office credit card. The dentist should not miss the payment due date. Most houses charge interest if they do not have payment in hand by the due date. The invoice gives terms of payment. The most common is "Net/30," which means the net payment is due 30 days from the time the invoice was issued.

Some suppliers, especially those that a dentist orders from infrequently, will post "pay from this invoice' or similar words on the invoice. This means that a dentist will not receive a separate monthly statement and that he or she should pay the vendor as stipulated on the invoice.

Laboratory Case Management

The dentist or staff can do all laboratory procedures in the office. However, many dental offices find that outsourcing these procedures is both convenient and cost effective, if the dentist has additional patients to see instead of doing the laboratory procedure. These may be procedures that the dentist does not have the materials,

machines, or knowledge to do; they may be procedures that the dentist can outsource for financial reasons; or they may be procedures the dentist simply does not enjoy doing. Regardless, the dentist needs a system to monitor work that goes out of the office to ensure timeliness, quality, and cost effectiveness.

Choosing a Laboratory

Deciding which laboratory to use for various procedures is an important decision from several perspectives. The dentist needs to have a good working relationship with the laboratory technician who does work for him or her. The dentist might need to call the lab and discuss problem areas with the case or ask questions about procedures or techniques. The lab is the expert in the area of materials and techniques, so the lab workers can help the dentist decide if a particular type or brand of material will work in a given situation. A healthy, open discussion is often necessary to gain optimum results for a patient. The dentist should visit the labs in the area and interview them as if they were a potential employee (which is really what the dentist is doing).

The dentist might have several different labs for different procedures. This may be based on their history of quality, their price, or the special materials and techniques that they employ. Lab A may do excellent porcelain work; Lab B does wonderful denture cases; and Lab C may work with the dentist in coordinating implant cases. Use each lab for its strength to gain the best result for patients.

Laboratory personnel may change over time. The technician who had been doing the work for a certain dentist may leave for another lab or retire. Often the only way the dentist knows if there is a noticeable change in the returned work. If the dentist sees a problem, he or she should be sure to call the lab to discuss the issue. If the lab cannot resolve the issue, the dentist may have to investigate a different laboratory.

Processing Cases

There is a cost trade off for most procedures. The dentist can send many impressions to the lab for model pouring and preparation, or he or she can do these procedures in house. This allows the dentist to save money and check the work before sending it out. The dentist should decide which types and what degree of cases that he or she processes internally. There are digital impression systems that currently allow the dentist to send an electronic image of the preparation to the laboratory for preparation and construction of the restoration.

Most states require that a dentist writes a paper prescription or authorization for the work that he or she wants the lab to do. This authorization lists the exact procedures that the dentist wants completed and any necessary material, shades, or special instructions. The state may require the dentist to retain a copy for a certain number of years.

When the case (all impressions, opposing casts, bite registrations, prescriptions, etc.) is ready, it should be sent to the laboratory. If the lab is local, it may have a courier who will stop by the office to pick up the case and deliver it when complete. If the lab is distant, the dentist should be sure to box the material so that it will not be damaged in transit. Further, the dentist should be sure to note on the authorization when the case is needed back in the office for try-in or seating. The dentist should note on the schedule that he or she requires a lab case for the appointment. The dentist should check at the morning huddle the day before the appointment to ensure that the lab has returned the case. If not, call the lab to be sure that they will deliver the case on time.

Part 5: Dental Insurance Management

Beaver: "Gee, there's something wrong with just about everything, isn't there dad?"
Ward: "Just about, Beav."
Leave It to Beaver

Objectives

At the completion of this part, the student will be able to:
1. Discuss the purchaser, provider, and patient relationship regarding payment for dental services.
2. Discuss the assumption of risk.
3. Describe common payment mechanisms.
4. Define various utilization incentives.
5. Describe the historical origins of third-party payment plans.
6. Recognize the role of the dental practice in third-party management.
7. Describe the carrier's responsibility to the practitioner and the patient.
8. Discuss the patient's role in the third-party process.
9. Recognize the different areas of the ADA claim form and discuss the importance of each.
10. Describe various techniques that can maximize benefits for the patient.
11. Discuss effects on office finances of the following payment mechanisms:
    Medicaid
    Medicare
    Indemnity plan
    Service corporation plan (Delta Dental)
    Health maintenance organization (HMO)
    Capitation plan (Cap plan)
    Preferred provider organization (PPO)
    Contract dental organization (CDO)
    Independent practice association (IPA)
    Direct reimbursement
12. Describe contract provisions of interest to practitioners
13. Discuss how the practitioner might effectively use third-party plans to his or her advantage

Key Terms

adverse selection
any willing provider
assignment of benefits
cafeteria (flexible) benefit plans
capitation plans (cap plan)
closed panel
contract dental organization (CDO)
cost shifting
dental health maintenance organization (HMOs)
dental maintenance organizations (DMO)
diagnostic-related groups (DRGs)
direct reimbursement (DR)
employee benefits
fee for service (FFS)
first party
fourth party
freedom of choice
indemnity insurance
independent practice association (IPA)

least expensive alternative treatment (LEAT)
managed care
managed dental care
medical loss ratio
Medicaid
Medicare
most favored nations clause
open panel
overall reimbursement rates
pacing
plan utilization controls
preferred provider organization (PPO)
relative value unit
second party
table of allowance
third party
table of allowances
traditional dental insurance
two-tiered treatment plans
unbundling
voluntary provider networks

Goal

This part introduces the various forms of third-party plans that dentists encounter when in practice. Their conceptual background will be discussed as well as how they affect the private dental practitioner.

A dental practice has several stakeholders, or parties, who have an interest in the care the dentist provides in the dental office. The "first" party is the dentist and the "second" is the patient. For many years, these were the only parties who had a vested interest in the

---

Box 21.6 Stakeholders of a Dental Practice

First Party: Dentist
Second Party: Patient
Third Party: Insurer
Fourth Party: Employer

---

dentistry. However, when insurers began to reimburse for dental services, they became an interested "third" party. The employers who purchased the insurance contracts soon realized that they were the "fourth" party and had an important interest as well. Depending on their contract, the price they paid and the services that they bought for their employees were entirely different. It is important to remember that there are four different perspectives on the issue of third-party reimbursement for dental care (Box 21.6). The dentist has one set of desires; the patient, the insurer, and the employer each have a different set of wants and needs in these programs. Each group lobbies in the marketplace for provisions that are beneficial for their group. The "ideal" third-party program balances all these perspectives.

Benefits for routine dental services are unlike traditional insurance in some important respects. Dental need is almost universal, unlike house fires, automobile accidents, or major surgery. So a dental plan, especially the component that pays for routine dental services, is more of a simple prepayment plan than a true insurance policy. There is less risk of a loss but much more certainty of one.

Employee benefits, such as dental plans, are typically bought by employers to increase employee compensation and, hopefully, morale and productivity. Plan administrators place bids with the employer for the dental plan contract. The employer (possibly in concert with union or worker representation) then picks a contract that best meets everyone's needs. The plan may be financed them through an employer contribution, employee contributions, or a combination of the two. In traditional indemnity insurance contracts, the carrier does actuarial studies to determine how many people will probably use the services and at what level. The insurers use that information to establish utilization estimates and policy rates.

Payment Mechanisms

Dentists customarily see four basic types or methods of payment for services.

Fee for Service

Fee for service (FFS) is simply an out-of-pocket expenditure by patients for the care that they receive. This still accounts for a large portion (approximately 45 percent) of the dental care payments in this country today. The obvious advantage for the practitioner is least interference in the dentist–patient relationship. The down side for both patient and practitioner is that consumers will purchase less dentistry because the cost to the consumer (patient) is higher than if someone assists in paying.

Traditional (Indemnity) Dental Insurance

Indemnity insurance pays the patient for the financial loss he or she has from receiving dental care. The plan estimates how much care that a given population (e.g., the employees at XYZ Corp.) will need. The insurer then pays the patient for part of the financial loss (dental care) that he or she has. If the insurance company has estimated too low, the insurer loses money. If their estimates are correct, then the insurance company makes money. The insurer carries the risk of overutilization of services. Traditional dental insurance stimulates demand for dental services because the patient's out-of-pocket expenditures are lower than FFS.

Managed Dental Care

Managed care is a system where the third party (insurer) contracts with dentists to provide a certain level of dental care. Instead of insurance, managed care is really a form of prepayment for services. It is the dentist's responsibility to decide the amount and type of care that the patient requires. However, the contract may stipulate the amount that the practitioner can charge the patient for the service. Because the dentist contracts ahead of doing the services, he or she carries the risk that patients may overutilize by demanding more services (either in type of services or number of services per patient). If, on the other hand, patients underutilize services, the dentist stands to profit.

Government Payment Plans

Government plans are a small part of the dental marketplace in the United States. Dental care is viewed as a consumer service (rather than a true health service) and so individuals are responsible for their own services. The government directly provides some care to special populations at the federal level (e.g., Indian Health Service,

National Health Service Corp., Uniform Military Services) and state and local health departments. The government also pays for some care in private offices, primarily through the Medicaid, and to a small degree, the Medicare programs.

Policy Limitations

Each third-party plan has certain incentives (and disincentives) for patients to use dental services. The provider (dentist) looks for maximum reimbursement, maximum coverage, minimum administrative expense, and no interference in the dentist–patient relationship (including closed panels). The patient wants maximum reimbursement and coverage, giving the lowest out-of-pocket expense. Patients want "freedom of choice" but are willing to forego this if the savings are substantial enough. The purchaser (employer) wants an adequate plan at low cost. Employers are concerned with providing a satisfactory benefit for employees with a minimum of administrative costs and problems. They do not care about freedom of choice unless employees complain that they can not find adequate dental providers. The third-party carrier is looking to reduce its own risk and maximize profit for its owners and shareholders. Carriers are looking for a small payout (low medical loss ratio) and minimum administrative expenses. Balancing all these different perspectives and needs is an impossible task. To try to balance these needs, insurance plans use many different mechanisms to encourage or discourage patient treatment.

Exclusions are procedures that the plan does not cover. Most insurers exclude experimental procedures. As those procedures become more commonplace, insurers begin to include them as covered procedures. Some plans may exclude orthodontics, temporomandibular disorder (TMD), or other treatments as cost-limiting measures.

Limitations are limits to payment of benefits for procedures or the number of times a procedure is paid for. Most plans limit prosthetic replacement to once every 5 years, regardless of who does the procedure. Many will limit payment for orthodontic treatment to once in a lifetime. Others limit recall exams to every 6 months (to the day). Patients often do not understand limitations, so it is in the dentist's interest to have a staff member (receptionist) who understands each plan.

Annual maximums are the maximum amounts in a given calendar year that an insurer will pay in total benefits for a person. Most plans set an annual maximum (or payment cap) near $1000, an amount that has not changed (even with inflation) in many years. Dentists often plan treatment so that is occurs at the end of one year and the beginning of the next. In this way, they can help the patient to maximize insurance coverage from 2 years.

Deductibles and copays limit the third-party's benefit payments. The patient is responsible for part of the costs, either the first dollar amount (deductible) or a percentage of the cost (copay).

Open panel plans allow covered patients to receive care from any dentist and allow any dentist to participate. They often call these "freedom-of-choice" plans. Closed panels allow covered individuals to receive care only from a certain group (panel) of dentists who have signed contracts and agree to terms of participation with the third-party carrier. Closed panels allow managed care organizations to limit the number of providers, and by that, guaranteeing a group of patients for each of those who do participate.

Method of Reimbursement

Third-party plans have developed many ways of determining reimbursement for services. If a dentist understands these methods, it will allow him or her to help patients to maximize their benefits and allow the dentist to evaluate the financial impact of third-party plans.

Usual, Customary, and Reasonable (UCR)

The UCR is a fee the dentist usually charges for a certain procedure. The customary fee is determined by the insurance company based on what dentists in the same area are charging for similar procedures (Box 21.7). A reasonable fee is used to justify special circumstances that may affect the fee usually charged for the procedure. Wide differences between commu-

---

Box 21.7 "Usual, Customary, and Reasonable" Fee

A patient's plan pays 80 percent of the UCR or dentist's fee, whichever is less. The dentist charges (and submits) a claim for a filling for $100. The insurance company compares that fee to their UCR for the area.

If the UCR is more (say, $120) then the insurance company pays 80 percent of the charge, or $80 (80 percent of $100).

If, however, their UCR for the procedure is less (say $90), then the insurance company will pay only 80 percent of this lower fee, or $72 (80 percent of $90).

nities have made this system controversial. Third-party carriers generally reimburse based on a percentage of the lesser of the dentist's usual fee or the fee that the third-party has determined is customary for the area. The fee that the carriers use as their "customary" fee is a closely held corporate secret. This causes problems between dentists and patients who feel they are being overcharged, based on insurance carrier information.

Table (Schedule) of Allowances

In this method, the insurer sets a maximum dollar limit for each covered procedure, regardless the fee that the dentist charges. They pay the fee charged (or a percentage of it) up to a specified amount from a table that lists the allowable (maximum) charge. Above that, the dentist may (or may not) charge the patient the difference, depending on the rules of the insurance contract.

Least Expensive Alternative Treatment (LEAT)

The LEAT method states that the third party will reimburse for what they decide is the least expensive method of correcting the patient's problem. For example, a dentist might replace a patient's missing tooth with an implant, a fixed bridge, or a removable partial denture. The dentist can recommend to the patient and do any service the dentist wants. However, the third-party payer will only reimburse for the LEATs (i.e., the removable). Others may "downcode" a posterior composite restoration to a less-expensive amalgam restoration. This obviously keeps their payout lower and places the burden to justify treatment choice on the dentist.

Capitation (per Capita)

Capitated plans reimburse a dentist a given amount for each participating patient that has signed up to be a patient of the practice. The dentist is then responsible for providing a certain level of care because of receiving the capitation payment. Patients are responsible for paying for (or a portion of) procedures not covered by the plan. The theory is that the dentist makes enough money on capitation payments, based on the panel of patients, to cover the preventive services of those patients who actually come for dental care. In fact, capitation plans have implied financial incentives for the dentist not to see patients or do extensive dental work on them.

Other Insurance Terms

A couple of additional insurance terms are important to understand. *Adverse selection* occurs when only high-risk individuals sign up for a particular insurance. The insurer is not able to spread the risk over a sufficient number of people. The insurer then either has to increase rates dramatically or suffer a loss. This often happens with voluntary participation plans such as flexible (cafeteria style) employee benefit plans. Only the employees who plan to use the plan sign up and pay for participating in the plan.

Insurers speak of a *medical loss ratio*. This is the percentage of premiums that the third party pays out (to the medical provider) for covered services. It is a loss for the insurer. It is income for the provider. The ratio typically runs from 50 to 90 percent paid out as medical (or dental) benefits to providers. Obviously, the providers prefer a higher percentage payout. The insurers prefer a lower ratio, retaining as much as possible to convert to profits.

Coordination of benefits applies to people who are covered by more than one insurance plan. (For example, both husband and wife receive different dental insurance through their workplaces.) Dentists must be careful about plan rules to help patients maximize their entitled benefits. As an industry rule (called the "birthday rule"), a person's primary carrier is through their work, the secondary is through his spouse's. The kids' primary insurance is whichever parent's birthday occurs first in the calendar year. Dentists submit reimbursement for the dental procedure to the primary carrier first. Once dentists have received payment, they submit the remainder to the secondary carrier. Some carriers have special rules concerning dual coverage. The dentist should not assume anything and should call the insurer or ask for a pretreatment estimate of benefits for the patient.

Predetermination is a system under which a dentist submits the proposed treatment plan to the insurer before beginning work. After review, the plan administrator will determine the patient's eligibility, covered services, patient's copay, and maximum benefit. This is intended as an aid for the dentist so the patient knows in advance how much the insurer will pay and what his or her portion will be. Some insurers require predetermination before treatment that exceeds a given dollar amount. Many dentists set in-office limits in which they send claims for predetermination. Dentists also call this pretreatment estimate, prior authorization, or preauthorization. The insurers claim that they are not authorizing treatment, only payment for the treatment.

Bundling occurs when the insurer combines several procedures together into one procedure, generally to lower the total payout. For example, a typical recall visit may consist of a periodic oral exam, bitewing radiographs, and a dental prophylaxis. If the insurer combines these procedures into a new code, lowering the cost over separate billing of the procedures, then "bundling" has occurred. Similarly, *unbundling* occurs when the dental practitioner takes a common procedure and breaks it into component parts, increasing the total fee. As an example, a composite restoration is generally understood to include acid etching, bonding, and placing of common liners. If the dentist charges separately for these procedures, by that raising the total fee, then "unbundling" has said to have occurred. The profession does not like bundling because it lowers reimbursement. Third-party payers do not like unbundling because is raises reimbursements. Both sides charge fraud against the other when it occurs.

Characteristics of Third-Party Plans

Each of the various types of plans has its own characteristics that are more or less valuable to each of the interested groups. The major types of plans and their characteristics are listed in Table 21.7.

Fee For Service (FFS)

FFS is not a third-party plan (Box 21.8). It only involves the first two parties to the transaction (dentist and patient). It is described here because it is the baseline or reference point for comparing all other reimbursement plans.

FFS is the oldest form of payment for dental services and still accounts for nearly half of all dental payments. Patients pay the dentist directly for their dental care. Reimbursement is based on an agreed price between the dentist and the patient. Patients are not reimbursed by any third party for their financial loss. If they have a large amount of work done, they (the patient) pay individually for the above average use of dental service. In theory, those who most value dental services will pay for them. FFS is an open panel system; a patient can go to any dentist who agrees to see them.

FFS dentistry is not without its problems. Dental care is expensive. Only those who can afford dental care receive its benefits, leading to large disparities in oral health between those who have adequate finances and those who do not. Dentists must be especially diligent with their credit and collection policies to ensure that they collect the amounts owed from patients. The amounts that patients pay for services are generally not tax deductible. (Medical-dental expenses greater than 7.5 percent adjusted gross income are deductible for those people who meet the limit and itemize deductions.)

Table 21.7 Major Plan Types and their Characteristics

Type of Plan	Contract Is Between
Traditional fee plans	
FFS	Dentist and patient
Indemnity insurance	Insurer and patient
	Dentist and patient
Direct reimbursement	Patient and employer
	Dentist and patient
Managed care plans	
CDO	Dentist and insurer
Capitation plans	Dentist and insurer
IPA	Dentist and IPA network
Medicaid	Dentist and government
	Patient and government

CDO, contract dental organizations; FFS, fee for service; IPA, independent practice associations.

Box 21.8 Characteristics of a Fee-for-Service Plan

- Not a third-party plan
- Generally not tax advantaged
- Reimbursement based on agreed price
- Patients carry risk of overutilization
- Open panel
- Leads to disparities in oral health

Most third-party plans offered through an employer are tax deductible. This means that the government covers some of the cost of the plan, giving more "bang for the buck" than nontax–deductible plans.

Dental Insurance Plans

Dental insurance plans are plans that provide for a reimbursement to patients for the cost of dental care that they incur. This reimbursement is usually from the employer, as a form of employee benefit. The money may flow directly from the employer to the employee (patient) in direct reimbursement, or it may flow through an insurance company, as traditional indemnity insurance.

Traditional Indemnity Care Plans

Traditional indemnity insurance is also known as "regular" or traditional dental insurance (Box 21.9). As with any insurance products, it "indemnifies" or pays for a loss. (Here, the loss is the patient's cost for the dental procedure.) The contract is between the patient and the insurer. No contractual relationship exists between the

> **Box 21.9** Characteristics of Traditional Indemnity
>   Care Plans
>
> Insurer reimburses (indemnifies) patient for financial loss
> Open panel
> Reimbursement based on:
>   Table of allowances
>   Usual, customary reasonable fee
> Insurer carries risk of overutilization
>   Plan control (deductibles, copays, maximums)
> Needs groups of subscribers
> Leads to overtreatment

> **Box 21.10** Characteristics of Direct
>   Reimbursement
>
> Promoted by organized dentistry
> Open panel
> Most similar to fee for service
> Dentist charges and collects from patient
> Employer reimburses patient for financial loss
> Reimbursement based on
>   Table of allowance
>   Usual, customary, reasonable fee
>   Annual maximum
> Patient carries risk of overutilization

insurer and the dentist. Dentists often agree to process forms, accept assignment of benefits, and send pretreatment estimates as a convenience for the patient. The patient owes the dentist for the service, no matter his or her reimbursement from the insurer. These plans often try (and succeed) in placing the dentist between the patient and the insurer, by requiring documentation and mediation of disputes for services or fees.

Indemnity insurance is an open panel product. The agreement, again, is between the insurer and the patient. The insurer does not care where the patient receives treatment because the insurance reimburses the patient. Employers purchase these insurance contracts from major insurance companies. They generally provide them as a benefit to all employees because allowing freedom of participation would lead to adverse selection.

Indemnity insurance reimburses the patient, not the dentist. The dentist charges the patient for the procedure. The employee (patient) sends a receipt to the insurer for reimbursement of his or her financial loss. The insurer pays the patient an agreed-upon amount. The dentist (the provider) may accept "assignment of benefits" in which the patient agrees that the reimbursement (benefit) is sent (or "assigned") directly to the dentist instead of to the patient first. The insurer agrees (through the contract) to reimburse the entire cost of the service, part of the cost through patient copays or a portion through a table of allowances, in which they will reimburse a certain amount for a given procedure, regardless the fee charged. (The patient is then responsible for the remainder of the charge.) The insurance company may have internal limits for employees (either family or individual) or exclusions for certain services.

From the patient's perspective, traditional indemnity insurance is simple, there is freedom of choice of a dentist, and it lowers out of pocket expenses significantly. Most researchers believe that traditional insurance leads to overtreatment when compared with uninsured patients.

Practitioners like indemnity insurance because it is an open panel with freedom of choice. Therefore, dentists see minor interference in the dentist–patient relationship. Traditional insurance stimulates demand for services and, once systems are in place, is relatively simple because there are standard forms to complete. Practitioners may experience cash flow problems waiting for the carrier to reimburse and may have traditional patient collection problems for the copayments and uncovered procedures.

From the employer's perspective, indemnity insurance is an expensive benefit to provide. Employers generally do not care about freedom of choice, only about providing a cost-effective benefit for their employees. They often believe that they can get more bang for the buck out of a capitation plan or preferred provider organization.

Direct Reimbursement (DR)

Direct reimbursement (DR) is also known as "paid dental." It is a plan that the dental associations are supporting as an alternative to managed dental care. It is being promoted through the professional press, by giving advice to employers and dentists, and by giving assistance through computer programs for employers to monitor and administer the program. It is promoted especially to smaller employers who do not have traditional insurance plans. There are several third-party administrators who will set up and administer a plan for a business.

DR is an open panel with complete freedom of choice (Box 21.10). It is a contract between the employer and the employee (patient). The employee goes to any dentist and has dental work done. The patient pays for the work. The patient then takes the paid receipt to their employer's benefits office. The employer then reimburses the employee for cost of care. This reimbursement may be total, involve copayments, or be based on a table of allowances. The employer may set individual maximums, or overall company maximums, use a "first come first served" basis, exclusions or other methods to limit their potential cost. A typical DR plan might pay for 100 percent of the first $100 spent on dental care, 80 percent of the next $500, and 50 percent of the next $1,000 for a total annual amount of $1,500.

From the patient's perspective, DR is simple. There may be increased out-of-pocket expenses or limitations when compared to other types of plans. The patient can go to any dentist. Depending on the particular limitations of the plan, patients may view it more or less favorably than other types of plans.

Practitioners support DR because of its open panel character and no interference in the dentist–patient relationship. DR stimulates demand like traditional insurance. It is simple for the practitioner (no forms to complete), but the dentist may have collection problems similar to FFS patients.

From the employer's perspective, there may be employee disenchantment from internal limits and such. Employees then complain to the employer rather than an insurance company. Employers often would rather contract out the administration of their dental plan rather than self-administer one. They can often get more bang for the buck out of a capitation plan or preferred provider organization.

Managed Care Plans

A managed care plan is any plan in which the dentist signs a contract to provide services for a contractually set fee. To make managed dental care plans work effectively, insurers, or managed care organizations (MCOs) must exercise control over the participating dentists, in contracts and guidelines for treatment (Box 21.11). An open panel arrangement allows a patient to go to any dentist and receive the same level of reimbursement for a given service. (This is also called freedom of choice for the patient.) A closed panel, on the other hand, denotes that patients may only go to a certain "panel" of dentists if they wish to receive full benefit from their dental plan. (Depending on their plan, patients may receive either a reduced reimbursement or no reimbursement at the nonparticipating dentist's office.) Most patients have a price at which they will switch providers. Closed panels are effective at moving patients to participating providers. Some programs require the participating dentist to be a member of the panel but accept "any willing provider" as a member of the panel rather than limit the number of providers in an area. It is not then truly a closed panel but requires that participants agree to the terms of the contract, if they participate.

Dentists claim several problems with managed care programs. These generally revolve around the issue of the managed care plan reimbursing at a lower level than

---

Box 21.11 Characteristics of Managed Care Plans

Trades groups (blocks) of patients, not individuals
Costs and benefits are calculated in the aggregate
Contract is between provider and insurer
Uses provider networks (closed panels)
Shifts financial risk (overutilization) to providers
Emphasizes cost-efficient care
    Optimal versus adequate care
It is a secondary market
    "Brokered care"
    Dental health care opportunity

Box 21.12 Characteristics of Preferred Provider Organizations (PPOs)

Also known as a contract dental organization (CDO)
Trades blocks of patients for contractually reduced fees
Dentist charges and collects from patient for service
Reimbursed based on table of allowances
Closed panel
Dentist carries risk of overutilization
    Tendency to undertreat
May have (limited) nonplan participant reimbursement

---

other plans, and dentists' efforts to manipulate the system to avoid the problem without compromising patient care. One common problem is a temptation for "two-tiered treatment plans." FFS and traditional insurance patients receive one plan, managed care patients receive another, less aggressive plan. Dentists often spread treatment out, "pacing" treatment based on payment plans rather than patient needs. They claim a loss of control of the dentist–patient relationship. These problems create new ethical dilemmas. (They do not create "poor dentistry.") Managed dental care offers many new opportunities to exercise poor judgment through the apparent no-win situations faced by dentists.

Preferred Provider Organizations (PPOs)

Preferred provider organizations (PPOs) are also called contract dental organizations (CDOs). The dental profession uses CDO because they claim that there is nothing "preferred" about these providers, except that they have signed a contract. Calling them preferred providers infers a difference of quality that simply is not there.

CDOs work on a table of allowance payment method (Box 21.12). They are often weighted toward preventive services. The contract is between the insurer and the participating provider. The dentist must sign a participating agreement (contract) if he or she participates. When the dentist signs the contract, he or she agrees to accept their schedule of allowance as the full payment for services. The dentist may not legally charge the patient more than the contracted price. Nonsubscribers may react negatively to reduced fees offered to plan patients.

From the practitioner's perspective, CDOs trade the reduced fees for the guarantee of patients for the practice. CDOs are closed panels. Only a certain number of dentists are contracted to participate. This keeps the numbers of patients per dentist at agreed levels. The advantage for the practitioner is that "warm bodies" are available, especially during practice start-up and building phases. This contributes to paying some of the fixed cost of the office, if the office has slack chair time. The level of the discount may not cover office overhead expenses. The practitioner should run the break-even point or other financial analyses to assess the financial impact of participation. The disadvantages to CDOs are that the practitioner receives less than their usual fee for many procedures. Dentists may also lose patients to participating providers if they are not a plan participant. It may be difficult for practices to enter or leave the plan because of contract provisions.

From the patient's perspective, economic incentives encourage him or her to receive care from a participating provider. (If the patient does not go to a participating provider, reimbursement is limited.) This reduces the cost of dental care. As a trade off, the patient may lose some freedom of choice if his or her traditional dentist is not a plan provider.

Point of service (POS) plans are a hybrid type of PPO. In the POS plan, the patient has the option of remaining in the network or going to a provider outside the network. There are strong financial incentives for the patient to remain in the network (higher reimbursement rates, lower copayments, etc.). However, POS plans allow patient choice of provider at a cost. Exclusive provider organizations (EPOs) allow covered patients to receive care only from their list of providers. If a patient receives treatment from a dentist who is not on the EPO panel, the services will not be covered by the plan. (Usually some allowance is made for out-of-area emergencies).

Capitation Plans (Cap Plans)

Capitation plans are also known as Cap plans, dental maintenance organizations (DMOs), and dental health maintenance organizations (HMOs). These are managed care plans (Box 21.13). They are a contractual arrangement between the dentist and the plan. Cap plans pay dentists a monthly amount per person enrolled in the plan through the dentist's office. This becomes a monthly "per capita" or

---

> **Box 21.13** Characteristics of capitation plans
>
> Trades blocks of patients for contractually reduced fees
> Dentist receives:
>   Monthly "per capita" reimbursement (PMPM)
>   Charges and collects reduced fee from patient for services
> Reimbursement based on table of allowances
> Closed panel
> Preventive oriented (in theory)
> Dentist carries risk of overutilization
>   Tendency to undertreat

per member, per month (PMPM) payment. In exchange, the dentist agrees (generally) to provide a dental exam, radiographs, and prophylaxis twice per year at no charge to the patient or plan. The dentist then provides other needed services at a reduced fee, similar to a PPO. Cap plans, then, are closed panels in which a portion is a per capita fee, and a portion is a table of allowance fee structure.

These plans have a preventive orientation. In theory, they encourage more preventive treatment, when dental care is most effective and least expensive. Once dentists get patients to a maintenance level of care (the theory goes) then they require less work and become more "profitable." The theory breaks down in several areas. Patients do not all stay long term with the program. People move and are transferred. They enter and leave the plan for their own reasons. And the high degree of personal responsibility inherent in preventive dental services requires high patient compliance.

There are several advantages for practitioners. The dentist can budget a more stable cash flow and plan resources for expenditures. These programs may provide additional patients during the practice building phase. However, these patients can overwhelm a practice if their numbers are not controlled. Because the plans end up reimbursing at reduced rates (from a full fee), they often only cover costs. There is inadequate profit built into the system to operate with traditional dental practice systems. Dentists shoulder the risk of increased utilization in this plan. The plans become most profitable to the dentist when patients do not come in for treatment, an idea that is anathema to many practitioners. Many patients view these plans as traditional "dental insurance." They may have difficulty finding a provider that is acceptable to them.

Independent Practice Associations (IPAs)

IPAs are also known as voluntary provider networks. In this form of a reimbursement plan, providers band

> **Box 21.14** Characteristics of Independent Practice Associations
>
> Providers band together and bid on blocks of patients
> Trades blocks of patients for contractually reduced fee
> Eliminates "middle man"
> Must compete in marketplace with other plans
> Dentist's payment type depends on the plan
>   Capitated
>   Table of allowance
> Closed panel
> Dentists carry risk of overutilization
>   Tendency to undertreat
> Problems of restraint of trade

> **Box 21.15** Characteristics of Referral Plans
>
> Trades blocks of patients for contractually reduced fee
> Eliminates "middle man"
> No third-party payments
> Dentist's payment is table of allowance charges
> Closed panel

together to compete for contracts (Box 21.14). These are contracts to provide services for groups of potential patients. The providers attempt to eliminate the "middle man" (in this case, the insurer) by negotiating directly with the employer or purchaser. This allows higher reimbursements for providers or more competitive prices for the purchasers. It is conceptually similar to a DR managed care program.

The program reimburses on any basis that the IPA negotiates. This may be indemnity, service, or capitation based. Most are service based, although capitated IPA plans are increasing in number. From the patient's perspective, these are closed panels, so there is limited choice of providers. Other than that, reaction depends largely on the structure of the plan.

The advantage for practitioners is that they have some control over contract provisions because the provider network negotiates the contracts. However, if the contract is not competitive with others in the marketplace, it will not be bought by the plan purchasers (employers). So IPAs, with time, end up being comparable to other third-party plans in the area. These plans generally have less than full reimbursement. There are also potential problems with the Fair Trade Commission and price-fixing from dentists banding together to negotiate prices. There are many of the same problems as other managed care plans, although these plans are more practitioner friendly. There is also often practitioner disillusionment because practitioners think they will have more control over contract provisions than they actually have.

Referral Plans

Referral plans are not truly a third-party reimbursement plan, but they are viewed by the public as a type of dental insurance (Box 21.15). A referral plan contracts with the practicing dentist to do dental services at a reduced fee. In return, the patients who are signed up with the plan are sent to the participating providers to receive the discounted cost dental care. (This is a closed panel arrangement.) Patients who sign on with the plan pay a nominal fee (a few dollars a month), which is used for administration and profit for the plan. No money for service flows through the plan. Dentists still must collect from the patient for the care rendered. Dentists gain patient base for the reduced fee that is contractually obligated.

Government Payment Plans

The government pays for a limited amount of dental service in private offices, mainly through two programs, Medicare and Medicaid.

Medicare

Medicare is also known, erroneously, as Social Security. (They are two different programs.) Medicare is a federal program. It is health insurance for older (older than 65) and disabled Americans (Box 21.16). It is essentially a major medical (hospitalization) policy. Participants can buy additional, optional coverage for physician's services. Medicare reimburses based on diagnostic-related groups (DRGs), which are actually tables of allowances for hospitals, based on the disease, rather than on hospital cost.

From the patient's perspective, Medicare is medical insurance for retired people. (Often older Americans cannot get any other health insurance when their medical needs are the highest.) It does not cover long-term (nursing home) care and does not cover many "optional" services, such as dental care. The typical dental practitioner sees little impact from Medicare. Some hospital practitioners (such as oral surgeons) may see some impact if a covered person has a disease or accident involving the jaws. This program profoundly affects the way physicians practice. It is mentioned here so that it is not confused with the Medicaid program.

> **Box 21.16** Characteristics of Medicare
>
> Government sponsored health insurance for:
>   Older (+65) Americans
>   Disabled Americans
>   Certain other categories
> Very little dental coverage or impact

> **Box 21.17** Characteristics of Medicaid
>
> Qualification based on family income below poverty level
> Provides payment for indigent care
> Varies from state to state
>   Coverage for dental services
>   Type and amount of reimbursement
> Open panel (but a contract must be signed)
> Usually preventive oriented

Medicaid

Medicaid is known by many other names including medical assistance (MA), medical assistance plan (MAP), "The Medical Card," and "The Card." It also has individual state associated names, such as "MediCal" (California) and "KMAP" (Kentucky Medical Assistance Program) in Kentucky. Medicaid is a combination state and federally funded program. Coverage varies from state to state. Some states pay for more comprehensive dental services than others. Some states have no dental component at all. The federal government reimburses the state a given amount for each state dollar spent.

Medicaid is a health subsidy for poor people (Box 21.17). Although each state's dental program is different, they often reimburse preventive care for younger people. They often reimburse emergency and diagnostic services for adults. Each state reimburses differently, but a typical method is to reimburse the UCR up to 75th percentile (allegedly) for the geographical area. These programs often pay relatively well for kids, especially preventive and diagnostic procedures. The theory behind this is if kids are treated early and given dental care, they will not need much work as adults. This increases the state's effectiveness in spending scarce resources (money for indigent dental care). Some states are moving to managed dental care programs for their dental Medicaid programs. This is in an obvious effort to hold down costs to the state and receive the maximum amount of indigent care for a dollar.

From the patient's perspective, patients often assume Medicaid is complete coverage. (Generally, it is not.) Often the services are also limited. But Medicaid provides dental care for many people who simply could not otherwise afford it. In some areas, it may be difficult for patients to find a practitioner who accepts patients who have Medicaid.

For the practitioner, Medicaid fulfills a social responsibility. At the professional level, dentists have a monopoly, granted through the state licensure mechanism, to do dentistry. (No one can legally do dentistry except dentists.) Dentists must keep the public trust or risk losing the monopoly. That public trust involves some method of responding to the dental needs of all the public, both the unfortunate and the fortunate. Medicaid brings several disadvantages to the practitioner as well. States often set unrealistically low reimbursement rates. Dentists may not legally charge the patient the difference between what Medicaid reimburses and the UCR fee. Dentists may, however, charge patient for procedures that Medicaid does not cover. These patients often show a low appointment consciousness.

Processing Insurance Claims

The ADA has developed a standard numbering system for the treatments that dentists do. It is called the *Current Dental Terminology* (CDT) code. This "Code on Dental Procedures and Nomenclature" is standard across the industry. The ADA periodically updates the code to be sure that dentists can code current procedures and materials for payment and reimbursement. Notice that these are treatment codes (based on the treatment that dentists do). They are not based on the diagnosis, as are most medical insurance codes. Dentists can purchase a book from the ADA that explains the code. Office management programs have these codes incorporated into their programs and update the codes as needed through software updates. Nearly all third parties accept these standard descriptions of treatments.

Insurance Code Categories

Insurers generally group procedures by type for reimbursement purposes. The specifics are not industry standard but vary somewhat from insurer to insurer and plan to plan, depending on the details negotiated with the purchasing employer. Insurers group procedures into one of four categories: preventive, basic, major, and other (Box 21.18). The insurers then reimburse a certain percentage of the cost of each procedure in each group. Typically, they reimburse well for preventive service, less for basic services, and even less for major and other services. Often they do not apply deductibles to preventive services. Because of the large variation between insurers

Box 21.18 Insurance Code Categories

Preventive Services
Diagnostic
Radiographic
Preventive
Basic Services
Restorative
Endodontic
Basic surgery
Major Services
Crowns
Removable prosthetics
Fixed prosthetics
Periodontics
Other Services
Orthodontics
Implants
Adjunctive services

and among specific plans by insurers, dentists need to have the patient bring their insurance booklet (from their employer's benefit office) with him or her to the appointment. They booklet will list the specifics of the plan, so that the dentist can enter the information into the office management system for more accurate estimates of patient payments and insurance benefits. Each plan also has a contact point (telephone, fax, or Internet) where the staff can ask about coverage for a specific patient. Box 21.18 illustrates how different indemnity plans can result in different reimbursements and patient payments.

Table of allowance reimbursement plans differ in that the insurer gives a list of allowable procedures and payment associated with each. Depending on the plan, the insurer reimburses part or all of the charges, and the patient is responsible for part or all of the allowable charges.

The ADA Insurance Form

Almost all third-party plans accept the ADA's standard Dental Claims Form for submission of dental benefits. This is a paper form but is also the basis of claims that dentists submit electronically. The form can be completed by hand, writing the information on a preprinted form and mailing it to the insurer. The only time dentists do this is when they do not use an office computer management program. Most management software will print a paper form (on plain paper) based on the information the dentist entered into the program. This form can then be mailed to the insurer. Currently, the most common method is submitting claims electronically. In this method, front office staff members use the management software at the end of the day to process claims for the day. The software checks the claims to be sure that the dentist has entered needed information. It then accumulates all claims and sends them via the Internet to a claims-processing company. This clearing house company checks all the claims for completeness, returning any that need additional information. It takes the rest and combines them from all subscribed providers. It then sends batches of claims to each individual insurer. In this way, the insurance carrier receives the claim the day it is submitted. The clearing house has checked it for completeness, so processing is quicker. There is a cost associated with electronic claims processing. However, it is generally no more that the time, paper, and postage associated with traditional processing.

A key element in speeding reimbursement (and therefore cash flow) from the carriers is to properly complete the insurance form. If the dentist is mailing forms, he or she should be sure to complete all of the information on the form. If filing electronically, the submission process will check that the dentist has entered all required information (but not that it is correct). Regardless how the dentist submits, several keys keep claims from being delayed. The CDT codes should be updated in the computer whenever the ADA updates them. Many plans have limitations on frequency or recency of replacement of crowns and bridges. The dentist should be sure to show if this is an initial placement or the date of prior placement. If this is not an initial placement, the dentist should include an explanation in the narrative and should only use the "Notes" section for notes regarding treatment needs. Most carriers remove claims with notes from the automatic process to have an adjustor look at the claim. So notes like "Please pay promptly" or "Have a nice day" may slow the claims payment process.

When the dentist completes an insurance form, each section has important information. All fields on the form should be completed. The insurer will return the claim if fields are left blank. Some common problem areas on the form are detailed here.

1. *Header Information* The dentist should check whether this is a statement for work that he or she has done or a request for predetermination of benefits. The insurer processes them differently.
2. *Policyholder/Subscriber Information* The insurer needs to verify eligibility of the subscriber to be sure that the insurance plan covers him or her.
3. *Patient Information* The insurer must verify the eligibility of the patient. If the patient is a dependent (e.g., a child), then the insurer needs to know the age of the patient to verify eligibility.

4. *Other Coverage* If the patient has secondary insurance, then the insurer needs to know to check for coordination of benefits.
5. *Record of Services Provided* This is the section where the dentist enters the services completed, along with other information (e.g., date of service, procedure code). The insurer pays based on the patient's plan's requirements and the procedures that the dentist submits.
6. *Authorizations* This section authorizes the dentist to file the claim (by the patient's signature) and authorizes the insurer to send payment to the dentist, instead of the patient (assignment of benefits). Both signatures may be kept on file, for electronic filing. In this case, the program prints "Signature on File" in these spaces. The dentist should have the signature on file.
7. *Ancillary Claim or Treatment Information* This section has information that the insurer may use to allow or deny the claim. Orthodontics often has a lifetime maximum. Insurance usually pay for prosthetics once every 5 years. If this claim was done for treatment resulting from an occupational injury, then the patient's workers' compensation insurance is probably responsible for the claim. If it is the result of an accident, then another insurer (health or automobile) may be responsible for paying the claim.

Insurance Company Processing

When the insurance company receives a claim, it then begins its processing process. The first step is for computers to check the forms and verify eligibility of the patient.

If the form is a predetermination of benefits, the computer program checks the procedures and patient eligibility. If the case has a questionable prognosis, or is beyond normal procedures, then the company sends the claim to a consultant who reviews the case. The dental consultant reviews the case (including any pictures, models, radiographs, or explanations that the dentist has sent) and decides eligibility of the procedures and appropriateness of the care. (This has been a problem with many practitioners.) They then issue an estimate of benefits or similar form that describes what they will reimburse. Depending on the complexity of the case and the backlog at the insurer, this may take several weeks.

If the form is for payment of services, then the computer calculates allowable amounts for the patient's specific plan. The insurer then writes a check for reimbursement and prints an EOB or similar form that describes how much is paid for each procedure. The insurer often accumulates several patients on one EOB and bulk payments form several patients into one check.

How to Manage The Traditional Indemnity Insurance Plans

Traditional indemnity insurance is a contract between the insurer and the patient. The insurer has agreed to indemnify ("make whole," or reimburse) for losses suffered because of dental care. For the patient, those losses are the financial cost of paying for the care. As the dentist/provider of services, dentists have a contract (written or implied) that if the patient agrees to have the recommended work done, the patient will pay for the service (as a FFS patient). If the insurer will reimburse the patient for financial loss, so much the better for the patient (and the dentist because it encourages people to "purchase" care). But there is no contract between the insurer and the provider, only between the insurer and the patient. As a convenience to the patient, dentists may agree to let the insurer send their reimbursement check (the insurance benefit) directly to them, instead of the patient.

This procedure (assignment of benefits) lowers the patient's cash outlay and apparent out-of-pocket expense but does not change the fundamental agreement between the patient and the dentist, or the patient and the insurer (Table 21.8). The patient owes the dentist the full fee charged, regardless the reimbursement of the insurer. Many savvy dentists send letters to their patients in the last quarter of the year informing them of their insurance benefits remaining for the year and any needed dental treatment. Because the insurance is a "use-it-or-lose-it"

Table 21.8 Example Indemnity Plan Reimbursement Schedules
The following two indemnity plans reimburse according to the following schedules:

	Plan #1	Plan #2	
Preventive	†100%	*100%	*Deductible applies to preventive
Basic	80%	50%	
Major	50%	50%	†Deductible does not apply to
Other	50%	25%	preventive
Deductible	$250	$100	
Annual Max.	$1,000	$1,500	

The patient has agreed to the following treatment plan.
The cost for the patient and insurers under each coverage are:

Service	Fee	Plan #1 Patient	Plan #1 Insurer	Plan #2 Patient	Plan #2 Insurer
Initial Exam	$75		$75	$75	
FMX rays	$85		$80	$25	$60
Prophylaxis	$90		$90		$90
Restore #2	$60	$160		$80	$80
Restore #7	$110	$110		$55	$55
FPD #3 X #5	$2,000	$1,035	$965	$1,000	$1,000
TOTAL	$2,420	$1,520	$1,000	$1,235	$1,285

proposition, many patients will schedule their treatment to maximize their benefit for the year. Many dentists will also schedule large cases at the end of the year, so that some of the work will be covered by this year's insurance, and some will be initiated and covered by next year's. In this way, they can help to maximize the patient's reimbursement.

How to Manage the Managed Care Plans

Participating in limited reimbursement insurance plans is similar to driving a car down the highway at 75 miles per hour in second gear. The person is getting where he or she needs to go but is working very hard to get there. At some point the person needs to shift to a higher gear or risk burning out the engine. To manage these programs in the office effectively, dentists need to understand the problems involved from both a financial and a practice philosophy perspective.

Overall Reimbursement Rates

The basic problem with managed care programs from the practitioners' perspective is not the concept of capitation, prepayment, risk shifting, or method of payment (Box 21.19). It is simply that the overall reimbursement rates are too low to maintain profitability. To track this reimbursement rate, the accounting system needs to be customized to give the dentist the needed information. For the practitioner who uses a pegboard style accounting system, he or she should use the "Business Analysis" section on the right-hand side of the day sheet and set up columns for each plan's charges and adjustments. Computerized offices can easily set the program to track these charges. These number should be tracked over the month. The total reimbursement rate is the total plan charges (at the prevailing full fee rate) divided into the total plan billings (charges less adjustments plus any capitation payments).

The overall reimbursement rate is where the cost controls hit the practitioner. It is also where the plan administrator sells the plan to various employers. If the administrator has to sell a plan that reimburses 80 cents on the dollar, it will obviously cost him more than a plan that reimburses 60 cents on the dollar. Prices to employers for the plan must reflect this difference in reimbursement rate. The employer is more concerned with the cost of the plan to the employer, rather than the percentage payout. The only time the employer cares about payout is if employees complain about poor performance by the plan.

The reimbursement rate should be tracked over time. Plan administrators will change the payout amounts. As

Box 21.19 How to Calculate Reimbursement Rate

Example #1
Last month, this preferred provider organization plan resulted in $8,000 of charges. The dentist adjusted $2,000 because of the plan's requirements. The overall reimbursement rate was 75 percent.

Charges	$8,000
Adjustments	–2,000
+ Cap Pmt (if any)	+0
Amount Realized	$6,000
Reimbursement Rate	75%

Example #2
Last month, this capitation plan resulted in $6,000 of charges. The dentist adjusted $3,000 because of the plan. The dentist also received a capitation payment for $1,000 for the month. The overall reimbursement rate was 67 percent.

Charges	$6,000
Adjustments	–3,000
+ Cap Pmt (if any)	+1,000
Amount Realized	$4,000
Reimbursement Rate	66% of full fee

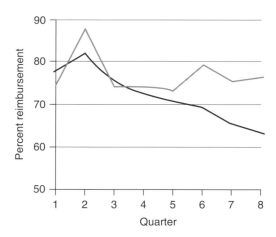

Figure 21.5 Tracking reimbursement rates over time

fees and procedure mix changes, the reimbursement level may change. The dentist should not assume that because the reimbursement rate was 85 percent of UCR that it will remain there. Figure 21.5 shows two plans over time. One plan has had steady reimbursement rates (with monthly fluctuations). The second plan shows a steadily decreasing reimbursement rate. Dentists should carefully consider whether they should continue to participate in the second plan.

Working on the Margin

A detailed analysis of office costs shows that many costs (e.g., rent, staff etc.) are fixed, regardless the number of patients seen in a given time. The only costs that vary directly with production are those associated with dental lab, supplies, and office supplies. These are the marginal costs of seeing additional patients. The decision on participation in these insurance plans can be stated simply: If the question is "Do I go in the back and read a newspaper or see a managed care patient?" the financial outcome is better if the dentist sees the patient. If the question is "Do I see a managed care patient or see a private, full fee for service patient?" then the outcome is better to not see managed care patients. So if there is empty chair time, then it is financially worthwhile to fill that chair time with the less lucrative managed care patient than to leave it empty. If the question lies between, "Do I add an operatory and assistant (or associate) to see managed care patients?" the answer gets to be much more complex. The dentist probably need to discuss that with an accountant or management or financial advisor to investigate the answer thoroughly. The dentist should try to limit the amount of managed care in the practice mix. If the practice is more than 25 percent of a single plan or 50 percent of the total practice production, then the dentist may be in the dangerous position of "needing" the managed care programs. Then, the administrator may change the rules or reimbursement rates, and the dentist has no choice but to stay because the practice now depends on these plans.

Plan Utilization Controls

The risk that traditional indemnity insurance programs face is that more people than planned will use services and file claims. In other words, there will be "overutilization." Traditional indemnity insurance companies use many techniques to limit this risk and the resulting amount of payout. Because the plan administrator in alternative payment plans has shifted the risk onto the provider, there is little incentive for the administrator to control this risk. As a result, many of these plans are offered to the public and to employers without these risk reducing factors built into the program.

A common method of control is to place a yearly maximum on the amount that the plan will pay to any given individual for any given year. Preexisting condition clauses, copayments, deductibles, and other methods that force patient out-of-pocket expenditures all accomplish the same goal. Because as practitioners dentists are assuming the risk in many of these managed care programs, they should likewise have controls built into the contract to protect themselves from large losses associated with overutilization. When negotiating with a plan administrator, the dentist should be sure to insist that they have yearly maximums, copays, and other loss, prevention measures written into the plan before the dentist agrees to participate.

Poor Patient Understanding

Insurance contracts are complex. The old adage that the "The large print giveth, and the small print taketh away" must have been coined by a sage who was studying his own coverage. When the complexities and vagaries of a host of managed care programs are thrust upon the public, it is little wonder that they do not understand them.

Good third-party reimbursement programs, both traditional insurance and managed care programs, go out of their way to explain their programs to the subscribers. It is really their obligation to fully inform their clients of the coverage, limitations, and rules associated with the various plans. However, they are not always diligent in their efforts, and patients do not always listen. So most of the population does not understand their plan but makes assumptions about their coverage. This may be based on misinformation or incomplete information provided by the plan administrators or on historical coverage of the patient that he or she assumes apply to the new program. When negotiating a contract, the dentist should ask to see the information that the plan provides to their potential subscribers and the information that they provide once they are participants. Check to see the accuracy of the description of the plan. It is not the dentist's obligation to explain insurance or managed care plans to the subscribers, but it is often in his or her best interest to do so. The dentist should have a copy of the plan's information and coverage brochures handy so that if a question of coverage should arise, he or she can easily show to the patient the rules of coverage.

Cost Shifting

If a dentist is using managed care patients to augment the schedule, working on the margin, then the managed care program patients are not really contributing to the overall office overhead. Instead, the dentist shifting that cost onto the full pay and traditional insurance patients or taking home less income.

How to Reduce Managed Care in Practice

Given these problems, why would anyone participate in managed care? Practitioners' needs change over time. When the practice is young, it is time to gain as many new patients as possible, even if they are not all excellent full-paying clients for the practice. As the practice growth progresses, the practitioner may begin to "shift gears" by holding steady the number of managed care patients and then gradually eliminating the programs as full-pay clients begin to fill the practice. Other times, dentists may feel the need to participate from a defensive strategy. If many patients are leaving the practice because of changing plan type, the dentist may feel the need to preserve that patient base through participation. If there is a major employer in the area that accounts for a large portion of the patient pool, the dentist may need to participate if that employer shifts to a managed care plan.

If a dentist is taking several managed care plans and wants to drop out of them, he or she should do some analysis before jumping. The dentist must maintain or improve practice volume and profitability and must be sure that he or she has potential patient visits to take the place of the lost managed care patients. The dentist should increase marketing expenditures (both internal and external) in anticipation to drive new patient visits. He or she should also look at the entire practice philosophy and operation. The dentist may be moving from a high volume, lower fee practice to a lower volume, higher fee style. If so, he or she should closely examine the type and scope of services that are provided, case presentation technique, patient financing options, and staff competencies to ensure that a higher-end clientele is catered to.

The dentist will probably eliminate plans one at a time rather than all at once (Table 21.9). He or she will, therefore, need to decide the order of plan elimination. All plans in which a dentist participates should be ranked by their total reimbursement rate and by the percentage of practice production. The dentist should eliminate the worst-performing and smallest plan(s) first. If a plan accounts for a small proportion of the practice revenues (less than 5 percent), the dentist can eliminate it fairly easily. With larger plans, a dentist may need to stop accepting new patients (called "going on hold") before eliminating the plan entirely (assuming the plan allows this process). This allows the dentist to gradually wean the practice off of the reliance on the plan. By continually (quarterly) reviewing and

Table 21.9 Assessing Managed Care Programs
A dentist participates in three managed care programs, two preferred provider organizations (PPOs) and a capitation (Cap) plan. The numbers for the latest quarter are given. Which plan(s), if any, should the dentist eliminate from the practice?

	PPO1	PPO2	Cap plan
Charges	$7,000	$14,000	$7,000
Adjustments	−490	−2,300	−2,500
Cap Payments	$0	$0	+ $1,000
Total Return	$6,510	$11,700	$5,500
Return (%)	93%	83.5%	78.5%

If a dentist has empty chair time, then the dentist should not eliminate any of the plans. All three contribute more than the variable costs of production (about 21%). If there is not a lot of empty chair time, then the Cap plan should be eliminated first. Its reimbursement is least, and it is a relatively small part of the practice. Next, the dentist should eliminate the worse-paying plan (PPO2) if there are enough patients to fill the majority of the empty time slots. (It is a relatively large portion of the practice). If not, the dentist may need to eliminate PPO1 and build the practice until he or she can afford (from a patient visit perspective) to eliminate PPO2.

These options are based on purely financial considerations, without regard to personal belief about managed care, how hard a dentist wants to work, or other personal concerns that may influence the decision.

eliminating the poorest-performing plans, the dentist should be able to completely remove his or her participation in managed care plans.

The dentist should have a strategy in place for how to handle current patients who are members of discontinued plans. The dentist should decide what he or she (and the staff) will tell patients. Some patients will remain with the practice even after the change. The dentist should let the patients know if he or she is going to make any special arrangements for payments if they remain in the practice. Other patients will leave, even though the dentist has treated them for years. The plan cost-saving incentives are too strong for them to refuse. The dentist should decide if he or she is going to refer the patients to another participating practitioner or let them "fend for themselves." The dentist needs to make sure that the staff knows the policy (and the state law) regarding transfer of patient records and radiographs.

Managing Risk in the Office

chapter 22

Part 1: Office Risk Management

*I'm built for comfort; I ain't built for speed. But I got
ev'rything that a good girl need.*
Willie Dixon

Objectives

At the completion of this part, the student will be able to:
1. Describe the methods of managing risks in the office.
2. Describe the common types of office insurances.
   Business liability insurances
      Business premises and personal injury insurance
      Professional liability insurance
   Loss of use insurances
      Property insurance
      Building contents insurance
      Business overhead expense (BOE) insurance
   Employer insurances
      Workers' compensation insurance
      Unemployment compensation insurance
3. Describe the elements needed to prove professional liability.
4. Define standards of care and their use in dental practice.
5. Differentiate between poor work and poor outcomes.
6. Describe the common areas of professional risk exposure for practicing dentists.
7. Describe the common elements of a patient record.
8. Describe the use of patient records in a possible malpractice action.
9. Describe the possible avenues of resolution for poor work or poor outcome.
10. Describe the typical dental malpractice insurance policy.
11. Define the National Practitioner Data Bank and its affect on dentistry.

Key Terms

board of dentistry	experts	managed care
carrier	failure to diagnose	negligence
causation	fee disputes	occurrence
claim	indemnity	ownership of dental records
claims made	infection claims	patient abandonment
contingency basis	informed consent	patient records
covered loss	capacity	peer review board
damages	loss exposure	peer review process
duty	malpractice	periodontal disease claims
exclusions	malpractice litigation	policy

(Continued)

Business Basics for Dentists, First Edition. David O. Willis.
© 2013 John Wiley & Sons, Inc. Published 2013 by John Wiley & Sons, Inc.

Key Terms *(Continued)*

poor outcomes
poor work
    equipment failure
    failure to diagnose
    failure to refer
    poor technique
    premium

professional liability
reasonable and prudent
risk control (risk avoidance)
risk management
risk (loss) prevention
risk reduction
risk transfer

standards of care
swallowed object claims
wrong tooth claims

Goal

The goal of this part is to make students aware of common risks encountered in the dental office and to develop plans to minimizing those problems.

The Risk Management Process

Risk management is the process of identification and minimization of the possible sources of negligence to which dentists are exposed. These may develop from a dentist's role as a practitioner or as the owner of the business. In the risk management area, the best remedy is prevention. So the major task of a practicing dentist is not simply to buy insurance (although that should be part of the whole risk management package). Instead, the major task of the practitioner should be loss prevention. Risk management is an ongoing process. The owner and manager of the practice must see that the practice examines the sources of risk and works to decrease them as much as possible. The risk management process can be divided into the following steps.

Identification of Potential Loss Exposure

The initial task is to evaluate a practice to detect liability exposures. Dentists need to decide why patients might sue them. They should examine the dental procedures that are done. Removing a deep bony third molar impaction that wraps around the mandibular canal exposes a dentist to more risk than if he or she refers that procedure to an oral surgeon. Emergency department patients are notorious for failing to follow-up treatment, resulting in poor outcomes of treatment and possible claims of professional negligence. If a dentist collects accounts aggressively, he or she may encourage retribution (through a lawsuit) by dissatisfied patients. If a dentist has inadequate or outdated patient record systems, he or she may have a difficult time proving that an event or conversation took place. If a dentist does a procedure so seldom that he or she is not proficient at it, or if he or she continually has less-than-optimum outcomes with a

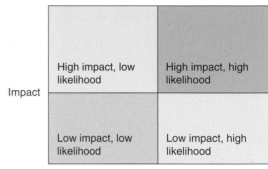

Figure 22.1 Risk Assessment Matrix

particular procedure (e.g., an endodontic technique), the dentist may be opened up to a claim of bad work. If a dentist has an older facility, he or she must be sure to keep it in good repair. The ultimate risk avoidance technique is simply to quit practicing dentistry. Nobody will sue a dentist for dental malpractice or business negligence then. Most practitioners agree that they can accept a certain amount of risk, if they can manage it effectively.

Risk is often expressed as a combination of two variables, likelihood and impact. Graphically, this is shown in Fig. 22.1.

Some risks may be likely but carry a low impact. For example, the possibility that a patient may inadvertently walk out with a pen is high, but the financial cost is low. On the other hand, the possibility of a fire destroying the office and a dentist's livelihood is low, but the impact is extremely high. Dentists would have a different way of managing the two risk exposures. The area of most concern is the area of high impact and high likelihood. Risks in this quadrant need immediate attention and review. Dentists should try to lower the impact, the likelihood, or both. Risks in the high impact, low likelihood often involve purchasing insurance to cover the loss. Dentists often manage risk of low impact and high likelihood by using risk management techniques (such as staff training) to lower the likelihood of occurrence.

Identification of potential loss exposure requires that dentists evaluate themselves and their staff members' skills and abilities honestly. Occasionally, that evaluation may identify problems or deficiencies that the dentist does not want to confront. (These may be clinical, interpersonal, or management related.) However, it is critical that dentists face them. Dentists should remember that recognizing areas of vulnerability to a liability claim is the first step to reducing the likelihood and severity of a claim against them.

Evaluation of Risk Management Control Techniques

A control is a mechanism that ensures that a dentist's process is working as designed and intended. Several categories of control techniques exist, including:

- *Risk avoidance* negates a potential loss because a dentist avoids or does not do the risky procedure. If a dentist refers all bony third molar impactions to an oral surgeon, he or she avoids the risk associated with that procedure. The oral surgeon accepts that risk because of his or her generally higher level of skill, training, and expertise in that specialized area. Dentists often use this technique for risks that have a high impact.
- *Risk (loss) prevention* reduces the possibility that a loss will occur. This technique occurs before a potential loss, and is, therefore, preventive in nature. If a dentist keeps excellent patient records, including notes of clinically relevant telephone conversations with patients, he or she may find that a malpractice action was prevented. Removing snow from steps in the winter prevents this as a source of negligence. Using this technique moves a risk from a high likelihood to a lower likelihood category.
- *Risk reduction* is similar to prevention but instead decreases the severity of a loss. If dentists decrease the impact that a loss may have, then the resulting patient damages will also be less. If the dentist has a current emergency kit, he or she should know how to use the drugs and materials in it. If the dentist and staff members are currently trained in CPR and other emergency protocols, then they have reduced the risk of a claim of negligence by a patient in case of a medical emergency. Dentists taking continuing professional education courses sharpen skills and knowledge in difficult clinical cases. In both examples, proper preparation has decreased a potential loss. This technique moves a risk from a high impact to a lower impact category.
- *Risk transfer* implies assigning the risk to someone else. The most common form of transfer occurs when a dentist buys insurance coverage for a possible professional negligence suit. Here, the dentist has contractually transferred the financial loss to the insurance company in exchange for annual insurance premiums. Risk transfer can also work against the dentist. If he or she participates in managed care contracts that require the dentist to sign a "hold harmless" clause, then he or she has increased the liability exposure to the practice by not allowing a transfer of risk to the managed care company. This technique is often used for risks that have a high impact but low likelihood.

Selection and Implementation of Control Techniques

Once a dentist identifies the risks associated with the practice, he or she should decide which techniques can prevent, reduce, or avoid the liability and resulting loss. This selection and application depend on the dentist's assessment of the effectiveness and cost of each technique when applied to a potential loss. Examples of controls include:

Training staff in medical emergencies and cardiopulmonary resuscitation (CPR).
Transmitting electronic data in a secure way.
Locking sensitive paper documents in a cabinet.
Using password protection and encryption for computer files.
Buying appropriate insurances.

Reassessment and Reevaluation of Techniques

Dentists should regularly reassess and reevaluate risk exposures and techniques for managing them. As a dentist grows professionally and financially, and as the practice grows, he or she will need to adjust methods and techniques to manage risk exposures and potential losses.

Office Insurances

Dentists should secure several office-related insurances, if they are the owner of a business. If the dentist is an employee, he or she will not need to carry business insurances (e.g., office liability and workers' compensation), but the dentist still needs a professional liability policy. If he or she is an independent contractor, the dentist is an independent business person and the owner's policies usually do not cover him or her. Here, the dentist should be sure to have general liability, workers' compensation (if employees are hired), and business overhead insurances. This book contains a separate section on personal insurance needs, although the two obviously overlap.

Business Liability Insurances

As the owner of a dental practice, a dentist should have two major types of liability insurance. These insurances cover him or her in case that the dentist is negligent, leading to someone's injury. Some practitioners advocate not carrying general or professional liability insurance, hoping not to get sued or trying to hide assets so that the injured party is not be able to collect significant amounts. This is a dangerous strategy. Lawyers and judges are adept at piercing through these veils of protection. The dentist may find himself or herself facing large legal and damage payments. The cost of insurance is insignificant compared with the cost of the loss of a liability suit.

Many insurers will develop packages of liability insurance for practitioners.

Business Premises and Personal Injury Insurance

A general liability policy (GLP) for the office covers the dentist in the event he or she is negligent and that action leads to a patient or other person being injured in the dental office. This is often called "slip and fall" insurance, from the common occurrence of someone slipping on ice or water, falling, and getting injured. As explained in the chapter on legal issues, a dentist must first be found to have been negligent before he or she can be liable for damages. As a rule, $2 million per occurrence and $4 million aggregate coverage is presently adequate.

Dentists can buy many additional coverage policies or "riders" for liability insurance. A dentist probably wants to be sure that his or her policy covers employees in their cars or in the dentist's while doing work-related errands. If an employee runs a case to the lab and has an accident, it is the dentist's accident. Many states allow a liquor legal liability rider. If a dentist entertains where liquor is served (such as a staff Christmas party or drinks after a continuing education course), the dentist may be liable if that person has an accident. The dentist may also purchase a business umbrella liability policy, similar to the personal excess liability coverage. Like all these riders, a dentist has to decide how much risk he or she is willing to take and how much he or she is willing to pay to sell that risk to an insurance company.

Professional Liability Insurance

Because the professionals have a special relationship with their clients (i.e., the dentist–patient relationship), a dentist should carry professional liability (malpractice) insurance to cover this possibility. Professional liability (malpractice) insurance is separate from a general (slip and fall) liability. This is a specialized field of insurance, so few companies will write this type of insurance. A later section in this chapter discusses this insurance in more detail.

Loss of Use Insurances

A couple of insurances cover dentists in case they lose the ability to practice in this location. These are beyond a personal income disability policy, which is described in the personal insurance chapter of this book.

Property Insurance

If the dentist owns the building in which he or she practices, the dentist must insure the physical structure. Commercial property insurance covers the building in much the same way that homeowner's insurance covers a home. The dentist should be sure to insure the replacement value of the building. The price of constructing a new space can appreciate quickly. If the building is in an area prone to floods or earthquakes, the dentist should be sure to include coverage for these events.

Building Contents Insurance

Dentists should insure the physical contents of the practice whether they own or lease the space. This type of insurance covers dental equipment, supplies, leasehold improvements, patient records, furniture, and fixtures in case they are damaged or destroyed. What could damage them? Fire, water damage from fighting a fire, theft, explosions, broken water pipes, or any of a host of problems that cannot even be named can damage property. Building contents insurance seems like an expensive luxury until a dentist gets to the office and finds that a water pipe has burst, flooding the reception room and business office. Often lenders will require that dentists purchase this insurance to cover them in case of loss.

Dentists have the option of covering the equipment at present (current) value or at replacement value. Present value is the value of the equipment when the loss occurs. Assume a dentist purchases a dental chair for $10,000 and insures it for the present value. If the chair is destroyed the day after it is insured, the present value is what the dentist paid for it. However, assume that the accident causing the loss did not occur for 5 years. That same dental chair may now have a present value of only $3,000, yet to buy a new one (replacement value) would cost $12,000. Although replacement policies are more expensive, they are generally worth the extra premium paid.

Business Overhead Expense (BOE) Insurance

If dentists are unable to practice because of a disability or other reason, office costs continue regardless. Although the landlord is a pleasant fellow, he or she is not going to forgo the rent because a dentist cannot practice. Likewise, the banker needs the loan payment, and the staff still need to be paid, if they are to stay in a dentist's employ. An office, or business, overhead expense (BOE) policy helps a dentist to pay many office costs if he or she is unable to work. The dentist should carry personal disability income insurance to be sure that he or she provides for the family budget in case of disability. BOE policies do much the same for the office costs. Premiums are deductible, so benefits are taxable. Because the benefits go to pay deductible expenses, the deductible expense offsets the additional taxable income.

Business interruption coverage is the core of the BOE. This coverage pays the dentist either direct costs or a set amount if he or she must shut down the business. If a dentist a major loss (such as a fire), he or she may have many months without practice income while the office is being repaired. The dentist should ensure that the policy covers him or her for interruption causes that are outside the building, such as a citywide power loss. Many do not.

Some practitioners opt not to carry BOE insurance. Instead, they plan to use their accounts receivable to pay office costs if they are unable to work. This is a risky plan. Typical accounts receivable may equal 1 1/2 to 2 months' billings. If the disability last longer than this (and many do) then the dentist would run out of money to pay the bills. At that point, the dentist would need to tap into personal savings or income to make regular payments. If the dentist does not keep the staff on the payroll, the staff will probably leave, looking for employment elsewhere. Even if the dentist weathers this storm, he or she will then have a cash flow problem when the office is opened again. The dentist will have used up his or her accounts receivable so no cash flows into the office. It will be just like starting up again. The dentist will need to go to the bank and borrow working capital, and then pay off the loan.

Insurances Provided for Employees

Dentists need several insurances to provide for employees. If a dentist does not have any employees, then he or she obviously does not have to provide these insurances. As a proprietor or a partner in a partnership, dentists do not cover themselves (or receive any benefits from) these insurances. If a practice is a corporation, then the dentist is an employee of the corporation. The corporation must provide these insurances for the dentist, the same as all other employees and may also receive the benefits, if qualified.

Workers' Compensation Insurance

This is an insurance that dentists must, by law, carry on all of employees. (It is optional in some states, but dentists are still responsible for any claims.) It covers a dentist case an employee is injured on the job. This insurance covers medical expenses that are injury related and provides some disability payment (lost wages) if the accident disables the worker. Workers' compensation is a pure no-fault system. It does not matter whose fault the injury was, workers' compensation pays for it because the injury occurred while the person was on duty. In return for the no-fault provision, workers' compensation laws have virtually eliminated the ability of the injured worker to sue the employer for negligence.

Specific workers' compensation rules vary state by state, but they all have several common elements including:

1. Workers' compensation provides benefits for accidental injury while on the job. The definition of an injury includes repetitive trauma, such as carpal tunnel syndrome. The compensation also includes occupational diseases, such as black lung disease for a coal miner or hepatitis for a dental worker who contracted it through an accidental needle stick.
2. Benefits include lost wages (about one-half to two-thirds of weekly wages), medical benefits, and death benefits.
3. This is pure no-fault insurance. Even if the employee's actions caused the accident or if the employer did nothing wrong (had no fault), the insurance still pays benefits.
4. The employer pays the entire cost. The compensation may not pass to employees because stiff fines are levied if this coverage is not provided.
5. Employees give up the right to sue employers for negligence if workers' compensation insurance covered the accident. This is called the *compensation bargain*.

Workers' compensation provides four types of benefits:

1. Medical payments pay for physician services, durable medical equipment, prescriptions, and most other conventional medical treatment, such as psychological therapy. This is without a limit and without a waiting period or copay.
2. Rehabilitation services may be physical or vocation rehabilitation and are beyond medical payments. The worker may also receive disability benefits during the rehabilitation phase of treatment.

3. Death benefits go to survivors of someone killed in a work-related accident. These include both a lump sum and a weekly income benefit.
4. Disability payments pay a worker who is disabled while on the job.

A dentist's payment (or premium) for workers' compensation insurance is based on the number of employees and the annual payroll. Workers' compensation is a federally mandated system operated by the states. Each state, therefore, has different rules concerning eligibility for benefits, costs, and owner requirements. A dentist can find an insurance company that writes these policies. Many office liability carriers will include workers' compensation policy in a package of insurances. These packages may be more expensive, but they are easier for the dentist. The question becomes a cost versus convenience trade off.

If a dentist is a proprietor or a partner, he or she is an owner, not an employee. Therefore, in most states the dentist does not fall under the workers' compensation laws. The dentist does not pay premiums on himself or herself, and he or she is not eligible for benefits. If a dentist practices as a corporation, he or she is an employee of the corporation (though also an officer) and must be part of the workers' compensation system, unless he or she opts out. The compensation generally includes limited liability company (LLC) members and family member employees, unless they opt out. The compensation does not include independent contractors. Again each state is different and specific application of the rules is confusing. Dentists should check with their workers' compensation carrier in the state of practice to know how these specifics apply.

Unemployment Compensation Insurance

Unemployment compensation is really a tax, but it operates like an insurance product. This is another joint federal-state program. Dentists pay two unemployment taxes, State Unemployment Taxing Authority (SUTA) and Federal Unemployment Taxing Authority (FUTA). Dentists pay state "contributions" (taxes) monthly. At the end of the year (January 30 the following year), the state checks to see how much the dentist paid into the state unemployment pool the previous year. If the amount were less than the federal requirement, he or she makes an additional payment to the federal government to make up the difference. So dentists only pay FUTA once a year, and the amount depends on the amount he or she has paid to the state (SUTA).

The system is complex. However, the total amounts paid are not large. Payments will vary depending on the history the practice has regarding staff unemployment. The gross FUTA tax rate is 6.2 percent on the first $7,000 of workers' earnings. Generally, the employer can take a credit against FUTA for contributions to state unemployment funds up to 5.4 percent of the first $7,000. The net FUTA tax rate then is 0.8 percent (0.008). An accountant or payroll manager will provide this information. If a dentist's staff has many claims, the dentist becomes a higher risk and rates go up. Few or no claims, rates and payments go down.

Other Insurances

Dentists may also provide other forms of insurance for employees as employee benefits. These may include medical, disability, or life insurance. Dentists should check the sections on employee benefits in this book for a detailed look at those insurances.

Professional Risk Management

This book has previously discussed the ideas of risk management as it relates to personal and business risks that dentists face. These are the same risks that all Americans or all US business people face. However, professionals face an additional risk that most other business owners do not. That is the risk that dentists may be negligent in their performance of their professional duties. This risk is special to the practice of dentistry, and so its management is different as well. Most practitioners have adequate malpractice insurance, believing that this satisfies the problem of risk management.

Professional Negligence and Liability

Professional risk management is closely aligned with quality assurance in the office, although risk management takes a more practical view of the problem. Dentists should identify potential sources of professional risk exposure, train themselves and staff to reduce the number and impact of these exposures, and continually work to improve the quality of the dental care delivered in the office.

Negligence is the failure to act as a reasonable and prudent person in a similar situation would act. As described in the chapter on legal issues, this definition is not absolute and opens the door for interpretation and changing definitions as social customs change. If a dentist's negligence causes an injury to someone, then he or she is liable or must restore that person's loss. This generally means that a dentist must financially reimburse the injured person for the damages that the dentist's negligence caused.

Elements to Prove Professional Liability

The same cause-and-effect relationship exists in professional liability issues. If a dentist is negligent in the delivery of health care, he or she can be found liable for the damages that result. These damages may include repair of the problem, lost earnings from missing work or reduced performance or ability, and pain and suffering experienced by the injured patient. (Obviously, significant discretion is available for judges and juries in awarding damages.)

In professional liability, an additional level must be satisfied to prove professional negligence. The idea is similar, but with a different "twist." Someone must prove each element to established professional liability.

1. *Creation of Duty*   When a professional agrees to treat a patient, he or she creates a practitioner–patient relationship. When this relationship exists, the practitioner has a legal duty (obligation) to act according to the standards of care for the profession. These standards involve using the required skill, knowledge, and care that members of the profession display. If a practitioner does not accept a person as a patient, he or she has not created a practitioner–patient relationship and, therefore, no has no duty.
2. *Breach of Duty*   If a practitioner fails to possess or use the skill, care, and knowledge that a reasonably well-qualified member of the profession would display under similar circumstances (i.e., fail to live up to the standards of care), then he or she has breached the duty owed to the patient. This is equivalent to the idea of negligence in a civil liability case.
3. *Causation*   If the breach of duty leads to an injury or harm to the patient, then causation has been proved. The connection between the breach and injury must be both "actual" and "foreseeable."
4. *Damages*   The patient must establish that an actual loss occurred from the injury. That loss may be either monetary (e.g., lost wages) or personal (e.g., disfigurement, pain, and suffering).

Standards of Care

Malpractice actions do not hinge on the absolute notion that any injury is a malpractice. Instead, these actions are based on what a "reasonable and prudent" professional in a similar situation would have done. This is known as a *standard of care*. These standards involve knowledge, skill, care, and judgment of the practitioner. They involve the technical level of expertise needed to complete a procedure successfully, the knowledge of how to interpret signs and symptoms, the behavioral accomplishment of treatment, and the ability to diagnose and properly plan for a patient's treatment. So the standard of care involves both the technical performance of an extraction and the knowledge and judgment of when an extraction is and is not appropriate therapy.

There are no written standards of care published by the American Dental Association (ADA) or other professional organizations. (Some organizations are trying, with mixed success, to compile them.) These standards evolve over time. The technology and knowledge of the profession influence them and well as the wants, needs, desires, and sophistication of the public. Posterior composites, gold foil restorations, silicate restorations, and implant prostheses all enter current standards of care in a dynamic interchange. Standards are not an absolute definition or "prescription" for how dentists should handle every patient procedure. Instead, they are a set of expectations for how a "reasonable and prudent" dentist would behave in a similar professional situation.

Although the standards of care are constantly evolving, they are determined by a consensus of "experts" in the field. Experts are individuals who have background and training that gives them a real or inferred level of professional expertise. In a malpractice case, both sides bring experts to the trial to bolster their point of view. The experts who interpret the prevailing standards are often specialists in their field. To this extent then, the law holds generalists to the level of standards that a specialist would hold. For example, if a case involved extraction of an impacted third molar, the experts would usually be oral surgeons. The courts would then hold the generalist to the same standard of care as the surgeon.

Standards of care vary by state or region of the country, although these differences are becoming smaller with time. Some practitioners in rural, inner-city, or poverty-stricken areas claim that the standard of care is different in those areas. The standard of what is proper care is probably the same in all areas. Patient acceptance of treatment may be different. With the increased speed of communication, ease of travel, and increase in third-party payers, these arguments are becoming less viable as well.

Common Areas of Professional Risk Exposure in Private Dental Practice

Several areas of common professional risk exposure show in the dental office. These may result in resolution through any of the avenues described previously.

Poor work

Poor work is a simple failure to do a procedure at the level of the standard of patient care. It can occur for a variety of reasons, even to competent dentists.

- *Poor technique* occurs when the technical aspects of a case are not up to the standard of care. If a dentist leaves an overhanging margin on an alloy or crown that can lead to future caries or a periodontal problem, he or she has committed bad work.

- *Failure to diagnose* a disease or problem is a common source of poor work. A dentist should give the patient a diagnosis of any disease within his or her area of expertise. If he or she fails to diagnose periodontal disease and fails to inform the patient of the problem and likely outcomes, he or she can be found liable for the results. Often a dentist may claim that he or she did a proper exam and found everything to be within normal limits but did not document that fact. An example is an oral cancer screening. If a dentist finds no oral cancers in an intraoral exam, his or her record should note that fact. This will protect the dentist from a future claim of "failure to diagnose" if an intraoral cancer is later found on a patient. The dentist giving a patient a reminder of needed or suggested treatment at each recall visit supports the diagnosis.
- *Failure to refer* to a specialist is another form of bad work. Although the courts understand that some diagnoses or technical procedures are out of the scope of a typical generalist, they also understand that dentists should recognize these cases and refer them to a specialist for evaluation and possible treatment. Dentists should be most interested in improving the health of patients, not their personal pocketbook.
- *Equipment failure* may be outside the control of the dentist, yet still be the responsibility of the dentist. If a dentist is doing an endodontic procedure and the file becomes lodged in the canal and breaks, he or she has had an equipment failure, which is considered poor work. As a rule, the dentist is responsible for any equipment or supplies that he or she should have known might be defective.

Poor Outcomes

A poor outcome does not involve poor work, merely a patient who is not satisfied with the result. Dentists have all seen denture cases in which the technical denture is clinically acceptable. The patient is simply not satisfied with the results. (The dentist might have had a suspicion when the patient walked into the office with a bag of seven other dentures that did not "work right.") The dentist may have also seen the opposite case of a patient who has an anterior crown that looks terrible to his or her eye, yet the patient is completely satisfied with the outcome, although the technical work was poor. This category of risk exposure is difficult for many dentists to accept. Yet the courts have ruled that is real and valid.

Poor outcomes are especially common in cases that involve patient values, such as esthetics. A dentist's notion of what is acceptable may be entirely different from the patient's. Patient communication is a critical issue in these cases.

Patient Communication Problems

Communication is a two-way street. Dentists may believe that they have adequately expressed their side of the issue, but the patient either did not truly understand or did not adequately express his or her side of the issue (Box 22.1). These patient communication problems can be grouped into the following categories:

- *Lack of treatment plans* is the basis of most patient communication problems. Without a treatment plan, patients do not know what to expect and may be surprised by the treatment or the cost of the treatment. Detailed and written treatment plans are one of the best methods of avoiding dental malpractice litigation.
- *Unrealistic patient expectations* often lead to liability problems. These expectations may be the result of the patient not adequately expressing goals and desires concerning his or her dental treatment or may be the result of the dentist making implied or actual promises of treatment that he or she do not fulfill. Either way, it is in the dentist's interest to ensure that the patient has realistic expectations of the outcomes before beginning treatment.
- *Lack of informed consent* becomes the basis of many dental malpractice lawsuits. Informed consent is the ethical and legal doctrine that requires that dentists give patients sufficient information so that they can make a free, rational treatment choice. This also implies the right of informed refusal. Informed consent relates to the treatment planning and patient communication issues discussed previously. For a dentist to have true informed consent, he or she must prove each of the following points concerning the treatment:

1. The patient must have the *capacity* to make health care decisions for himself or herself. From a legal perspective, this means (in most states) that the patient must be at least of legal age (18 years old) or an emancipated (married) minor. From an ethical standpoint, the patient must have the mental ability to decide. These decisions can be difficult for the patient who is in emotional turmoil or physical pain or a

---

Box 22.1 Communicating with Patients

- Personally discuss benefits and risks
- Personally discuss alternatives and consequences
- Encourage the patient to ask questions
- Use lay or common terms
- Get a commitment from the patient to proceed
- Keep well-documented records

patient who is approaching senility and is intermittently capable but at other times totally incapable.

2. The dentist must provide *information* concerning the proposed treatment. This includes the nature of the treatment, the proposed time, and the cost to complete the procedure. Treatments that are within the general understanding of the patient from past treatment history do not need to be explained. The patient's treatment decisions will take into account consideration of the risks involved in the treatment. To that end, dentists should discuss complications that commonly occur because of the procedure. They should also inform the patient of reasonable alternatives to the treatment proposed and the risks associated with those alternatives. Dentists do not need to discuss every alternative and every risk of every alternative. However, dentists should discuss the material and foreseeable risks in which a reasonable person would be interested. Obviously, there is some room for interpretation in what is "material," "foreseeable," and "reasonable." That is what juries are for.

3. The patient must *comprehend* (understand) the information provided. Dentists should use uncomplicated language to discuss the treatment and alternatives, not technical dental terminology or jargon. If the patient does not understand the language, the dentist must get an interpreter to ensure that the person understands the oral description and has a chance to ask questions about the proposed treatment. Dentists may use written communication and other visual aids as appropriate to supplement (not replace) oral discussions.

4. Agreement must be *voluntary*, without coercion, deception, duress, or other influence. A patient cannot be tricked or coerced into agreeing with the agreement. Oral agreement is adequate. Written (signed) agreement supplements an oral agreement, but it is not an ironclad defense for the dentist. (All the patient has to say is "I didn't really understand what I was signing.")

5. The patient must positively *authorize* the treatment. The patient must positively say, in effect, "Yes, do the treatment." If he or she is uncertain or does not affirm the desire for treatment, the dentist has not gained informed consent. The dentist should not do anything the patient has not authorized, even if the dentist believes that it is in the patient's best interest. The law says that what to do with a patient's body is his or her decision, not the dentist's. If a dentist does dental work that the patient did not authorize, the dentist would be guilty of not only malpractice but also assault.

A patient may not legally consent to malpractice. If a dentist advocates or does a procedure that he or she knows is not within the standard of care, then the dentist has committed malpractice. This happens whether or not the patient has consented to the treatment or agreed not to hold the dentist responsible. So if an 18-year-old patient with healthy teeth and periodontium requests full-mouth extractions and dentures and the dentist does the requested service, he or she is committing malpractice and is liable for the results, even if the patient signed in the record their understand this and will not hold the dentist responsible. This extreme case is easy. The problem comes in interpretation of the standards of care in borderline cases.

Dentists must also allow informed refusal. Informed refusal means that the patient fully understands the treatment, the alternatives, and the outcomes. The patient refuses the dentist's advice for treatment. If the patient truly is making an informed decision, then the dentist must accept that decision. The dentist should explain the possible outcomes of the lack of treatment. If the patient still refuses the dentist's advice (even after adequate explanation), the dentist should document the advice and refusal in the patient's record. Even after this initial refusal of treatment, the dentist has an obligation to again recommend treatment at subsequent follow-up or recall visits, for as long as the condition remains and the dentist–patient relationship exists. Some dentists dismiss patients from the practice who do not accept the full advice of the dentist. The dentists believe that this opens them to charges of "supervised neglect," in which they know of a problem and are guilty of negligence because they contributed to the problem by allowing the patient to continue to decline under the dentist's care. If a dentist adequately expresses and documents his or her recommendations, he or she will be on sound legal footing. A dentist's preferred practice pattern may encourage dismissal of nonaccepting patients.

- *Poor work or outcomes by another dentist* these issues often arise from fee or third-party problems. One dentist is going to redo poor work from another dentist; however, the third-party carrier will not pay to have the recent work redone. The patient then seeks various methods to have the second dentist pay for the poor work. Dentists are understandably reluctant to criticize their fellow practitioners. They really do not know the circumstances, decision process, patient compliance, or a host of other issues that can negatively affect treatment outcomes. So dentists should avoid saying or giving the patient the impression that the previous dentist did faulty or poor work.

  If a dentist encounters poor work by a previous dentist (either negligent treatment or undiagnosed disease), three options are available. The first is to contact the other dentist directly. Often the other dentist can inform the present dentist of problems or circumstances affecting treatment that the patient either could or would not discuss. The previous dentist might also offer to respond directly to the patient in an attempt to correct the problem. The second avenue is to discuss with the patient various professional methods, such as peer review or mediation, that are available for resolution of the problem. However, when a dentist sees grossly or continuously faulty work, he or she has an ethical obligation to report the problem to the appropriate body of the local dental society or to regulatory boards or bodies.

- *Fee disputes* fee disputes often arise from patients who are not completely satisfied with the dental work they have received. When the dentist then pursues aggressive collection techniques, the patient responds with a malpractice complaint. The job of the dentist is to balance the right that he or she has to collect the money owed with the possibility of triggering a lawsuit. Before sending anyone to a collection agent or attorney, the dentist should be confident that the work done is clinically acceptable. Most states have a statute of limitations of 1 year from the date of discovery for malpractice actions. (The patient has 1 year from when he or she knew or should have known about a problem to sue.) Many experts recommend waiting until after 1 year to pursue aggressive collection techniques. The dentist should check with an attorney in the practice state. Many nuances about these laws might affect the dentist's decision.

- *Auxiliary treatment problems* The dentist is responsible for the actions and work of the auxiliaries employed in his or her office. If the dentist has committed acts of malpractice, he or she is also liable, through the doctrine of agency. So if a hygienist accidentally injures a patient by dropping an instrument in his or her eye, both the dentist and the hygienist will be liable.

- *Patient abandonment* Once a dentist–patient relationship is established, the dentist must continue that relationship for the care of the patient. The patient may end the relationship at anytime. The dentist may end the relationship but only under certain conditions. He or she may not end the relationship in the middle of treatment. (What constitutes the "middle of treatment" is obviously open to interpretation.) The dentist may end the relationship if the patient is in stable condition and will not be harmed by a delay in treatment while he or she seeks care elsewhere. If, for example, the dentist is in the middle of root canal therapy, he or she must complete the endodontic treatment and probably place an adequate provisional restoration. If the dentist has done a surgical procedure that normally involves follow-up appointments for dressings, suture removal, or other follow-up care, he or she must complete that course of treatment. If a patient owes the dentist money, the dentist still must complete the procedure and ensure that the patient is dentally

---

Box 22.2 Ending a Relationship with a Patient

1. Reason for termination
2. Date it becomes effective
3. Treatment remaining
4. Referrals or source of new dentist
5. Method of continuing emergency care
6. Offer to transfer records to new provider
7. Office policy regarding record transfer.

---

stable before ending the relationship. The notion here is that dentists should not harm (or even potentially harm) the patient by ending the relationship. If a dentist simply refuses to continue to treat a patient, he or she has violated the duty to treat that was established in the initial relationship, opening the dentist up to charges of abandonment.

When a dentist ends a relationship with a patient, he or she should inform the patient verbally and in writing (Box 22.2). (The dentist should keep a copy of the written correspondence.) The dentist's letter should state why the relationship was ended and ensure patient health through referral, emergency care, and an offer to send records to the new dentist.

- *Insurance problems* Insurance problems have led to a new set of malpractice issues. Although managed care itself does not cause poor ethical decisions and malpractice by the practitioner, it causes new problems in the dentist–patient relationship that can lead to accusations of malpractice. The single biggest influence is the temptation to perform less-than-optimal care. The pressure for minimal treatment may come from the dentist, the plan administrator, the patient, or the employer. Despite the pressure, the dentist is still responsible for the treatment rendered.

The dentist should remember that the best treatment for a patient is the best treatment, no matter how much money he or she makes (or does not make) when doing the procedure. The dentist is obligated to recommend and do treatment that is at least at the standard of care, regardless the method or amount of payment. If a dentist can not abide by the rules as established in the managed care contract, then he or she should not participate in the managed care program.

Patient Treatment Records

The patient treatment record is the official document of all treatment procedures, referrals, professional communications, recommendations, and advice that the dentist renders to patients in the dental office. The written treatment record (or its computer equivalent) is the basis of knowledgeable patient treatment and serves as the recorded history of treatment and recommendations in case of professional liability issues.

Components

Patient records may be paper or electronic in form. They should have the following components:

1. *Identification Data* This information is the demographic information about the patient, his or her name, age, responsible party, Social Security number, insurance carrier, etc.
2. *Health Insurance Portability and Accountability Act (HIPAA) Disclosure* The patient should read and acknowledge receiving the office HIPAA disclosure.
3. *Consent Form* The doctrine of informed consent that is customary in this country requires that health care providers inform patients of the nature of the proposed services, the possible outcomes (positive and negative) of that treatment, and the alternatives to the proposed treatment in language that the individual can understand. Simply having a patient sign a consent form, therefore, does not adequately gain informed consent of the patient. The dentist must present the proposed treatment in a way that the patient can understand. The dentist should orally explain the procedure, give written explanations (especially if the procedure is difficult or complex), and gain written understanding of the patient in a "consent form." This may be a general consent for treatment or a specific consent for a procedure that has additional risks not present in common procedures, such as removal of a bony impacted third molar.
4. *Medical History* The written medical history should include an oral follow-up (consultations when indicated) of any abnormal conditions. The history should note drug usage (prescription and over the counter), allergies, substance abuse (including alcohol and tobacco), and family history of disease.
5. *Dental History* This section should include the patient's chief complaint and his or her past use of dental services.
6. *Clinical Exam* Dentists often note this section graphically as charts (caries, periodontal, and soft-tissue exam). Dentists may also include radiographs and photographs. A complete exam is standard for all initial patients; updates may be conducted on routine recall examinations.
7. *Diagnosis* The dentist should write the diagnosis of findings clearly in an understandable form. This is the basis of the treatment plan.
8. *Treatment Plan* The treatment plan is a written statement of the proposed treatment to address the defined diagnoses.
9. *Progress Notes* This section chronicles the patient's treatment visits to the office. Dentist should note any treatment or advice rendered to the patient and note any changes in the proposed treatment plan or sequence, laboratory services ordered, or medications prescribed.
10. *Completion Notes* A summary of treatment, including postoperative radiographs and photographs if indicated, concludes the record. Record recommendations concerning continued or follow-up care.

The Value of Good Records

The individualized dental record needs to contain all of the information concerning a patient's treatment. If many practitioners (e.g., partners, associates, hygienists) all make entries in records, the office depends on accurate entries by every member of the team. Even as a individual practitioner, the records become an indispensable source of information. Memories are notoriously faulty after months (or years) have passed. Most dentists can not accurately remember having an encounter with a patient, much less any specific diagnostic finding, treatment recommendations, or outcome of treatment that occurred during that encounter.

Patient records also are the cornerstones of any malpractice case defense. The old adage that "if it isn't in the record, it didn't happen" is, unfortunately, accurate. Because patient records are critical to prevention and resolution of patient problems and disputes, a few words concerning their use are in order.

All Entries Should Be Accurate and Thorough

Dentists should make entries at the time that the event occurs, rather than later. The patient's record is a legal document. When the dentist or staff writes in a record, it should only be in blue or black ink. (Colored chart notations are OK.) The dentists should not use slang or common language or use only objective, factual, and medically accurate information. The dentist should avoid disparaging or personal comments. ("Patient was a real pain in the butt today" is a highly inflammatory statement. "Patient appeared agitated, was demanding and uncooperative in treatment" says the same thing in a more factual way.) If a dentist has a shorthand system for chart notations, he or she should be sure to post a list for consistent use by all office personnel. If the dentist sends a record or copy to another office or expert witness, he or she should be sure to include a copy of the shorthand definitions, so nobody misunderstands them.

Never Attempt to Alter Records

Dentists should not delete or add to records if there is a potential legal action. Tampered records are more damaging to the professional than incomplete records. People can examine computer records forensically to learn when entries were added or altered.

Make Corrections Correctly

If a dentist makes an entry in error, he or she should make a single line through the entry, followed by the reason for correction and the correction itself on paper records. The dentist should not use correction fluids or tapes; should not scratch over an entry until it is a solid ink; or should not attempt to erase an entry. A note explaining an incorrect entry (besides the original note) should occur in a computer record. Finally, a dentist should never correct a record once a malpractice action has been initiated. Any changes that the dentist makes at that point will look at best, suspect, and purely fraudulent at the worst.

Records Should Be Neat and Legible

All entries should be typed or written legibly in ink and then signed or initialed by the person who makes the entry. If a staff member makes the entry, the dentist should review and countersign the entry. Computer records should be as complete as handwritten records and data should be backed up regularly.

Keep Separate Financial Information

Dentists should keep financial information separate from the treatment record, to the extent possible. The patient's ledger records all financial transactions and communications. If a dentist is using a computerized billing system rather than ledger cards, he or she should put a separate sheet in the patient's record to record financial issues (e.g., collection calls, agreements, etc.). Many programs have a "Comments" section of the program, or the dentist can add a new procedure code for various collection efforts. This should be added to the patient's ledger when it is used.

All Records Should Be Considered Confidential

Dentists should secure written patient consent before granting access to the records for any other party, except as required by valid subpoena. The original copy of the patient's record should never leave the office, unless by court order. Dentists may send photocopies to other health care providers, or other people may view the records (with permission of the patient) in the dentist's office. Remember, the dentist owns the physical record, but the patient also owns the information in that record. The dentist has an ethical and legal obligation to keep that information confidential, as dictated by HIPAA.

Patient Records Should Be Kept Indefinitely

Generally, dentists should retain patient records for as long as they are in practice. This serves two purposes. It improves patient oral health by providing a historical record of treatment, and it serves as the basis of defense in a malpractice action against the dentist. From a practical standpoint, the dentist will probably want to purge records of patients whom he or she has not seen in the office during the past year or two. When a dentist purges records, he or she should do not destroy them but move them to another area of the office where they can be retrieved them within a reasonable time. Some states have minimum times that the records should be kept, but it is a good idea to keep them as long as possible. If storage is a problem, then the dentist can microfilm or store seldom-used records off premises. The dentist should check with a lawyer and malpractice carrier before destroying any records.

Use Supporting Records, Where Appropriate

Photographs are excellent means of supportive record keeping; however, they should not replace the normal written record procedure. The dentist should keep casts for difficult or complex cases. He or she may substitute good photographs of casts in routine cases for satisfied patients. Casts and photographs are excellent means of documenting pre- and posttreatment oral conditions.

Format of Daily Entries

Several common formats exist for daily entries in a patient's record. The most common is a "SOAP" note (Box 22.3). These formats intend to ensure that dentists record important information about the patient visit in a systematic way, so that they do not miss anything important. These formats require that dentists include the date and a paragraph for each heading. The important thing is that the dentist is systematic in the way he or she enters information.

SOAP Notes

SOAP is an acronym for:

Subjective: What the patient said was their reason for the visit. The dentist may also include his or her observations about the patient.
Objective: The objective findings related to the patient's chief complaint. This includes the results of any tests or measurements.

Box 22.3 Example of SOAP Notes

Date:

S: Patient reports "a bad pain in my upper right jaw. It keeps me up all night. Nothing makes it stop hurting." (Patient points to tooth #3.) Patient appeared tired and agitated.

O: BP: 125/80, P: 62, R: 12, T: 100.7. Tooth #3 with large, cavitated carious lesion. PA radiograph shows extensive caries on M and D of #3 with large (2-mm) periapical radiolucency on palatal root. Tooth #3 percussion sensitive +++ (#2, 4 neg to percussion) Pos R cervical lymph nodes. Patient displays generalized gross caries.

A: Rampant dental caries. Tooth #3 irreversible pulpitis with periapical abscess, questionable restorability. Patient is febrile.

P: Discussed treatment options, risks, and benefits (RCT/Crown vs EXT with FPD or implant replacement). After discussion, patient desires extraction #3. Administered 1.8 cc lidocaine with epi 1:100,000. Simple forceps extraction #3. Rx: PenVK 500 mg #28 one q6h until gone. Patient instructed to return of further pain, fever, or swelling. Patient advised of need for extensive dental care.

Assessment: The assessment and diagnosis of the problem. The dentist may develop several diagnoses.

Plan: The plan and treatment for the patient. This includes any treatment done or medication prescribed, and patient recommendations, instructions or required follow-up.

For patients undergoing routine, continuing care, the SOAP note becomes simpler. The *subjective* section may be "Patient for routine dental care per treatment plan," or "Patient for periodic maintenance visit." The *objective* section consists of recording vital signs and "See patient data base." *Assessment* is "periodontal disease treatment," "preventive visit," "caries restoration," or other description. The *plan* section is then a listing of the treatment rendered.

Ownership of Patient Records

The dentist owns the physical patient record (including the radiographs), but the patient has a right to control the information that is in the record. HIPAA dictates how the dentist will safeguard this information. Personal and health information is confidential. The dentist may not give that information to anyone else without the written consent of the patient. (The dentist should be sure to maintain the written consent in the record.) Most states require a dentist to provide the patient a copy of the record within a reasonable time. The dentist should also note in the chart any time he or she sends a copy of the record to anyone outside the office. This can avoid confusion if, in the future, apparently multiple copies of a patient's record exit. The dentist should be sure to have on file a signature from the patient authorizing him or her to release information to a third-party carrier for claims processing. Access to records for quality assurance reviews should be limited to patients of an involved third-party carrier.

Telephone Calls

The dentist should document all telephone calls (and attempted contacts) that relate to patient treatment in the treatment record. This includes calls to follow-up treatment, advice to patients, referrals or specialist discussions, and calls from patients requesting information or clarification of treatment or advice. (The dentist should note financial calls, either to or from a patient or account guarantor, in the patient's financial file, ledger card, or computer financial file. Financial issues do not have anything to do with the patient's treatment and should be separate.) Documenting telephone calls that he or she receives or makes from home during nonoffice hours is also important. Many practitioners keep a pad of paper or "sticky notes" at the phone to jot down notes concerning patient conversations. If a dentist prescribes medications or recommends additional care, he or she should be sure to make a note and transfer it to the patient record the following day.

Avenues of Resolution of Poor Work or Poor Outcome

A patient (or the public) has four avenues to try to gain satisfaction for what they believe is poor work done by a dental practitioner (Box 22.4). State laws vary concerning when each avenue is appropriate, so the dentist should be sure to check with a local attorney or malpractice carrier if he or she faces a potential malpractice action. (For example, some peer review boards do not handle fee disputes.)

Individual Communication

The profession handles most complaints through individual communication between the dentist and the patient. Unfortunately, many dissatisfied patients are

---

> **Box 22.4** Common Risk Management Mistakes
>
> 1. No treatment plan
> 2. No medical history
> 3. Failure to document phone calls
> 4. Failure to dismiss noncompliant patients
> 5. Believing return of money is an admission of guilt
> 6. Critical second opinions or consults
> 7. Assuming patients are knowledgeable and correct about their previous treatment
> 8. Assuming patients know what they are talking about and always tell the truth

reluctant to discuss their perceived problem with the dentist. It becomes a self-fulfilling prophesy, that if a dentist has a problem that results from poor communication, the patient will not express this with him or her. However, communication is two-way street. It is important that the dentist establish an atmosphere of trust and openness so that patients and staff are not reluctant to bring problems to his or her attention. If the dentist can, he or she should resolve a problem while it is small.

Peer Review Process

Peer review is a system that organized dentistry has developed to resolve conflicts between patients and practitioners. Generally, it is a voluntary process. If a dentist does not want to participate, no one requires him or her to do so. (Some states require a peer review process before any malpractice litigation. In such cases, peer review is mandatory.) It is in the dentist's interest (and the profession's) to try to resolve problems fairly before they end in a courtroom. In this process, patients bring a problem to a peer review board, which is composed of members of the local dental society. (Many states have a statewide "appeal" board, as well.) Generally, each side of the dispute will give their side of the tale, in writing, so that the board can investigate or ask for additional information. In a hearing that follows, the patient voices his or her problem. The dentist gives his or her side of the story. The board may look at records, examine the patient, or ask for "experts" in the field to give opinions.

In most states, the peer review board's decision is advisory. It has no force of law, although it has the moral force of a professional imprimatur. (If the peer review board votes overwhelmingly that the work shows a problem, the dentist should take heed.) If a patient is not satisfied with the outcome, he or she can usually still pursue malpractice litigation. Peer review has helped to decrease the amount of professional litigation. Because organized dentistry runs peer review, in many states it is only open to members of the ADA (and its affiliate state and local societies.) Not all practitioners (only about 80 percent) are members of the organization. Those that are not obviously can not participate. The only disciplinary action that boards can generally take is expulsion from the professional society. For members, this may, or may not be significant. For nonmembers, it is obviously meaningless.

Malpractice Litigation

The best-known avenue for resolution of disputes is through malpractice litigation. In these cases, the dentist (the defendant) will be taken to court by the dissatisfied patient (plaintiff) who claims that the dentist was professionally negligent and therefore owes damages. In fact, most of the cases never reach the actual courtroom. The plaintiff drops some, and the defendant settles some, or the defendant's malpractice insurance carrier may negotiate a settlement. The plaintiff's lawyer handles most cases on a "contingency" basis. This means that the lawyer only gets paid a percentage (usually about 33 percent) of any awards collected. If the dentist wins, he or she gets nothing. This obviously makes plaintiffs' lawyers careful in choosing their cases. The lawyers will only take cases that they believe they can win and will likely result in large damage awards. This process helps screen out small nuisance type cases but encourages others where the plaintiff does not have enough money to hire an attorney on their own.

If a dentist receives any information from a lawyer or patient indicating that a lawsuit is possible, he or she should contact the malpractice carrier immediately. The carrier will help and guide the dentist through the process. The carrier is interested in paying out the least amount of money for damages, so carrier will do what it can to help the dentist in the case. The carrier will find (and pay for) an attorney to represent "the dentist's" interest in the case. (Actually, the attorney represents the carrier's interest in the case.) The carrier will also pay any damages from the dentist's case up to the limits of his or her coverage. Most carriers will vigorously defend the dentist's case so that plaintiffs' lawyers do not see dental malpractice as an easy area to get a settlement. A carrier may not spend $100,000 defending a dentist in a $20,000 suit, even if it believes that the case can be won. It makes economic sense for the carrier to settle the suit before going to trial. The dentist then, may continue the suit, but the carrier is no longer involved and will not pay any losses the dentist has as a result.

Licensing Agency Actions

Each state has some form of a "board of dentistry." This is the agency that the state charges with protecting the public from poor or fraudulent dental practitioners. The agency sets rules and regulations concerning the practice of dentistry in its individual state and then enforces those rules daily. The agency's job is to protect the public not to protect the dentist's ability to practice dentistry. State boards have the authority to grant dental licenses. They can also revoke or suspend licenses and reprimand, censure, or probate practitioners. Most boards have investigative powers. If they receive a complaint, they can require documentation of the dentist or conduct an inspection at the dentist's office. Many boards, by law, must investigate every patient complaint (or certain types of complaints) that they receive.

Boards enact disciplinary actions for several common reasons. They may be involved if a practitioner has been found to do work that is "grossly or continually faulty." (A single act or finding of malpractice *generally* does not lead to board action, unless it is "grossly" or "egregiously" faulty.) The boards are often involved in cases of interpretation of the state dental laws, such as proper auxiliary use and specialty designation. Boards often punish practitioners who are chemically impaired (alcohol or drugs) or who are guilty of improper prescription writing. Most state dental practice acts require "good moral character" of its dentists. Based on this rule, many boards can (and do) punish dentists for conviction of moral types of crimes. Obviously, if a dentist is involved in board of dentistry action, the results can be disastrous for the dentist and his or her practice. Because these are not malpractice actions, malpractice carriers will not represent the dentist in actions by the board of dentistry.

Malpractice Insurance

Despite a dentist's best efforts at managing the professional risk in the office, he or she may, at some time in his or her career be sued for dental malpractice. Those are the times for which the dentist has professional liability (malpractice) insurance.

Malpractice Insurance Terminology

Like general business liability insurance, several terms are common to all malpractice insurance contracts. The dentist pays an annual amount, or *premium*, to the insurance company (*carrier*). In return, the company writes a contract (policy) in which it agrees to indemnify, or repay the dentist, for any covered loss while the contract is in force. Covered losses are judgments of damages against the dentist, usually in a court of law, that arise from his or her professional negligence. The carrier usually puts stipulations in the contract that limits the maximum amount that it will pay. For example, the insurer may write a policy with limits of "$1 million/$3 million." This says that it will pay up to $1 million for a single claim (judgment) against the dentist and up to $3 million in total judgments per year. If the dentist is successfully sued for $2.5 million in a single case, the insurer will pay $1 million. The dentist is responsible for finding the other $1.5 million. Usually no deductibles are associated with these policies. Policies will have a long list of exclusions or cases in which the insurer will not pay. A claims made policy covers the dentist for any claim made while the policy is in force. If the dentist then leaves practice, he or she should purchase a "tail policy" to cover him or her for the work done previously after the claims made policy is no longer in force. An occurrence policy covers the dentist for the work he or she does during a given period, even if no one discovers the problem until many years later.

Some carriers will pay for the cost of medical follow-up care (often called "first aid expenses") for a patient of the practice. For example, assume a patient swallows a crown while the dentist is adjusting it before cementation. The dentist wants to send the patient to a physician or to the emergency department for a chest X-ray to ensure that the crown is in the stomach and not lodged in the patient's lung. Most malpractice carriers will pay for the cost of the follow-up care. (It is obviously in its interest to ensure that a more serious problem does not develop.) The dentist should check his or her policy before a problem arises.

What to Do in Case of a Suit

If a dentist suspects that a patient is so dissatisfied that they might sue him or her, the dentist should contact the professional liability agent immediately. The dentist should not wait until a summons, requiring the dentist to be present for a deposition, arrives. This is probably new territory for the dentist. The agent, however, has handled many such cases before. He or she can help the dentist through the process and give advice that will, hopefully, reduced the likelihood of a full-blown court case or even avert a claim being made. Conversely, inappropriate comments or actions by the dentist may hasten or intensify a claim. If a case does become serious, the insurer will find (and pay for) an attorney to represent the dentist's side of the case. However, the dentist should remember that the attorney works for the insurance company. Some policies say that if the insurer decides to settle the case without going to trial, the dentist does not have much say in the matter. (This is called a *hammer* clause, for good reason.) Even if both the dentist and the attorney believe that they will win the case, the insurance company may find it less expensive (from its perspective) to settle before trial, rather than going through a lengthy and expensive court trial. If that is the case, the company usually will settle. The dentist should read his or her policy carefully before signing. Not all policies contain such clauses. Some require the dentist's consent to settle. This can be a deciding factor for some practitioners in their choice of malpractice insurance carriers.

Factors that Affect Rates

Several factors affect a dentist's malpractice insurance rates. The area in which a dentist practices is one of the most important. Some areas experience many more malpractice cases that others. If a dentist practices in one of these high suit areas (e.g., California, New York, Florida), the rates will be higher than in other areas. A dentist's professional history plays a large role. If he or she has had previous malpractice cases, the insurer will see that dentist as a greater risk, and therefore, he or she will have to pay higher premiums. Each insurance company has a point at which it will simply refuse to write the dentist any more policies. The company may believe that the dentist is simply too great a risk for it to carry. Specialists do more complex and risky procedures than generalists. Their premiums are also higher. If a dentist uses deep sedation or general anesthesia, he or she will pay a much higher premium to compensate for the additional risk that those procedures carry. (Nitrous oxide analgesia generally does not lead to higher premiums.) Many plans will give a dentist a premium reduction if he or she completes a risk management seminar or quality assurance office review by the staff.

Coordination of Policies

Many malpractice insurers also carry general business ("slip and fall") liability insurance and workers' compensation policies. The dentist can coordinate the three to ensure that there are no gaps in his or her coverage. A patient falls while getting out of the dental chair, injuring themselves. Is this a general or professional liability problem? If the dentist coordinates his or her insurance policies, the dentist does not have to worry.

Many group practices require that all providers carry malpractice insurance through the same carrier. This decreases problems if a patient jointly sues several practitioners in the same practice over a case. It simply avoids a squabble between the insurers (claiming the other should pay) that leaves the dentist hanging out to dry.

National Practitioner Databank

The federal government has been concerned about tracking down health care practitioners who have poor malpractice records. Often these practitioners move from hospital to hospital or state to state. Their histories and backgrounds are not always adequately or easily checked. The problem is primarily with medical practitioners, although they have included dentists in the mix. To address this problem, the government has established the National Practitioner Data Bank. Any time a health care practitioner receives a judgment against him or her in which the practitioner (or a malpractice carrier) pays an award, he or she must notify the data bank. The data bank then develops a historical record of payments. Any time a practitioner applies for license, credentials, or privileges, the investigating agency can receive a report on the person's malpractice history.

The profession sees several problems with the data bank. The idea of what makes up a payment to a patient is in question. If a patient is dissatisfied with a denture and the dentist refunds his or her money, some contend that is a payment and must be reported. Peer review intends to avoid problems, but many in the profession see reporting to the data bank as punitive. Finally, right now, only credible investigators have access to the information. Practitioners are worried that the public may have easy access to the information and make false or uninformed decisions based on the information.

Information Security and Management

As practicing dentists, dentists deal with sensitive data every day. Modern dental offices contain a great amount of information that can be misused or abused by unscrupulous, dishonest, or incompetent people. This information consists of personal medical information of patients, personal and financial patient information, payment card information, and personal information about the employees and owners of the practice. With the instant dispersal of information through the Internet, dentists must proactively and zealously protect that information from intrusion.

It is both a moral and legal responsibility for use to ensure that this information does not fall into the wrong hands or be used improperly. HIPAA rules and sanctions govern protested patient information. Federal rules govern large organizations' handling of financial information. Many states have rules about disposing data that contains sensitive information. Finally, dentists as individuals would be incensed if sloppy security allowed their personal information to be used inappropriately. Dentists must take the same view on the other side to ensure that the information they have on others is well protected.

Types of Information

Data exists in many forms in the dental office. It may be physical (such as paper, film, or a computer screen), electronic (on a computer, Internet, office intranet, or fax), storage media (such as computer tapes, back-up drives). This data is at risk for being accessed by unauthorized people (both inside the office and outside) any time it is used, stored, transferred, or disposed. In the old days, the biggest concern was that someone might look through the trash (dumpster dive) and find sensitive information on discarded paper forms. This information could then use this for illegal purposes. Today, computer hackers and thieves are more inventive in ways that they can steal sensitive information, so the management of this risk needs to evolve similarly.

Elements of a Plan

Any plan for information security must be reasonable, yet protect patient, staff, and dentist's interests. As in all risk management efforts, the dentist should use a reasonable level of diligence to be sure that the data is secure and used as intended. Some data is more sensitive, or potentially more damaging than other data, and should be treated differently. Reasonableness is the key here. HIPAA sets the baseline on what dentists should do with patients' personal information. The data management plan describes how this and other forms of sensitive information are handled.

Computer Back Ups

Dentists should back up their computer database daily. They should be sure that their data backup uses data encryption techniques. To read an encrypted file, a data thief must have a secret key or password that enables

decryption. Many computer consultants call for redundant backups, one on a physical disc, the other on a secure offsite storage area. When a dentist makes back ups on physical media, such as a removable disk, drive, or tape, the best procedure is to take it off site. In case of an office fire or other catastrophe, the dentist must be able to access the information. If a dentist places media in a fireproof safe, he or she should be sure that it is rated for enough time and temperature to withstand a complete fire. The safe should also be water proof because fire departments use water for fire suppression. If the dentist takes the media off site, he or she should have the additional problem of securing the media to ensure that it is not stolen. Many people have found laptops or storage discs stolen from the cars while they took a brief stop in a grocery store on the way home. Off-site backups are secure, although slightly more expensive.

Destroying Data

When information is no longer needed, or when the storage media is changed, dentists need to destroy the information properly. Shredding any paper or film that has any sensitive information should be normal operating procedure. All cities have companies that will come to the office and shred documents and destroy computer discs. For large jobs, the cost is well spent. Most will give a dentist a certificate that guarantees the complete destruction of the media.

Data in Transit

Any time dentists move data, physically or electronically, it is a greater risk for being lost or stolen because it may be out of their control. Dentists need to take special precautions.

- For physical (paper and film) data, dentists should use approved couriers (such as UPS, FedEx, USPS, etc.) for sensitive data. For sensitive documents, the dentist should ensure that parcel tracking is available and that someone must sign for the package.
- For electronic data, the dentist should be sure that software vendors are compliant with HIPAA for information processing (most are). The dentist should use proper encryption techniques. If he or she uses a wireless network, he or she should be sure that it is effectively configured for security. If a dentist e-mails information, he or she should be sure that the provider secures the information properly.

Part 2: Regulatory Compliance

Badges? We ain't got no badges. We don't need no badges. I don't have to show you any stinking badges.
Gold Hat, *Treasure of the Sierra Madre*

Objectives

At the completion of this part, the student will be able to:

1. Describe the types of licenses that a dental practitioner needs to practice legally.
2. Describe the process of gaining a state dental license.
3. Describe the process of registering to write prescriptions for scheduled drugs.
4. Describe the purpose of the Occupational Safety and Health Administration (OSHA).
5. Define the owner–dentist's role in worker safety in the dental office.
6. Describe the office policies required by OSHA regarding blood-borne pathogens.
7. Describe the Hazard Communication Program required by OSHA for the dental office.
8. Describe fines and actions that may result from a dentist's failure to comply with OSHA standards.
9. Describe the purpose of HIPAA.
10. Define protected health information (PHI) and give common dental office examples of PHI.
11. Describe why it is important to protect a patient's PHI.
12. Describe the three broad HIPAA rules.
13. Describe the use of the common HIPAA forms in the dental office.
14. Describe present regulations and standards regarding disposal of medical wastes.

Key Terms

acknowledgment of receipt of notice
Blood-borne Pathogens Standard
board of dentistry
blood and other potentially infectious material (BOPIM)
business associate agreement
continuing education requirement
DEA number
Drug Enforcement Administration (DEA)
Electronic Transactions and Code Set Standards Rule
engineering controls
exposure control plan
general industry standards
general waste
hazard communication standard
hazardous material
Hepatitis B vaccine
Health Insurance Portability and Accountability Act (HIPAA)
infectious waste

license renewal
medical waste
minimum necessary information
narcotic registration
occupational license
Occupational Safety and Health Administration (OSHA)
operations
payment
personal protective equipment (PPE)
privacy notice
privacy rule
protected health information (PHI)
regional clinical examinations
security rule
state dental license
treatment, payment, and operations (TPO)
training program
treatment
universal precautions
work practice controls
written exposure control plan

Goal

The goal of this part is to prepare the new practitioner to be compliant with regulations that affect dental practice.

There are several mundane business needs that dentists should be sure that they have taken care of in their practice. These issues are not exciting, but they are important. They involve complying with governmental regulations.

With all these compliance issues, in the end it does not matter whether the dentist likes them or not, whether the dentist believes they are an intrusion into his or her life, or whether the dentist believes they are effective. The dentist needs to comply. The business owner is responsible for seeing that everyone in the office complies with the general intent and details of the regulations. Several steps will help to ensure that the dentist does comply.

1. *The dentist needs to learn the laws*   As the leader and manager of the practice, the dentist must be familiar with the regulations that affect the practice. He or she should take continuing education courses that tell how to comply with these laws. (The dentist should require staff to take these courses as well.) He or she should purchase material from the ADA or other sources that guide the dentist in developing office compliance policies. The dentist can often delegate compliance to a trusted employee and should encourage the employee to take his or her role seriously and remain involved. Many consultants will help the dentist to set up compliance policies and develop documentation.

2. *The dentist should train new and current employees about how to follow the law*   Each regulation describes the training that dentists must conduct with employees. Most require extensive training for new employees and retraining and certification for ongoing employees.

3. *The dentist should document office compliance*   If the dentist does the training and other compliance requirements, he or she must be able to prove it if proof is requested. The dentist must, therefore, document all of the training and other activities that have been done to support compliance. Often, the documentation (not the training itself) is what avoids a problem.

Much like patient records, if the dentist does not document it in the records, it did not happen.

4. *The dentist should do annual updates* Dentists often believe that once they have done something, they have complied with the regulations. Most regulations require that dentists update all staff members annually. People forget information if they do not use it regularly. Their perspectives change and the laws and regulations change over time. Annual refresher courses help everyone understand what to do and why they need to do it.

These regulations are not onerous. They are well-intentioned rules to be sure that dentists protect themselves, their workers, patients, private information, and the public. Each office needs to develop a culture of compliance. This culture says that the office does not grudgingly do the minimum of what has to be done but look for ways to ensure that all the people whom are affected are protected.

Licenses and Registrations

State Dental License

Completing a state or regional clinical board exam does not get a dentist a license to practice dentistry. The dentist still must apply for a license in every state in which he or she will practice. As a rule, the dentist must also pass an exam that covers the state's dental laws before the state will grant the dentist the license as well. By far, the biggest problem is the clinical exam. The rest is pretty much paperwork, although the dentist must know the state dental laws intimately.

The dentist should have a current state dental license certificate (the piece of paper) in hand before seeing the first patient. The dentist should not see a patient without it because he or she would be practicing dentistry without a license. This is a bad way to start a dental career. The dentist may have received notice at school, by phone, or any of several other ways that he or she has "passed," but until the dentist has the license in his or her, the dentist cannot see patients.

Some new dentists schedule patients based on the assumption that they will pass the licensing exams. Others assume the license will arrive by a certain date. These are bad gambles that can have serious negative results if the gambles do not pay off. Other new graduates hurry to have their names placed in the phone book, so that it will be there for the remainder of the year. This is another bad bet that can cause trouble for the dentist if someone complains to the board of dentistry that he or she is purporting to be a dentist before graduating or being licensed. The problem is that yellow page phone books are only printed once a year. If a dentist misses the deadline, he or she is not in the book for a year. People want to be sure to get a jump start. Sometimes they may be too quick. If a dentist has trouble with an exam or another unforeseen problem occurs (illness, etc.), he or she may have a yellow page ad claiming that he or she is a practicing dentist when in fact, he or she is not. These are all bad ways to start a dental career.

Many states require that the dentist registers his or her license at the county courthouse where he or she will be practicing. This seems like a silly contrivance to pad the wallet of the court clerk. Maybe it is. Nevertheless, if the state dental practice act says that a dentist should register, he or she should register. It is the law, despite how silly someone might think a particular requirement is. He or she should follow the law.

All states have a requirement for either annual or biennial license renewal. If a dentist fails to renew or fails to pay the renewal fee, he or she will forfeit the license. If there is a date for renewal (e.g., December 15 of the previous year), then the dentist should have it in on time. Many states require that dentists complete a certain number of hours of continuing education courses. Some states require particular types of certification (e.g., CPR or HIV education) before renewal. The dentist should read state laws carefully and follow them to the letter. A dentist's ability to practice is simply too important. If a dentist wants to make a statement about intrusion of government into his or her life, then he or she should write a letter to the editor of the newspaper and not use his or her dental license renewal as a forum to speak.

Many people hold dental licenses from several states, although they only practice in one state. Many states may accept regional board examinations for dental licensure. However, most states only accept those clinical exams for the first 5 years after they are passed. Consequently, many dentists will gain licensure in many states, using that as insurance in case they may want to move to that state in the future. The annual license renewal fees are seen to be cheap by comparison to the problem and expense of taking a new clinical exam at some time in the future. Besides, the cost of those licenses is a tax-deductible expense of doing business. This further decreases the out-of-pocket (after tax) expense for maintaining those licenses. The dentist should be sure to check with the states in which he or she holds licenses. Some states put time limits on how long they will license someone if that person does not practice in their state.

Local Occupational Licenses

Many municipalities have local occupational licenses. They are generally inexpensive but another requirement for a dentist to meet. These licenses are also often used as the basis of ad valorem, or property taxes, levied by the local municipality. Other areas may have local income taxes (occupational taxes) that they levy on people who work in their jurisdiction. They may use occupational licenses to track compliance with these taxes as well. The dentist should check with the local dental society, an established practitioner, or an accountant about these because they will know if the municipality has such a tax and where to sign up for it.

Drug Enforcement Administration (DEA) Registration

Before a dentist can write prescriptions for "scheduled" or narcotic drugs, he or she must register with the US Department of Justice, Drug Enforcement Administration (DEA). Many people call this a "license" although, in fact, it is only a registration. Dentists do not need to pass a test, only provide information concerning dental license, prescription writing needs, and send a fee. (Note that a dentist needs a valid dental license number before registering with the DEA, but he or she can request an application form before being licensed. This may save the dentist several weeks in the initial practice start-up time.) Each registration number is for a particular office. If a dentist has more than one office location, he r she must have more than one DEA number (and pay more than one registration fee). The DEA has a Web site (http://www.deadiversion.usdoj.gov/drugreg/) that allows practitioners to apply for registration.

When the Department of Justice issues a certificate, it contains a number that must appear on all narcotic prescriptions. Many practitioners have their DEA number printed on their prescription forms. (The dentist also needs this number to phone in a prescription to the pharmacy for a scheduled drug for a patient.) Some states require that the dentist use prescription pads that have special characters imbedded in the paper that make them difficult (or impossible) to photocopy. This is an attempt to keep patients from misusing prescriptions for narcotic drugs. Again, the dentist should check with the local dental society or practitioners to find the laws for the particular area.

Most dentists occasionally prescribe narcotics, especially analgesics, in their practices. Therefore, they will need a narcotics registration. A dentist can still practice without this registration; he or she just cannot dispense or prescribe scheduled drugs. If a dentist does not have this registration, he or she can still write prescriptions for nonscheduled drugs (such as antibiotics). All prescriptions must relate to dental treatment and must be for a patient of the practice. Many dentists run into trouble with their dental board or other law enforcing agencies for improper prescriptions. This is usually for

writing nondental related prescriptions or for writing prescriptions for people who are not patients (often self or family) medication.

Staff Certification

The dentist must keep his or her dental license current. Individual staff members may have license compliance issues as well. It is usually the dentist's responsibility to ensure that he or she does not hire someone the state has not properly licensed or certified. This includes the hygienist's license, expanded function assistant's certification, or radiographic safety certification. The dentist should keep current copies of these certifications. Some states require that the dentist post the certifications in a public area of the office.

Osha and the Dental Office

The Occupational Safety and Health Administration (OSHA) is a federally mandated program that intends to increase worker safety while on the job. Traditionally, unions were the source of worker safety rules. As the workforce became less unionized, the federal government began to develop these rules. President Richard Nixon developed OSHA in 1973. Originally, it only covered high-risk workplaces, such as construction sites and heavy manufacturing. It has gradually increased its sphere of influence to cover almost every possible workplace in the United States. Many federal laws that govern business only control the larger corporations. OSHA pertains to all businesses that hire employees, even if it hires only one employee.

Many dentists want to rant and rail against OSHA as an unnecessary intrusion into their sacred dental practices. However, these rules simply provide guidance on good workplace techniques and conditions. OSHA compliance is not a big problem, if the dentist takes a positive attitude and sees that it is done. The ADA has material that is useful for complying with OSHA regulations in the office. One of the big issues is to be sure that the dentist has documented all of the training and other compliance measures.

Purpose of OSHA

OSHA's goal is to protect the worker. OSHA does not concern itself with customer, client, or patient safety. (For example, OSHA would not cite a dentist if a patient does not wear safety glasses, but it could cite the dentist if employees do not wear safety glasses.) OSHA develops rules and regulations for each workplace environment.

They often depend on other federal agencies to make recommendations concerning the rules and standards to follow. For example, OSHA follows the Centers for Disease Control and Prevention (CDC) guidelines concerning transmission of blood-borne pathogens when developing OSHA guidelines for the workplace.

OSHA has an open definition of an employee. Anyone who receives pay is an employee. They may be full-time, part-time, or probationary. Professional employees, such as dental associates, also fall under OSHA rules. An owner–dentist may or may not be personally under these rules. If the dentist practices as a proprietor, or as a partner in a partnership, then he or she is an owner, not employees. OSHA is not concerned with owners, unless the owner is also an employee. This happens when the dentist practices as a corporation. Here, the dentist is both an owner and an employee of the corporation. OSHA rules then pertain to them.

OSHA became concerned with dental offices because of the possibility of spread of AIDS in the dental environment. Although this possibility is remote, other diseases, such as Hepatitis B and Hepatitis C, can easily be spread. Regardless, OSHA guidelines are now firmly in place in the dental workplace.

OSHA Requirements for Dental Practices

OSHA presently has three standards that apply to the dental office work environment. They are the Blood-borne Pathogens Standard, which is concerned with the transmission of blood-borne infectious diseases, the Hazard Communication Standard, which is concerned with hazardous chemicals, and General Industry Standards, which are not specific to dental offices but relate to safety rules for all places of employment.

Blood-borne Pathogens Standard

The Blood-borne Pathogens Standard intends to prevent employees from contracting infectious, blood-borne diseases while on the job. It is based on research conducted by the federal CDC in Atlanta. It is generally concerned with the handling of blood and other potentially infectious material (BOPIM). BOPIM consists of blood and blood-soaked materials, such as blood-soaked gauze. In dentistry, saliva often contains significant amounts of blood, so saliva (in dentistry) is considered potentially infectious. Finally, any unfixed tissues, such as biopsy specimens, extracted teeth, and gingival fragments, are considered potentially infectious.

The OSHA standard dictates that dental offices will:

Develop a written exposure control plan.
Carry out specific housekeeping, laundry, and labeling procedures.

Provide Hepatitis B virus vaccination and postexposure evaluation and follow-up.
Develop a training program for employees and keep records of their participation.
Provide adequate personal protective equipment and ensure that employees use it.

Written Exposure Control Plan
An exposure control plan assesses each employee's potential exposure to blood-borne pathogens and then lists specific things that the dentist will do to prevent or decrease exposure to these pathogens for employees. The first step is to decide which employees are likely to be exposed to these pathogens. In the dental office, dentists, hygienists, and assistants are all at risk (by nature of their jobs) to exposure. The receptionist may not be at any risk (unless they also help by taking radiographs or assisting occasionally.)

The next step is to decide the methods of compliance for employees. There are four general areas for the dentist to consider when developing this part of the plan.

1. *Universal precautions* amount to treating everyone as if they are infectious. In this way, the dentist protects himself or herself from the patient or staff member who is infectious. This means that the office staff needs to use personal protective equipment (PPE) on all patients, use rubber dams, sterilize all equipment, and perform routine disinfection procedures.
2. *Engineering controls* are pieces of equipment that force compliance with safety practices. Use of safety-engineered equipment is much more effective than simply telling someone to act in a certain way. For example, a self-sheathing needle (engineered control) is more effective at preventing needle sticks than simply telling employees not to use a two-handed recapping technique.
3. *Work practice controls* reduce the likelihood of exposure by changing the way tasks are done in the office. For example, dentists can require that employees not recap needles with two-handed techniques or that they restrict personal habits and eating in the work area. The problem with work practice controls is that the dentist must be diligent in following-up to ensure that the controls are always followed. The dentist must label all biohazards, sharps, and sharp containers and provide red bags for all potentially infectious material.
4. *Personal Protective Equipment (PPE)* is the equipment that the dentist provides for employees' protection. This includes gloves, masks, eye protection, protective clothing, and resuscitation equipment. It is the employer's responsibility to provide this equipment, repair or replace it, and to ensure that employees use

it appropriately. The dentist must provide protective outer garments for employees and see that the garments are properly laundered.

Housekeeping chores must be completed regularly. The dentist must have a written schedule of decontamination for operatories, written decontamination procedures, procedures for containing regulated wastes, and procedures for handling contaminated laundry. (Laundry must be cleaned in-house [by employees] or laundered off premises by a laundry company, or other nonemployees. The owner, if not incorporated, can take laundry home for cleaning.)

Hepatitis B Vaccine

Dentists must provide the series of hepatitis B virus vaccine injections for employees who are at risk of exposure to the disease. This is free (the dentist's expense) to employees who are prone to exposure. This must be available within 10 days of beginning employment. If the employee refuses the vaccine, the dentist should have him or her sign a form that acknowledges refusal; but the dentist must then provide it free if the employee ever changes his or her mind.

The dentist must have a plan in the event an employee is exposed to a blood-borne pathogen (e.g., through an inadvertent needle stick). This postexposure evaluation and follow-up plan includes documentation of the following elements:

1. Document the route of exposure
2. Inform and test source individual, if voluntary consent of the source is obtained
3. Test the employee
   a. If negative, use as a baseline for three-week, three-month, and 6-month follow-ups.
   b. If positive, end the series.
4. The dentist must have a health care professional's written opinion on the results.
5. This is free to the employee (i.e., the dentist pays the cost) and under supervision of a licensed physician
6. The dentist must maintain confidentiality

Communication of Hazards of Blood-borne Pathogens

This part of the plan requires that dentists provide training for all employees. He or she must provide this training to all new employees and annually to all continuing employees. Furthermore, the dentist must keep records of the training (initial and annual).

Hazard Communication Standard

The second OSHA requirement for dental practices is to protect employees from potentially hazardous materials in the workplace.

Definition Hazardous Material

Hazardous materials are any substances used in the workplace that could injure an employee. These are generally chemicals that can cause rashes, burns, or other physical distress. Many common products, when used in the workplace, have the potential of becoming hazardous. Common chlorine bleach is found in virtually every house in the United States. When it is used in the dental office (or other workplace), it is a potentially hazardous material. The dentist can not assume that employees should have the common sense to use these materials carefully and wisely.

Steps to Compliance

The four basic steps for a dentist to be compliant with this standard are:

1. Read and know the standard
2. Begin a written hazard communication program
3. Begin a training program
4. Maintain records

Hazard Communication Program

The first step in the process is to develop a list of hazardous chemicals. The list needs to specify where to find the material and how to prepare it for use. All hazardous materials now have Material Safety Data Sheets (MSDSs) prepared for them. These sheets tell about the product, what chemicals are in the product, and what to do if it is accidentally ingested or improperly used. (These are obtained from the supplier.) The dentist must maintain a file of these MSDSs that is open to all employees. If an employee, for example, splashes a bonding agent into his or her eye, the dentist can quickly pull the MSDS on that agent to give the physician at the emergency department information for treatment.

The dentist must also have a hazardous chemical training program for all staff. This program must contain the following elements:

1. Inform employees of the regulation.
2. Train employees in the use of MSDSs.
3. Label all hazardous chemicals according to certain labeling requirements.
4. Locate all chemicals in the workplace.
5. List where those chemicals are encountered.
6. List physical and health problems associated with chemicals.

The dentist must provide precautions to protect employees from any chemicals or other hazardous materials. These precautions include work practices, engineering controls where appropriate, PPE, and emergency procedures.

Record Keeping

The record-keeping requirement for hazardous materials is similar to that for blood-borne pathogens. That is to say, dentists must provide annual training and document that they had the training. The specific elements of the record-keeping requirement are:

1. Written description of hazard communication program.
2. List of hazardous chemicals.
3. Location and use of MSDSs.
4. Record of training sessions.
5. Employee comments on training.

General Industry Standards

General Industry Standards apply to all workplaces, not just dental offices. Many are common sense. But just because they are common sense does not mean that dentists have thought about them or informed employees about them.

Medical Services and First Aid

Dentists should have a first-aid kit available for employees. They should also have staff trained in cardiopulmonary resuscitation (CPR) and know how to handle medical emergencies. (The dentist should obviously have them trained for patient emergencies. Training for staff emergencies should be the same.)

Materials Handling and Storage

Most materials will be handled in the hazardous materials section of the dentist's compliance plan. However, there are other, nonhazardous materials that need to be processed and stored safely. For example, the dentist should be sure that employees know how to safely lift and store heavy boxes.

Building and Equipment

There are many local fire and safety codes for building and equipment incorporated into smart business practice. A partial list of these safety features in the office includes:

Automatic sprinkler system must be maintained (if the office is equipped with one).

Dentists must have a design with sufficient exits in case of an emergency.

Exits should be readily marked, even when dark or when electrical power is lost.

Exits must not be locked from the inside during working hours.

Compressed gas cylinders must be in a locked area and secured fastened.

Dentists must have an eye wash station.

Dentists must provide adequate sanitary waste receptacles.

Dentists must have a written fire safety plan.

Portable fire extinguishers must be maintained annually. Employees must be trained in their use.

If dentists have electrical cords, they need be sure that the cords are of adequate size and in good repair.

Dentists should be sure that they protect employees from ionizing radiation.

Dentists must have a fire evacuation plan.

Dentists must adequately ventilate or scavenge anesthetic gases (such as nitrous oxide).

OSHA Inspections

In the past, OSHA inspections were one of the most feared occurrences in a dental office. OSHA seldom conduct the inspections now. Instead, OSHA tries to work with the professional organizations to gain cooperation from practitioners. However, OSHA still has the right and responsibility to conduct individual office inspections. OSHA inspectors are usually busy with larger employers and accident inspections. If a dentist is subject to an inquiry, it will probably be an "OSHA Letter of Inquiry." About 1 in 10 of these letters leads to in-office inspections. They are seeking "probable cause." OSHA personnel realize that many complaints are unfounded or come from disgruntled (generally former) employees. Nevertheless, they are diligent about inquiring about complaints. If a dentist receives such a letter, he or she should explain why he or she is in compliance. The dentist should not "promise to do better" because that admits that the dentist was not in compliance. The dentist should not take a potential OSHA inspection lightly. Fines for noncompliance are substantial. As with most other office issues, prevention is the most cost-effective method.

Inspection Process

OSHA inspectors can come unannounced to the dental office. They may have (or the dentist can require) a warrant for entry to premises and a subpoena for any records. They can inspect the premises and interview any employee(s). They will have a closing conference in which they inform the dentist of any adverse findings. If the inspectors have any negative findings, they will send the dentist a written notice of citation and proposed penalty. This lists any violations, how and when to fix them, and any penalties. The dentist must post this notice for employees to see. The dentist has have 15 working days to contest the findings or penalties.

HIPAA in the Dental Office

HIPAA affects the transmission of information among all health care providers. This includes not only dentists, but also physicians, hospitals, pharmacies, optometrists, insurance companies, and even corporate personnel departments. Anyone who has access to health information about an individual must take special precautions to ensure that the patient's health information is used appropriately. The ADA has material that is useful for complying with HIPAA regulations in the office. Aa with OSHA, a big issue is documenting how the dental office has complied with the requirements.

HIPAA was enacted by then President Bill Clinton and affirmed by President George W. Bush. These rules address most aspects of documentation related to health care. HIPAA mandates that practitioners do the following:

I. Develop a privacy policy for the office.
II. Give a copy of this policy to all patients.
III. Obtain consent before releasing medical information or records.
IV. Allow patients to restrict the disclosure and use of their medical information.
V. Reveal only the minimum amount of health information that is necessary for the procedure.
VI. Allow patients to make corrections to their health information.
VII. Develop a formal complaint mechanism for patients who believe that practitioners have misused or improperly disclosed patient information.
VIII. Educate staff as to their responsibilities under this law.
IX. Ensure that business entities with which the practitioner subcontracts follow privacy policies.
X. Periodically review policies to ensure that they are effective.
XI. Use a standard identifying provider number in all electronic transactions.

There are stiff criminal and civil penalties (including monetary penalties and prison terms) if a practitioner fails to comply with these regulations. These rules are national minimums. If the practice state has stronger privacy rules, the dentist must follow those stronger rules.

HIPAA Rules

HIPAA contains three separate sections, with rules that defined each section.

1. The *Privacy Rule* protects individuals from wrongful use of their protected health information.

2. The *Security Rule* safeguards protected health information through security measures in the office.
3. *Electronic Transactions and Code Set Standards Rule* sets standard codes for electronic transaction involving health information.

The Privacy Rule

The privacy rule sets the standard for using someone's health information. It is based on the notion that information about a person and his or her health should be private and protected. There is a huge potential for abuse of an individual's health information. For example, if an employer knows that someone has a medical condition, the employer might be less likely to hire that person. A health insurer might refuse to insure that person, raise rates, or claim preexisting condition clauses if the insurer knows of a condition. A person could be slandered in the community if a neighbor knows of a medical condition. An insurer might deny someone life or disability insurance if the insurer found out that he or she did not have a clean medical history. Drug companies or other medical suppliers could badger someone with solicitations about their product based on medical history. All these abuses have occurred when someone released people's private health information. Especially in the age of large computer databases, it becomes easier to share information electronically and compile information from various sources on individuals. This leads to potentially invasive and abusive acts. That is what the privacy rule is intended to prevent.

Protected health information (PHI) is any information about a person that someone can track to that individual. It includes name and Social Security number, telephone number, and account number. An address and even zip code (along with other information) could identify an individual, so it must be protected as well. PHI includes any information about a person's medical condition, including disease diagnoses, treatment plans, regimens and options, tests, or treatments done, and consultations with other health providers. This information can be in any form, including paper (written forms, notes, photocopies, or photographs) electronic (fax, Internet transmission, computer discs, or back-up tapes), radiographic (film or electronic), or even oral communication (through the spoken word, telephone, or voice mail).

It is the practitioner's responsibility to ensure that the information given about a person is given only to the specific people or organizations that the practitioner has told the person who he or she will give it to. Even then, the practitioner must only give that organization as much information as it needs to complete its job.

A dentist may disclose PHI routinely for three major functions in the office, namely, treatment, payment, and operations (TPO). Treatment means conducting medical (or dental) procedures or tests that relate to the patients' medical condition. For example, if a dentist consults with the patient's physician regarding a medical condition, that is part of the patient's treatment and so the dentist may disclose it without specific consent. Payment involves information that the dentist provides to third-party payers related to a person's condition, so that the third party may accurately determine benefits and make timely payments. When the dentist submits an insurance form, the form contains a large amount of PHI (both personal and medical). However, the insurance carrier needs this information to process the claim. Therefore, dentists can routinely disclose this information. Operations involve normal health care business operations. Examples here include quality assurance programs, regulatory compliance procedures, or other uses that are normal health care operational activities. If the dentist has a quality assurance office review by a third-party carrier, he or she may reveal information to them (e.g., through chart audits) without specific consent.

Dentists may use PHI routinely for TPO without specific authorization of the patient. (The patient provides a general authorization in an acknowledgment of the dentist's privacy policies.) So after the patient gives general acknowledgment of the dentist's privacy procedures, the dentist does not have to ask for specific permission to submit insurance claims, consult with other practitioners, or respond to quality assurance reviews. The dentist may also use the information for other uses, if he or she declares them in the "Privacy Notice" and the patient acknowledges that he or she knows this. However, the dentist may not use or disclose a person's PHI for any other purposes without a signed authorization by the patient.

Providers must make a good faith effort to give every patient a written notice ("Notice of Privacy Practices") that explains the routine uses and disclosures of PHI. It must also explain the patient's rights and the dentist's responsibility in using and disclosing PHI. Dentists must give every patient (or their legal representative) a copy of the privacy notice as soon as feasible (usually at the beginning of the first visit). The patient must also sign an acknowledgment that he or has received and understands the policies. This acknowledgment should be kept in the patient's chart with other records. If the patient refuses to sign, the dentist may still work (and use the information). However, the dentist must document the patient's refusal and try to use the information in a way that is consistent with patient desires. If the dentist changes his or her policies, then every patient must sign a new acknowledgment.

The Security Rule

The second HIPAA rule safeguards PHI by mandating certain procedures and personnel in the office. It requires the dentist to name a security officer for the office that conducts training for employees and sets standards for office conduct regarding health information.

Security measures include defining "reasonable safeguards" for the protection of PHI. These are rules that all employees (and providers) must follow while in the office. These are self-defined and left to the imagination of the particular entity (office). They may include using a lowered voice in public areas when discussing treatment or conditions with a patient. If a provider talks on a telephone about a patient (e.g., when receiving a medical consult), he or she should do it in private or not use the patient's name or other identifying information. The provider should shred any paper that has any PHI on it (old forms, computer printouts, routing slips, etc.), rather than simply throwing it in the trash. Employees should be sure that they turn their computer screens from the view of patients. Dentists should strictly maintain chart security, either by storing them in secured area or by ensuring that only authorized people have access to them. (It is not appropriate, for example, to leave charts on counters, where nosy patients may scan them.) The staff should leave voice mail messages that do not reveal PHI.

The rule also requires that the dentist uses the "minimum necessary information" when disclosing someone's PHI. Minimum necessary information is only that information that someone needs to complete the procedure assigned to him or her. Again, this is a self-defined limit. As an example, dentists do not need to inform a dental laboratory of a patient's medical history, unless it, somehow, affects the work that the laboratory is doing. Conversely, a specialist's consultation may require complete medical information but no payment history information.

Dentists must establish sanctions and disciplinary actions for employees who violate their privacy rules. Besides notification to law enforcement officials and regulatory bodies (such as the board of dentistry), the dental office should have policies that violations may result in termination of employment or other sanctions appropriate to the breach. Dentists should clearly state this in their employees' handbook and reinforce these at HIPAA training sessions.

If a dentist subcontracts with any people or organizations, he or she must ensure that those subcontractors follow the dentist's rules concerning patient privacy. It becomes the dentist's responsibility (and problem) if a subcontractor abuses a patient's PHI. For example, a dentist hires a collection agency to collect his or her accounts. That agency now has a large store of PHI (personal and medical) on the patients of those accounts. If the collection agency then sends those patients' names and information to a financial planner to help them manage their debt loads, they have violated the spirit and letter of the HIPAA laws. Common subcontractors include collection agencies, software vendors, lawyers, and consultants. Dental labs are considered providers and therefore exempt from this rule through the "treatment" option of the privacy rule.

Dentists may reveal PHI to a subcontractor without patient authorization if they obtain satisfactory assurances that the business associate will use the information according to their rules. This will be as a written business associate agreement. The dentist must have a separate business associate agreement with each of those entities that subcontracts for him or her, although the contracts will be essentially the same.

Electronic Transactions and Code Set Rule

The final HIPAA Rule is the Electronic Transaction and Code Set Rule. This sets standard codes for electronic transactions, such as filing insurance forms. The vast majority of vendors use the ADA's CDT-5 code set for dental procedures. However, several third-party vendors (especially governmental organizations such as Medicaid) have unique code sets. This rule will standardize those organizations, requiring all insurance companies to use the ADA code set.

This rule has a small impact on dental offices. It affects vendors more, especially those that use proprietary code sets. The one big item in this standard for dentists is that they must obtain and use a National Provider Identification (NPI) number. This is a ten-digit number that will identify the dentist in al HIPAA standard transactions. All dental plans must accept the one standard number. There are two types of NPIs, Type 1 and type 2. Type 1 identifiers are for individual health care providers who act independently. Type 2 numbers are for organizations, such as a group practice or a corporation (including incorporated dental practices). If, for example, a dentist is in a group practice that bills procedures under the corporate name (e.g., "Anytown Smile Center"), he or she should use the entity's NPI on the claim form as the billing dentist and enter the individual's NPI as the treating dentist. The newest ADA claims form has a space for both numbers.

HIPAA Required Forms

The HIPAA regulations require all offices to have many forms for use with patients. Dentists will use several of them frequently. The dentist will use others seldom, but he or she still must have them, in case they are needed.

Dentists have developed the example forms from the ADA's forms in their *HIPAA Compliance Manual*. This is an excellent reference and starting point for those who are developing their office HIPAA compliance program.

Privacy Notice

Each practice must develop a notice that describes the office's policies regarding the privacy of patient information. The practice must give it once to each patient. If it is changed, it must be reissued to all patients. It must be given at the time of initial service, except in severe emergency cases. The dentist must also post it in a clear and prominent location in the office.

Acknowledgment of Receipt of Notice

A separate form signed by the patient acknowledges that he or she has received a copy of the privacy form. Besides that, the dentist must document reasonable efforts if he or she is unable to obtain the acknowledgment.

Patient Authorization

This form is different from the acknowledgment that the patient has received the privacy notice. It authorizes the dentist to use the information for purposes other than those specified in the privacy notice. For example, the dentist has interacted with a particularly effective diabetes support group. If the dentist wishes to send the name of a diabetic patient to that group so that he or she can send literature and solicitations. The dentist must receive a specific authorization for that release.

Patient Authorization to Transfer Records

If a patient transfers to (or from) a dentist's office, the patient will generally want his or her "records transferred" so that the new doctor is aware of the entire treatment history, radiographic findings, and other pertinent information. Before the transfer, the dentist must gain patient authorization. He or she will not send (or expect to receive) the original record. Instead, the dentist will send a copy of the record and radiographs. States vary in their allowance for reasonable charges for duplication of those records.

Patient Complaint

If a patient has a complaint about a dentist's privacy practices or compliance, he or she must have a means of registering that complaint. The office's compliance officer must respond within 30 days.

Health Information Access: Response/Delay

A patient may request access to the information in his or her record. This form tells the patient whether the dentist grants that information or not. There are few legitimate reasons for denying someone access to his or her dental records. Psychiatric records are another issue.

Request for Additional Restrictions

Patients may request additional restrictions on the use or distribution of their PHI. This form allows them to request these restrictions. If they are reasonable, the dentist must abide by them. For example, a patient may request that a dentist leave no answering machine messages (or post cards) because other people in the household may listen to or read them. The dentist should abide by the patient wishes in these cases.

Request to Amend Protected Health Information

A patient may request to amend his or her health information. This form registers the request. The dentist may agree to change the information or not. For example, a patient was in an automobile accident and claims that her front tooth was knocked out. She wants to remove the information from the record showing that the tooth had previously decayed through and through because she believes that she can get the automobile insurance to pay for an anterior bridge. The dentist does not need to (and should not) allow this request to change information.

Staff Review of Policy and Procedures

The dentist must train all staff in the office on his or her privacy rules. This form registers verification that the staff have received the training and will follow the policies.

Business Associate Agreement

The business associate agreement specifies for subcontractors how the dentist uses PHI and the dentist's expectations of how he or she will use the information.

Medical Waste Disposal

Regulated medical wastes (RMW) are also called *biohazardous* or *infectious medical* wastes. These materials are exposed to blood or other body fluids that can lead to a real risk of infecting someone else. In the dental office, this includes used needles, blood- or saliva-soaked gauze, discarded instruments, extracted teeth, or other materials used intraorally. In the office, the staff should separate infectious waste from general waste, and sharp waste from infectious waste. Fortunately, the majority of dental office waste is general waste (similar to household or general office waste) and requires no special handling.

Regulated medical wastes are defined and regulated at the state and local levels. These agencies may further classify medical waste as infectious, used sharps, hazardous, radioactive, or other general wastes. Because of the possible hazards to people collecting, transporting, or disposing of these wastes, the hazards must be disposed of properly. Depending on the regulating body, there may be specific rules or precautions for different types of medical waste. (Most states do not allow a used sharps container to be placed in the general trash, for example.) Regulatory compliance is further complicated by the fact that different wastes may be regulated by different agencies within a state.

Dentists should check with the state's dental association to find specific requirements and lists of acceptable vendors for medical waste disposal. Many states require disposal companies to be certified, licensed, or otherwise regulated. Vendors will provide appropriate containers and establish a schedule for disposal of hazardous material. Dentists should shop around for a vendor. Online and mail-order waste disposal companies also may be appropriate for the practice situation. Dentists also need to document how medical wastes were disposed of, in case a problem ever develops.

Radiographic Machines

Many states inspect machines that produce ionizing radiation (often annually). Others inspect when a machine is bought. This inspection ensures that the machine does not emit too much radiation. The dentist should check with the state dental board to see if he or she needs to have this inspection done. A nominal fee is generally charged for the inspection.

Part 3: Quality Assurance

The quality of a champagne is judged by the amount of noise the cork makes when it is popped.
Mencken and Nathan's Ninth Law of the Average American

Objectives

At the completion of this part, the student will be able to:
1. Define the three dimensions of quality and cite examples of each in dentistry.
2. Discuss the history of quality assurance activities in dentistry in this country.
3. Explain the difference between quality assessment and quality assurance.
4. Define standards of care and discuss why they are important.
5. Discuss commonly used standards for performing a facility review.
6. Review a record using accepted standards of care.

Box 22.5 Quality Assurance Terminology

Structure
Process
Outcome
    Effect of care
    Patient satisfaction

Key Terms

ADA's Commission of Dental Accreditation (CODA)	records review
	quality assessment
board of dentistry	quality assessment reviews
clinical licensing exams	quality assurance
facility review	quality of care
malpractice litigation	standard of care
outcome	structure
patient satisfaction	technical quality
peer review	total quality management (TQM)
process	

Quality of health care services is a major social issue. Activities directed toward the assessment and assurance of quality of dental care are receiving increased attention. Changes in reimbursement and payment plans, heightened competition, and a rise in consumer expectations have all contributed to the increased emphasis on the quality of patient care. Consumers, government, business, and insurance companies are scrutinizing the quality of dental care considering the billions of dollars that they spend annually for that care.

Quality Assurance Terminology

Quality is difficult for most people to define. When asked whether a given good or service is of high quality, people generally have an opinion but might have difficulty in stating the rationale for providing the opinion. In other words, it may be difficult to answer the question "What makes Burger King higher quality than MacDonald's?" It may be the way they cook the burgers. Or it might be the variety of menu items, the service or the cleanliness of the restaurants. It might simply reflect a personal preference or taste, or there might be other criteria used to judge.

Dentists often equate quality of care with technical quality—for example, does a restoration have smooth margins, proper dental anatomy, and adequate occlusion? In reality, quality of care encompasses a much larger domain than simply technical quality. It includes issues such as the appropriateness of care provided to patients, the ability of a patient to receive care when needed (access), and the timeliness of care provided. To include all these aspects when defining quality, health care professionals refer to the three dimensions of quality: structure, process, and outcome (Box 22.5).

The dimension of structure addresses the characteristics of the setting in which the dentist provides the care. This includes the infection control and radiation safety procedures followed in an office, the training and certification of dental office staff, the adequacy of office hours, and office cleanliness. For example, if Dr. Smith operates a dental practice that is roach-infested, a person would question the quality of her office, and therefore the care provided in that office, based on a structural concern. The dimension of process describes the activities that occur between the dentist and the patient. This dimension is the one most often thought of when discussing quality. It includes the actual technical quality of care plus issues such as the accuracy and documentation of oral examinations and medical histories, the status of the recall system to ensure continuity of care, and the frequency with which the dentist takes radiographs. For example, a practitioner who never takes radiographs for diagnostic purposes would not offer high-quality care. Finally, the outcome dimension of quality reflects the effects of dental care on the health and welfare of the patient. This aspect of quality is new and is still evolving. Dentistry contains two components to the outcome dimension. The first is the effect of the care on a person's health and functioning; does a person feel better, look better or eat better because of the care received? This component is difficult to measure, and little work has been done on refining approaches to measuring it. The second component is patient satisfaction with the dental care received. This is based on the belief that patients can accurately evaluate the quality of care provided by their dentist. From the consumer's perspective, if a dentist has met the patients' needs as a consumer, then the care is of adequate quality.

Several terms are important in any discussion of quality of care. The first is the term *standard of care*. Standards of care are precise statements outlining what makes up an acceptable level of quality. Probably the most commonly recognized standards of care in dentistry are those promulgated by OSHA, which define acceptable infection control practices. There have been some efforts to develop standards of care for other aspects of dental practice; however, presently no universally accepted standards govern quality in dentistry. *Quality assessment* refers to the measurement of quality of any good or service in comparison with a set of standards. An example of quality assessment in dentistry is the comparison of infection control procedures in a dental office with the OSHA standards. If it is common practice in a given office to reuse saliva ejectors, an assessment of the office would obviously show a deficiency. *Quality assurance* relates to quality assessment, but it includes an important additional idea. Quality assurance activities go beyond mere measurement and include any necessary changes needed to bring the quality of care into compliance with standards governing that aspect of care. In the infection control example, any policies, procedures, or actions that bring the office practices in line with OSHA standards (e.g., using a new saliva ejector for each patient) represents a quality assurance activity. *Total quality management* (TQM) is a system used in business that attempts to involve all producers of the goods or service in the identification and resolution of quality assurance activities.

History of Quality Assessment and Quality Assurance in Dentistry

The dental profession has always been involved in evaluating and ensuring the quality of dental care rendered to the public. As early as the 1700s, the profession encouraged states to develop a system for licensing dentists. By the 1860s, state dental boards became the entities legally responsible for examining and licensing dentists. Today,

clinical board examinations and licensure procedures show organized dentistry's commitment to quality dental care because they help confirm that a dental graduate is adequately prepared to provide that care.

During this time, dental education underwent significant changes in this country. It progressed from the apprentice system, through proprietary schools, and finally to university-based programs. Accreditation activities were founded on the dental profession's commitment to quality; that is, ensuring that dental schools give students the knowledge, skills, and abilities needed to render high quality care to the public. Today, all dental schools are subject to accreditation through the ADA's Commission of Dental Accreditation (CODA). This accreditation process requires schools to evaluate critically their curricula, facility, and educational practices. It culminates in a multiple-day site visit by CODA representatives. If a dental school loses its approval by CODA, its graduates will not be eligible for licensure in most states. This, then, is a virtual death penalty for the dental school.

Dental school accreditation and dental school licensure are important components in a quality assurance program. However, simply graduating from an accredited school and getting a dental license does not guarantee that a dentist will continue to provide high quality patient care. In an attempt to insure that practitioners remain current in knowledge and technique, many states have requirements that dentists participate in continuing education courses as a prerequisite for relicensure. These states often require a certain number of hours per year of participation in scientific course work by each dentist or hygienist. Although these courses expose practitioners to current materials, they offer no guarantee that participants will learn or use the material presented.

Each state has laws that govern the practice of dentistry in their state. Most have a board of dentistry or a similar oversight committee whose job is to protect the public from incompetent or unscrupulous practitioners. They have several methods to accomplish this end. They intend clinical licensing exams to assess the technical quality of an unknown practitioner, protecting the public from poor quality dentists. (In fact, nearly all dentists eventually pass a licensing exam, so they are not particularly effective at their job.) Boards may also revoke or suspend dental licenses for conduct that endangers the public. Examples of this conduct may be alcohol or drug abuse, continually faulty dentistry, or conviction of crimes that show poor moral qualities, judgment errors, or character deficiencies. There is obviously significant room for interpretation by the individual boards and state laws.

Another form of professionally developed quality assessment activities is peer review, which is a system operated by most dental societies. In these systems, a dispute between a patient and a dentist can go to a committee composed of dentists trained to evaluate the situation impartially. Disputes handled by peer review committees generally relate to the quality of treatment and the appropriateness of care. The peer review process reflects one basic tenet of a profession: the ability to "police our own" and thereby maintain high standards in the profession. It also has a couple of disadvantages that are worth mentioning. First, peer review is a reactive process, initiated only after the allegations of poor quality work exist. Thus, rather than raising the overall level of quality provided by the profession, the process is directed toward the few poor quality providers. Second, most patients who perceive that they have received less than optimal care simply change dental providers. They will not go to the time and effort of filing a complaint with the peer review board. Thus, peer review does not become involved in many situations where the care may warrant it.

Malpractice litigation is another form of quality assurance in the profession. A dentist who has several instances of successful malpractice litigation brought against them may have difficulty finding malpractice insurance and may lose patients as the public becomes aware of their incompetence.

The most recent step in quality assessment and assurance activities stems from third-party involvement. Insurers became involved with quality of care issues primarily as they related to efforts to contain costs. They began to review claims of the insured to detect patterns of overutilization, where particular patients or groups of patients consumed "too many" services. Traditional indemnity plans quickly became aware that "over treatment" was common among their involved providers. Third-party plans began requiring dentists to obtain a preauthorization from the plan to ensure that the services the dentist has proposed are, in the opinion of the plan, necessary and by that warrant coverage. Because of this concern with controlling the costs of care, quality of care issues, such as appropriateness of care provided and patient overtreatment, began to be addressed.

Current Focus on Quality Assessment and Assurance Activities

Today's health care arena has an increasing focus on the quality of care being provided. One needs only scan the daily paper to find an article about health care reform, with quality of care concerns being a central focus. Four trends in the health care system contribute to the public's concern with quality.

Third-Party Plans

By virtue of the reimbursement structure, many managed care plans (e.g., capitation plans, preferred provider organizations, etc.) provide incentives for a dentist to undertreat patients. For example, if Dr. Smith receives less than the usual fee for a crown for a patient covered by the local capitation plan, she may choose to reduce costs by using lesser quality materials, by providing less than ideal treatment, or by not treating the patient at all.

Health Care Costs

The costs of health care have risen dramatically over the last several years. Though dentistry is only a small component of the health care system, the costs have followed those in the medical community on their upward spiral. As patients, insurers, and employers pay more for the care received, they increasingly demand that their purchases be of high quality. If the old axiom that a person gets what he or she pays for is accurate, then "I better be getting the best health care in the world."

Consumer Involvement

Forty years ago patients accepted the advice of health care practitioners with no questions asked. After all, the doctor knows best. Today, however, patients are taking a more active interest in their own health and in the care they receive. Most want an understanding of what the problem is, explanations of treatment, a discussion of the options available to them, and a perception that the care they receive will be of high quality, before ever consenting to care.

Professional Litigation

People sue others for anything (or for nothing) because we live in a litigious society. This results in malpractice suits costing the system millions of dollars. To avoid or decrease the costs of a liability suit, dentists and their liability insurers are focusing efforts on monitoring quality to reduce risk. Many insurers conduct courses for students and dentists, which address the methods to monitor and document the care being provided in their offices.

Implications for Practicing Dentists

The current focus on quality of care has several implications for practicing dentists. First, if a dentist participates in a managed care plan, he or she will likely go through a quality assessment review of the office. To counter the allegations of undertreatment discussed previously, most managed care plans have written standards for their participating providers and conduct formal annual quality assessment reviews. The review format is discussed later in the chapter. Second, because of the increased focus on quality and increased consumer concern with quality, even traditional indemnity plans are becoming more involved in quality assessment. That means that, if a dentist participates with any third-party insurer, the chances are good that the insurer will review the dentist's office at some point.

Dentists generally have one of two responses to these reviews: either they are highly insulted that anyone would question their professional capabilities and resent the intrusion of the reviewer into the practice, or they view the review as an opportunity to learn something about their practice, welcoming reviewer comments and opinions. A word of advice: the second response may be one for which to strive. Usually, if an insurance plan has reached the point of reviewing a dental office, that plan wants to have the dentist work with them. In other words, the plan wants the review to go well. The dentist should remember that the reviewers are usually dentists who have reviewed hundreds if not thousands of offices and thus have a wealth of experience in what works and what does not. The dentist might learn something from the reviewer and should be open to suggestions for change!

Benefits of quality of care reviews for practitioners relate to professional liability premiums and practice marketing. The quality of care provided in an office, and the documentation of that care, is of obvious concern to liability insurance carriers. Like reduced health or life insurance premiums for nonsmokers, the day may come when liability insurance carriers will offer a decrease in the premium to practitioners who have participated in a quality assessment review and provide care according to professional standards. Participating in a quality assessment program and receiving the "seal of approval" from a recognized entity can also have implications for marketing a dental practice. Any patient who chooses a dentist would likely be drawn to a practitioner who has evidence from an independent reviewer that the care being provided in the office meets professional standards.

Quality Assessment Reviews in Dentistry

Third-party (especially managed care) plans conduct most quality assessment reviews in dentistry. Most of the quality assessment programs operated by those plans are similar in design. Quality assessment reviews generally contain five components. Those are facility review, records review, laboratory work review, patient examinations, and patient satisfaction surveys.

Facility Review

A review of a physical practice facility addresses the structural aspects of quality (Box 22.6). It entails an on-site visit by the quality assessment reviewer. The reviewer will tour the office and ask a series of questions of the dentist or of the office staff. This portion of the review looks at several structural aspects of the practice to find out whether they comply with professional standards. The reviewers look for specific facility issues. For example, third-party payers are usually interested in contracting with offices that have enough operatories to see the plan's patients efficiently. They will, therefore, examine the number and condition of the operatories compared with patient volume. If the dentist delegates clinical work to auxiliaries, those staff members must be duly licensed or trained to carry out the work legally and safely. Written policy manuals, regular staff meetings, and such suggest to the reviewer that the dentist is attentive to personnel issues. Constant staff turnover hinders continuity of care and decreases the satisfaction of patients and plan members. Are the dentist's office hours sufficient to handle the patient load, or is the waiting time for appointments prohibitive for patients? The dentist should be accessible to patients during hours when the office is closed or, if not, the dentist should arrange for someone to cover emergencies. Does the office have a recall system with a follow-up mechanism to ensure that patients do not get "lost?" Is there equal access to care for patients with different payment sources? This question is one that is critical to alternative care plans to ensure that their plan members are not limited in their access. The reviewer

---

Box 22.6 Facility Review Items

Office cleanliness
Equipment
   In good working order
   Clean
Layout of the office
   Number of operatories
Office staff
   Staff licensure and certification
   Personnel policies
Access to care
   Office hours
   Emergency coverage
   Recall system
   Access to care
Infection control
Medical emergency preparedness
Radiation safety

may want to observe infection control procedures in action and question the staff about their level of knowledge of proper procedures. The reviewer may also check to be sure that the office follows standard emergency procedures, OSHA guidelines, worker safety, and radiation hygiene practices.

Records Review

The quality assessment reviewer will likely ask the dentist to select a sample of records to review or will select them himself or herself. The reviewer will examine records of people who have been patients for some time, so that there will be sufficient treatment recorded to warrant a review. The reviewer will conduct the review at the dentist's office. If the dentist is concerned about patient confidentiality, many plans will ask that he or she make copies of the record and mask any identifying names, numbers, and such before the review. The reviewer will be a dentist who will be looking for specific features in the records (Box 22.7). Usually, the reviewer looks to be sure that the record is complete from a medical-legal standpoint. He or she checks that the dentist's progress notes are thorough, recording in some detail what has occurred at each appointment. The reviewer verifies that the notes are in ink and signed by the dentist. Obviously, technical quality is difficult to judge by simply examining patient records. However, some facets of technical quality become readily apparent by reviewing multiple records. For example, if the same poor margins or calculus are visible on radiographs year after year, while the bone level decreases. Extensive crown and bridge procedures are sometimes done on periodontally compromised teeth. Note that reviewers are looking for a pattern of work that may not meet professional standards, not for one or two patients.

Computer Review

Many third-party payers conduct computer reviews of a dentist's billing procedures. They do these in an attempt to find mistaken or fraudulent billing practices by practitioners. They know the service profile of typical general dental practices. They then compare the billing profile to the "average" dentist, looking for any area in which the dentist charges more or fewer procedures than their average dentist. For example, assume that an insurance plan knows that their "average" general dentist does about 4 percent of his or her billing as endodontic procedures. The dentist shows about 10 percent of his or her practice as endodontic procedures. The reviewer might question why the dentist does so many more endodontic procedures than the average dentist. On investigation, the reviewer might find that the dentist charges for the procedure when it is initiated instead of completed (when it should be charged), and that many of the patients did not return for the completion of their endodontic procedure. The reviewer would probably then ask the dentist to return to the insurance company the amounts paid for the procedures that were not completed.

Review of Laboratory Work

This component of quality assessment reviews is less common, but some plans include it. Usually it is informal because, to date, there have been no standards to guide reviewers. When it is conducted, reviewers (dentists) are examining cases for proper work orders, adequate mounting/articulation, and acceptable model preparation.

Patient Examinations

A few plans will conduct clinical examinations of patients in a dentist's office to decide the quality of care being provided (Box 22.8). Because of the intrusion into the practice and because of the logistics in scheduling, this component of a quality assessment review is seldom done.

Box 22.7 Record Review Items

Performance and documentation of:
Medical histories
    Complete oral exams
    Diagnoses
    Treatment plans
Radiographs
    Quality
    Frequency
Progress notes
Technical quality of work

Box 22.8 Patient Examination Review Items

Appropriateness of care
Timeliness of care
Cost
Lack of pain
Office cleanliness
Helpfulness of staff
Interpersonal interactions in the office

Patient Satisfaction Surveys

Patient satisfaction surveys are taking on increasing importance as a quality assessment mechanism. Recent research has shown that such surveys may even be the best predictor of quality of care. Therefore, most third-party plans will conduct surveys of their plan members to monitor levels of satisfaction and help detect concerns with individual providers. Patient surveys are also the one quality control mechanism that the dentist, independent of any third-party plan, can conduct in his or her own office. If the dentist wants to maintain his or her patient base and serve them optimally, knowledge of their perceptions is important.

Section 4

Practice Transitions

Career development is becoming more important for dental graduates in today's economic climate. Many students leave dental school with hundreds of thousands of dollars of student debt. Not only do graduates need immediate income to make student loan payments, but the large debt levels may also hinder their ability to secure loans at favorable rates. The increase in the number of corporate and franchise practices provides immediate employment opportunities, but it also increases competition in the local marketplace for start-up practices. Individual practitioners, who face increased competition as well, are often reluctant to take on an associate in the traditional role of owner and mentor. The complex dental insurance world makes practices less profitable than in the past, leading to further cash flow problems for young practitioners.

Because of these economic constraints, graduates need to plan their career development. In the past, the simple answer was to "set up a practice." Now the plan may involve working in a corporate practice for several years to increase clinical and management skills or to work in a public health setting to gain some student loan relief and build clinical skills. Most graduates still have the ultimate goal of practice ownership (either individually or in a group) but now must take an often winding road to get to their goal.

There are two general categories of income generation for new dentists. First, they can work for someone else (get a job). This option allows immediate income generation but does not provide long-term professional security. They can find employment with a private practicing owner\$en\$dentist as an associate dentist, with a dental management service organization (DMSO) as an employee dentist, or with the government through the public health or military systems. (This discussion does not look at opportunities in industry or academia, only practice opportunities.) The second option is to own all, or part of a practice. This option provides long-term security, but it is often expensive and risky to establish. With this option, dentists can buy an existing practice (buy out), start a practice from scratch (cold start), or buy into an existing practice (buy in) in a partnership arrangement. This section of the book looks at each of these possibilities.

Concerns of the Career Development Process

The financial planning process really is concerned with three major goals:

1. **Establishing Short- and Long-term Career Goals** Dentists each have a long-term career goal. They each take different paths to reach those goals. Their short-term goals contribute to achieving their long-term career goals.

2. **Understanding the Difference between Employment and Ownership Positions** Employment and practice ownership are two different concerns. Each has advantages and disadvantages that become decision factors in career planning.

3. **Planning for Career Transitions** As dentists move through their careers, they need to be sure that the transitions from one phase to the next are well planned.

Objectives of the Career Development Process

Given these three main concerns, the objectives of the career development process can be grouped into common categories. The issues that dentists should

Business Basics for Dentists, First Edition. David O. Willis.
© 2013 John Wiley & Sons, Inc. Published 2013 by John Wiley & Sons, Inc.

examine in their own career planning process include the following:

Chapter 23: Career Planning Dentists need to examine their personal wants, needs, desires, and abilities to develop a comprehensive career plan.

Chapter 24: Employment Opportunities Many new graduates will enter directly into employment situations, whether in private practice (associateship), corporate, or government situations. Dentists must understand the nature of employment and the advantages of each type of employment position to be a successful employee.

Chapter 25: Practice Ownership An ownership position (either individually or in a group) has an entirely different purpose from an employment position. The owner is trying to build personal wealth by increasing the value of the practice. There are several types of practice ownership, each with different constraints and opportunities.

Chapter 26: Practice Transitions Practice transitions involve changing employment or ownership positions. This may involve starting a new practice, buying out an existing practice, or buying into an existing practice.

Chapter 27: Valuing Practices If dentists purchase or sell a practice, they need to set a value so that they can borrow money to pay for the practice, without placing a large burden on practice cash flow.

Chapter 28: Securing Financing When dentists locate a practice to purchase and have a reasonable value associated with the practice, they need to find a lender who will lend them the money required for the purchase.

Chapter 29: The Business Plan Most lenders require that dentists complete a business plan for their new business before lending the money for the purchase. This business plan describes how the dentist plans to make his or her business successful.

Career Planning

chapter 23

Don't confuse having a career with having a life.
Hillary Clinton

Objectives

At the completion of this chapter, the student will be able to:
1. Describe the characteristics of dental practice as a career.
2. Define professional options available to the new dental graduate.
3. Describe career choice points that affect the career path.
4. Describe personal and professional factors that affect the location decision.

Key Terms

career decision points   career path

Goal

The goal of this part is to describe common career planning decision points and processes.

Characteristics of Dental Practice

Dental practices are unlike many other service businesses. Most dentists are still in individual practices, with few colleagues with whom to confer. They must personally deliver the service, which involves hard physical work. They can not delegate most procedures and must be personally present for the procedures that are delegated. This means that there is little managerial leverage, so the dentist cannot play golf while the office operates. There is no managerial progress. The dentist can not work his or her way up the management line to become regional manager or vice president. Most new graduates come to the workplace with high educational debt and must include that in their practice debt finance plan. Dentists' earnings typically peak at 45 to 50 years of age. After that, the physical nature of the work causes them to decrease patient visits. Often dentists then look to add associates or plan to sell their practices. Their quandary is whether to sell at the peak of the income-generating potential (and therefore at the highest price) or to "milk the cow" and take income from the practice as they continue to slow down.

Common Myths About Dentistry

There are several misconceptions about that dentistry that will influence career choices.

Dentistry Is Easy Money

Many people outside the profession view dentistry as an easy way to make a lot of money. Although dentistry is still one of the more lucrative professions, those in the profession know that it is not an easy way to make money. Dentistry is physically demanding work. Dentists often work long hours and in contorted positions to try to make patients comfortable. Back and neck problems, repetitive motion injuries, and eye strain are common problems of seasoned dental practitioners. Dentistry is also emotionally demanding work. Many patients are fearful of dental procedures or have unrealistic expectations about the outcomes they want. Staff members may have personal problems or interpersonal disagreements that affect the work environment.

A Dentist Makes More Money Owning a Practice

Dentists might make more money if they own their own practice. Practice ownership requires knowledge, skills, and abilities that not all dentists have. Additionally, owner–dentists need to spend time and emotional energy to operate an effective practice. Not all dentists want to do this. Some are excellent clinicians but do not want the extra problems of ownership. They want to treat patients, not worry if the hygienist and assistant are having interpersonal problems or fret about the changes in a local employer's dental insurance plan. These dentists are best off working for someone, letting the owners worry about the management of the practice. If they work with someone who is good at managing a practice or a network of practices, they can make more money treating patients. The dentist who is excellent clinically, behaviorally, and managerially, and loves all aspects of running a practice can make more money owning his or her own practice.

Bigger Is Better

Many dentists believe that a bigger practice is better. Personal wants needs and desires might lead a dentist to a smaller, more intimate practice that is a better fit for his or her temperament. A larger practice is not necessarily a more lucrative practice. Profits come from using the resources of the practice to the maximum amount possible, regardless of the size. A small practice can be as profitable as a large one. However, a large, well-run practice does have some advantages, if the owner has the managerial expertise to make this larger and more complex business entity use all of its resources effectively. A larger practice might show a higher profit, if well run. A bigger practice may weather economic downturns more easily. When sold, larger, more profitable practices bring a higher price, although sometimes finding a buyer for these large practices is difficult.

Student Debt Makes It Impossible for a Dentist to Borrow Money to Buy a Practice

Dental graduates are carrying higher levels of student debt than before. Changes in the student loan programs have made it more difficult to consolidate these loans at low interest rates. Tax law changes have limited the amount of student loan interest that graduates can deduct. Nevertheless, dentistry is still one of the higher income professions. Banks and other lenders who make start-up and buy-out loans to dentists understand these problems. They will work with dentists to develop loan packages, if the practice can support the cash flow needed to pay all expenses, including student loans. Not all practices will be profitable enough at a price that can support the cash flow required to make all of the payments. This can be the result of the practice price being set too high, high overhead in the practice, or financial characteristics of the potential buyer. A graduate who does not have a high loan burden or who has a spouse who earns a significant income may show cash flow needs that are much lower. This dentist may qualify to borrow for a practice purchase when another dentist would not.

Public Health Is for Dentists Who Can Not Make It in Private Practice

It has become part of the professional culture that "good" dentistry is exquisitely done (expensive) reconstructive dentistry. True, dentists in the public care sector may not do a significant amount of complex reconstructive dentistry because the organization's purpose is to provide more basic services to a larger clientele. This in no way makes the dentistry or the dentist's application of their hard-earned skills any less quality or less important. The public sector provides valuable services to a large segment of the population. Many dentists find satisfying and rewarding careers by devoting their skills to this style of practice.

A Dentist Does Not Have to Take Insurance Plans in Practice

If a dentist is in a private ownership position, then he or she makes all of the management decisions. Long-term, the insurance-free practice is the goal of many practitioners. However, most do not get there. It takes a combination of location, clientele, management, clinical expertise, and time to develop a practice that does not participate in any dental insurance plans. The dentist may take plans in the short term with the plan to wean off them as he or she builds a private clientele. As the economic environment and insurance industry change, more practices find the need to participate with insurance plans.

A Dentist Will Be in the Same Office His or Her Entire Career

This used to be more true than it is today. In the past, the graduate would open or buy a practice and then build it over the years. He or she would be in an ownership position immediately after graduation. New graduates today may work in several professional situations before arriving at their final practice setting. With the increasing number of employment opportunities, many dentists never reach an ownership situation, choosing, instead, to do clinical work in nonownership positions for their entire career. The old notion that the only good form of dentistry is private practice is dying out.

Professional Options

Dentists have many professional options to use their skill and training. Some involve ownership, whereas others are employee situations. In this book, only the practice-related options are discussed.

Employment
    Private sector
        Private associateship (nonowner)
        Corporate employee (nonowner)
        Industrial research
        Corporate support
    Public sector
        Military or Veterans Administration
        Public health patient care settings
        Dental education
Ownership
    Private individual practice (owner)
    Private group practice (owner)

Career Paths

Dentists now talk about career paths, in which they have an ultimate, long-term goal but may take several steps to reach that goal. Short-term goals then support long-term goals. Each step in the short-term should support the long-term intention. For example, the traditional path would be to finish dental school, go directly into a pediatric dentistry residency, and then open a practice. A new graduate who has high student debt may take a different career path. In this path, he or she may graduate and join a public health practice that offers loan forgiveness. He or she can build speed and confidence while working on young patients in the clinical setting. The dentist then attends residency and joins a group pedodontic practice. Career paths are different for each individual depending on their individual circumstance. Graduates who have an immediate family member who has or had a career in dentistry or other health care profession are at an advantage. They generally have a deeper understanding of what a health care career involves and often have a built-in entrance into a practice situation. Graduates who have a history of working in private industry or government use that knowledge to advantage.

Career Choice Points

Each person makes career path decisions based on his or her own situation at the time of the decision. Certain decision points direct and influence decisions.

The Desire for Income

If a dentist has a desire for a high income (as opposed to an adequate income) then a long-term plan should include a private practice ownership option. Specialist dentists' incomes are higher than generalists. Short-term options might include associateships or military practice to build skills and knowledge while debt is paid down and assets are accumulated. If a high income does not drive a person's professional needs, then other desires can be driving forces.

Debt Load

If a dentist has small or no student debt load at graduation, then he or she is in the fortunate position of being able to take on debt for a practice purchase or personal needs. A heavy student debt may limit the possible practice options to those that show an excellent cash flow. Short term, a dentist might need to practice in an associateship or corporate practice for several years to pay down debt or find a public health practice that includes loan payment or forgiveness.

The Desire to Be the Boss

Most dental students claim to want to "be their own boss," but when they come face to face with the reality of the debt load, managing the business, and the extra time necessary, many decide that the trade-offs are not worth it. Part of the old culture of the profession was that the ultimate form of professional effort was a private individual practice. That notion has changed. Currently, many corporate and public practices offer full use of a dentist's professional skill, care, and expertise without practice ownership. If a dentist is fiercely independent and wants to make it or break it on his or her own skills, then private practice is the place.

The Desire to Live in Different Locations

Some people enjoy the idea of moving and living in different places. Others know where they want to settle and live the rest of their lives. If a dentist fits into the first group, then practice ownership is a problem. Practice ownership is a long-term commitment. It takes many years to fully recover the investment (time and financial) that is made when establishing a practice. The dentist may not find a willing buyer for a practice when he or she wants to sell it or have licensing problems in a new location. Network practices, the military, and public health practices are all more conducive to moving to different areas and experiencing different cultures.

The Desire for Personal or Family Time

Some people love dentistry and would do it 24 hours a day, if they could. Others enjoy time away from the office for personal or family activities. Some like to take time every week, others prefer to take periodic blocks of time off for travel or other similar activities. Where a person falls on this continuum is important in helping to decide career points as well. It is difficult to take a lot of time off in a individual ownership position and maintain a high income. Patients want work done, staff members want to get paid, and income stops when the dentist is not there. The dentist can set his or her own hours and take time during the week but taking many extended blocks of time is more of a problem. It is easier to take time in a group practice situation in which others can cover for a dentist and share costs. The easiest way to take blocks of time is to work in an employment situation with guaranteed time off (such as military or public health). Often the dentist will work more hours during the week but will have the flexibility of blocks of vacation time.

Other Decision Points

There are many other career decision points. If a dentist enjoys doing research, then he or she obviously will be in a situation in industry or academia where this activity is done. Where a dentist wants to live influences the path as well. If a dentist wants to live in a particular rural area, the only option may be a private ownership. Some people prefer working in an organization with many other people; some prefer working alone.

Location Decisions

Regardless of a specific career option, the dentist's first decision is where he or she wants to live. Several factors contribute to this decision.

Professional Factors

The single most important professional factor is the dentist-to-population ratio. This ratio describes the number of dentists to treat a given population in the area. It is used as an indicator of the potential viability of a dental practice. It is usually expressed as "1:2,300," which says that there is one dentist for every 2,300 people in the service area. A dentist may need to modify the ratio because it is a general number. The dentist should check that the ratio represents the area in which he or she is interested. (The numbers may be for the entire county or part of an urban area.) It includes specialists and generalists. If a dentist is a generalist, he or she probably want to take the specialists in the area out of the equation. The ratio also includes a simple count of all licensed dentists. This includes retired, part-time, and nonpracticing dentists. If the dentist can, he or she should play with the numbers to arrive at the number of full-time equivalent (FTE) generalists per population. (A dentist who practices half-time represents 0.5 FTE dentists.)

Healthy ratios are generally between 1:1,800 and 1:2,500. The military has traditionally believed that one dentist can treat 800 soldiers. (But the military has 100 percent utilization.) Higher income areas tolerate lower ratios as people in the area buy more dental services. Rural areas traditionally have a lower utilization rate than urban areas. A ratio of 1:2,500 or 1:3,000 may be required in these areas to suggest enough patients. The dentist can get these ratios from the American Dental Association (ADA), which has several publications that summarize economic factors for dentists across the country. In smaller communities, the dentist can get a phone book and talk to people in the area. With information from the chamber of commerce, a dentist can probably develop an accurate ratio.

The number and type of other dentists in the area are a decision factor. The dentist should feel comfortable with the professional community. These are people he or she will work with in the local dental society and civic organizations. The dentist should also be sure there are there adequate specialists for referral and should consider the availability of staff. A dentist may need to train staff or there may be training programs nearby.

Personal Factors

Personal desires are probably the most important practice location decision. The dentist should decide where he or she wants to live and move there. If he or she is not personally satisfied, then even excellent professional opportunity will not make up for the lack of personal fulfillment. The dentist should consider his or her personal aspirations, career, and life plans. He or she should decide the preferred lifestyle. Each person has preferences for climate, culture, and recreational opportunities. Some want a rural lifestyle, where hunting, fishing, and hiking opportunities abound. Others would not live anywhere that does not have a full arts community and excellent country clubs. The dentist should be sure to reconcile his or her preferred practice pattern with his or her preferred personal style. The dentist may want

a crown and bridge style practice but prefers a remote rural location. The two might not be compatible. Therefore, the dentist should be realistic in his or her assessments.

The single biggest factor in most dentists general location decision is spouse and family desires. Where a dentist wants to go is only part of the lifestyle decision. If he or she is married, a spouse is generally involved in the decision process. A professional or working spouse needs personal growth opportunities as much as the dentist does.

Economic Factors

Once the dentist has decided one, or several, general areas to live, he or she should then look at the economy of the area. As a service provider, the dentist is dependent on other businesses to provide employment so that people have money and insurance to afford dental care.

The dentist should examine the economic base of the area. He or she should find out the sources of income for people in the area. Primary industries, such as mining, farming, and manufacturing bring money into the local economy. (Each primary industrial dollar circulates eight times in a local economy before dissipating.) From there, the money flows to the secondary industries that support the primary industries, such as construction and retail stores. Tertiary industries, such as dentistry, provide service to the employees of the other industries. The dentist should look for broad-based primary industries in a selected location. Several industries in town provide a strong economy. If an area has a single primary industry (such as one large manufacturing plant or a mining-based economy), the dentist should be prepared for a boom-and-bust economy. When the mines (or other primary industry) are busy, then everyone has money. If the mines shut down, then miners do not buy shoes or build houses, and construction workers and shoe salesmen do not go to the dentist. A well-diversified primary industrial base can absorb an individual sector shut down without leading to a general economic collapse.

Several indicators help to gauge the economic health of a community. Most patients consider dental care to be a deferrable expense, rather than a medical necessity. As such, it is highly dependent on disposable income. (Disposable, or discretionary, income is what is left over after people have paid for necessities, such as food, housing, and clothing.) Higher disposable incomes generally mean a better dental economic location. Economic growth in an area means that people's incomes are growing and that more people are moving into an area. These people will need a dentist. High growth areas are also good locations. Some areas have a high turnover rate (people move frequently). Others are more stabile.

It is easier to establish a practice in an area that has high turnover than to break into a stable area, in which most people already have a dental provider. However, in the high turnover area, a dentist will need to continually grow the practice, as patients that were attracted move out of the revolving door.

There are many places to find this information. A call to the area chamber of commerce is an excellent place to start. The chamber's job is to encourage commerce in the area. They already have much information about the potential town. Census data is useful for comparisons. The problem with census data is that it is usually old by the time a person can get to it. Many states have state data banks that the dentist can call to find the information needed. Additionally, much of this information is readily available on the Internet.

Employment Opportunities

A man's got to know his limitations.
Harry Callahan, *Magnum Force*

Objectives

At the completion of this chapter, the student will be able to:
1. Describe common methods of compensation for dentists.
2. Describe common associate–owner arrangements in dentistry.
3. Differentiate between an employee and an independent contractor.
4. Describe advantages and disadvantages to working as an associate in a private practice.
5. Describe advantages and disadvantages of working for a corporate practice.

Key Terms

associateship
dental management service organization (DMSO)
draw against future earnings

employee
employment contract
independent contractor
percent of collections

percent of production
salary
wage

Goal

The goal of this part is to describe common issues in employment situations for dentists.

Business Basics for Dentists, First Edition. David O. Willis.
© 2013 John Wiley & Sons, Inc. Published 2013 by John Wiley & Sons, Inc.

Many new dental graduates take employment positions initially out of dental school. This may be to hone clinical skills, pay down debt or build assets, improve practice management knowledge, or because they do not want the involvement of practice ownership. Regardless of the reason, the important point about employment is that the dentist is there to make money for the employer, whether a private practitioner, network practice, or governmental organization. If the dentist does not make money for the employer, he or she will not be there long. So the dentist should understand that employee positions are not about him or her, they are about the organization. The dentist is valuable so long as he or she contributes to what the organization does.

Methods of Compensation

There are as many compensation formulas as there are employment opportunities. Most involve some variation of a salary or per diem (daily) rate or a percentage of collections or production. Each has advantages and disadvantages, but any system should provide profit and incentives for both sides (Box 24.1). Here only direct monetary compensation is discussed. Employee benefit plans may increase the total compensation significantly. A dentist may take an initially lower compensation with the hope or expectation of higher earnings or ownership later in the relationship.

Salary

A salary is a negotiated amount that the employer pays, regardless how much work that the employee does. The salary may be based on a weekly or daily (per diem) amount. Salaries are easy from a bookkeeping sense. Salaries provide a known budgeting amount for both the owner and associate. This provides substantial financial security for the associate. There is no problem of allocating or dividing accounts receivable in case of break up because all of the accounts are the owner's. The owner does not pay the associate based on the accounts. However, salaries provide no incentive for the

---

Box 24.1 Tips for Compensation

1. Allow reasonable profit for the owner
2. Allow reasonable compensation for the employee
3. Provide incentives for the employee to produce
4. Provide incentives for the employee to collect
5. Provide incentives for both to be efficient
6. Be fair to both

---

employee to produce or collect. Employees soon realize that if they see 2 or 20 patients a day, their remuneration will be the same. The owner takes a risk that the employee–dentist may cost more than they produce, leading to a financial loss for the employer. This loss may be from employee abilities, inadequate patient base, excessive insurance plan adjustments, or unrealistic expectations of the parties involved.

Wage

A wage is similar to a salary, but it is based on the number of hours that the employee works. This limits, to a degree, the loss that an employer might suffer in that if there are inadequate patients; then the employer can limit the employee's hours (and, therefore, compensation). This obviously transfers some financial risk from the employer to the employee.

Percentage of Production

Many employers base compensation on a percentage of production. This may be gross production (the total dollar value of the dentistry done) or net production (the value of the dentistry less any required insurance plan adjustments). Most practices use the net production as the basis for compensation.

This method has the advantages of quick cash flow (and therefore more security) for the employee and provides an inducement for the employee to produce because this directly ties compensation to the amount of dentistry that he or she does. Because the employee has no control over the credit and collection policies of the office, this method adds fairness in that he or she is not held accountable for collection failures. Some owners who base compensation on this method simply lower the percentage paid to take into account the uncollectibles or charge back uncollectible amounts to the associate when they write off the bad account. There is no problem of accounts receivable if there is a break up because the employee–dentist has already been compensated for production.

Percentage of Collections

Another common method of compensation involves paying the employee a percentage of the amounts collected from what the employee produced. Many established private dentists like this method because it is similar to the problems of collection and cash flow faced by the established practitioner. This method also provides obvious incentive for the associate to produce and

Table 24.1 Example – Draw Against Future Earnings
Assume that the employee will be paid 33% of production as a commission. He or she will be paid a monthly salary of $5,000 as a draw against future earnings. The financial result is:

Month	Employee Production	Employee Commission (33%)	Employee Compensation	Monthly Shortage/ Overage	Total Shortage/ Overage
1	$5,000	$1,650	$5,000	–$3,350	–$3350
2	$10,000	$3,333	$5,000	–$1667	–$5017
3	$15,000	$5,000	$5,000	$0	–$5017
4	$20,000	$6,600	$5,000	$1,600	–$3,417
5	$25,000	$8,250	$5,000	$3250	–$167
6	$30,000	$10,000	$9,833	$0	$0

collect. The owner, in this situation, is less likely to lose. However, this method involves more complex bookkeeping methods. The office must specifically allocate the work done by each provider to him or her. (The problem is not difficult, especially if the office has a computerized office accounting system.) The employee has a problem of delayed compensation. This means that it may be several months after the production that the money comes into the office. This makes it difficult, especially for a new practitioner, to develop a family budget. A significant, related problem is the disposition of accounts receivable in case of break up. If the employee is paid based on collections, then he or she must have access to the patient financial records to verify that the owner has made appropriate compensation payments. The owner may not be as diligent as the associate would like in making collection arrangements. A common solution for this is for the owner to pay the associate 80 percent of all of their (associate's) accounts receivable. The owner then collects the accounts.

A common point of negotiation is whether to credit the employee with production attributed to the dental hygienist that he or she "covers." Employers claim that they are paying the salary and other costs of the hygienist, and the employee is seeing these patients to generate additional work that leads to compensation. Employees claim that they are using their clinic skills, knowledge, and abilities in doing the exam and reviewing the hygienist's work. A common resolution is to credit only the exam portion of the visit to the employee's production.

Combination Methods

There are many combinations or variations on these methods. Some have a base salary with a bonus for production. Many charge back laboratory charges to the employee. Many offices use a variable commission, which provides incentives for the associate to produce at higher levels. Because the employer has already paid fixed costs, these higher production levels are more profitable for them as well.

Some employers offer new dentists an initial salary to develop personal cash flow and then switch to a commission basis when the employee has developed sufficient patient base and clinical skills. Other employers help new practitioners to weather initial cash flow problems by offering a draw against future earnings. In this arrangement, the owner pays the employee a percentage of production or collections. The employer pays an initial fixed monthly amount, similar to a salary, regardless the employee's earned compensation. Once the employee's commission is above the "salary" amount, the employee pays back the difference by continuing to take the same draw until they make up the difference. (Table 24.1 gives an example of this arrangement.)

Employee Benefits

Benefits are things of additional value besides money that the employer offers to the employee as a condition of employment. These may be as various insurances (medical, disability, life, malpractice), paid time off (holidays, vacation, personal, or sick days), additional compensation (bonus plans), or financial inducements (retirement plan contributions or dependent care allowances). Benefits are valuable for the dentist from a financial perspective because the whole value of the benefit comes to him or her free of income or social security taxes. Benefits cost the owner the cost of the benefit, although the owner offsets part of the cost through the tax-deductibility of the benefit. (The chapter on employee compensation discusses benefits in more detail.)

There are two ways to fund benefit plans: either the owner can pay the entire amount of the benefit or they can share the cost with the employee. The more the employer pays, the richer the benefit becomes for the employee. Whenever a dentist evaluates an employment situation, he or she should remember to include the value of the benefits offered in the total compensation.

Associate–Owner Arrangements

An associateship occurs when one dentist (generally a junior dentist) works for another dentist (generally the senior dentist) who owns the practice. The essential characteristic of this arrangement is that the practitioners are not equal. One controls the workplace or the work of the other. The owner–dentist may be a proprietorship or corporation. The nonowner dentist may be an employee of the practice or have an autonomous practice within the owner–dentist's practice (independent contractor arrangement).

Many associateships are part-time. The owner–dentist knows that he or she has more patients than can be seen, but he or she does not have enough patients to keep two dentists fully busy. In these cases, the new dentist often works a second associateship or salaried position the times he or she is not at the primary office. These dentists need to be sure that they do not violate restrictive covenants or other agreements in the primary office.

There are several common scenarios of owner–dentists seeking associates. Regardless the specific scenario, the best associateships are in which the owner can provide adequate patient pool to keep the employee busy.

1. *The owner–dentist has many "extra" patients and extra office capacity (space and staff).* This scenario is the best for both parties. The owner–dentist can refer new patients to the associate. The office has unused capacity, so the associate adds few additional costs.
2. *The owner–dentist has an unused operatory (s) for the associate.* The key to this scenario working is adequate patient base for the owner to share with the new associate. That means that the owner–dentist must be as busy as he or she wants to be, with excess patient flow.
3. *The owner–dentist is not busy and wants the associate to help share costs.* This common situation leads to many problems, often the result of the two practitioners competing against each other for patient base. If the owner–dentist is not busy, he or she needs to increase his or her own patient base through marketing or other methods, rather than trying to decrease costs through an associate.
4. *The associate can use the office during time when the owner is not there.* This scenario works for the new dentist to build patient base. It works well if the new dentist wants to continue to work the "off" hours (evenings and weekends). Once the new dentist establishes patient base, then he or she looks for a new office (or establishes an office) to work more reasonable hours. Often the owner–dentist simply provides space and materials. The associate generally provides staff.
5. *The owner has a second office for the new dentist to work in.* The owner may have established or purchased an office in a nearby town. He or she wants someone to work the practice, often with potential buy-in opportunities. There is not much mentoring in these situations, each dentist (owner and employee) is busy working his or her respective office. These are usually good opportunities to do a large volume of dentistry under the management tutelage of a senior dentist.
6. *The owner provides basic care or managed care patients for the associate.* In some associateships, the owner–dentist gives the associate all of the excess insurance patients or assigns the associates to do all of the basic care, with the owner doing the advanced (and costly) complex restorative care. The only way this scenario works is if the owner pays a salary to the associate. If the associate's compensation is based on production or collections, he or she finds that there is simply not enough profit in these situations to fund the associate's lifestyle adequately.

Ownership

A true associateship arrangement involves a senior owner–dentist and an employee dentist. This takes one of two forms.

Employer–Employee

One associate form is the pure employer–employee relationship, in which the associate is a professional employee of the practice (proprietorship, partnership, or corporate). As an employee, the associate participates in office benefit plans like other employees. The practice withholds income taxes and matches Social Security taxes the same as other employees. The owner is in clear control of the situation. A restrictive covenant (covenant not to compete) is common in employee situations.

Independent Contractor

The second type of relationship called an "independent contractor." In this arrangement, the associate dentist contracts, independently, to do dentistry for the owner–dentist. Several advantages exist for the owner–dentist for this arrangement. Because the associate is independently employed, he or she is a proprietorship and files his or her own Schedule C. The owner does not pay matching Federal Income Contributions Act (FICA) tax and pays no unemployment tax on the associate. The owner does not withhold income taxes. Instead, the associate estimates and prefiles quarterly like any other proprietorship. The associate does not participate in any office retirement plan or benefit plans offered to other employees. The down side for the employer–dentist is that a restrictive covenant is virtually nonenforceable in an independent contractor arrangement. By definition, if the associate is *independent*, then he or she can work for any dentist (or self) where and when they see fit. If the associate leaves the practice, he or she ethically and legally obligated to inform patients so that the patients can receive continued care. Otherwise, this may put the associate in a position of being forced to abandon the patient. (The owner can have a nonsolicitation clause for employees and patients not under the care of the associate.)

Many owner–dentists want to have the best of both situations. They want to avoid the tax consequences of the additional employee, but they also want the advantage of a restrictive covenant. It simply does not work that way. The IRS has several guidelines for determining if a relationship is an employee–employer relationship or an independent contractor relationship. As Box 24.2 shows, most dental associateships are employer–employee relationships. The only true independent contractor relationships are space- and time-sharing arrangements.

Costs

Most associateship arrangements result in increased costs for the owner. The owner must hire additional clinical assisting staff for the employee practitioner. The front office staff often needs to expand, especially if hours are offset, so that the junior dentist is in the office hours the owner is not. Office space may even need to increase. The new dentist is usually not as productive as the owner–dentist, leading to decreased relative revenues. Often the owner–dentist spends time with the new dentist that they formerly spent seeing patients, decreasing income further. For all these reasons, associateships often lead to decreased income for the owner–dentist for the first year. By the second year, the younger dentist's production should increase, and cash flow should improve enough that the owner–dentist begins to see some profit from the arrangement.

The practice typically pays costs for the associate with a couple of exceptions. (This varies by geographic area.) The owner generally deducts the lab bill and extraordinary costs (such as implant parts) from the production (or collection) amount before applying the percentage. This results in a sharing of these costs on a percentage equal to the percentage income split. (Box 24.3 gives an example lab bill allocation.) Direct professional costs (such as malpractice insurance and continuing education expenses) are paid by either owner or associate. The owner usually pays other costs (supplies, staff, etc.).

Box 24.2 Characteristics of an Independent Contractor

- Worker personally delivers the service
- There is a continued (ongoing) relationship
- Worker must work on employer's premises
- Worker uses employer's equipment or materials
- Owner controls employees (hiring, firing, and paying)
- Worker cannot work at other locations
- Worker cannot suffer a loss

Box 24.3 Example Associateship Arrangement

This example assumes: $1,000 procedure, $200 lab bill, 65/35 split, $300 overhead costs. There are three scenarios:
1. Associate pays the lab bill after the split
2. Owner pays the lab bill, after the split
3. The lab bill is subtracted from the gross ("off the top"), before the split.

	Associate Pays		Owner Pays		Split (Off Top)	
	Associate	Owner	Associate	Owner	Associate	Owner
Fee		1,000		1,000		1,000
Lab						200
						800
Split(a)	350	650	350	650	280	520
Overhead costs		300		300		300
Lab	200		200			
NET	$150	$350	$350	$150	$280	$220

Advantages

There are many advantages to associateships for both the owner and junior dentists. The associateship can act as a trial period before a partnership or buy-in. This gives both sides a chance to decide if they are compatible enough to establish a long-term professional relationship. The junior dentist invests a minimum amount of money. These people often have high educational debt loads and probably cannot borrow enough money for a practice purchase or start-up. If they require expansion, then the owner–dentist has the financial resources to be able to afford the expansion. There should be few ego conflicts because there is a clearly delineated hierarchy. Associateships should be excellent learning opportunities. The senior dentist can learn new techniques and materials from the new graduate. The associate learns practice management, patient interaction skills, and clinical efficiency in practice. As a result of economies of scale, the now-larger practice can afford equipment and personnel that would not be profitable or feasible in a smaller practice. If the associateship leads to a buy-in or buy out, the owner sells, and the associate buys the practice at the peak of its income-generating potential.

Disadvantages

Associateships have no incidents of ownership for the associate. It is a job, pure and simple, not a co-ownership arrangement. Associates often believe they have "helped build the practice," increasing the value of the practice through their efforts. They believe the owner should give them some consideration in compensation or a buy-in valuation. On the other side, owners contend that they have paid a good wage for the work that the associate has done. The associate has no more claim on the increased value of the practice than a hygienist or assistant. This conundrum has led to more than one associate buy-in offer failing to complete. The answer lies in communication and openness from the beginning.

Associateships face many of the same difficulties as other group practices. With more than one dentist in the office, staff can become disoriented, not being sure who to go to for what problem. There are increased management problems for the owner because the practice now is larger. These occur in accounting, staffing, and scheduling issues. Often owners see a drop in income for the first year of an associateship. This is because of increased expenses, extra time required helping the associate (fewer patients seen), and possible decrease in the patient pool because the owner shares patient pool with the associate.

Most associateships (80 to 90 percent) end without a partnership being formed. When they end, many associates find that a restrictive covenant that they signed as part of the employment agreement excludes them from an area. The prospective associate should be sure that if he or she can not live by the restrictive covenant, he or she should not sign it. (This may mean that the dentist does not do the associateship.) This problem is especially acute in associateships that have lasted for several years. When there is no realistic buy-in, the restrictive covenant forces the associate to uproot from the area, though he or she has established ties in the community and want to stay.

Working for Corporate Networks Practices

Rather than have one practice with 50 dental practitioners, networks of practices may have 50 practice locations, each with one practitioner. In these, the owners attempt to gain the savings of large groups but retain the intimate nature of the individual practice. There are two common forms of organization. One is a dental group practice (DGP), in which the practices are owned by nondentists. The other is called a dental management service organization (DMSO), in which the parent company owns most of the assets of the practice and provides support services to the practice under a strict contract. State laws regarding ownership of professional practices plays a large part in which form is common in each state.

Corporate networks claim to be more efficient than individual practitioners. Much of this comes from their size, which allows them to negotiate volume discounts aggressively that the small, individual practitioner cannot. The networks negotiate lower costs (volume discounts) for dental supplies and office products. They often establish a corporate laboratory or negotiate volume discounts with existing dental labs. Their knowledgeable background ensures that they negotiate favorable leases and find the better locations for new practices. They develop competitive staff compensation packages that are market driven, but not too generous. The parent company can also negotiate higher reimbursement from third-party carriers (insurers). If they control a large share of the dental marketplace, they may threaten to leave the insurer's network of providers if they do not increase reimbursements for their practices.

Ownership

A common form of ownership is a DGP in which the parent organization owns the individual practices directly. Here, the dentist is an employee of the parent corporation. The parent corporation (DGP) compensates the individual dentist for the dentistry that they do. Supply and demand determines the pay scale. The DGP pays what it must pay to get enough skilled dental providers. Often the parent will provide significant employee benefits as part of the total compensation package. Some DGPs allow more senior dentists to buy an ownership interest in the parent through employee stock ownership programs (ESOPs) or other form of ownership involvement. They often offer these through retirement plan or bonus options. Some DGPs have a co-ownership arrangement with the individual practitioner. The parent organization may own a controlling portion (say 51 percent) of the practice and the practitioner may own the remainder. When the practitioner leaves or retires, there is a ready buyer for the practice.

ADMSO is an arrangement that is common in states that require dentists to own dental practices. Here, the parent company owns most of the tangible assets of the practice (e.g., dental equipment and the building). Depending on state law, the dentist continues to own the intangible assets. The DMSO then has a contract (business service agreement [BSA]) with the dentist to provide management and other services for the dental practice. These services often include purchasing or leasing office space and equipment, scheduling, billing patients, filing insurance claims, hiring employees, marketing the practice, and managing bank accounts for the practice. The contacts often have strict buy-out and restrictive covenants that make it difficult and expensive for the dentist to leave the practice and compete directly with the former DMSO. These arrangements vary by state depending on the individual state's laws.

Compensation

In corporate network arrangements, dentists often earn a percentage of production or collections. If production is the basis of compensation, then net production (production less adjustments) is often used, especially in areas where a large portion of the dental market includes managed care (reduced payment) plans. Supply and demand in the area determines the specific percentage. The parent company often offers employee benefits (such as health insurance, paid vacation, or retirement plan contributions) that add to the total compensation value. Typical percentage of compensation run between 25 and 28 percent with employee benefits added to this. Because there is no ownership interest for the provider, the difference between this and the office profit ratio (typically 40 percent) is income to the parent company. The parent company deducts corporate costs (administrative, training, etc.) from this to calculate corporate profit. The cost of doing the dentistry (i.e., hiring dental practitioners) is a cost of doing business for the parent company. It is income for the individual practitioner.

Advantages

There are advantages over practice ownership to both the new and experienced practitioner for working in a corporate network. The practitioner makes no investment, nor is there a long-term commitment to the practice location. The arrangement can be a good learning experience if the parent company values clinical and management training for practitioners. The practitioner has an immediate "paycheck" without worrying about debt repayment or cash flow. A practitioner might make a higher income than in a privately owned practice because the parent company uses their management systems and expertise to manage the practice. The dentist spends time seeing patients, which helps to generate additional income. There is less of an emotional and time commitment for the practitioner. If the hygienist quits, the parent company will find temporary coverage and hire a replacement. The dentist's free time is left for personal use, without worrying about the business of the practice. The dentist can often move within the network's practices without losing income or benefits.

Disadvantages

There are also disadvantages (when compared to practice ownership) to working in a corporate network. First, it is a job; the owning parent company is the boss. Many dentists enter the profession to enjoy self-reliant independence, which does not occur in this practice form. Often the practitioner will work more hours and work the less-desirable weekend or evening off hours than in an established practice. The parent company may place unrealistic production quotas (overt or hidden) on the practitioner. This may lead to ethical dilemmas as the practitioners balances quality of care with production. If a dentist wants to leave the network, a restrictive covenant may severely limit his or her practice opportunities. The dentist has no ownership interest, therefore no equity build-up. The dentist then has no practice (asset) to sell at retirement or leaving. A corporate opportunity may not be available where and when the practitioner wants. If the dentist is managerially, clinically, and behaviorally competent, then he or she can make a higher income in an ownership situation because he or she gains the value of ownership (both profit and equity build-up). Finally, the parent company may fail or be bought by another management company with a different philosophy.

Employment Contracts

Whatever employment situation a dentist is in, a parent organization will probably ask the dentist to sign an employment contract. (In the private practice associateship, these are called *associateship contracts*.) These contracts define the expectations the employer has of the employee. They also list what the dentist can expect from the employer. Good contracts are written. A verbal contract is legal, but it can be difficult to define exactly what was agreed between the two people.

Every contract is negotiable until it is signed. If a dentist has questions or qualms about the wording or intent of a section of the contract, he or she should resolve it with the employer before signing. If the dentist and the employer are adamant about a particular piece of the contract, then maybe the arrangement is not a good one. The dentist needs to know this sooner, rather then later. Individual private practices have more leeway in the contract negotiation process. Often the larger chains and networks have standard contacts that they use with all their dentist providers. These can be "take-it-or-leave-it" negotiations.

Generally, the associate and owner discuss issues and resolve differences. Then the owner has an attorney draft the contract, including the points that have been resolved. As the potential employee, the dentist should have a separate lawyer review the contract, looking out for the dentist's interests. It is a few dollars well spent.

Several points are commonly included in employment contracts:

1. The duration of the contract.
2. Whether it is an employee or independent contractor arrangement.
3. The compensation mechanism, often giving examples for clarity.
4. How the office will allocate patients.
5. Employee benefits (if any).
6. Amount of time off (paid or unpaid).
7. What happens in case of death or disability of either party.
8. How a dissolution is handled.
9. How to modify the contract.
10. If there are any buy or sell provisions.
11. If there is a restrictive covenant, and if so, the terms of that covenant.

Practice Ownership

My son is now an "entrepreneur." That's what you're called when you don't have a job.
Ted Turner

Objectives

At the completion of this chapter, the student will be able to:
1. Describe the characteristics of dental practice ownership.
2. Differentiate between the two ways to make money in dentistry.
3. Describe advantages and disadvantages of individual practice.
4. Describe advantages and disadvantages of individual group practice.
5. Describe advantages and disadvantages of true group practice.
6. Describe advantages and disadvantages of franchise practice ownership.

Key Terms

compensation for doing
dentistry
incidents of ownership

individual practice
individual group practice
ownership compensation

relative value unit
true group

Goal

The goal of this chapter is to describe common issues in practice ownership for dentists.

Business Basics for Dentists, First Edition. David O. Willis.
© 2013 John Wiley & Sons, Inc. Published 2013 by John Wiley & Sons, Inc.

Owning a dental practice is the dream of most dental school graduates. However, that ownership comes with many costs and advantages. A dentist will spend additional time managing the business of the practice. Most dentists get into the profession because they want to treat patients, not realizing the time and emotional energy that must be devoted to running a successful business. But the upside of ownership is the pride, happiness, and financial return that come from running a successful practice.

In the past, the only type of practice ownership was the independent individual practitioner in a cottage industry business. Now there are large and small groups, franchises, and network practices. This opens many more possibilities to new graduates than were available previously.

Characteristics of Practice Ownership

Doing dental services does not require owning a dental practice. Likewise, dentists can own a dental practice and not personally do any dental services, instead hiring another dentist to do them. If dentists separate, in their minds, owning a practice from doing dentistry, they can understand better the characteristics of practice ownership.

Incidents of Ownership

Business owners have certain rights in the business that nonowners, such as employees, do not. These incidents, or rights, of ownership are the result of a dentist putting his or her capital (money) at risk in the business (Box 25.1). Because the dentist has taken on the risk associated with ownership that workers have not, then he or she has the benefits that result, whereas workers do not. Dentists can make a profit (or incur a loss) from business activities, whether they personally do dentistry or not. This is the basis of network practice entities. Dentists may choose (through a profit-sharing plan) to share those profits with workers, but it is not necessary. If the business shows a loss, workers will not accept paying for a loss; they will go elsewhere to work or not

---

Box 25.1 Rights of Business Owners

- Ability to make a profit from the business
- Decision-making authority (may be delegated)
- Increased responsibility and liability
- Pledge assets (for a loan)
- Gain in the value of the business

---

work at all. Because a dentist owns the business, he or she can decide how the business will operate and who will be hired to do the various business functions. The dentist has the responsibility for ensuring that the business is operated effectively. He or she also has liability in the case that the business (or someone working in the business) injures someone, or if the dentist directly injures someone through his or her negligence. Because the dentist owns the assets of the business, he or she can pledge them as collateral for a loan or other purposes. If the business gains or loses value because of a dentist's management abilities, then the dentist (as the owner) will enjoy the gain or suffer the loss in value. Workers do not share in this gain or loss. Associate dentists may not understand this difference clearly. They often feel that they have contributed to the growth in the value of a practice and should not, therefore, have to pay for that growth when they purchase (or buy-in) the practice.

Making Money in Dentistry

There are two ways to make money in dentistry. The first is to do the dentistry itself. The second is to have an ownership interest. If a dentist owns the practice and sees patients, then he or she makes money both ways.

Compensation for Doing Dentistry

Whether a dentist is the owner of a practice or an employee, he or she will earn money for doing dentistry. If a dentist is a proprietor or a partner, then he or she is an owner. The dentist takes a draw on the assets of the practice (one of which is the office checking account), estimates his or her income tax liability, and prepays it quarterly to the IRS. If the dentist is an employee of an organization (such as a health center) or a practice corporation (even if he or she is the sole stockholder and provider), then the corporation will pay him or her as an employee. The corporation will estimate the dentist's personal tax liability (based on IRS tables), withhold that amount, and send it to the government in his or her name as prepaid taxes. The dentist receives the amount left after the corporation has paid estimated income taxes for him or her.

If a dentist practices in a corporate structure, then he or she will earn pay for doing dentistry as any other employee. That is, the corporation may pay the dentist a commission (based on production or collections), salary, wage, or a combination method. If a dentist is a proprietor or a partner in a partnership, he or she pays himself or herself through taking a draw on the assets of the practice. Some dentists simply take any money left over in the checkbook at the end of the month as a draw. Others take a fixed amount (similar to a salary) for budgeting purposes and to ensure enough cash in the practice to pay normal bills. A dentist does not pay tax on how much money is taken out of the practice (as draw) but on how much profit the practice generated. Whether the dentist took any of it for personal expense is irrelevant.

Compensation for Ownership Interest

If a dentist is an owner, he or she may have a profit left in the business (practice) after he or she has paid all expenses (including paying dentists to do dentistry on patients). This is often called *entrepreneurial profit*. If the dentist is an excellent manager, his or her entrepreneurial profit will be larger than if he or she is a mediocre or poor manager. The dentist may distribute that profit to employees (as a bonus) or to the owners of the practice as a reward for their investment in the practice. The dentist may also combine the methods.

Bonus

The dentist may distribute any profit to any employee as a bonus. The IRS considers this taxable income. He or she can distribute it by shares, based on production, or any other means that the owners(s) choose. For example, a dentist may distribute profits only to certain dentists (owner or nonowner). It is entirely up to the owners what they do with the profits from the business.

Box 25.2 Example of Paying for Equity (Ownership)

A group practice has three dentists, one associate (nonowner) and two owner dentists. Dentists are paid 25 percent of production, dividing any money left over (profit) equally between the owners. The practice produced $1.8 million last year. Total costs (not including payments for doing dentistry) were $1,150,000. The resulting compensation for the three dentists is shown here.

Practice production	$1,800,000
Less payments for production	−$450,000
Less office costs	−$1,150,000
Equals business profit	$200,000

	Total	Owner #1	Owner #2	Associate
Production	1,800,000	700,000	600,000	500,000
Compensation for production (@25%)	450,000	175,000	150,000	125,000
Compensation for ownership	200,000	100,000	100,000	0
Total compensation	650,000	275,000	250,000	125,000

Ownership Interest

A dentist may distribute any profits to the owners of the business to compensate them for their ownership. If a practice is a corporation, then the distribution is based on the number of shares owned. Dividends are from the corporation's profits. If the practice is a C corporation, then the corporation must pay taxes on the profits first and then distribute them as dividends (where they are taxed again as personal income). To avoid this double taxation, C corporate practices usually pay out profit as bonuses, so they are only taxed once. Often these bonuses go only to the owner(s). S corporations (or "pass-through" corporations) do not have this problem. They pass dividends through to the owners without paying tax at the corporate level. Because these dividends are unearned income, the individual does not pay Social Security, Medicare, or self-employment taxes on them. Box 25.2 gives the results of how a hypothetical practice might divide income and profit.

Individual Practice

An individual practice involves the greatest investment of a dentist's time and emotional energy. It also provides the greatest personal rewards when successful.

Ownership

One person owns an individual practice. From a management perspective, the business entity is not important. It may be a proprietorship, a limited liability company (LLC), or a corporation in which the only stockholder is the owner. This means that the owner has complete control and responsibility for the business.

Compensation

The owner takes all profit from the business as compensation. This can be separated into compensation for doing dentistry and business profit if the owner wants. In the proprietorship practice, the difference is not meaningful because the owner is the business. In an individual corporate practice, the owner can characterize profits from the business as dividends, which the IRS taxes differently than earned income.

Advantages

In the individual practice, the owner exercises complete control over the operational and strategic direction of the practice. It is the dentist's practice. He or she can make the practice what he or she wants, without having to compromise with other owners. If the practice increases in value, the dentist enjoys the gain.

Disadvantages

As an individual practitioner, the dentist has additional time commitments to manage the business. Often the dentist may want an additional trusted practitioner to discuss clinical or management problems. (Study clubs and mentors help to solve this problem.) The dentist is responsible for the financial health of the practice. If he or she wants to borrow money for a practice purchase or expansion, the dentist has his or her credit rating and borrowing power to use.

The individual practitioner may find it more difficult to take time from the office for vacations or personal reasons. If the dentist is not there seeing patients, his or her income decreases. If a dentist finds a substitute, he or she pays the substitute most of what the owner would have taken as compensation for doing the dentistry, leaving only the entrepreneurial profit for the owner. When the dentist is gone, patients still want to be seen and staff still wants to be paid. Without a large cash cushion, cash flow problems can occur with time away from the office.

Solo Group Practices

This arrangement consists of independent practices physically located under one roof. Each dentist practices as a single practitioner (proprietorship or corporate) and may provide for common overhead expenses. This form of practice has also been called space sharing, time sharing, a cluster group, or a condo arrangement. Individual autonomy is high. One dentist may own and rent the office space to another (time share) or the participating dentists may jointly own the property (real estate partnership). The general purpose is to increase net income through a reduction in overhead, by using facilities, equipment, and possibly staff more efficiently than the traditional individual practitioner. This is accomplished while maintaining the nature of separate practices that many dentists cherish. For these reasons, this has become a popular method for established dentists to merge their existing practices.

The essential nature of an individual group is that the practices remain separate. This means that each practice has separate patient pools, (clinical) staffs, billing, decision-making authority, and responsibility. This form of practice requires a strict cost and income accounting because there is really little sharing of authority or responsibility, only division of costs. The individual

practices within the group may be proprietorships, corporations, or even partnerships.

Ownership

There are many possible arrangements for individual group ownership based primarily on the control of the facilities:

- The facilities may be owned or rented by one dentist who then sublets space to another during his or her off hours (time sharing).
- The facilities may be owned or leased by one dentist who rents space to another dentist during the same office hours (space sharing).
- The facilities may be jointly owned or leased by two or more dentists who have separate treatment areas, yet share business office and reception areas and the costs associated with each (condo arrangement or real estate partnership).

Some or all practice participants may own the facilities as a management company, which provides, for a fixed or percentage fee, common management services such as scheduling, billing, and collections. The equipment may be owned jointly by an equipment leasing consortium of members who lease equipment to the various practices. These umbrella organizations allow for practitioners to enter or leave the group more easily. They also allow dentists who dislike management functions to concentrate on clinical patient care. They are usually formed as some form of a pass-through entity so that expenses (e.g., depreciation) may pass through to the individuals.

Compensation

Because each dentist operates a separate practice, compensation is based on collecting fees for individual services. Separate accounting systems are generally used, so calculating compensation is easy. The individual dentist then pays his or her own practice costs and then pays any shared costs to the individual group.

If common business personnel and billing are used through a management company, the management group collects fees and allocates them to the individual practitioner. The group then deducts expenses and the practitioner receives compensation directly from the management company. If a percentage of production compensation system is used instead of a collection-based system, the group either applies a standard collection ratio or charges back bad debts to the individual dentist's account. This prevents members of the individual group from sharing in the bad debt.

Owners of the management company receive a proportional share of any profits generated by the group be based on the percentage equity interest of each partner.

Costs

Efficiency in the individual group practice comes from sharing expenses for common concerns. These may include rent, utilities, supplies, waiting room, receptionist, business personnel, or any other mutually agreed-on common expenses. The more expenses shared, the more the savings. The individual dentist is responsible for any other costs associated with his practice such as production (clinical) staff, associated lab bills, or professional education costs. These common costs are allocated among participants on several bases.

Fixed-Fee Basis

Under a fixed-fee basis, the owner or owner organization rents the office and other agreed-on services for a fixed dollar monthly. This method is simple to administer and easily understood. However, this method charges the lower-producing members of the group more and typically benefits the higher producers.

Percentage of Production

In this method, the contract specifies the percentage of total monthly production that the renter pays for the privilege of using the owner's office and supplies. Often dentists include a minimum or maximum dollar amount to protect parties for unexpected production levels.

Cost Ratios

Here, the individual's production is related to the entire group's production. Costs are then assessed proportionally to each individual according to the ratio of production. For example, if a dentist is responsible for 32 percent of the entire group's production, then that dentist would be responsible for 32 percent of the costs for the month. This allocation assumes that the use of supplies and other common expenses vary in concert with the production.

Combination Methods

Some dentists combine the preceding methods. Fixed costs may be allocated on a straight percentage with an addition of variable costs based on production or a ratio of fixed costs.

Advantages

An individual group arrangement has several advantages over a "true" group practice or individual, freestanding practice. Because these practices are separate, there are fewer management disputes. The arrangement may be easy to administer because each practice maintains separate dental and financial records. Professional consultation and companionship are available, which can lead to improved emergency coverage shared between the patients. Patients may even perceive the group as a more modern practice. Finally, the common costs, such as rent or business manager, may decrease increasing the individual practitioner's net income.

Disadvantages

An individual group arrangement also has several disadvantages. Competition may arise for patients and staff among the practices. This is particularly evident for new practitioners who participate in this type of group. The solution is a clear system of allocation for walk-in emergency or nonreferral patients.

Because the public may perceive a dentist as practicing with another dentist, his or her reputation may be either enhanced or tarnished by the acts of the other dentist. The courts may even hold a dentist to the liability requirements of a partnership if they offer themselves as a group practice. Disagreements over common areas and staff may develop. One dentist, for example, may feel that he or she should reprimand a receptionist for job deficiencies, but another does not. Similar problems may arise as to the purchase of new equipment or costs associated with redecoration of the reception room.

The individual group generally does not benefit from the advantages of partnerships and true groups, such as shared treatment areas and clinical staff. Real savings typically come at the expense of autonomy and independent decision-making ability. Individual groups do not increase efficiency unless the dentists share space or offset hours. If a dentist does not want to practice evenings and weekends, an office rotation system may be unacceptable.

True Group Practices

True group practices are two or more dentists who have a legal arrangement in which they share common space, patient records, income, expenses and personnel in patient treatment, and business management of a common dental practice. The true group may be either a partnership or corporation. A proprietorship is incompatible with a true group practice. The individual's autonomy and control are low, in deference to group control. True groups share expenses and compensate dentists based on a previously agreed formula. The essential nature of the true group is that the individual subordinates his or her managerial authority and decision making to the group. Clinical decisions are affected to a lesser degree. True groups may consist of either one or multiple specialties.

The true group is a single practice entity, with the group in control of staff, patients, and expenses. (Many groups assign patients to particular doctors for continuity of care.) The important point is that the group is the primary entity, rather than the individual practitioner as in the individual group. The practitioners share responsibilities, equipment, records, and even patients. The group then compensates the dentists for doing dental or other practice-related services, based on production, collections, or even hours worked. There may be different degrees of ownership: associate nonowner, management, equipment, or real estate umbrella partnerships as in the individual group.

From the patients' perspective, true groups differ from traditional individual practices:

1. Patients may identify more with the group then the dentist. This eases or eliminates the direct monetary relationship between provider and patient that exists in individual practice.
2. Patients can usually use emergency and nontraditional hours more easily.
3. There may be less choice regarding specialist referral but the patient can get care in one office. If the group is multidisciplinary, policies of the group may dictate that specialty referrals are conducted internally.
4. The patient also perceives a greater continuity in care in case of death or disability of the practitioner and can get comfort from consultation that may occur within the group or complex care.

Ownership

True groups show many different forms of business organization. The practice, its management of the practice, the equipment, real estate, or the laboratory may each have distinct organizations that are a part of or separate from the practice. They may act either as umbrella organizations or as subcontractors for the practice itself. Each of the separate units may be a profit center and charge the other units reasonable fees for the services provided.

The practice itself is either a corporation, LLC, or partnership. All of the participating dentists are not necessarily owners of the practice, nor are the necessarily equal owners. They also may be simply employees compensated for doing dentistry but do not share in the risks associated with ownership.

Compensation

Compensation in dentistry involves accounting for income from doing dentistry, specific costs associated with producing that dentistry, and specific costs for the individual dentist. Any money left over is considered entrepreneurial profit, which is allocated among the owners, usually on a pro rata ownership basis.

Compensation for Doing Dentistry

Total compensation for doing the dentistry is a combination one of the income determination methods and a cost method.

Methods of Income Determination

There are several common methods of establishing income from doing dentistry.

Salary
One method is to pay either a monthly salary or an hourly wage. It provides easy bookkeeping and gives income security but lacks any production incentive. The group may lose money if the individual is not self-motivated or feels unjustly compensated. If, for example, all members receive the same salary but have significantly different production levels, then the higher producers may become upset and feel inadequately compensated. Compensation by a salary encourages non patient activities such as management duties, community activities, or part-time teaching in a university. Some groups structure a salary drawn against an average or minimum production levels. This forces the participants to produce enough to at least "make their salary." For example, a dentist in the group may draw $10,000 per month salary. If the overhead averages 66.7 percent, then the dentist must produce $30,000 per month to "make salary." If he or she only produces $20,000 one month, the salary would remain the same, but the dentist would need to produce an additional $10,000 in subsequent months to offset the underproduction.

Payment for Production
Payment can be based on a percentage of production or collections. This is probably the most common method. Bookkeeping is more complex in this arrangement. However, management computer systems simplify this activity. The nonowner practitioner has little incentive to spend time in nonproduction endeavors. If production is used as the income method, either a standard collection ratio (e.g., 96 percent of all charges collected) to estimate collections is applied, or bad debts are charged back to the individual practitioner.

Salary with Commission

Another common system is a salary base with commission based on production. Often a practice establishes a minimum for bonus compensation. This gives the participants the security of a fixed-base income but encourages and rewards production by the individual. This case presents an example of the salary or commission compensation.

Relative Value Units

A final variation is to set relative value units for each procedure. Relative value units assign values to procedures other than the traditional dollar amounts associated with individual services. These units may be based on the expected time required to complete a procedure, a dollar figure based on costs, specific practice incentives, or some combination of all of them. The practitioner is rewarded on this relatively established value. Relative value units encourage participants to do procedures that may be less profitable or more time consuming, such as doing a simple alloy as opposed to a cast restoration. The practice then takes any efficiencies as profit. For example, a typical three-surface alloy may take 30 minutes of chair time and generate $150 of income. A casting for the same tooth may take 60 minutes of chair time but generate $1,000 of revenue. A pure dollar relationship is 6.6:1 (1,000:150), whereas the pure time ratio is 2:1 (60:30). A relative ratio may be arbitrarily set at two units for the alloy and seven units for the casting. Their relative value ratio is then 7 : 2. If the unit is defined as $50, then the dentist would be compensated $350 for the crown procedure (7 units × $50/unit) or $100 for the alloy procedure (2 units × $50/unit). This makes the casting somewhat less valuable for the provider (from a remuneration standpoint) and the alloy more valuable.

Methods of Production Cost Allocation

The basic methods for cost allocation involve deciding how two broad classes of expenses will be charged to each practitioner. These are the fixed office costs and variable costs of production. The importance is evident in practices in which the practitioners' production numbers are significantly different. If Dr. A has a large production, relative to Dr. B, then Dr. A would prefer costs to be divided equally; Dr. B would prefer costs to be divided according to the production ratios because this would lead to a lower cost (and higher profit) for Dr. B. There are common methods of allocating costs.

Equal Shares

Sharing expenses equally makes all costs fixed for the practitioners. The more costs that they share equally, the more the higher producing members of the group are helped financially.

Based on Production

Sharing expenses based on a pro-rata share of production assumes that different practitioners use supplies and common services equally. Strict production-based cost accounting favors the lower producing members of the group. Some procedures, for example, periodontal therapy, use fewer lab and supplies than others, such as crown and bridge procedures. Practices often charge laboratory charges to the individual provider as a specific charge.

Individual Expense Accounting

Fixed expenses may be shared based on equal shares, with costs of production (variable expenses) based on production.

Specific Cost Allocation

Specific costs for a practitioner are generally charged to that individual practitioner. These are costs that the individual might take is income but instead decides to take as a business expenses. Examples include retirement plan contributions, personal insurance benefits, automobile expenses, professional dues and publications, continuing professional education, and professional meeting expenses. Exceptions may include costs that all practitioners share equally. Here, examples might be dental association dues or standard malpractice insurance policy premiums.

Compensation for Ownership Position

Compensation based on the ownership position of the participants leads to incentives for owners to see the group succeed, incentives to control costs, and incentives to produce. Any money left over after paying for producing dentistry is business or entrepreneurial profit. This is then split based on ownership interest of the practice.

The compensation formula must leave enough after paying for production to have meaningful compensation for ownership (Box 25.3). Usually 10 to 15 percent should be left for equity payment. What associates in the area typically earn dictates the production compensation amount. (This would be the cost to the practice for hiring someone to produce the dentistry produced by the owner(s).)

Advantages

There are several advantages for dentists who practice in a true group.

Professional consultation is readily available. In a true group, individuals succeed when the group succeeds. Concentrating on an area of particular clinical interest may be easier.

Box 25.3 Example Specific Costs Allocation

A group practice has three dentists, one associate (nonowner) and two owner dentists. Dentists are paid 35 percent of production, less specific charges for their production (lab and implants) and personal expenses (auto, retirement plan, etc.). All common costs are paid by the practice, dividing any money left over (profit) equally between the owners. The practice produced $1.8 million last year. Shared costs were $1,061,000. The resulting compensation for the three dentists is shown here.

	Total	Owner #1	Owner #2	Associate
Collections	1,800,000	700,000	600,000	500,000
Gross production payment (@ 35%)	630,000	245,000	210,000	175,000
– Specific Charges	141,000	52,000	48,000	41,000
Net Production Payment	489,000	193,000	162,000	134,000
– Office (Shared) Costs	1,061,000			
Business profit	250,000			
Divided by ownership		125,000	125,000	
Total compensation		318,000	287,000	134,000

A potential for greater individual incomes exists because costs are shared and greater efficiency develops with a larger practice.

The practitioner has greater flexibility for personal time because other practitioners can share the patient load. However, group needs may temper individual autonomy in such time requests. An additional benefit of financial security exists for the practitioner in case of sickness, accident, or other disability. Other dentists are available to maintain the production of the disabled practitioner.

Many creative buy-in, buy-out, and retirement options are available to a group practice. There is a ready-made buyer in the group and generally a predetermined price. A group may be better able to offer financing for the purchase amount than an individual practitioner. No lag in patient treatment occurs if there is the death or disability of one practitioner. The quality of patient care may improve if active peer review and sharing of techniques and information take place. The quality of patient care may improve if active peer review and sharing of techniques and information take place.

Disadvantages

Some disadvantages exist for the practitioner who is contemplating a group practice.

There are differing personalities to adapt to in the group. The dentist who seeks a high degree of autonomy should not consider a group arrangement.

The individual generally loses some independent decision-making authority. This loss increases with larger groups.

The dentist may lose the direct production–compensation relationship. Depending on the circumstances, this may be either an advantage or a problem. If a dentist is interested in doing nonclinical duties (such as management of the practice, community work, or teaching), then this can be an advantage for that person.

There may be a loss of the dentist–patient relationship in favor of a practice–patient relationship. This new relationship may be based on financial responsibility, treatment responsibility, or interpersonal relationships.

Franchises as Ownership

A franchise is a business arrangement in which the individual business (practice) is owned by an individual who contracts with a parent organization for business guidance in an ongoing relationship. The owner must adopt the franchiser's methods and materials. It differs from a consulting relationship in that a consulting relationship offers advice for a short time. The owner is free to carry out the advice or not and can generally end the consulting contract whenever he or she wishes.

Ownership

This allows the individual to retain ownership, while tapping into the expertise of a proven organization. An individual owner (franchisee) must pay the parent organization (franchiser) both initiation ("front-end fees") and ongoing management fees for use of the trademark, training, and advisory services. The parent then provides name recognition, management expertise, and a proven business formula for success.

There are no federal requirements for franchise information. Generally, states enforce laws and regulations on the franchises that operate in their state. So the individual owner must enter these relationships cautiously and only with expert advisors.

Compensation

Because the practice is individually owned, the dentist's compensation is based on his or her practice's profit. The franchisee may pay significant fees to the parent company (franchiser) for the ongoing guidance and use of the trade name.

Advantages

The advantages of joining a franchise include:

- Name recognition of the parent organization. Everyone in the United States knows the McDonald's corporate name. The individual franchisee benefits through that corporate image. Although not as prominent in dentistry, franchises can advertise on a region level, increasing their presence in the dental consumer's mind. As patients move, they may seek out franchise dentists in their new locations.
- The franchiser has management expertise that the individual practitioner does not. (Dentists are trained to do dentistry!) The franchiser brings management expertise, proven systems, and tested methods of doing business to the individual franchise. The inexperienced individual franchisee would struggle for years to achieve this level of expertise.
- The franchiser offers training for staff and dentist. This shares the knowledge of how to do business and patient procedures with the people who are doing them.

The dentist keeps an ownership interest in the practice. Many dentists want to be practice owners for the autonomy and income that ownership offers.

Disadvantages

Franchises have several disadvantages for dentists as well.

A dentist is locked into a long-term relationship with the franchiser. Many dentists believe that once the practice "up and running," he or she will cancel the franchise arrangement. That is not so. Most franchise contacts have large costs associated with ending the relationship. After many years of practice, the ongoing franchise fee becomes a sore point for many practitioners.

If other franchises have problems, he or she may be guilty by association. For example, if another dentist in the franchise is found guilty of drug charges, the public may associate "all of those dentists" in the franchise together.

The parent franchiser company may fail. This may leave the franchisee with significant legal and financial problems. The parent company may be sold to another who then changes terms of contracts or does not offer the same level of services. Restrictive covenants may prohibit the franchisee from opening another practice nearby.

Practice Transitions

For many people a job is more than an income—it's an important part of who we are. So a career transition of any sort is one of the most unsettling experiences you can face in your life.
Paul Clitheroe

Objectives

At the completion of this chapter, the student will be able to:
1. Differentiate between a buy-in, a buy-out, and a cold start.
2. Describe the types of buy-in arrangements.
3. Describe the types of dental practices that are typically for sale.
4. Describe factors in locating a new dental practice.
5. Describe various methods of financing the practice transfer option.
6. Describe transfer considerations for each type of practice transfer option.
7. Describe tax implications for each type of practice transfer option.
8. Describe the typical process for each of the practice transfer options.
9. Describe the typical process that banks go through when evaluating a loan application.
10. Describe the information that loan officers will require for loan processing.
11. Define the more important factors used in evaluation of the economic state of a community.
12. Describe the typical series of events in negotiating a practice transition.

Key Terms

bank financing
cold start
depreciation recapture

immediate buy-in
intrafamily transfers
sweat equity

walk-away sale

Goal

This chapter will provide guidelines for the dentist to use when deciding practice options. Factors that affect a practice's transfer will also be discussed.

Business Basics for Dentists, First Edition. David O. Willis.
© 2013 John Wiley & Sons, Inc. Published 2013 by John Wiley & Sons, Inc.

Life transitions are a difficult, confusing, and exciting time for people. Most dentists now make several transitions in their professional careers. Often these are moves from one employment situation to another. This chapter looks at the transitions involved in changing practice ownership: starting a practice, buying an entire practice, or buying into a practice becoming a partner.

Selecting among these ownership transitions is in part a financial decision and in part a management decision. The buyer's quandary is, do I set up a practice or buy an existing practice? If I buy a practice, I buy an ongoing business with existing staff, location, patient base, and cash flow. If I set up a practice, I have complete control over site and location, new equipment, and a facility that is what I want. I have to hire staff and generate patients, but both will be the ones I want. I will need to borrow additionally for working capital, but I am not paying fro patient base. From a purely financial perspective, spreadsheets can be developed that purport to show the outcome of the buy or start-up decision. These are based on the assumptions that the spreadsheet creator uses. They can show either outcome as superior. Generally, in more competitive dental marketplaces, purchasing a practice comes out ahead financially because of the built-in patient base and resulting immediate cash flow. In a less competitive area where the dentist can be busy from the first day, he or she does not need the additional cost of buying patient base. It becomes less expensive to establish a practice.

Most dentists will hire a consultant to help with the valuation, purchase, and transfer of a practice. A dentist may do this once or twice in his or her lifetime. A transition consultant does it many times each year. Usually the seller will hire a broker to value, advertise, and sell the practice. Most brokers charge a percentage of the sale price to the seller as a commission. (Some charge a flat fee.) Some brokers claim to work for both sides in a transfer. It is difficult to represent both sides when one side is paying the broker and the other is not. The buyer has a different advisor work with him or her. Although an added expense, it is worth it (financially and emotionally) to have someone looking out for the buyer's interests in the process.

Starting a Dental Practice (Cold Start)

Advantages

Starting a practice is often called a *cold start* because the person is, literally, starting from the beginning. The advantages of a cold start relate to the fact that the dentist can make the dental practice exactly what he or she wants it to be. It is his or her practice, including business systems, practice philosophy, and managed care participation. The location, the design of the office, and the staff all will be what the dentist wants, not what a previous owner wanted. New offices and equipment need less maintenance and repair. New practices may be less expensive than comparable existing practices because the dentist is paying someone else for any "goodwill." If the area chosen is in a high need of dentists, then the newcomer does not need to buy goodwill. If a dentist can be relatively busy from the beginning and grow at an acceptable rate, then he or she should not pay someone else for a patient pool.

The dentist controls the regional and specific site location of the practice. He or she may want to buy into a practice in a certain area, but if no dentists are interested, then he or she obviously can not buy in. Not so with a practice set up. Similarly, a dentist's office design and equipment selection fits his or her individual criteria, not what is existing in the facility.

When a dentist starts a practice, he or she can grow professionally with the patient pool. Initially, the clinical speed will not be as great as later. (Clinical speed comes from decisions making, not just hand skills.) So clinical speed increases as patient pool and practice "busyness" increase.

Disadvantages

On the down side, starting an office from scratch can be more expensive because a dentist is are generally buying new equipment and supplies. Establishing a new practice takes time, often as much as 6 months from the idea to the first patient visit. If a dentist is not working or in school during this time, he or she has lost a half year's income, adding to the expense. New offices take much time, effort, and headaches to develop.

A new practice has a lack of patient base. Depending on the area, it may be easy or difficult to market and build a patient base. Because of this, new dental practices generally have cash flow problems. New practitioners must borrow additional working capital (often about 3 months' expenses) to weather this problem. Insurance plan participation currently drives dental marketing in many areas. These plans result in lower income from plan-fee requirements. This leads to lower cash flow and lower profit in new practices in these areas. Because of this, bankers are more wary of financing a practice that does not have a demonstrated cash flow.

Locating the Practice

The first problem a dentist faces is finding a location for a new practice. This is really two separate problems. The first is finding a general region. The second is finding a specific site.

Regional Location

Many new dentists have already decided when they entered dental school where they plan to practice. They are from a specific town or area and have always wanted to return to that area to practice. Their decision is easy. The tougher decision is for the dentist who has no pre-established region to move into. He or she has to examine his or her own desires and then do a lot of homework to find an area that meets his or her needs.

Site Location

Once a region, or general area in which to practice, is selected the next decision involves picking a specific site for the practice. Marketing gurus say that there are only three factors to consider in developing a successful business: location, location, and location. Although this is an oversimplification, it points to the importance of the specific site selection in practice development.

Visibility

The dental office should be easily seen by as many people as possible. The dentist should try to find a busy street or major thoroughfare to place the office. He or she wants to be seen often enough that he or she lies in the back of people's minds. When people decide to look for a dentist, that dentist that they have passed by frequently is one of the first names that pop up. People have to know where the dentist is.

The dentist should invest in a good sign. He or she wants the sign to "cut through the clutter" of the other signs that compete for people's attention. That is not to say that the dentist's sign has to be the biggest, but it has to be as large as the others. That also does not say that he or she needs a flashing neon sign, unless the office is found on the strip in Las Vegas. Here a dentist would need flashing neon simply to be noticed. Signage is even more important if the office is tucked into a retail center or an office building. In these cases, the sign is the dentist's drive-by visibility.

Accessibility

The dental office must be easy to get to. The dentist should imagine how a receptionist telling people how to find the office. He or she should be able to describe the location in fifteen words or less. "Right across from the hospital in the Doctor' Park Office Building, Suite 221" is easy for most people to find. "Take Main Street south to the third light; right on Oak for 2 blocks, then down the alley on the left for 200 feet" is not easy. The dentist should be sure there are adequate parking and easy entrance and exit from the street. (Adequate parking is simply expected by modern dental patients.) If a dentist will practice in an urban area, he or she consider the location of public

Table 26.1 Types of Locations for Dental Offices

Location	Set-up Cost	Lease Cost
Strip Mall	Medium	High
Major Mall	High	Very High
Medical Office Building	High	High
Individual Office Building	Very High	High
Leased Building	Medium	Low

transportation. The dentist should also be sure that there are no physical barriers to entry (e.g., steps without a handicapped accessible ramp). In a new office, the dentist must meet building codes regarding disabled accessibility. The architect or designer will know the codes.

Type of Site

There are many types of locations for dental offices, each with pros and cons (Table 26.1). Freestanding buildings, either owned or leased, are becoming less common as commercial real estate becomes more expensive. Medical office buildings are easy for the public to find, have ample parking, and lend an air of professionalism. The landlords are used to the specific needs of professionals, which can be helpful. These sites are expensive. Many of these are condominium-type arrangements, in which a dentist purchases the office and then pays a fee to the condominium association for maintenance and repairs to the building. Strip-type shopping centers have adequate parking and are generally on a major road, giving high visibility. They are relatively expensive. The landlord is usually responsible for snow removal and other common maintenance items, although the landlord generally charge the lessee (dentist) a maintenance fee to cover these items. The lessee usually must purchase and maintain heating and air-conditioning units. The dentist should check the types of businesses to which the landlord caters. The dentist probably does not want a pawn broker, tattoo parlor, or head shop opening next to his or her office. Large shopping malls are the highest cost location. Set-up costs are high because most retail space is not set up for plumbing, electrical, and other dental office improvements. Malls often charge high rent and sometimes a percentage of gross sales. The dentist should try to negotiate this out of the lease. Like strip centers, the dentist is usually responsible for utility upkeep. General office buildings may be the least expensive alternative. Location and parking may or may not be optimal. The advantages of these sites are on a case-by-case basis.

Zoning

Before a dentist signs for any property, he or she should be sure that the zoning will allow a dental office in the site. The dentist should take care, particularly in residential areas, that he or she has the go-ahead before committing any money. Zoning changes do not always go as expected. Legal fees can mount quickly if a citizen's action group or another developer wants to challenge a zoning request.

Developing the Facility

Once a location has been decided on, the dentist must develop the facility in which he or she will practice.

Lease versus Buy

Most dentists today lease space for their office. Many who do own are owners in a condominium arrangement. Many owners believe that owning their own building insulates them from problems of landlords. That is true, but it brings the problems of ownership. When the plumbing breaks down, the dentist is responsible for fixing it. Tax laws have been change to reduce the value of ownership.

If a dentist is going to lease, he or she should be aware that most commercial property is priced on a square-foot-per-year basis. "Thirteen dollars a foot" for a 1,000-square foot office is $13,000 a year, or $1,083 per month. Depending on the state of commercial real estate in the area, the dentist can negotiate specific clauses into the lease. He or she wants the landlord to pay as many ancillary costs as can be negotiated. These include general maintenance, plumbing, heating and air conditioning, snow removal (if appropriate), and cleaning of the common areas. Leasehold improvements (improvements that the dentist makes to the landlord's property) are expensive for a dental office. This is largely because of the extensive plumbing needs. (Each operatory requires hot and cold water, waste, air, vacuum, nitrous, oxygen, and electrical outlets.) Many dentists have negotiated a given amount (e.g., $10,000) for leasehold improvements. Others have gotten several months free rent while the improvements are being completed. When a dentist negotiates any of these items, he or she should be sure that these items are written into the lease. The landlord may be noble and true. However, if the landlord sells to another party, there is no record of verbal agreements. Many landlords want a professional office in their space. Dentists are excellent, high-class, long-term tenants. So the dentist does have some bargaining leverage.

Designing the Office

The dentist should get a book on dental office design and visit as many offices as possible, asking the dentists for suggestions to improving their space. The dentist is going to have to live in the space for many years to come, so he or she should make it a place with which he or she is comfortable. The dentist should consult an interior decorator or designer to assist with color and wallpaper selection.

If the dentist is building a freestanding building (shell) from scratch, he or she should probably will use an architect or construction engineer that is familiar with the needs of dental office construction. Most full-service dealers have one or more people on staff who are familiar with dental office design. Most will work with the dentist and do the design free (or a nominal cost) with the understanding that the dentist is going to buy the equipment from that dealer. These dealers may also help a dentist find space. They know the building codes related to dental offices and the requirements for inspection and certification for a particular state. They may even have several general contractors who they have used that are familiar with dental practice construction.

The dentist should let the designer know what he or she wants in an office design. The designer will probably bring a couple of preliminary design for review. The dentist should study the designs to find the features of each that he or she does and does not like. The dentist should then take suggestions back to the designer. The dentist should continue doing this until he or she is happy with the design. Once construction begins, changes become *very* expensive. The dentist will probably want a general contractor if he or she is making substantial changes to an existing office space. The equipment dealer can help the dentist find one.

General Design Decisions

There are special design criteria for operatories and X-ray areas. The dentist should decide if he or she wants open operatories or closed rooms. Either one works, depending on the dentist's style. Pass-through X-ray heads save costs, if they can be designed to reach chairs in both operatories. They often can not. The type of equipment that a dentist buys may determine, in part, the design of the operatories and support areas. Traffic patterns should be made convenient for patients, staff, and the dentist. The dentist should be sure to place high traffic areas near the front, making patient traffic patterns as short as possible. This also relieves congestion in hallways. The hygienist probably will see more patients a day than the dentist. Therefore, the hygienist's operatory should be nearer to the patient reception area.

The dentist should have a centrally located sterilization area. He or she will need a large counter space for breaking down trays and cassettes; a deep double sink is used to wash instruments; another counter is used for packaging and autoclaving; and more counter space is needed for preparing and storing sterile trays and cassettes for use in the operatories. A dentist will need a minimum of 10 to 12 feet of counter space for efficient instrument sterilization. If the dentist has cabinets below and above the counter space, he or she should have enough space for office sterilization procedures. Many people use the lab for this space. Separate areas, however, are a better idea.

Some areas are low-use areas. These should be kept away from high-traffic areas. Staff lounge areas and mechanical room are often noisy and smelly; those should be kept away from patient treatment and traffic areas. Private offices are luxuries and should be kept out of the traffic flow as well. If a dentist is in a stand-alone building or a freestanding office, he or she needs public restrooms. These restrooms should be near the patient waiting room but under control of the staff. (It is amazing what kids try to flush down the toilet.)

Most designs do not have a large enough business office area. A dentist needs significant counter space for electronic gadgets, such as a computer, printer, fax, copier, answering machine, and maybe an old-fashioned typewriter. The more storage, the better off a dentist will be. As patient chart numbers increase, so do storage requirements. Front office personnel should not make collection or other private patient calls within hearing of patients in the reception room or treatment areas. The dentist should have a separate room, near the business office but closed off with a door, for making these telephone contacts. There should be a counter, at elbow height near but out of the patient flow, for patients to write checks. It should also include a pen.

The reception area should be just that. Patients should be received there, not made to wait there. If the dentist and patients are both on time, there is minimal waiting. Rural practices and practices that see many children will often have family members waiting for the patient receiving treatment. In these cases, a larger waiting room is useful. The dentist is the best judge of the practice area. The lab is a seldom used area, and so should be put in a peripheral, low use area. The same goes for the private office. If a dentist is sitting at a desk, he or she is not seeing patients or generating any money. The office should be a low-priority, low-use area as well. Many dentists like a consultation area for patient treatment plan presentation and financial arrangements. If the dentist wants one, it should be a separate room near the patient traffic flow area.

Ordering Equipment and Supplies

If a dentist purchases new operatory equipment, he or she should be sure to order it at least 2 months before it is needed. Most of the equipment will be in stock, but there may be one critical piece (like a compressor) that is back ordered. The equipment supplier will help the dentist by providing lists of instruments and materials. The dentist will also need to order business office equipment and supplies, including accounting packages (peg board or computer), patient records, and office stationery.

Staffing the Office

The dentist should begin to staff the office at least 6 weeks before opening. This assumes that it will take him or her 3 weeks to find the right people, 2 weeks before they can come to work, and a week of training and preparation. Friends and family should be used to have mock patient visits and phone calls to prepare for the first day of patients.

The dentist should try to find an experienced front office person at the beginning of practice. An experienced person can help to set up the office systems and remember forms and procedures that the dentist does not know. Eventually the person may leave, but by then, the office will be functioning smoothly and the dentist will be much more knowledgeable of how he or she wants to operate.

Financing the Office

Most banks and finance companies will qualify a dentist for a line of credit. The dentist then taps into this line any time a bill comes due. The dentist should be sure to establish a line of credit for working capital as well. As a rule, he or she should plan on 3 months' expenses as needs for working capital.

If a dentist is going to own his or her own building, he or she will probably need to arrange financing. Banks are generally willing to lend 80 to 90 percent of the cost of appraised real estate. The dentist will need to come up with the remainder as a down payment. If he or she is also buying a practice or equipping an office, the dentist may be entering more debt than the banks will allow. The mortgage is generally paid off in 20 years and the building depreciates over 30 years. The dentist will proportion the cost of land and building. Building is depreciable. Land is not.

Buying an Existing Practicing (Buy-out)

Types of Practices for Sale

Dentists who sell their practice typically fall into one of six groups. Understanding these groups is important so that the buyer can negotiate more effectively for the practice.

Retiring Dentists

Retiring dentists make the first group. These older dentists are usually more concerned with finding the right person to care for their beloved patient pool than in getting an excellent price. Depending on their personal practice style, they may have a large portion of the patient pool that needs advanced periodontal and restorative needs. The new owner–dentist will need to continue carefully with these patients to introduce them to the advantages of modern dentistry without appearing to insult the former dentist as providing out-of-date dentistry.

Young Dentists Changing Career Paths

Many dentists who have been in practice for several years decide to change their career paths. This often involves going for specialty training or may involve moving to the military or public health career options. Depending on the history and price of these practices, they can be an excellent opportunity. The buyer should be careful if the practice has shown good growth and profitability because sometimes these young practices show good gross income, but because of managed care and other write-offs show poor profitability.

Dentists with Personal Problems

Often, dentists who have significant personal problems may be selling their practices. This may involve a nasty divorce, depression over the death of a loved one, personal bankruptcy, or other personal problems. The buyer should approach these practices with caution. The potential buyer might be buying a host of problems, such as the reputation of the dentist in the community, unpaid tax liens, future divorce court problems, or competition from the former dentist who clears up his or her problems.

Dentists with Health Problems

Occasionally, the potential buyer may find a practice available from a dentist who has a disabling health problem. This may be as the result of an accident or disease. The negotiations for many of these practices can be difficult. The owner does not really want to leave practice; he or she is being forced out. Here, the buyer needs to be careful that he or she does not pay too much through sympathy for the dentist's condition. But the buyer also does not want to offend the dentist by being insensitive to his or her needs. If the dentist has accepted his or her condition, the buyer can generally find a reasonably priced, valuable practice.

Death of the Dentist

If the owner–dentist dies unexpectedly, the most critical issue for all concerned is time. The longer the practice remains closed, the more patients will find another provider. After about 3 months of inactivity, there is really no goodwill value left in the practice of a dead dentist. All a buyer will pay for at that point is the equipment and other hard assets. If the buyer is fortunate enough to buy and practice in the office soon after the other dentist's demise, he or she will get a fair value and save the estate a significant amount of money. Although it sounds cold, contacting the estate soon after the dentist's death helps to preserve the value of the practice for the estate. It can get complicated, but it is absolutely in the survivor's best interest to sell the practice as quickly as possible.

Entrepreneur Dentists

Some dentists think highly of their business and clinical skills. They believe that no one can establish a practice like they can. They then establish practices with the notion of selling it to a young dentist. Although these may be fine practices, they often overvalue them. Nevertheless, the selling dentist is quite a businessperson and can sound quite convincing in discussions with him or her.

Types of Buy-outs

Buy-outs fall into three general classes.

Walk-Away Sale

In this type of sale, the (previous) owner walks away from the practice when the buyer purchases it. In this scenario, the buyer owns the practice upon closing the purchase deal. The next day, the dentist is in the practice and the previous owner is not. The dentist needs arrangements to handle accounts receivable, patient questions, and staff concerns.

This is not to say that this type of transition is always a complete surprise. Often negotiations are done in private, with the announcement when the deal is signed and completed. Two interested groups are the staff and the patients. Staff members want to know that they will still have a job under similar terms and conditions as they did previously. The dentist should hold a staff meeting with the outgoing dentist to assure staff members that this is the case. Patients may have a long-trusted relationship with the previous practitioner. The owner should write a letter to patients of record, informing them of his or her intention and urging patients to remain in the practice to see the new dentist for their dental care.

Transition

In this buy-out, the (previous) owner works a short time to help in the transition. This may be from a few weeks to 6 months. This type of transition helps to comfort the new dentist by knowing that he or she has someone to ask questions of and to help with clinical or management problems. Sometimes, the new dentist pays the outgoing dentist a consulting fee (as part of the purchase price). Generally, the new dentist finds that he or she does not need the outgoing dentist as much as he or she thought. Instead, the outgoing dentist begins to be a burden. Staff is not sure who to report or complain to, patients often still want to see the outgoing dentist, and some departing dentists give unwanted opinions about changes the new dentist wants to make.

Trading Roles

In this buyout, the (previous) owner works long term as an associate in the practice for the new owner. Problems are similar to a transition, in that staff and patients may show allegiance to the former owner. This buy-out works best if the new owner has done an extended associateship before the buy-out. In this way, patients and staff members become familiar with both dentists.

Reasons to Buy an Existing Practice

There are reasons that make sense to buy an existing practice rather than starting a practice from scratch. Some of these reasons relate to a dentist's particular style. A decision that makes good sense for one dentist does not fit the personality, style, or goals of another. Other reasons are financial. A particular purchase deal might make better financial sense than starting a practice. A dentist should explore both areas before making an informed purchase decision.

All these discussions assume that the dentist can maintain the practice's production level at the current level. A new practitioner looking at a large, established practice simply may not have the skills and professional maturity to handle a large practice. It would be foolish to pay top dollar for a productive practice when the production would decrease dramatically the first day he or she took over. So purchasing a practice is a bigger advantage for an experienced clinician who can maintain high production levels.

Advantages to Buying a Practice

From a financial perspective, purchasing a practice may allow the dentist to make more money than a cold start. This occurs more in areas where the competition for patients is higher because a dentist has a built-in patient pool. The dentist will have a full book of patients from the first day. He or she will have a more immediate cash flow because of those immediate patient visits. When starting a practice from scratch, a dentist may lose time that the office is not open because of construction delays or equipment delivery schedules. The dentist is generally buying new equipment for a new office. Although this

equipment needs fewer repairs, it also costs more for the initial outlay. If a dentist purchases accounts receivable, he or she will not need as much working capital or start-up cash. The dentist probably will not need to immediately recruit staff for the office. Hopefully existing staff will remain when the new dentist takes over.

From a personal perspective, purchasing a practice may decrease stress. The dentist knows that the practice can succeed. He or she does not have to worry about construction problems and delays. There is an immediate cash flow. The dentist has the reputation of the departing dentist to rely on. Often, the new dentist may gain the departing dentist's expertise as well, by using a long-term consulting agreement. When a dentist purchases a practice, he or she buys the ongoing business systems; the accounting, inventory, or patient billing systems do not have to be set up.

Disadvantages to Buying a Practice

All of the advantages come with a price, and the financial price is called *goodwill* or the value of the ongoing business concern. (The chapter of practice valuation discusses goodwill in more detail.) The dentist is paying the departing owner extra money, above the cost of the readily apparent assets of the practice, for the expectation that the practice's profit will flow to the new dentist. If the new dentist pays too much for the practice, then the payments for the practice will eat up any increase in the long-term money generated over a cold start. Similarly, if a dentist does not get a good transfer of patients (at least 90 percent), then the price for the practice may be too high. So from a financial perspective, buying a practice gives the new dentist higher costs than starting a practice from scratch, but an immediate cash flow to help cover those costs. The value (cost) of the practice is obviously a critical factor in the decision. If the area is in need of dentists and a dentist can be busy when he or she opens the door, then it generally makes financial sense to start, rather than to buy out a practice.

As a dentist ages, the patient pool typically ages with him or her as children grow up and move away. If a dentist is buying the practice of an older dentist, then he or she may need to do significant marketing to gain a younger patient pool. Many older dentists have not updated equipment in many years. If a dentist buys such a practice, the cost of significant facility and equipment updates should be included.

From a personal perspective, the dentist buying the outgoing dentist's reputation, good or bad. It takes many years to change a community's perception of a dental practice, even if the practitioner has changed. If the previous dentist's style was simply to fix holes in people's teeth, then it will take a considerable amount of time for a new dentist to change the character of the practice to one of comprehensive periodontal and restorative services. If the new dentist is completely changing the character of the practice, why buy it? The immediate cash flow advantages simply may not be worth the extra effort.

What a Dentist Is Buying

When a dentist purchases a dental practice, he or she is paying for the hope that the profit that the practice has shown in the past will comes to him or her. The dentist buys dental equipment, charts, goodwill, and other assets because he or she believe that they can be used to make money. He or she does not buy them because they have any intrinsic value or because they are collectors' items. The assets are only instrumental to what the dentist is purchasing and that is the demonstrated profit of the ongoing concern of the practice as a business entity.

The dentist hopes that the profits of the practice will transfer to him or her. To help this, the new dentist wants to make few changes to the office until the patients have transferred their allegiance to him or her. (Generally this is one or two recall cycles.) The more alike the new dentist and the departing dentist are will increase the possibility that patients will transfer and remain. Patients select practice for their reasons, not the dentist's. The patient pool that the departing dentist has built over the years selected that dentist for their reasons; the new dentist should try to cater to them.

Financing the Purchase

Many buying dentists become too concerned with the simple price of the practice. Instead of asking "How much is the practice?" they should be asking "How much will I make when I buy the practice?" The method of financing the practice sale dramatically affects the financial outcome of the practice transfer. The chapter on securing financing discusses these options.

Transfer Considerations

There are several special issues to consider in transferring practices from one owner to another. A brief discussion of several of these issues follows.

Buying a Practice and Real Estate

Some practices are located in freestanding office buildings. If a dentist buys the practice, he or she needs assurances that the practice can be kept in the same location, for transfer of income-generating potential. The departing owner may want to sell the building to the buyer, or the owner may want to continue to own the building but offer a long-term lease. The owner may retain and lease the building to add to retirement or investment income. The new owner should be sure to have a long-term lease included in the purchase of the practice. An advantage for the buyer is a right of first refusal to purchase the building if the owner decides to sell it.

If the owner insists on selling the building with the practice, the buyer faces additional financial problems. Valuing the building is relatively easy; a reputable real estate appraiser can appraise the real estate. Securing financing for the real estate may be more difficult. Many buyers are financially stretched to purchase the practice. They have little collateral to pledge and are concurrently borrowing to buy homes, cars, and other personal items. Buying a piece of real estate may increase the new dentist's debt level beyond what a banker believes is prudent. Understandably, the banker might not finance the loan. On the other hand, real estate is tangible. Bankers may be willing to finance a higher percentage of the value of a real property than intangible property such as goodwill. (Bankers will often require 20 percent of the property value as down payment, financing the remaining 80 percent.) Here, the dentist should perform careful cash flow and pro forma income analyses. If the numbers look right, the buyer might work with the bank for the real estate loan and use owner financing for the practice purchase (or vice versa). If the dentist purchases the real estate, then he or she must allocate the price to land and building. Buildings are depreciable over 31 years. Land is not depreciable. The buyer obviously wants to allocate as much as possible to building.

Price and Other Considerations

The price that a dentist negotiates should be based on the true value of the practice. Whether or not he or she can afford the price may be determined by other considerations thrown into the equation. For example, the whole deal may be contingent on the owner financing half the practice. Part of the price may be paid in consulting fees that the buyer pays to the seller. These fees come out of practice profits over time, and so do not really enter the stated price for the practice. They do affect the extended price of the practice. The owner may agree to stay for a certain length of time to aid in the transfer by introducing patients to the new owner and even by doing some work on those patients for a reduced (or no) fee to the buyer. All these types of side deals can help to justify the price or make the buyout work; they should not be overlooked. But the dentist should also not allow them to sell a bad deal. If the practice is overvalued, the dentist should simply not purchase the practice.

Intrafamily Transfers

Intrafamily transfers are looked at closely by the IRS. They realize that many small business owners might want to transfer a business to their children or other relatives at less than its true value to avoid taxes. The IRS rule in these cases is called "substance over form." This rule means that the reality of the transfer governs how it is taxed, not merely what the dentist says the form is. If the transfer is a gift, then the value of the practice is included in the Uniform Gift and Estate Tax and the transfer is taxed as a gift. This most frequently happens when a dentist sells their practice to a child for much less than actual value and reports the transaction as required by tax law. It is difficult for the IRS to track the dentist who simply closes the doors to the practice and then his or her child establishes a practice the next day in the same location under a new name.

Accounts Receivable

The issue of purchasing accounts receivable is often contentious in practice purchases. The seller believes that the accounts receivable should be valued higher than the buyer. The buyer would like to have the immediate cash flow without having to get additional line of credit for working capital, but only if the price is right. Buyers have the additional trouble of educating patients about an account receivable purchase. Many patients want to pay the departed dentist, not the new one. Others do not want to pay either one. The buyer can not aggressively pursue these accounts without risking offending the patient pool, which he or she has just paid a considerable amount of money for as goodwill.

It is generally easiest to keep the accounts receivable out of the purchase price of a dental practice. (The buyer will usually need to borrow working capital in this case.) The owner can collect the accounts as aggressively as he or she wishes. The new owner is relatively immune from patients' anger in this situation. The other common method of handling these accounts is for the buyer to use normal collection methods to collect the accounts for the seller. (The buyer generally has use of the seller's name for 1 year.) The seller then deducts a nominal amount, such as 10 percent, for the cost of collecting the accounts and then sends the remainder (90 percent) to the seller. After 6 months, the dentist may turn over any uncollected accounts to a collection agent.

Minimizing Change

As a rule, dentists should make as few initial changes as possible in the practice. They should not rush in to paint or put up wallpaper. He or she has paid for the patients, and the dentist wants them to think that nothing has changed until the patients become accustomed to the new practitioner. If there are changes required for safety reasons (e.g., the previous owner did not take adequate health histories), then the new dentist should do what needs to be done to be safe. But if a picture is not straight on the wall, the new dentist should let it remain crooked for a year. After the patients have bonded with him or her, then the dentist should make cosmetic and structural changes. The new dentist should try to keep staff for the initial period as well because many patients are as close to the staff members as the dentist.

Length of Overlap

Many new dentists want a long period when the seller remains in the office. The belief is that this period of overlapping clinical time helps the transfer of patients. In fact, it only helps a small amount. (If other factors have been taken care of the patient transfer will take place.) What often happens is that the buyer, because of insecurity in his or her management and patient relations abilities, wants the seller to stay on a crutch. However, after the first month, the seller will be getting in the way. Patients will want to continue to see the seller if they think there is a choice. Staff will take problems (real or perceived) to the former owner. By the second month, the seller will be a problem. By the third month, the dentist simply wants the former dentist out of the office. The dentist should use a good letter of introduction and other methods to encourage an immediate transfer and then get the seller out of the practice quickly.

Patient Records

Sellers need access to records if a former patient sues them. Otherwise, the buyer generally buys the records. That really means that the buyer has bought exclusive business rights to the information in the records. The medical information in the record belongs to the patient. If the patient requests that their records be sent to another dentist, the new dentist has an ethical obligation to see that the information (written and radiographic) is sent so that the patient's health is not compromised. The dentist does not send originals, only copies. (Many states allow the dentist to charge a nominal amount for copying records.) The dentist may not refuse to send a copy of the record because a patient still owes money (that is a separate issue) or because the dentist does not like the other dentist. The dentist may (in most states) require the patient's signature to release medical information.

Typical Order of Business

Practice purchases follow similar patterns. The details of the individual practice purchase are different in each purchase, but the dentist must resolve many common issues for the purchase to work. The first thing to decide is if the seller *really* wants to sell the practice. Often practitioners feel pressure from family or peers to retire or sell for other reasons. The owner, however, really does not want to sell. It may even sound like a good idea initially, but as the dentist draws closer to making the deal, the owner begins to get cold feet and backs out of the sale. Other times, a retiring dentist may visit their accountant and find out that the deal being negotiated simply does not leave enough money, after taxes, to fund the retirement as envisioned by the owner. Regardless the reason, many sellers decide late in the process to back out of the sale. The buyer should try to be sure that this dentist wants to sell.

In all negotiations, the buyer must remember that he or she must produce at the seller's level, or higher, for the numbers to make sense. Otherwise, the profitability of the practice goes down. The dentist is buying the income generation of the practice. For example, assume a seller is producing $600,000 per year. The dentist buys the practice, but can only do $400,000 of production. The dentist has suddenly turned that practice making $600,000 into a practice producing $400,000 overnight. Would the dentist have bought the practice for the same amount if it were producing $400,000? Probably not. The dentist must also keep the overhead at the seller's level. Otherwise, profits go down. If the owner's spouse worked in the office free, profits will go down when someone is hired to replace the owner's spouse. (Unless the spouse agrees to work long-term free for the new dentist, which is a unlikely scenario!) The dentist will also have increased costs, from equipment and supply changeover and from making a large mortgage payment to the bank.

Locating a Practice

The most difficult step may be simply finding a practice for sale in the area a dentist wants to buy. In some area, there may be only a few dentists. None of them may want to sell. Metropolitan areas offer more dentist wanting to sell at any given time, but more new dentists looking to buy. A dentist may not find a practice where he or she wants when he or she wants to buy it. Often the selling dentist does not want anyone else (like patients or other dentists) to know that they are selling their practice. They generally will use a practice broker or local accountant to develop confidential leads for them. If a dentist has not expressed an interest with that particular broker, he or she may miss the opportunity. (Even if the dentist has, the broker may choose someone else as the "chosen one" for this practice.) Equipment dealer and supply representatives often know who is looking to sell a practice. Many new dentists have found practices when working for tempo-

rary agencies. The truth is that the best way to find a practice is to network with other dentists; a dentist should let other dentists know that he or she is looking in an area. The dentist should be diligent and attend the local dental society meeting, join a study club, or become a member of the local professional community. If a dentist has a practice broker, he or she can help the dentist find and develop possible practices. The dentist should talk to everyone he or she can and let his or her intentions be known.

Investigating the Practice

When a dentist finds a potential practice to buy, he or she needs to do some homework. He or she probably wants an accountant, management consultant, or other professional familiar with transitions to help with the analysis. Initially, the dentist will meet the selling dentist and examine the office. He or she should ask questions about the organization and operations of the practice. The dentist should look at the schedule book an determine numbers of patients available for transfer. During the initial visits, the owner probably will not give the dentist access to detailed financial records because the owner wants the dentist to be sure that he or she is serious about the practice before showing tax returns and other important financial information. The selling dentist will decide if the buyer is the person that he or she wants to take over the practice. Part of his or her assessment is an appraisal of the buyer's financial condition. The owner will want to know if the buyer has money or collateral to arrange financing or if the he or she will need to offer owner financing.

Some selling dentists have brochures developed describing their practice. Others have a few numbers jotted down on the back of a napkin. Regardless, when a dentist is seriously discussing buying the practice, the seller must provide a couple of key things. One is a recent equipment appraisal done by a reputable supply house. Secondly, the seller will need to provide the last 3 years' tax returns for the office. (The buyer will need this for his or her financial analysis and for the banks to make theirs.) The notion is that anyone can put numbers on a piece of paper. What they report to the IRS is usually the truest information. Some practice, particularly if the dentist owns multiple practices grouped onto their tax return, will have an accountant's report that breaks this practice's numbers out from the others. Some dentists will require that a buyer signs a nondisclosure form. This says that the buyer agrees not to share this information with any except his or her professional advisors. This is reasonable because this often contains sensitive personal financial and tax information. Other dentists ask the buyer to sign a form of a restrictive covenant that says if they show their financial information, he or she agrees not to set up a competing practice in the same area. The buyer should avoid these, if he or she has any interest in staying in the area. They are often promoted by dentists who think much more of their practices than they should.

The buyer may want to have help in negotiations. Often the selling dentist will have professional help in developing a practice value and identifying potential leads. These people may claim to be able to represent both sides. That is difficult for anyone to do. The seller is usually paying the broker anywhere from 5 to 10 percent of the purchase price as a sales commission. The buyer knows where the broker's loyalties lie. The buyer should have an accountant or management consult with him or her to ensure that someone looks after his or her interests. (The dentist will pay this person a reasonable amount for their time, effort, and knowledge.)

Making an Offer

The owner–dentist should state a price that he or she is asking for the practice. The buyer can then accept or reject the offer or make a counteroffer. A counteroffer says, "No, I don't accept your offer, but I would buy the practice at this price and for these terms." Any offer should be in writing to be sure that all points are clearly understood. At this point, the buyer begins negotiations. He or she probably does not want to make a really low counteroffer, but the buyer also does not want to make one that the owner instantly accepts. The buyer is negotiating what he or she believes is the honest value of the practice. He or she can not worry if the seller is going to lose money. That is his or her problem. The buyer does not want to bail the owner out because he or she made bad business decisions in the past. On the other hand, a buyer does not want to foul a deal that really does make sense by insulting the seller with a low ball offer.

Most offers contain contingencies. These are qualifiers that the buyer or the owner must meet before the deal can proceed. Some common contingencies in offers include:

1. The buyer must be able to gain acceptable (to seller) financing from a bank.
2. The buyer must gain a dental license for the state of practice.
3. The equipment must be in good working order at the time of transfer.
4. The owner will agree to a restrictive covenant of X miles and Y years.
5. The owner will write a letter (acceptable to the buyer) to all the current patients of the practice informing them of the transfer and urging them to continue patronage of the practice.

When the buyer has negotiated a deal that is acceptable for both sides, he or she should send a letter of acceptance. (The buyer can consummate the deal with a handshake, but many people have been disappointed by final contracts or sales because of what one side "thought" was in the offer. It should be written down.) This letter spells out the buyer's offer and conditions. It is written, so it carries more force than the handshake deal. At this point, some sellers want the buyer to put down some "earnest money" to show that he or she is serious; others do not because they figure that the buyer has done this far, so he or she must be serious.

Securing Financing

The dentist should not wait until this point to talk to a banker. As soon as the buyer finds a desirable practice, he or she should begin discussions with a banker to find out what is needed to make a loan. (Some dentists begin talking with a banker before they find a practice.) Bankers can also act as an advisor in the process and ensure that a buyer does not make too many mistakes. The dentist should talk with colleagues to find out which banks are making loans to professionals and should talk with more than one bank. Different banks have different strategies regarding the types of clients they are trying to gain. One bank may not be seeking professional clients, whereas another may. The chapter on securing financing describes the typical types of loans that a dentist can find for practice purchases and the type of information that a banker will want to have.

Making the Transfer

Once the details have been ironed out, the transfer itself is almost anticlimactic. The buyer will get together with the seller, often at the banker's office, sign a few papers, and, voila, the buyer is a practice owner! But the buyer's job is not over. (Actually he or she should have done these tasks before the closing date.) The dentist should find an accountant that he or she is comfortable with and who has other dentists as clients. The seller should transfer the lease for the office from him or her to the buyer. The dentist should contact the various utilities (water, gas and electric, telephone, etc.) to be sure that the account will be in the buyer's name. The buyer will need to pay any deposits as well. (Often the cost of the deposit is included in the practice purchase price. The buyer simply pays the seller, and he or she calls the utility and transfers the deposit to the buyer's name.) The dentist should call insurance agents (workers' compensation, business liability, malpractice, and office overhead) to ensure that his or her coverage is in effect. The dentist should secure a federal tax identification number if he or she does not have one. He or she should check to see if a state or local tax number or account is needed. The dentist should find out if he or she can convert any reserve in the seller's unemployment account into his or her name. The dentist should call his or her software vendor to change the name in the office computer system and the support contract, if there is one. The dentist should open an office checking account at a local Federal Reserve bank and get an office checkbook. He or she should call the disability insurance agent to be sure that he or she is covered for the new expected level of income. The dentist should take his or her spouse or significant other to dinner and celebrate the accomplishment and contemplate the future.

Buying Into an Existing Practice (Buy In)

Buying into a dental practice is similar to buying out a practice. The dentist should select a location and specific practice in the same way. The practice is valued similarly. The issues of transferring ownership are comparable. However, there are a couple of major differences that change the game dramatically:

- The dentist is only buying part of the income-generating potential of the practice. When he or she purchases a practice outright, the dentist buys all of the income generation of the practice. When buying into a practice, the dentist must be sure that there are adequate patients for the new number of practitioners.
- The dentist is forming or joining a group practice. Group practices have problems and advantages that are different from the individual practitioner's. (See the chapter on group practices.) When a dentist puts money on the table for a buy-in, he or she makes a decision that is difficult to undo. The dentist must, therefore, be sure that it is a correct one.

Types of Buy-Ins

There are several types of buy-in arrangements.

Immediate Buy-In

An immediate buy-in is rare. Because a buy-in implies some form of a group arrangement, most dentists want to be sure that they are compatible. They often use an associateship to test the compatibility of personalities, practice styles, and philosophies. The times that immediate buy-ins occur are generally either family members buying into a family practice or former (or present) employees who have completed dental school.

Associateship Leading to Buy-in

The most common scenario is an associateship that leads to a buy-in. Many associateships are established with this intent. However, both dentists need to understand that the associateship is not a guarantee of a buy-in. It is a trial period to see if the practitioners are compatible and to see of the practice can sustain two practitioners. The associateship trial period makes sense because a decision to buy-in is difficult to change.

Trading Roles

The most difficult type of buy-in occurs when the new dentist buys into a practice (or buys out the entire practice), and the former owner then works for the new owner. This usually occurs after an associateship. The original owner–dentist often wants to begin slowing down in anticipation of retirement, but he or she also wants to keep professionally active. The greatest problems come from staff disorientation. The staff members have a history of dedication to the former employer. Changing those allegiances can be difficult, especially when the new owner makes significant personnel changes.

Advantages to Buying into a Practice

When a dentist buys into a practice, he or she knows that the owner–dentist believes in the practice. Otherwise, he or she would not plan to stay. Like buying an entire practice, the dentist has the advantage of an ongoing business, with ongoing cash flow, staff, patients, and equipment. If the price is right, then the dentist should make more money, in the long run, than establishing a practice from scratch. New practitioners have the advantage of an experienced practitioner on the premises for clinical and management advice. The dentist also has all the advantages that a group practice shows.

Disadvantages to Buying into a Practice

The biggest disadvantages of buying into a practice relate to the group that results. If a dentist does not want a group practice situation, or he or she is unsure about future partners as co-professionals, then he or she should not get involved in this type of relationship. When the other owner(s) decide to retire or leave, the dentist must find another person to buy his or her part of the practice or else the dentist has wasted money by purchasing too much dental practice. This means that once a dentist establishes a group practice, he or she will probably be involved in a group for the rest of his or her career.

The second major problem occurs if the dentist decides that he or she wants to end the professional relationship. Who is going to buy the dentist's part interest in a dental practice? He or she will probably discount the value of his or her portion of the practice to make up for the uncertainty that a new owner has about moving into an established practice. If the dentist tries to split the group up, the contract will probably have significant restrictions and covenants to the future practice.

What the Dentist Is Buying

Like an outright practice purchase, the dentist is buying the ability to make money from the practice. That takes two forms: producing dentistry and from ownership in the practice. The dentist essentially has an investment in equipment, intangible assets, and financial assets. He or she expects, and deserves, a reasonable return on those assets. This is the pure "profit" that the practice generates.

When there is one owner–dentist, the dentist has 100 percent of the decision-making authority. When there are two equal partners, then each has 50 percent decision-making authority. It is possible to reach an impasse on important decisions if the two disagree. (In a publicly traded company, the dentist can easily sell his or her share in the market. Not so with closely-held companies.) If there are three or more owners, then the dentist can essentially lose decision-making authority if the other owners "gang up" against the lone disagreeing owner. Ownership interest is then worth less when there are many dentists because one owner's decision-making authority is diluted. Typically, practices decrease about one third in value in these cases. The problem with this scenario is that now the other owners can force a dentist out at the discounted price, leaving them with a more valuable practice than they paid for. Obviously, this becomes a complex and potentially expensive proposition. So, the dentist should be sure to work with an experienced transition consultant and lawyer when buying or selling partial interests in practices.

Financing the Purchase

Financing a partial practice purchase is different from a total buyout. The existing owners will remain and ensure that the practice remains profitable. There are two options commonly available for financing buy-ins.

Bank Financing

Banks are usually willing to finance a significant part of a buy-in if several conditions are met. Bankers are more comfortable lending money when a buyer can show a strong cash flow. If a dentist has been an associate in the practice, he or she can generally show a production level and cash flow that satisfies the banker's risk aversion. Bankers also know that many groups do not last. They want to see a well-crafted partnership agreement.

Sweat Equity

Generally, the dentist only needs to have a portion as a down payment for this option. He or she will pay the rest over time through his or her practice profits. This is the more common form of buying into ongoing practices.

Corporate Practices

When a dentist buys into a corporate practice, he or she buys stock as the ownership indicator. The corporation owns the assets, and so the corporation claims the depreciation and other deductions. The stock that is purchased is considered a capital asset. It is neither depreciable nor deductible. Instead, the dentist pays a capital gain or loss on the stock when it is eventually sold. (This may be 30 years from the date of buy-in.) For example, if a dentist buys half a $500,000 practice, he or she will pay $250,000. If the entire purchase amount is for stock, the dentist has $250,000 committed that he or she can neither claim as a deduction nor depreciation. If that same purchase were a proprietorship, the dentist would have most of the cost that he or she could have claimed as a depreciation deduction, decreasing taxes significantly. To avoid this tax whammy, most corporate buy-ins are structured differently. A nominal amount for the value of the stock (e.g., 10 percent of the practice value) is established. The buyer pays this amount up front as a down payment. The remainder is financed through an employment agreement with the corporation, whereby the dentist takes a decreased income, allowing that money that he or she would have made to go to the selling doctor(s) as income. The decrease is determined so that after a set time, the dentist has paid off the difference in purchase price. In the preceding example, the buyer is buying into a practice for $250,000 and pays the present owner $25,000 for half the corporate stock. The remainder ($225,000) will be paid over 5 years by the buyer decreasing income by $45,000 per year for 5 years. This arrangement makes the payments tax deductible for the buyer. The seller must claim them as ordinary income. Often a nominal interest rate will be included in the buy-in package (e.g., prime plus one percentage point) and the buy-in payments determined incorporating interest rate computations, or amortization. This is essentially a sweat equity arrangement. At present, the IRS is allowing this buy-in arrangement. They might not in the future.

When a dentist buys stock in the corporation, buying the stock from individual stockholders is generally best, rather than from the corporation itself. This gives some immediate cash to the seller(s) as a return on their investment. Buying from individuals is cheaper as well. Assume that a dentist wishes to buy half an existing corporate practice, whose value is $50,000. If he or she buys stock from the existing stockholder, he or she pays $25,000 for the other stockholder's half. If the dentist buys an equal share from the corporation, he or she must buy $540,000 from the corporation to have an equal portion of the stock. However, if the table is turned and the stockholder is leaving (because of death, retirement, etc.), and the corporate practice is ongoing, then the stock repurchase is generally made by the corporation. This allows the ratio of ownership to remain the same, with the purchase being accomplished with pretax money from the corporation, as opposed to spending personal funds to buy the stock of the departing member.

Transfer Considerations

Merging an Associate into the Mature Practice or Partnership

This arrangement implies that a dentist who has been working for another dentist (without ownership privileges) is offered ownership in the practice. The associate generally does not have the same level of financial resources and as a result this process is different from merging mature practices. The concept of taking a junior partner is a dynamic process that often stretches over several years. It begins with the realization of mutual need, usually progresses through an associateship or trial period arrangement, then a partial buy-in of the new partner, and finally culminates in a partnership.

There are many advantages to this process of partnership evolution. In the trial period, no future financial commitments are usually made. There are minimal financial investments, yet mutual financial benefits. Because there is clearly a junior-senior relationship, there may be fewer ego conflicts and an opportunity for a positive, mentoring relationship. If problems arise, they are usually about personnel issues and patient disposition in case of a breakup. In addition, the junior partner may find that their income goes down when the buy-in begins. This is the result of a new monthly practice purchase payment.

Both owner and associate must remember that an associateship is not a guarantee of future ownership. An associateship is an employment situation. At best, associateships only express the intent of the parties to form a partnership. Associateships are trial periods to see if the practitioners are compatible enough to form a group and to see if the practice can sustain the practitioners. The owner–dentist looks at several factors regarding the associate when considering a partnership:

Did the Associate Earn His or Her Salary?
Unless a partnership is being contemplated for nonfinancial reasons such as a merger with a relative, the associate should prove that he or she has sufficient income. When the buy-in begins, the associate will be paying a significant amount to his production to the lender to pay off the purchase. The associate must be sure that his or her potential income is high enough during the buy-in period to maintain an acceptable personal living standard.

Are the Two People Compatible Personally?
One of the most common reasons partnerships break up is over personality conflicts that escalate into major business disagreements. The dentists should be sure that there is both a behavioral and philosophical compatibility before a long-term commitment.

Is There a Sufficient Patient Base for Two Productive Practitioners?
Usually, an associate does not reach full productive potential for several years. Often established practitioners know that they have more patients than they need but do not really know if they have enough for two practitioners. In these cases, the practice patient base must increase to allow adequate patient flow for both practitioners.

Did the Associateship Meet Its Patient Treatment Objectives?
Part of the initial reason for an associateship may have been to retain referrals within the practice, to add new techniques to the service mix, or to serve a new population base. Did this happen as expected or will a partnership need to develop a new and different set of objectives?

Has It Been Enjoyable and Professionally Rewarding?
Some people thrive on the camaraderie and interaction involved in sharing space with another practitioner; others consider it bothersome. The practitioner should make an honest appraisal about the professional nature of a partnership.

Steps in Forming a Group Practice

Taking a junior partner involves the same problems as forming a group of established practitioners. There are several steps that the owner–dentist should take.

1. **Determine the form of the new group** Decide whether the group will be a partnership or corporation, individual group, or true group.
2. **Have the practice valued** Until both parties know how much money that they will need, it is impossible even to decide if the buy-in is feasible. Dentists who are unsure how to proceed with the valuation should secure sound professional counsel.

3. **Decide all the issues that are important in group practices** These issues include which advisors to use, how to divide income, how to allocate costs, any ancillary agreements, required physical changes in the facility, required staff changes, disposition of present and future accounts receivable, and what happens in the dissolution of the practice.
4. **Write a partnership agreement** Consult with an attorney to develop a document that covers the issues in detail.
5. **Determine the percentage to sell** If all dentists will be equal partners, then the new dentist will buy a proportional share. If the existing practitioners(s) wish to retain control, then they will sell less than a proportional share. The partnership and its attending aspects (i.e., when the papers are signed) control when the transition begins not when a dentist makes the last payment. The senior dentist should immediately expect to share authority.
6. **Determine the amount of down payment required, if owner financing** If the owner finances part of the sale, the buying dentist typically must make a down payment. The owner may ask for a minimum of 10 percent or $10,000 on up to 25 to 25 percent. If the buyer borrows the down payment from a bank, it may require a first mortgage on part of the practice, subordinating the debt of the seller in case of default.
7. **Determine interest, terms, and term of note if seller financing** If the seller finances the sale, he or she will usually give the buyer an interest rate that is similar to the bank rate. This will often give the seller an acceptable rate of return while compensating for the risk. The owner should also decide if there will be a prepayment clause and if the loan

will be assignable to another party. Decide what happens if either party wants to end the relationship before the note is completed. Should accumulated cash and interest be repaid or are penalties appropriate? Terms will not alter the value of the practice, but they may make it easier for the buyer to finance the purchase.
8. **Have all documents drafted** An attorney should draft all of the necessary legal papers.

In a partnership buy-in, the list of legal documents would include:

1. Bill of sale that transfers a share of the titles of assets being sold.
2. Sale contract (contract of purchase) that stipulates the terms of the sale of the assets. It should include any covenants, restrictions, hold harmless clauses, and an allocation of the assets bought.
3. Promissory note (of security interest) that is the buyer's promise to pay for the assets and offers security or collateral in the event he defaults on payments.
4. Partnership agreement that specifies the rights and responsibilities of the members in the new partnership.

In a corporate buy-in, the papers required include:

1. Buy–sell agreement (or stock purchase agreement) that defines how shares in the corporation are bought or sold.
2. Employment agreement that specifies the job the new dentist will have with the corporation. It includes income determination formulas, work schedules, benefits, and other duties and rights that come with the job.

Valuing Practices

chapter 27

Price is what you pay. Value is what you get.
Warren Buffett

Objectives

At the completion of this chapter, the student will be able to:
1. Describe the basic approaches to practice valuations
   Summation of assets
   Capitalization of income
   Cash flow feasibility
   Comparable sales
2. Discuss the advantages and disadvantages of the various methods of asset valuation.
3. Describe factors that contribute to the valuation of a practice's "goodwill."
4. Describe two common methods for valuing accounts receivable in practice transfers.
5. Briefly discuss the tax implications of practice assets for the buyer and seller.
6. Describe the method of valuing corporate practices.
7. Describe the three classes of assets purchased in practice sales.

Key Terms

book value
corporate ownership
fair market value
goodwill

intangible assets
minority interest discounts
practice price
practice value

replacement value
value and price

Goal

This chapter will provide guidelines for the dentist to use when evaluating a practice for purchase options. Factors that affect the practice's price will be discussed.

Business Basics for Dentists, First Edition. David O. Willis.
© 2013 John Wiley & Sons, Inc. Published 2013 by John Wiley & Sons, Inc.

Dental practices have a value for dentists who want to begin a practice. They can avoid start-up problems and gain an ongoing business, complete with patients and cash flow. The problem is to decide how much they will pay to buy an ongoing practice as compared to other professional options. In this sense, the actual price is irrelevant. So the wrong question to ask is "How much does the practice cost?" The right question is "How much will I make while I pay off the practice compared to other options?" If a practice is fairly valued, then a dentist can live comfortably while paying off the practice loan.

Why Value Practices?

There are several common reasons that dentists might want (or need) to set a value for a dental practice. Unfortunately, the most common is to figure out the value of common assets in a divorce settlement. As a rule, all assets gained in a marriage are common assets and spouses must divide the value in a divorce. (Some states consider them personal assets.) The dental practice is often an important and contentious marital asset to divide. A dentist may also want a value attached for buying (or selling) the entire practice or buying into a practice as an owning partner. The third common reason for valuing practices is for general financial and estate planning purposes. If, for example, a dentist wants to know how much retirement income to expect from the sale of a practice, he or she needs an accurate estimate of the value of the practice.

A dentist will probably use someone who is an expert in the field of practice valuation to help with setting a price and the practice transition. He or she will do this once or twice in a career. The experts do it many times a year. They know how to set reasonable values and how to find buyers and set up financing plans and tax compliance. The dentist should concentrate on his or her area of expertise, doing clinical dentistry, and hiring a consultant to use his or her expertise for the dentist.

General Rules of Practice Valuation

There are several general rules to remember when valuing practices.

Value Does Not Equal Price

The value of the practice is an estimate of the financial worth of a practice. The value, then, depends on the formulas used to determine the value. The price for the practice is determined by how badly the seller wants to sell and how badly the buyer wants to buy the practice. If a practice is in an isolated rural area, few people may be willing to move to and live in the area. The seller, in this case, would be much more willing to sell the practice for less than the financially determined value.

The Buyer Is Buying the Income Producing Capacity of the Practice

The buyer does not really buy dental chairs, handpieces, X-ray processors, or patient charts. What the dentist buys has the proven ability of the practice to make money. All of the assets are incidental to (though supportive of) that purpose. A practice that makes no profit has a value of zero (0). A buyer might purchase the physical assets, but there is no value placed for the ongoing concern of the practice. Gross production, then, is not a good determinant of the value of a practice. Net income as shown on tax returns is a much more useful determining factor. A common pitfall is the departing dentist who claims that the practice is really much more profitable because they have consistently taken a certain amount of cash per year out of the practice in unreported cash. The seller claims that the price should be much higher than the numbers warrant. The purchaser has no way of verifying these illegal activities, and so he or she has to disregard them in the valuation estimate.

The Practice Value Is the "Fair Market Value"

The IRS definition of fair market value (FMV) of any transaction is the "price that property would sell for on the open market. It is the price that would be agreed on between a willing buyer and a willing seller, with neither being required to act, and both having reasonable knowledge of the relevant facts" (IRS Pub 561). This says, essentially, the value is whatever the seller can get for it. The price paid becomes the value. The FMV is related to the motivation of both the buyer and the seller.

A Dentist Does Not Buy the Practice's "Potential"

A buyer purchases the expectation that the present, or historical, profits will be transferred to them. Future profits are uncertain and depend, largely, on the abilities of the buyer to improve the practice. Many new practitioners end up overpaying for practices based on the misguided belief that they should pay for the practice's potential. If a new dentist doubles the profit in a practice, he or she should reap the rewards of that increase, not the departing dentist. So a purchaser only buys the profits proved from the practice.

Methods of Valuing Assets

Several different methods help to determine the value of the various components of a practice. Each has strengths and weaknesses. The fairest method is the FMV. The FMV is an estimate of the willing buyer and willing seller method described previously. Another way of thinking of FMV is to think of an estimated price that someone would give at an auction, with interested, informed people participating in the auction. There are no "blue book" values. There are rules of thumb for determining FMV, some useful, some less so. Until the asset trades hands, the purchaser does not really know its value. *Replacement value* is the cost of replacing the equipment with a new, similar asset. This method overstates the value because the asset being sold generally is not new. Used assets need more repair and maintenance than new ones. A problem with this method is that there may not be a new similar asset to learn the value. Accountants often use the "book value" to calculate value of assets. Book value is the purchase price reduced by any depreciation or amortization charges taken against the asset. For example, a dentist has a dental chair that he or she bought new for $20,000. After 3 years, the dentist has taken $13,000 in depreciation expense. The value "on the books" (book value) is $7,000 ($20,000 − $13,000). The problem with this method is that it is determined, largely, by the method of depreciation used. This is determined by the IRS estimate of a "useful lifetime," which may bear only passing similarity to the actual useful lifetime of the asset. Some methods speed up the depreciation deduction for tax purposes. To solve these problems, some accountants use an "economic depreciation" figure, which tries to account for actual useful lifetimes and depreciation methods. Although better than a straight book value method, it is still subjective, although accountants claim that it is less so than appraisal methods. In the preceding example, the dental chair may have an actual useful lifetime (economic lifetime) of 15 years, although the IRS lets the owner depreciate it (for tax purposes) over 7 years. The "economic depreciation," based on a useful economic lifetime of 15 years, is 3/15 × $20,000 or $4,000. The "adjusted book value" of this asset, based on this economic depreciation then, is $16,000 ($20,000 − $4,000). If the adjusted book values of all the assets in the office is added up, an estimate of the value of the tangible practice assets can be derived. Similar calculations for financial assets, such as accounts receivable, can also be derived.

Four Asset Classes

In valuing practices, a value on each of four classes of assets may need to be placed (Box 27.1).

Physical (Tangible) Assets

These assets include in-place physical assets such as equipment (dental operatory and office), leasehold improvements, and furniture and fixtures. (This is usually a small part of the value of a practice.) Any of the methods can be used to value these assets, but the best is to have a reputable equipment dealer give an estimate of the FMV of the assets. Consumable supplies (inventories) can be valued by taking the purchase cost less useless supplies (taking into account shelf life). This is easy but time consuming. Another estimate of FMV of supplies is $5,000 per dentist. This is also a small part of the purchase price, so the dentist should not worry about it (i.e., do not count matrix bands). Placing a value on the leasehold improvements of the office is a disagreement in many practice purchases. Some advisors claim that leasehold improvements are a separate tangible asset and should be valued, either by appraisal or estimated through a useful lifetime of 20 (or 30) years. Most valuation experts claim that leasehold improvements are part of the ongoing concern value of a business and are, therefore, included in the value of the goodwill of the business.

Intangibles

These assets generally make up the largest part of the total value of a dental practice. Because they are intangible, they become difficult to value (Box 27.2). These

---

Box 27.1 Four types of assets

Physical (Tangible) Assets
  In-place physical assets
  Leasehold improvements
  Furniture and fixtures
  Consumable supplies
Intangible Assets
  Goodwill
  Restrictive covenants
  Ongoing concern value
Financial Assets
  Cash on hand
  Security deposits
  Accounts receivable
Real Estate
  Land
  Building

Box 27.2 Types of Intangible Assets

1. Goodwill
   a. Ongoing concern value
   b. Workforce in place
   c. Information base
   d. Know how
   e. Customer-based intangibles
   f. Supplier-based intangibles
   g. Franchise, trademark, or trade name
2. Covenant not to compete

Table 27.1 Value of Accounts Receivable

Status	Minimum Multiple	Maximum Multiple
Current	85%	90%
30–60 day	75%	85%
60–90 day	50%	75%
90–120 day	0%	30%
120+ day	0%	0%

assets are called "Section 197 Assets" because that section of the IRS code defines them and how they are treated from a tax perspective. All Section 197 assets are depreciated over 15 years, regardless of the actual or expected useful lifetime. Box 27.2 details these assets. Goodwill is the major intangible asset to be valued. It is an estimate of the expectation of future profits or transferability of the income generation of the practice. The more likely the income will transfer to a new owner, the higher the value of the goodwill for the practice. This obviously depends on the present owner of the practice, the new owner, the patient pool, and the other practitioners in the area. Other intangible assets, such as the use of the office telephone number, use of logos and letterhead, and right to patient records are included in the value for "ongoing concern" as a subset of goodwill. A restrictive covenant, or a covenant not to compete, is a separate asset in a practice transfer. Any restriction must describe the particular area and duration. They may have restrictions on solicitation of patients and staff ("nonsolicitation" clauses), and conditions of redress (what happens if the covenant is broken). These are used in both buy-in and buy-out situations. When valuing the ongoing concern value of the practice, include a reasonable (market) rate of rent as an expense because this affects practice profitability. The dentist should ensure that the lease will transfer to him or her for at least 5 years under similar terms as the seller. If not, the dentist should adjust the price downward.

Goodwill is generally the largest part of the value of a dental practice, often representing two-thirds to three-quarters the total value. These are many factors that go into the valuing of goodwill for a dental practice, but the single most important one is practice profitability. Often a smaller grossing practice that has higher profitability will be more valuable than a higher grossing practice that shows lower profitability. Some of the highest-producing practices may be the most difficult to sell because the prospective pool of buyers who can manage such a practice decreases as the value increases. The location of the practice may also affect goodwill value. Areas that are more competitive paradoxically command a higher price for a similar practice. This is because the buyer needs to buy patient pool in the more competitive area. In the less competitive area, the buyer does not need to buy the patient pool. If it is relatively easy to generate it, then there is no need to pay someone else for something that can be gotten for free.

The high proportion of value assigned to goodwill often leads to borrowing problems for prospective practice purchasers. Banks are under strict guidelines from regulatory bodies as to the amount and percentage that they can lend for unsecured and intangible assets. The bank may not be willing or able to lend the large amount required for a borrower to purchase a practice outright. Owner financing may be the only option to finance a large amount of goodwill.

Financial Assets

This type of asset is only valued if it changes hands. Many practice transfers do not involve any financial assets. If the sale does not include accounts receivable, then the buyer needs to borrow additional funds for working capital. Cash on hand is obviously valued dollar for dollar, as are security deposits.

The value of accounts receivable are often contentious. The problem is that the buyer must spend money to collect the account, in postage, paper supplies, and staff salaries. The older the account, the less likely that the buyer will collect anything from the account. So the accounts must be discounted from their face value to set an actual value. The question is how much to discount them. One common method is to use 80 percent of the value of all accounts 90 days old and less. All debt more than 90 days old is considered "bad" or uncollectible. More specifically, it will cost the dentist as much to collect these accounts as will be gained in their collection. Table 27.1 gives another common, though more complicated, accounts receivable valuation method. This second method looks at the age of the account and the historical collection effectiveness of the office to set a multiple for each age category of account. An office with an excellent history of collections (overall 98 to 99 percent) would be at the maximum multiple. An office at the other end of the scale (93 percent) would be at the low end of the multiple scale. (The two methods generally come out with similar values.)

To solve the dispute in the value of the accounts, transfers often require the seller to collect his or her own accounts receivable, using his or her own time, money, and resources. This effectively removes the accounts receivable from the purchase. Other transfers have the buyer collect the accounts as normal, allocating payments to the seller or buyer's account for a given time (often 90 days). After that, the buyer turns all uncollected accounts to the seller for whatever continued action the seller desires. Sometimes the buyer charges the seller a reasonable fee (e.g., 10 percent) as a cost of collections.

Real Estate

The final category of asset is real estate. Often the real estate is not part of the practice sale. If the practice leases office space, then obviously the seller cannot sell the real estate. (The seller may be able to transfer a lease at favorable rates to the buyer.) The owner may not want to sell the real estate, preferring instead to retain the property and gain rental income from the buyer. In either of these scenarios, the buyer should be sure that he can keep the lease with a favorable price and conditions for at least 5 years.

If the real estate is part of the practice sale, then a separate appraisal and loan is used for this class of asset. Real estate is easy to appraise. The loan for real estate is often easy to secure because it is a tangible asset.

Methods of Practice Valuation

Practice valuation is an inexact science at best. A comprehensive valuation uses several different methods to set values. Each method should begin to close in around a final value. There are four basic methods of valuation.

Summation of Assets Method

This method adds everything the practice owns (assets) and subtracts what it owes (liabilities) to set a value (Box 27.3). It answers the question "What things of value does this practice have that I would want to buy?" Tangible assets, such as equipment and supplies, are relatively easy to value. Most dental supply houses have people who are knowledgeable and capable to do this. If real estate is to be sold, the buyer can get an appraisal. Banks and real estate appraisers do this routinely. Accounts receivable (if they are sold) can also be valued,

---

Box 27.3 Summation of assets method

Value of equipment and supplies
+ Goodwill
+ Financial assets
+ Real estate
− Liabilities
Practice Value

Box 27.4 Profit capitalization method

$$VALUE = \frac{Entrepreneurial\ profit}{Capitalization\ rate}$$

Income risk-free interest rate
− Cost of services
+ Illiquidity premium
− Overhead
+ Risk specific premium
− Depreciation
− Other expenses
Capitalization rate
Profit before tax
− Taxes
"Entrepreneurial" Profit

---

based on the practice's collection history. The problem then becomes how to set the value of the intangible assets. There are several methods that are frequently applied to estimate goodwill value. These include variations on gross production and net income, often averaged over the past several years to account for practice growth or decline. A common (and useful method) is the weighted average of practice net income from the past 3 years. The value of leasehold improvements is generally included as a component in this estimate of goodwill, and so it is not valued separately.

Profit Capitalization Method

This method is commonly used to value other types of businesses. It compares the dental practice (or other business) to other investment opportunities (Box 27.4). It answers the question, "How much would a reasonable business person be willing to buy this practice for as an investment?" It did not ask how badly a dentist wanted to practice in this office. But if someone else were investing in this as a money-making venture, how much would he or she pay for it? It assumes that the owner would hire a dentist (maybe self) to produce the dentistry (cost of services), pay the bills, pay taxes, and then have some profit left over. This "entrepreneurial profit" is the result of business acumen and savvy management technique. That profit is then given a risk-adjusted investment value by dividing by the cost of money, or "capitalization rate." The actual computations take some understanding of finance principles, but the method is coming into more frequent use as business people enter the health care arena. This method is less useful in professional settings because the practice success is tied closely to the individual practitioner's reputation and abilities. The reputation and abilities do not automatically transfer to the new owner as other branded products or services do.

Comparable Sales Method

This method is often used to value houses and other real estate. If a dentist is looking at a three-bedroom house in a particular area of town, he or she looks at the price the other, comparable houses brought. Dentists can also find what other, similar practices sold for, and say that this practice should sell for a similar amount. The problem with this method is to determine a "comparable" practice. Many practice brokers and consultants belong to a trade organization that compiles all of the reported practice sales. This helps their members to determine comparable practices based on gross and net income, location, and many other factors. This method does not show if the cash flow supports the price (that takes another calculation) but does say what price the practice will probably sell for on the open market. A broker or advisor has access to the practice sales data. Often this is used to value the goodwill, with hard and financial assets valued separately.

Cash Flow Feasibility Method

This method gives an idea of the maximum a dentist could afford to pay for the practice or the maximum theoretical price for the practice (Box 27.5). It answers the question, "Can the practice meet normal business

---

Box 27.5 Cash Flow Feasibility Method

Professional income (revenue)
  – Normal business expenses
  – Taxes
  – Family budget expenses
  – Retirement plan contribution
Income available for debt service

---

expenses, produce a regular income for the family budget, pay taxes, provide future financial security, and have enough left over to service the debt?" If the answer is "yes," then the practice is fairly valued. This method depends on the prevailing interest rates, the finance terms, and the specific family income needs. Many people believe that this is not really a method of value a practice as it is a method of assuring the buyer of his or her choice. But it does ensure that the value makes economic sense.

Corporate Practices

The value of a practice is the same, regardless the form of business. (That is to say, a practice has the same value whether it is a corporation, a partnership, or a proprietorship.) However, there are a couple of special issues to consider when transferring corporate practices.

The ownership interest of a corporation is its stock. In the perfect world, the value of the total shares of stock should be the value of the practice. In the real world, dental practice shares often must be owned by dentists. No one openly trades them on the stock markets, so their value is difficult to set through normal supply and demand, open market methods. Shares of stock are neither depreciable nor deductible for the buying dentist. Instead, a capital gain or loss on the shares is realized only when they are sold, possibly many years in the future. For these reasons, most corporate practice sales do not place the full value of the practice into the shares of stock. Instead, some nominal value is given and the cost of the practice is made up to the seller through employment agreements or other methods of income transfer. This improves the tax advantages for the buying dentist.

If a dentist buys out or buys into a corporate dental practice, the new owner shares in not only the assets, but also in any corporate liabilities. For example, if a former employee sues for unjust dismissal, he or she sues the corporation, regardless who the present owners are. If there are unpaid tax liabilities or penalties, similar consequences occur. Consequently, buying dentists need to protect themselves from assumption of potential liabilities. There are two ways of doing this. One is to buy the assets of the practice from the corporation, leaving the corporate shell with the previous owner(s). Any undiscovered liabilities are then the responsibility of the original corporate owner. The previous owner can then dissolve the corporation when he or she chooses. (This method is generally used when buying out an existing corporation.) The new owner can then form a new corporation or operate as a proprietorship, as they choose. The second method, which is more frequent with buy-ins, involves a side contract in which the selling dentist agrees to be responsible for any undiscovered liabilities. This method is not as clean as the first because the

Table 27.2 Percentages of Referral By Specialty

Specialty	Percentage
Endodontist	95%
Oral surgeon	90%
Prosthodontist	80%
Periodontist	75%
Orthodontist	35%
Pediatric dentist	20%

Box 27.6 Tax Treatment of The Various Types of Assets

Seller
    Capital gain over basis
    Depreciation recapture
    Ordinary income
Buyer
    Deductible
    Depreciable over useful lifetime (hard assets)
    Amortizable over 15 years (Section 197 assets)

original owner can contest the details of the contract. Although this problem is not frequent, it can be significant when it happens.

Speciality Practices

Specialty practices are valued in much the same way that general practices are valued. However, the referral basis of many specialty practices makes their valuation problematic for many buyers. The more that a specialty practice depends on referrals, the lower its transferability of income generation is, and therefore, the lower its value. That is to say, if an endodontist depends on referrals as the lifeblood of a practice, most of those referrals were generated because of that practitioner's relationship to referring dentists. The generalists may not continue to refer patients if a new endodontist buys the practice. A buy-in is less of a problem in this regard because the new co-owner should retain most of the referral base and income generation. Time that the selling specialist remains with the practice to assure a smooth transition becomes important for the new practitioner.

Different specialties have different percentages of referral and self-generated business (Table 27.2). Most pediatric dental practices generate the vast majority of their patients the same ways that generalists do, through direct contact with the public. A small percentage is referred from other practitioners. Few people, on the other hand, call an endodontist because they need a root canal.

Tax Implications of Practice Sales

Tax laws change frequently. The tax implications of a practice purchase therefore also change frequently. The tax implications given here could change tomorrow. The dentist should have an accountant or tax attorney involved in any practice purchase. Box 27.6 gives a synopsis of the tax treatment of the various types of assets.

From the seller's perspective, there are two types of money received in a practice sale. One type is ordinary income and is subject to ordinary income tax. Depending on the seller's income tax bracket, that might be as high as 38 percent, plus any state income tax. The second type of money is a capital gain. Capital gains occur when a person buys a long-term asset (such as a dental chair) and then sells that asset for more than it is worth, thereby showing a gain on the capital investment. (There can also be a capital loss.) Capital gains are presently taxed a lower rate than ordinary income. In addition, capital gains are not earned income and so are not subject to self-employment or Social Security taxes. Sellers then would obviously prefer for the maximum amount of the sales price to be considered a capital gain.

One kink in this basic interpretation occurs when a seller has reported a substantial amount of depreciation on an asset. If, for example, a dentist purchased a dental chair for $10,000 and has claimed, over time, $7,000 as depreciation on the chair, he is now telling the IRS that the chair is worth $3,000. If he sells that chair for $5,000, he has made a capital gain of $2,000. Because the gain is a result of depreciation deduction, he must "recapture" that depreciation. The $2,000 is therefore considered ordinary income for tax purposes. Ordinary income is the more highly taxed type of income for the seller.

From the buyer's perspective, the money that is used to purchase a practice is two types of money (again, from a tax perspective). Some assets that are purchased, such as supplies, will be used up within 1 year. They are an immediate deduction for tax purposes. When a dentist first purchases a practice, he or she has many deductions. Often this results in using the tax deduction against income taxed at a lower (15 percent) rate. Some assets are long-term (capital) assets. The dentist can not deduct his or her cost immediately but must spread the cost over the useful lifetime of the asset and take the tax deduction through depreciation. Hard, tangible assets have shorter useful lifetimes (from 3 to 7 years). According to the IRS, all intangible assets (such as goodwill or restrictive covenants) have 15-year useful lifetimes. Buyers then are less concerned with the allocation of the sale price than the seller is but would generally prefer to have the maximum amount allocated to tangible assets to take the more rapid depreciation deduction.

Usually, the buyer and seller will come to an agreement on the total price for the practice. After that, they will negotiate how they will allocate the assets for tax purposes. Depending on how they structure the deal, usually they will characterize the soft assets as capital assets, and hard assets will be taxed as ordinary income. Sellers want to allocate more to goodwill because this is subject to capital gains tax rates, currently 15 percent for the seller. The IRS taxes hard assets as ordinary income (currently up to 35 percent) for the seller. Buyers want the opposite. More money allocated to hard assets allows the buyer to speed expense and shorter depreciation deductions (5 to 7 years). Goodwill amortization is spread out more than 15 years, slowing the deduction for the buyer. The objectives of the buyer and seller are then often at odds. Whatever amount is negotiated must be "reasonable," and reported to the IRS. The dentist must file that form with the IRS when a business is purchased, such as a dental practice. This form describes the assets transferred and what price was given to each of them. In that way, the IRS can check to be sure that both the buyer and seller have correctly declared the value and type of assets sold.

Securing Financing

A banker is a person who is willing to make a loan if you present sufficient evidence to show that you don't need it.
Herbert V. Prochnow

Objectives

At the completion of the chapter, students will be able to:

1. Define the common sources of loans for dentists.
2. Discuss these types of debt instruments with respect to the purposes, types, benefits, limitations, and uses for dental practitioners:
   Bank note
   Line of credit
   Promissory note
   Signature loan
   Installment loan
   Credit
   Mortgage
   Home equity loan
3. Define loan security and how it affects loans for dentists.
4. Describe the various types of interest rates.
5. Discuss the tax implications of debt for practitioners.
6. Describe how to control debt.

Key Terms

accounts payable
amortization
  installments
  amortization schedule
arm's length transaction
balloon payment
bank note
banks
business plan
collateral
consumer debt
  charge account
  credit
  credit cards
  line of credit
  debit card
cosigner
credit unions
debt-to-income ratio
down payment

first lien position
home equity loan
  after-tax interest rate
  marginal tax rate
  nontaxable interest rate
  personal debt interest
  real after-tax rates
  tax deductible
  taxable interest rate
installment loans
interest
  APR
  compound
  fixed rate
  interest rates
  prime
  principal
  simple
  term of the loan
  variable rate

interest-only payments
lien
lien holder
lines of credit
loan committee
loan security
mortgage
owner financing
payment schedules
private banking
pro forma financial statement
promissory note
qualifying for a loan
second mortgage
secured loan
signature loan
Small Business Administration
unsecured loans
working capital

Business Basics for Dentists, First Edition. David O. Willis.
© 2013 John Wiley & Sons, Inc. Published 2013 by John Wiley & Sons, Inc.

Goal

The purpose of this chapter is to understand the structure and use of various types of debt. Specific types of loans are discussed. Their use in personal and professional situations is detailed.

Table 28.1 Allowable Debt Levels

Type of debt	Rule of Thumb
Consumer debt	20% or less of gross monthly income
Housing costs	28% or less of gross monthly income
Total debt	36% or less of gross monthly income

Debt can be a valuable financial tool, allowing a person to purchase goods or assets he or she could not otherwise afford (Table 28.1). It can also be a huge drain on resources, especially if not managed properly. Usually, debt is used for large purchases (such as home or practice purchase) when obtaining the item for cash would be difficult or impossible. The problem is, assuming debt means that a person must pay interest, adding to the cost of the asset, and he or she must pay off the principal, reducing the funds that are available for other purchase or investment purposes.

Bankers and loan officers have several rules that they go by when qualifying a client for a loan (and, therefore, debt). These rules are not simply made up by the bankers; they are often required by the agencies that underwrite the loan. For example, the Federal National Mortgage Association (Fannie Mae) requires that total monthly payment on all debt should be no more than 36 percent of the family's gross monthly income. These debt payments include monthly housing costs, including taxes and interest, payments on installment credit, alimony, child support or maintenance payments, and any other payments on nonincome-producing property. Although some of these items (like taxes) are not really debt, they are a required periodic payment, and so lenders treat them as if they were debt.

Most professionals incur debt at some point in their career. Generally, this is during the initial phases, when practices, houses, and new automobiles are bought. Often professionals enter the marketplace with a large amount of preexisting debt needed to finance their education. This student debt may be so large that it impairs their ability to secure additional personal or professional loans. Most bank loan officers understand the large potential earning power of professionals and work to develop them as clients.

Box 28.1 Example Bank Loan

Dr. Jones buys a dental practice, securing an installment note for the amount shown. Her annual (estimated) payments are given. This shows only annual estimates. Loans are actually amortized monthly.

Principal = $400,000
Term = 7 years
Rate = 9.0%

Year	Total payment	Principal	Interest	Remaining principal
1	77,228	42,971	34,256	357,500
2	77,228	47,002	30,225	310,497
3	77,228	51,412	25,816	259,086
4	77,228	56,234	20,993	202,851
5	77,228	61,510	15,718	141,342
6	77,228	67,784	9,443	68,179
7	77,228	74,062	3,637	0
	$540,593	$400,000	$140,593	0

As professionals move through their professional lifetime, the need for debt usually declines, as loans are paid off and assets are accumulated. So it is during the first several years that managing debt become crucial. Mistakes made early in a career can haunt a person financially for many years.

Sources of Loans

Banks are the best-known source of loans for the professional. However, there are many other potential sources of funds. Each has specific advantages and disadvantages.

Banks

Banks are the most common source of funds for new practice loans. Bankers are in the business of lending money to people that they think will repay it. So a dentist will need to convince the banker that he or she will repay the loan (Box 28.1).

There are two types of banks, national and local. National banks have an entire division dedicated to working with professionals. A dentist will work with a special internal group called "private banking." The private banking section manages small business and other special banking concerns. Large banks may have people within their private banking group that manage only professional (or even only dental) practice loans. These people are knowledgeable about practice financing issues. The dentist may need to establish all professional (and often personal) bank accounts within the private banking section. However, it works well because the banker will know the dentist personally. Local banks, on the other hand, are variable as to their understanding of dental office finance. Some small banks do not have private banking sections. Instead, a dentist may need to educate the banker about the specific problems faced by dental practices. (Bankers do not like to take risks they do not understand.) The larger local banks have private banking sections and individuals who service professional clients. Many of these people are also knowledgeable and helpful.

Owner Financing

Many professional practices finance some portion of the cost through the previous owner. If the bank is unwilling to lend the entire amount, then the owner may finance the remainder of the purchase price. The seller does this by allowing the buyer to pay part of the price over time to the owner, rather than the lending institution. The seller will generally charge a comparable interest rate and require a promissory note, which details all of the terms of the loan. Owner financing carries additional risk for the owner over simply getting the entire purchase price as cash up front. If the buyer runs the practice into the ground, becomes disabled, dies, or is unable, for any reason to pay off the loan, the owner may not receive the entire purchase price. Generally, the bank will require a first lien position on all tangible (hard) assets of the practice, which means that it gets to sell the assets to satisfy its. So the owner may be left holding an empty bag. This may be the only way that the owner can sell the practice for the price that he or she wants. If so, then the buyer can expect to pay the owner a reasonable interest (comparable to a bank rate) for the portion that is financed. The buyer may need to finance the down payment through a bank and arrange the rest of the purchase price as owner financing to make the buyout work.

Dental Supply Companies

Most of the major national supply companies (e.g., Patterson, Sullivan-Schein, Benco) have arrangements with banks or finance companies that allow the dentist to borrow money to establish a professional practice. There is an obvious advantage for the supplier (the dentist buys equipment and supplies through them). The advantage for dentist is that he or she may qualify for financing through these organizations when he or she may not qualify at the local bank. The down side is that the dentist often pays a higher interest rate than he or she would at the local bank. The finance company may also have significant prepayment penalties and other disadvantageous loan clauses. The dentist generally must buy his or her equipment through the particular supply company as well. Some only finance new practices, not buy-outs of existing practices. Others only offer financing for equipment purchases or upgrades. However, these companies know the dental marketplace, and if a dentist is unable to gain financing through a bank, they may offer a method of financing the establishment of his or her practice.

Family Members

The dentist may be fortunate enough to have family members who have sufficient assets to lend him or her for practice or personal needs. If this is the case, the dentist should structure the loans as an "arm's length" transaction. This means that this is a bona fide business transaction, similar to what another would negotiate at arm's length, or without the benefit of the family ties. The IRS considers family loans to be partly a gift if they are not negotiated at arm's length. This infers a definite interest rate and pay back schedule.

A more common occurrence than an outright loan is the case in which a family member guarantees the security of a loan by pledging assets or cosigning a loan for the young professional. Here, the family member has not provided the direct funds but has agreed to pay the cost of the loan if the borrower defaults and is unable to pay.

Mortgage Companies

Previously, the professional has used mortgage companies primarily when purchasing a home. They generally have not entered into the commercial loan market. In the past several years, mortgage companies that cater to young professionals have emerged. They have found a niche in lending to professionals who are establishing their practices. Many of these clients have high student and other personal debt and so do not qualify for traditional bank loans. They are still good long-term lending risks because of their high expected incomes. Traditional banks may be unable to lend money to these people because of banking regulations. However, the finance companies are not under the same guidelines. They may charge a higher interest rate and include prepayment

Table 28.2 Sweat Equity

Buy-in Details			No Buy-In		With Buy-In	
			Owner	Associate	Owner	Associate
Cost	$400,000	Collections	$600,000	$300,000	$600,000	$300,000
Term	7 Years	Payment for Service	$200,000	$100,000	$200,000	$100,000
Interest	6%	Equity Buy-In			$70,121	–$70,121
Payment/Month	$5,843	Business Profit	100,000	0	50,000	50,000
Payment/Year	$70,121	Total Compensation	$300,000	$100,000	$320,121	$79,879

This example assumes the associate will buy-in for the given amount. The associate will become an immediate equal owner. Providers receive 33% of production as compensation. Business profit is divided equally among owners. When the buy-in is complete, the equity payment ends.

penalties that make these loans less attractive when compared to a traditional bank. Despite these shortcomings, many young professionals are using them as a source of start-up financing.

Small Business Administration (SBA)

The SBA is an agency of the federal government whose charge is to help developing businesses secure start-up financing. They do not actually provide the loan proceeds but instead guarantee the loan through a local bank or lending agency. Usually, two or more banks must have turned a person down for a traditional business loan. A dentist may then contact an SBA officer who may help arrange financing. Often, the SBA will only guarantee a loan for a start-up, rather than a buy-out (because the latter is not really a new business). The SBA often requires substantial down payments that young professionals can not make. There is a considerable amount of paperwork involved in securing these loans. Some banks will not work with them. Because the federal government funds them, the borrower is subject to the whims and attitudes of Congress and other governmental bodies. Availability and rules change constantly. Some young professionals have found success in this source of loans. Dentists should not count on them as the best opportunity for practice finance.

Sweat Equity

Sweat equity occurs when a dentist works for another dentist, taking less pay but building up an equity or ownership position in the practice. The dentist shifts the decreased salary to the seller who takes the amount given up as additional compensation. The practice is valued and an imputed loan (with interest, term, principal, and possible down payment) is developed. These arrangements occur more frequently in buy-in situations. There are substantial risks for the owner–dentist in this arrangement.

The purchasing dentist may decide during the buy-in that he or she does not like or want the practice. He or she may not be able to handle the load. Or the purchasing dentist might decide that he or she does not need to pay extra for this practice because he or she can easily start his or her own. Because of these risks, these arrangements are tightly structured (from the seller's perspective), which leave the buyer little room to change their mind. Table 28.2 gives an example of a sweat equity buy-in.

Credit Unions

Credit unions are similar to banks and savings and loans, except they serve a specific clientele (e.g., teachers, public employees, dental association members). Their loans are usually for smaller personal purchases (automobiles, boats etc.), rather than for business purposes. Credit unions often offer better interest rates than traditional bank loans, but they generally do not finance large business loans.

Credit Cards

Every time that a consumer makes a credit card purchases, he or she essentially borrows the money from the issuing card's bank. Depending on the conditions associated with the card, there may be no interest accrued until the payment due date. Any balance left unpaid is subject to interest, often nearing 2 percent per month on the unpaid balance. (This is equivalent to approximately 24 percent per year.) Credit card debt is ab expensive way to borrow money.

Effect on Credit Rating

A persons' credit history affects whether he or she qualifies for a loan and the interest rate charged for the loan. A credit score is generally used as the indicator of a

Table 28.3 Credit Rating Impacts Interest Rate and Total Payments over the Lifetime of a Loan

Credit Score	Interest Rate	Monthly Payment	Total Loan Cost
720+	5.55%	$856	$173,438
675–699	6.21%	$920	$194,063
620–674	7.36%	$1,034	$230,000

Difference = $56,562
Example: $150,000 principal, 30-year mortgage.

credit rating. It is based on past use of credit and history of paying it back in a timely manner. The higher a credit score, the better a credit risk a person is, and the lower the interest rate a banker is going to charge because they are surer that the person will repay the loan. Table 28.3 shows how a change in credit rating can make a huge difference in interest rate and total payments over the lifetime of a loan. Before asking for a loan, the dentist should check his or her credit rating and repair any problems in his or her credit history before applying for the loan.

Types of Professional Debt

Debt incurred by professionals typically is in one of the following forms.

Bank Note

A bank note is the normal type of credit extended to professionals for business purposes. Bank notes are generally based on compound interest and amortized as in other compounded loans.

Lines of Credit

Often, a borrower is unsure exactly how much money he or she needs to borrow and when he or she will need it. Bankers solve this problem by establishing a line of credit. A line of credit allows a person to borrow up to a certain amount of money any time that he or she decides it is needed. It is essentially a prearranged loan that does not start until the borrower uses the money. For example, when a dentist starts a practice, he or she makes an estimate of cash needs. Depending on the accuracy of cash flow projections, he or she might need more or less cash to pay the bills at any given time. Rather than borrowing a set amount (e.g., $20,000) and beginning interest payments on the entire balance immediately, the dentist will generally establish a line of credit, so that he or she will only borrow as much as is needed, when it is

needed. If he or she uses $5,000 the first month, then he or she is charged interest on only $5,000. The remaining $15,000 (of the initial $20,000) remains for the person to borrow when needed. It is in the bank, waiting, but not being charged interest.

Promissory Note

A promissory note is an agreement between two people, saying that one agrees, or promises, to pay a certain debt to the other. In the professions, promissory notes are often seen in practice purchases in which the owner finances all, or a part of the purchase price. As a separate contract from the contract to purchase the practice, the seller will usually require the purchaser to sign a promissory note, which sets the terms for the payment of the principal and interest.

Signature Loan

As mentioned previously, a signature loan is secured only by a signature and promise to pay the entire loan. It is generally used for short duration loans (1 year or less) in which the borrower has an immediate cash need. Bankers will usually give signature loans to customers that have shown they have an excellent repayment history and then only for limited amounts.

Accounts Payable

An amount that is owed to someone else is an account payable. For example, if a dentist orders several hundred dollars worth of dental supplies and the supplier send a bill, the dentist has agreed to pay that debt. When the merchandise is accepted, the dentist owes the vendor for the supplies. The dentist has an account payable until the account is paid in full. If the dentist does not pay it by the stipulated time, the vendor may charge interest or a service charge. Charges that are made on a professional credit card for meals, entertainment, or other professional expenses are considered a form of an account payable.

Tax Implications of Debt

The way that the federal tax code views debt affects the cost of debt and how to manage debt. The IRS views the interest on certain types of debt to be tax deductible. Notice that this is only the interest portion of the debt payment and only for certain types of debt.

The types of interest presently considered tax deductible include home mortgages, second mortgages, business

Box 28.2 Tax Implications of Debt

Nontaxable (tax-deductible interest) debt
Consumer
1. Home mortgage
2. Mortgage on second home (e.g., vacation)
3. Home equity loan
4. Certain student loans

Business
1. Business debt interest (including rental property)
2. Business credit interest
3. Certain investment interest

Taxable (nontax–deductible interest) debt
Consumer
1. Credit cards
2. Automobile loans
3. Certain student loans

Business
All business interest (that is a bone fide cost of doing business) is *deductible* (not taxable)

Table 28.4 Real After-Tax Rates

Tax bracket					
Interest rate	0%	15%	28%	33%	40%
8%	8%	6.8%	5.8%	5.4%	4.8%
9%	9	7.7	6.4	6.0	5.4
10%	10	8.5	7.2	6.7	6.0
11%	11	9.4	7.9	7.4	6.6
12%	12	10.2	8.6	8.0	7.2
13%	13	11.0	9.4	8.7	7.8
14%	14	11.9	10.1	9.4	8.4

"Tax bracket" is the marginal tax rate. This is the percentage of tax paid on the next dollar earned. It consists of federal, state, and local income taxes.

loans, business credit interest, certain student loans, and certain investment interest expenses. Most personal debt interest is not tax deductible. This includes credit card interest, personal lines of credit, auto loan interest, and any other personal loans. (Tax law is under the control of Congress. These lists may change anytime.) Box 28.2 summarizes these categories.

The important element of deductibility of interest is the resulting, after-tax interest rate. By allowing the deduction of the interest portion of the payment, the federal government, in essence, pays part of the interest. Assume that a person is in a 33-percent marginal tax bracket (that is to say, 33 percent of the next dollar earned will go to taxes). If that person has $1,000 in interest payments that is deducted from income before paying taxes, the taxable income by is lowered by $1000 and taxes are paid on that lower income. In fact, that person saves $330 (33 percent of $1000).

In other words, the $1000 of interest actually only cost $670 ($1000 – $330). This decreases how much tax is paid, which in turn affects the actual after-tax rate that is paid.

Real after-tax Rates

Real interest rates, after-tax consideration, then depends on the nominal rate and the marginal tax rate of the individual. Table 28.4 gives common combinations of interest rates and marginal tax rates. A table such as this one helps to make the comparison of dissimilar loans or investments much easier.

Negoitiating with Lenders

Bankers are in the business of lending money. However, they want to lend to people that they believe will repay their loans as agreed. So a banker will naturally ask many questions and gather much information to "qualify" a person for a loan (or to decide whether he or she is a good loan risk). The borrower should show the banker that he or she knows what he or she is doing from a business perspective so that the banker will be more comfortable with the loan. The borrower will probably need a formal practice valuation done by a reputable consultant, cash flow projections, and often a complete business plan. (Developing a business plan is covered in another chapter.) The banker may have specific items, such as tax returns and the seller's tax returns from the past 3 years, that are wanted in addition. These are not simply hoops to jump through. The banker must take the loan application to the bank's loan committee to gain approval. Maybe the banker does not understand professional practices or a particular arrangement. More than likely, he or she does. The borrower should listen to the banker. If he or she does not believe that the borrower can finance a practice at a given price and make it work, he or she should seriously reconsider the potential arrangement.

Most of the issues discussed in this chapter are negotiable. That is to say, the lender has some discretion in setting the rates, terms, and conditions of a loan. However, the banker must also gain approval for the loan from the bank's loan committee. This is a group of senior bank officers who act as a supervisory board, making the final decision on whether or not a loan is acceptable, from the bank's point of view. Because the banker must represent the borrower in this meeting, the borrower should provide the bank as much positive information as possible. The bank might ask the borrower to develop pro forma financial statements or a complete business plan. Other times the loan application process may be a mere formality. If a person is buying into the practice of a family member who is a longstanding, excellent customer of the bank (and will cosign the loan), the borrower may only need to complete a few forms to qualify for a loan.

A borrower might negotiate the specific conditions of the loan. It is common practice to negotiate "interest only" for the first 6 months to a year. This means that the borrower only needs to pay interest on the loan, or even let the interest accumulate on the loan. This decreases payments in the first, critical portion of the loan, when start-up costs are high and the cash flow may be at the lowest. If the dentist does not purchase accounts receivable, he or she will need to negotiate a line of credit for "working capital." The borrower might negotiate variable rates, longer term, or even lower interest rates. His or her bargaining position depends on the history with the bank and how much the bank wants to gain the borrower as a long-term customer. If the borrower has presented a loan request to other banks or financial institutions, he or she might even be in the position of having one bank match or exceed another bank's offer to gain the business.

The bank may not lend the borrower the entire amount of the purchase price of a practice. Instead, the bank may require that the borrower pay part of the total purchase price as a down payment. (Common amounts are 10 to 25 percent of the total purchase price.) This ensures that the person has a personal stake in the practice. Bankers assume that the borrower might work a little harder and be a little more serious about the practice if he or she has some of his or her own money at stake. If the borrower does not have the money or assets for a down payment, he or she might convince the seller to lend the down payment in the form of a "second mortgage" or owner financing. The borrower might also have a parent or other family member cosign a loan or pledge specific assets to secure the loan, and by that, qualifying the borrower for the loan.

At larger banks, professionals usually deal with a bank employee in the private banking section. Private banking is the division of the bank that works with wealthy clients. (The starting dentist may not be wealthy yet, but the bank expects that he or she will be.) Few professional practices file bankruptcy, and few professionals default on loans. Private banking is much more personal than public banking. The dentist will have a specific loan officer assigned to his or her case. The

---

Box 28.3 Loan Factors

1. Meet normal business expenses?
2. Produce an income for the family?
3. Service student loans?
4. Service the practice debt?
5. Pay taxes?
6. Provide future financial security?

---

dentist can often work with the specific loan officer if cash flow or tax problems develop in the practice. Some banks extend additional credit for the purchase of a home or other consumer purchases through private banking. In return, the bank usually expects that the dentist will maintain personal and professional accounts with that bank.

Different banks place different importance on loan factors (Box 28.3). Many bankers value cash flow above all else. They want to be sure that the borrower will have enough cash flowing through the practice to pay the practice's bills, service the debt, pay taxes, and support a family (including student loan payments). If the dentist can show the cash flow, then the loan is a good one. Others require a down payment to ensure that the borrower has some "skin in the game." Others may require a formal business plan. Some will look at production history to be sure that the dentist can handle a practice of the size being contemplated. Still others place a high value on collateral and loan security. Bankers that understand dental practices realize the high load of student debt many graduates carry. They will look at the cash flow (especially within a family budget) to ensure that the practice can support this payment as well.

Bankers will look at the use of the loan differently. If the dentist is using the proceeds for a practice purchase, they will generally secure the hard assets through a lien (Box 28.4). The soft assets can not be secured by a lien. Instead, the banker may ask for other security (such as a consigner). Similarly, working capital is not secured. Most practice loans will include a line of credit for working capital wrapped into the overall loan package. If a dentist is borrowing money to purchase real estate along with the practice (e.g., an office condominium), the bank will usually make a separate loan for the real estate portion. The bank may require 10 to 20 percent of the value as down payment. The bank generally extends this loan over a longer period (such as 20 years) to match the lifetime of the asset and lower the monthly payment. This is a secure loan because the banker files a lien on the real estate until the loan is paid in full.

Box 28.4 Considerations for Loans

1. Personal Financial Statements
   a. Balance sheet — Required
   b. Family income statement — Usually required
   c. Past year's tax returns — If appropriate
2. Practice Financial Statements
   a. Formal practice appraisal — Required if buy-in or buy-out
   b. List of assets to be bought — Required
   c. Pro forma cash flow — Usually required
   d. Pro forma income statement — Occasionally required
3. Other Practice Information
   a. Past tax statements (3 years) — Required if buy-out or buy-in
   b. Partnership agreement — Required if buy-in
   c. Lease — Usually required
4. If Buying the Real Estate
   a. Real estate contract — Required
5. If Doing a Cold Start
   a. Contractor's estimate for build out — Usually required
6. If a Cosigner Is Needed
   a. Cosigner's personal financial statement — Required
   b. Cosigner's credit report — Bank will do this
7. Other Forms
   a. Loan application — Depends on the bank
   b. Business plan — Nice to have, often required
   c. Credit report — Bank will do this

The Business Plan

It's not the plan that is important, it's the planning.
Dr. Graeme Edwards

Objectives

At the completion of this chapter, the student will be able to:
1. Describe the typical process that banks go through when evaluating a loan application.
2. Describe the information that loan officers will require for loan processing:
   Loan application
   Personal balance sheet
   Pro forma income statement
   Cash flow analysis
   Business plan
3. Define the sequence of investigation of practice opportunities.
4. Define the more important factors used in evaluation of the economic state of a community.
5. Define the more important factors used in evaluation of the worth of a dental practice.
6. Describe the typical series of events in negotiating a practice transition.

Key Terms

business plan

cash flow analysis

Goal

The purpose of this chapter is to prepare students to effectively interact with bankers, loan officers, and other representatives of financial institutions during the practice transition process.

Business Basics for Dentists, First Edition. David O. Willis.
© 2013 John Wiley & Sons, Inc. Published 2013 by John Wiley & Sons, Inc.

Starting and running a successful dental practice has never been easy. In the volatile and competitive marketplace the profession now faces, this task has become even more difficult. One common trait of all successful dentists (and small business people generally) is that they have a solid plan of what they want to do with the business. A dentist's financial, personal, and emotional energies will be tied to the success or failure of his or her practice. The dentist will invest a lot of his or her soul into a dental practice. The sad truth is that some dental practices never succeed or only barely "scrape by." Many of these unsuccessful dental practitioners are there by their own devices; they have simply failed to plan the small business adequately. Particularly during these competitive economic times, trying to start a business without a plan is akin to going to sea without a chart or compass. Rational people would want to know where they are going, whether sailing the ocean or the financial seas. A business plan is a chart of a dentist's practice voyage. It is a plan of where he or she wants to go or what he or she hopes to accomplish with the business.

Most new dental practitioners will need to secure some financing from a bank or other lending institution. Bankers are in the business of lending money to people that will repay them. One of the best ways to help convince a loan officer that a person is a good business risk is to present a business plan with a loan application. Much of the information that is required in the loan application is also included in the business plan, so the additional work is not as formidable as it first appears.

Strictly speaking, a business plan is a document that is a dentist uses to project the future performance of the practice. It begins with general statements and conditions and moves through a more detailed explanation, ending with numbers that the dentist projects to represent the financial outcomes of the practice, based on previous conditions. The process of developing the business plan is important for more than just the pieces of paper that result. The dentist learns about his or her business through the process of writing the plan. This is where the dentist writes down concisely what he or she expects his or her financial health to be in a year and why. So developing a business plan forces the dentist to decide in an organized way, rather than just letting things happen and responding to them in a crisis fashion. The banker, or loan officer, then will be interested to see that the dentist has thought out these problems, determined solutions, and committed them to paper. He or she may have specific forms that the bank needs to be completed to process the loan application. Once the business plan is completed, the borrower will generally only need to shift information from one form to the other. The additional work is well worth the effort when the bank approves the loan!

The format of the business plan given here is an adaptation of the standard business plan format used for any small business. Many bank loan officers, especially in rural areas, may never have processed a dental practice loan. This business plan format makes a special focus on dental practices. Often the dentist's job, as applicant, will be to educate the banker to the special business needs that the dentist, as a practice owner will have. The banker, or loan officer, usually can not make the final decision on a loan. Instead, he or she must take the package of information that has been developed to the bank's loan committee, which is composed of senior bank officers, owners, or board members. They are the ones who make the final decision on a loan. The loan officer is the borrower's spokesperson in this process. The chances of a dentist gaining a loan under favorable terms will obviously increase if the loan officer is in his or her corner. The best way that a dentist can do that is by showing the loan office that he or she has done background work, is well prepared, and has provided all of the information that will be needed to represent the dentist in front of the loan committee.

The Written Part of the Plan

The written part of the business plan or loan application details the information and ideas the dentist has developed when considering a possible practice opportunity. The overall purpose of the plan is to convince the banker (or other lending entity) that the dentist and dental practice are a good place for the bank to invest its money. The plan should lead the bankers down a logical path that shows the reader that the dentist will use their money wisely and that the borrower is likely to repay as agreed. The dentist should anticipate any significant questions a lender might have about the application or plan and answer them before he or she asks them. The dentist should be absolutely honest in the planning process. If there is a significant potential problem in the business, the borrower should bring it in the open and offer potential solutions. If he or she lies about or tries to hide a problem, the bankers will probably reject the whole application. Bankers understand that there are many problems involved in running a business; they are primarily interested in knowing that the dentist understands them and has a good idea how to craft a solution to the problem.

The following section gives a brief idea of what should be in each section of the written plan. A more detailed description and checklist will appear in subsequent sections.

A. **The Cover Sheet** The cover sheet identifies the applicant and the institution or organization from whom the dentist is asking for funds. This sheet also gives contact numbers so that the banker or lender knows how to reach the dentist.

B. **Table of Contents** The table of contents gives the reader the overall organization and locating specific sections of the plan.

C. **Statement of Purpose** The statement of purpose may be the most important single page in the document. It tells the reader, in a paragraph or two, why the dentist is applying for this loan.

D. **Description of the Community** The description of the community defines the area in which the dentist is planning to establish a practice. A dental practice is a small business and will respond to economic variables like any other small business. This section describes those variables and the planned response to them. The dentist should show that he or she has "done homework" regarding the background of the community. If there are problems in the local economy, then those should be noted along with the strengths that are seen in the business climate of the area.

1. **Demographic Considerations** Demographic considerations in the community include all of the "numbers" that have gone into the decision to locate in the area. These include the population, age and income distributions, location of the town or city, per capita savings rates, or other specific numbers that the dentist believes will have an impact on the small business.

2. **Economic Considerations** Economic considerations are similar to demographics and are often included in that section. This section should describe economic factors that the dentist believes will lead to the success of the practice. The major employers in the area, the amount and type of third-party coverage, and projected housing and industrial growth are all economic factors that will influence the business.

3. **Competition** The dentist should detail competition in the area, concerning numbers and types of practitioners. If some are practicing part-time, then an adjustment for full-time equivalents is in order. These numbers should be compared with national, regional, or state averages to give the reader a better frame of reference.

E. **Description of the Practice (Business)** The previous section has given the reader an overview the practice's geographic and economic base. This section gives specific information regarding the practice opportunity. If a dentist is purchasing an ongoing practice, he or she should use the existing operation as a basis for the practice, describing any modifications that he or she plans to make in operations. If this is a new practice, national averages or prevailing methods of operation are in order. A banker probably understands general business concepts and problems very well; however, he or she may be ignorant of the specifics of dental practice administration. The dentist may need to use this section as an educational tool for the banker or loan officer.

1. **Nature of the Profession** Dentistry has opportunities and problems that are specific to the particular industry. For example, how does dental service marketing differ from fast-food or dry cleaner marketing? What causes patient loyalty and how does the dentist hope to gain the loyalty of the existing patients? These professional business considerations about dentistry need to be addressed to help the banker understand the problems will be faced in the business.

2. **Overall Strategy** This section should briefly describe the overall strategy the dentist plans to take in running the business. This is where the dentist should describe where he or she plans to take the practice in 5 or 10 years. Does the dentist plan to use aggressive marketing efforts, increasing patient visits, or raise fees, thereby increasing revenues in the short run? Is the dentist going to base the practice on new patient visits or on periodic maintenance (i.e., recall) visits? Does the dentist plan to bring in a partner or an associate in the future? If this is presently a successful practice, the overall strategy may be to maintain the success previously proved. How is the dentist going to do that?

3. **Marketing** The market section describes who the potential (and existing) patients are, how many of them there are, and how the dentist plans to appeal to their wants and needs.

4. **Location** Location is one primary factor in business success or failure. The dentist should describe the location of the particular practice opportunity and any strengths and weaknesses from that particular location. If this is a new practice, the dentist should describe why he or she chose this location for the business.

5. **Operations** This section explains how the dentist will run the practice on a day-to-day basis. The dentist should let the banker see that he or she has a realistic idea of the numbers and types of patients that are needed to be successful in the practice.

6. **Personnel** The dentist should describe the types of personnel he or she is going to need to accomplish his or her strategy. The dentist should also state how much qualified employees will need to

be paid. He or she should be sure to include the legal implication of the duty delegation laws of the particular state.

F. **Description of the Applicant** This is where the dentist lets the banker know about him or her. The dentist should strive to show himself or herself as knowledgeable and responsible and the kind of person to loan money to!

1. **Professional Qualifications** The dentist should list his or her professional history in this section. If he or she has received any scholastic or clinical awards, they should be highlighted here. If he or she has worked in dental offices after school hours or during an extramural rotation or have other nondental, business experience it should be emphasized here.

2. **Personal Information** Personal information is an important factor for the loan officer to consider. A family can be an asset, in that it shows a permanence and commitment that a single person may not have. The single person, on the other hand, must prove that he or she is stable and plans to make the practice a lifelong commitment. A loan officer will be reluctant to give money to someone who may be pursuing practice on a whim or a trial basis.

G. **Application and Expected Effect of Loan** This section tells where the dentist anticipates getting funding and it will be spent on. If the dentist has other sources of money, they should be highlighted in this section. These factors will be critical for the banker to decide if he or she wants to "invest" the bank's money in the business venture. However, this section should be just as important for the dentist because he or she is investing not only personal money, but also his or her time, life, and soul in the venture. The dentist also needs to be confident that he or she will be successful.

1. **Sources and Amounts of Funding Required** This section describes how much money is required to begin the business and make it profitable and where it is going to come from. One commonly used source of money is owner financing. If a dentist will have a family member or another person cosign the loan, it should be noted here. Bankers generally like to see the dentist have an investment in the practice as well. If the dentist does not personally have assets to pledge, then the next best thing is for the family to pledge assets as collateral.

2. **Uses of Funds** This section is often combined with the previous one. It describes what the dentist plans to spend the money on, the assets that will be bought, and the expenses that will be paid with the secure financing.

The Financial Part of the Plan

The financial part of a business plan quantifies the ideas that the dentist has presented in the written part of the plan. Businesses (and bankers) use several standard formats when evaluating the financial health of the practice and the applicant. The following section gives a brief synopsis of the various forms that will need to be developed to present to a banker. The dentist will generate most of these using a spreadsheet program.

A. **Personal Financial Considerations**

Personal financial considerations are especially important if the dentist plans to operate the business (practice) as a proprietorship or partnership because in these forms of business, the dentist is personally liable for any business debts. If the dentist is planning to incorporate the practice, the banker will probably ask to personally pledge assets for any financing above the corporation's hard assets. After all, the bank needs to protect itself in case the dentist defaults on the note payments.

1. **Personal Balance Sheet** The personal balance sheet takes the familiar form of Assets − Liabilities = Net Worth. The dentist will need to sign a balance sheet to make it "official." Anyone cosigning a loan (pledging assets as collateral) also needs to send the lending institution a balance sheet as well.

2. **Family Budget** The banker will want to know how much money the dentist needs to support a family. This logically affects how much money the dentist plans to take from the practice monthly. If the dentist is the sole support for a family with children, this will obviously be more than if he or she is childless with a working spouse. The dentist is attempting this venture to provide for the family's well being; this is the place to detail those needs. The dentist should include any upcoming loan payments (such as student loans) that will become due when he or she is out of school.

B. **Professional Financial Considerations** The dentist's professional financial considerations show what he or she expects the practice to generate in the future. A pro forma statement is one that estimates what the given form will look like as of some future date.

1. **Financial Analysis of Present practice** (if any) If the dentist is purchasing an existing practice, he or she should analyze the last 3 years (if available) of Schedule C (Profit or Loss from a Business) or the corporate equivalent. The dentist should point out any particular strengths or weaknesses in the schedules, showing any changes that he or she plans to make.

2. **Professional Capital Equipment List** Capital equipment is the aggregate of the tools and equipment the dentist is buying so that he or she can practice. These are hard assets. Generally, the dentist will pledge them as collateral for the loan to buy them. A large part of the value of many dental practices is the soft-asset base of the practice. These include a restrictive covenant, goodwill, and other nontangible items of value. The dentist can not pledge them as assets because there is really nothing the banker can repossess and resell in the event the dentist defaults on his or her loan payments. The dentist should list all of the assets of the practice in this section. If he or she is purchasing an ongoing practice and has had the practice valued, the dentist should include the professional valuation as an appendix to the plan, giving a brief synopsis in this section.

3. **Cash Flow Estimate** Cash flow differs from an income statement in one important aspect, in that it takes into account only cash expenditures and income. In this sense, it is essentially a checkbook register rather than a tax-expense statement because it records cash money taken in and spent. Bankers are interested to see that the cash flowing through the practice will support the expenditures. Cash flow projections are also important for determining how much working capital a dentist will need to arrange in the bank loan.

4. **Pro Forma Income Statement (optional at banker's request)** The pro forma income statement shows what the dentist thinks an income statement will be in the upcoming years. These pro forma statements are only as accurate as the data used for the projection. However, the dentist should strive to make them as accurate as possible for both the banker's information and his or her own peace of mind. Like the pro forma balance sheet, the income statement is generally initiated for the calendar year, to make it compatible with tax returns. This means that, if a dentist buys a practice beginning July 1, then the initial period will be only 6 months. After that, the dentist will be on an annual, calendar basis.

Checklist for Business Plan and Loan Application

I. Written part of the plan

A. Cover sheet
   1. What is the name of the practice?
   2. Who is this plan or application going to?
   3. How does the banker get in contact with the borrower?
   4. Who are the "principals"?

B. Table of contents
   1. Do the entries on this page correspond with the sections of the document?
   2. Are the page numbers correct?
   3. Have all referenced material included in the appendix?

C. Statement of purpose
   1. What is the overall mission of the practice or business?
   2. What is the borrower asking for? Is this a policy guide or a request for financing?
   3. Is this a start-up, buy-out, buy-in, or expansion?
   4. When was the practice started? By whom? Why is it being sold?
   5. What form will the practice take? Proprietorship, Partnership, C-Corp (PSC), Subchapter S (PSC), PLLC
   6. What is the total amount of money required? What will this money be used for?
   7. Why would the banker (or an investor) want to invest in the practice?
   8. What is the plan to repay, over what term?

D. Description of the community
   1. Demographic considerations
      a. What are the demographics of the practice area (age, sex, family status, income levels [per capita or family based] dental utilization patterns)?
      b. Where was this information found?
      c. How are those trends changing? Is there a net in- or out-migration?
   2. Economic considerations
      a. What is the base of the local economy?
      b. What is the forecast for the local economy? Is it expanding? Contracting? Cyclical?
      c. Are major employers planning to come into or leave the area?
      d. How many employers have dental insurance? How much poverty or Medicaid is in the area? What effect will those have on the practice?
   3. Competition
      a. How many other dentists are there in the area? Are they full or part-time?
      b. What is the full-time dentist equivalent, given their ages, expanded function usage, and so on?
      c. Are the dentists busy? How far ahead are they booked?
      d. What is the dentist-to-population ratio? What are national figures? Are there important factors that affect this number?
      e. What types of services do they provide?

E. Description of the practice (business)
1. Nature of the profession
   a. Describe dentistry as a service- versus product-based industry.
   b. Is dentistry, as a profession, growing? How fast?
   c. How does dentistry respond to general economic factors?
   d. What are common practices like?
   e. Will the practice follow dental practice conventions or will it set new trends?
2. Overall strategy
   a. What is planned for the practice in 5 years? 10 years?
   b. Is the plan to bring in an associate or partner?
   c. Is this a maintenance (cash cow) or growth strategy?
3. Marketing
   a. How large is the market? What share of that market is expected to be gained?
   b. How are patients from the existing practice going to be retained?
   c. What is the fee schedule and typical fees in the area? What is the pricing strategy?
   d. How are new patients going to be attracted to the practice?
   e. How effective are the strategies expected to be?
   f. What will the practice offer that others in the area do not?
4. Location
   a. Where will the practice be located?
   b. What are the strengths and weaknesses of this location?
   c. Is there adequate traffic, parking, public transportation, sign space, and handicapped access?
   d. Where are other referral sources and specialists located in relation to this practice?
   e. Where are patient housing areas or neighborhoods located in relation to the office?
   f. Are any special licenses, permits, or zoning changes needed for the practice?
   g. Describe the facility. Is there room for expansion, if desired?
   h. If renovations are required, what are they? How much will they cost? (Attach a builder's estimate in the appendix)
5. Operations
   a. What are the anticipated hours of operation?
   b. Any insurance plan participation?
   c. What is the anticipated credit or collection policy? What is conventional in the area?
6. Personnel
   a. How many and what types of staff will be initially hired?
   b. What are the expected duties of these staff members? What is their expected contribution to the team?
   c. What are the duty delegation laws in the state? How will they affect staffing decisions?
   d. What are typical pay levels for staff in the area? What is the staff going to be paid?
   e. What are the long-term expectations regarding personnel issues?
   f. Are needed personnel available in the area? How much training will be required?
   g. What advisers or professional consultants or services are planned to be used?

F. Description of the applicant
1. Professional qualifications
   a. Where was education completed?
   b. Any awards or recognition? Any honorary society memberships?
   c. What other business experience?
   d. Worked in any other dental offices?
   e. Dental extramural rotation experience?
2. Personal information
   a. What personal attributes does the applicant have that will make this practice a success?
   b. What is the personal family situation?
   c. How will this affect business decisions?
   d. Will more or less money be needed from the practice?

G. Application and expected effect of loan
1. Sources and amounts of funding required
2. How much money is needed?
3. Where will this money come from?
   a. Bank
   b. Equipment dealers or leasers
   c. Personal savings or assets
   d. Family loans or gifts
   e. Cosigners
4. Uses of funds
   a. Practice purchase
      i. Depreciable assets
      ii. Nondepreciable assets
      iii. Practice expenses
   b. Working capital
   c. *Personal expenses

II. Financial Part of the Plan

A. Personal financial considerations
1. Personal balance sheet
   a. Include personal assets
   b. Personal liabilities, including student loans
2. Family budget
   a. Include other sources of funds (e.g., spouse's employment)
   b. Realistic estimate of family financial needs

B. Professional financial considerations
   1. Financial analysis of present practice (if any)
      a. Last 3 years' Schedule C (or comparable Schedules)
      b. Analysis of important features of these schedules
   2. Professional capital equipment list
      a. What are the hard assets that are owned or bought?
      b. What is the useful life of each (for depreciation purposes?)
      c. What additional equipment do is expected to be purchased?
   3. Cash flow estimate (practice)
      a. Projected cash flow for year 1 by month
      b. Projected cash flow for years 2 and 3
      c. When will the practice will be profitable?

   4. Pro forma income statement (optional, at banker's request)
      a. Projected income statements for years 1, 2, 3, 5

III. Appendix

A. Fee schedule
B. Practice appraisal
C. Credit and collection policy
D. Builder's estimate of renovation costs
E. Balance sheet for cosigners (if any)

Index

account aging, 210, 288
account guarantor, 200
accounts payable, 407
accounts receivable, 165, 207, 288
active listening, 233
ADA (Americans with Disabilities Act), 93
AD&D (Accidental Death and Dismemberment) Policy, 22
adjustments, 164, 284
administrative regulation, 88
advertising, 222
amortization, 122, 132
AMT (Alternative Minimum Tax), 48
annuity, 37, 39, 115
antitrust laws, 97
any occupation policies, 20
appointment plan, 183, 184
arbitration, 88
assets, 31,103, 106, 117, 397
assignment of benefits, 203
associateship, 364

balance sheet
    corporate, 106
    personal, 102
balloon payment, 123
bank deposit, 286
bankruptcy, 8, 96
banks, 6, 404
barter, 130
board of directors, 66
body language, 231
book value, 397
branding, 218
break-even analysis, 244

budget, 8, 117
bundling, 306
business
    cycle, 80
    entity, 62, 137
    plan, 412
buy-in, 390
buy-out, 383

C Corporation, 67, 69
capacity, 278, 326
capacity utilized, 280
capital assets, 117
capital gain (loss), 130
capitation plans (cap plan), 306, 310
career path, 8, 357
cash basis accounting, 130, 138, 282
cash control, 201, 287, 292
cash discounts, 204
cash flow, 5, 409
cash flow statement, 107
CDO (Contract Dental Organization), 309
chairside assistant, 175
charging interest, 96, 203
checkbook, 289
civil law, 89
claims made policy, 333
closed panel, 305
cold start, 380
collateral, 120
collection agency, 211
collection policy, 207
collection ratio, 164, 166
collection techniques, 208, 210

Business Basics for Dentists, First Edition. David O. Willis.
© 2013 John Wiley & Sons, Inc. Published 2013 by John Wiley & Sons, Inc.

common law, 88
communications, 220, 230
compensation for doing dentistry, 362, 370
compensation for ownership, 371
compounding, 32
constructive discharge, 275
contractor, independent, 364
contracts, 89
contribution limits, 36
core values, 155
corporate ownership, 366
corporation, 65
cosigner, 120
cost
   allocation, 164, 242
   shifting, 316
CPI (Consumer Price Index), 81, 196, 197
credit, 284
credit bureau, 6, 200
credit card, 7, 11, 202, 287, 406
credit check, 6, 200
credit rating (FICO score), 6, 406
credit union, 406
criminal law, 89
cross purchase agreement, 22

DEA (Drug Enforcement Administration), 338
debit, 284
debit card, 202
debt, 10, 404
deductible expenses, 26, 131
defined benefit plans, 36
defined contribution plans, 36
deflation, 82
delegation of duties, 177, 179, 182
delinquent accounts, 210
demand, 75, 77
dental assistant, 175
dental hygienist, 174
dental license, 337
depreciation, 131
   recapture, 132
DMO (Dental Maintenance Organization), 310
DMSO (Dental Management Service Organization), 366
down payment, 120, 203
DR (Direct Reimbursement), 308
draw against future earnings, 363

economic indicators, 81, 359
EDDA (Expanded Duty Dental Assistant), 175, 180
EEOC (Equal Employment Opportunity Commission), 95
EFDA (Expanded Function Dental Assistant), 175, 180
effectiveness, 218, 278
efficiency, 278, 280
elimination period, 20
embezzlement, 292
emergency
   fund, 5, 19
   patients, 189
employee, 362, 364
   compensation, 255, 265
   exempt, 257

   leave, 258, 259
   non-exempt, 258
   salaried, 256
   terminating, 273
employee benefit programs, 258, 260, 363
employment
   application, 249
   contract, 368
   interview, 250
   process, 248
   at will, 254
End of Day (EOD) procedures, 285
End of Month (EOM) procedures, 286
End of Year (EOY) procedures, 286
engineering controls, 339
entrepreneur, 143
environment, 149, 155
environmental analysis, 154
equipment replacement plan, 119
equity theory, 268
estate planning, 54, 55
executor, 54
expenses, 102, 105

fair market value, 397
Fed (Federal Reserve system), 84
fee, 165, 191, 219
fee setting objectives, 191
felonies, 89
FFS (Fee for service), 307
FICA (see Social Security), 19, 30, 39, 94, 259, 262
financial policies, 200, 220, 235
financial statements, 102
fiscal policy, 83
fixed costs, 242
flexible benefit plan, 261
FLSA (Fair Labor Standards Act), 92
40-40 Rule, 221
401(k) plans, 37
franchise, 376
freedom of choice, 305

GDP (Gross Domestic Product), 79
goodwill, 398
gross lease, 125

health care cards, 202
HIPAA (Health Insurance Portability
   and Accountability Act), 324
holdback (discount), 287
human resources, 145

incentive plans, 269
incidents of ownership, 370
income, 102, 105, 130
   unearned, 130
income statement
   corporate, 105
   personal, 102
income tax, 130
   Schedule C, 44, 131
   state, 44, 48

Individual Retirement Account (IRA), 34
inflation, 33, 82
informed consent, 326
installment loan, 122
instruments, 296
insurance, 5, 26
   automobile, 9, 24, 27
   benefit, 27
   dental, 196, 203, 219, 304
   disability (income), 18, 27
   homeowners', 25, 27
   life, 22, 26
   malpractice, 333
   medical, 17
   office, 321
   term, 23
   universal life, 23
   variable life, 23
   whole life, 23
interest, 120
   fixed rate, 121
   variable rate, 121
interest only payments, 122
invoice, 290, 302
IPA (Independent Practice Association), 310
IRS useful lifetime, 119

Job application, 249
job description, 248
joint and severable liability, 64
JTWROS (Joint Tenants/Right of Survivorship), 57

labor substitution, 176
laboratory, dental, 302
laboratory technician, 175
leadership, 264
lease, 123
leasehold improvements, 125
LEAT (Least Expensive Alternative Treatment), 306
Leverage, 120
Liability(ies), 10, 91, 103, 106, 324
Lien, 119, 409
line of credit, 407
litigation, 88
living will, 56
LLC (Limited Liability Company), 68, 71
loan amortization, 122
loan security, 120
loss exposure, 320

macroeconomics, 79
malpractice, 332
managed dental care, 66, 304, 309, 315
mandates, 134
marginal cost, 223, 316
marginal tax rate, 131
market equilibrium, 76
market segmentation, 217
marketing, 169, 214
   external, 221
   incentives, 204
   internal, 218

mediation, 88
Medicaid, 302
medical waste, 345
Medicare, 301
microeconomics, 74
mid-level practitioners, 174
misdemeanors, 89
monetary policy, 84
money factor, 124
mortgage, 119, 120, 405
motivation, 266

need theories, 267
negligence, 90, 324
net lease, 125
net worth, 33, 103

occurrence policy, 333
office hours, 280
open panel, 305
operating lease, 127
operating statement, 105
optional benefits, 260
OSHA (Occupational and Safety Health Administration), 93, 338
outlining the appointment book, 182
outsourcing, 177
overall reimbursement rates, 315
overhead percentage, 167
overtime, 92, 258
own occupation policies, 20
owner financing, 405
ownership, 370

PA (Professional Association), 62
PAR (performance appraisal review), 271
Partnership, 63, 69
pass through entity, 68
patient abandonment, 328
patient records, 328, 350
patient schedule, 174, 181, 280
pay equity, 268
payment methods, 284, 286
payment plan, 202
peer review, 332, 347
periodic maintenance, 224
personal checks, 201, 287
personal excess liability policy, 26
personal outline, 56
PHI (Protected Health Information), 324
piercing the corporate veil, 69
plan utilization controls, 305
poor outcomes, 326
poor work, 325
power of attorney, 56
PPO (Preferred Provider Organization), 309
practice
   mission, 155
   philosophy, 144, 155
   planning, 154
   stages, 148

pre-appointing, 237
predetermination, 306
pre-heating, 225
prime rate, 121
principal, 120
private banking, 404
probate, 54
probationary period, 254
problem solving purchases, 238
production
  gross, 64, 284
  net, 64
professional courtesies, 204
professional liability, 65
profit, 105, 134, 164
profit and loss statement, 105
profitability formula, 164, 167, 195
proforma financial statement, 110
progressive discipline, 272
promissory note, 407
property lease, 126
proprietorship, 44, 69
proxemics, 232
PSC (Public Service Corporation), 62

qualified plans, 32
quality assessment, 346
quick call list, 190

ratios, 166
recall, 169, 220, 224
recare, 220, 224
receptionist, 175
referrals, 221, 311
reorder point, 301
replacement value, 397
required benefits, 259
residual clause, 21
residual value, 124
retirement planning, 31
returns and allowances, 134
risk management, 16, 320
risk/return relationship, 32
Roth IRA, 35
routine purchase decisions, 23

S Corporation, 67, 71
salary, 256, 362
SBA (Small Business Administration), 406
Schedule C, 105
SECA (Self-Employment Contributions Act), 49
SEP Plans, 36
signature loan, 120, 407
SIMPLE plans, 37
small claims court, 211
social security, 19, 30, 39, 94
sole proprietorship, 63
solo group practice, 372
solo practice, 371
staff, 174, 279

standards of care, 325, 347
statement, 208
statement of financial position, 103, 106
sterilization, 298
stock, 65
student loan, 8, 356
supervision, 176
supplies, 300
supply and demand, 75, 76, 78
sweat equity, 406
SWOT analysis, 155

table of allowances, 306
target market, 217
tax(es)
  ad valorem, 137
  audits, 50
  credits, 46, 135
  deductible debt, 11
  deductible savings, 32
  deferred annuity, 37
  rates, 46
  sheltering, 32
temporary placement services, 136
term of a loan, 119, 121
termination, wrongful, 94, 275
testamentary letter, 56
theory x, theory y, 267
time codes, 183, 228
time value of money, 112
torts, 89, 90
total compensation, 257
treatment plan, 182, 235
triple net lease, 125
true group practice, 373
trust, 57

UCR (Usual Customary and Reasonable), 305
unbundling, 307
unemployment compensation insurance,
  93, 274, 324
unjust dismissal, 94, 275
unwithheld expenses for the employer,
  135, 260

valuation, 399
variable costs, 242
vesting, 36

wage, 256, 362
wage and hour laws, 274
web sites, 222
will, 55, 56
work ethic, 266
worker's compensation insurance, 92, 135, 323
working capital, 409
working interview, 254
writing off accounts, 212

0-2-10 Rule, 217